SECOND EDITION

Pharmacology
for Nurses

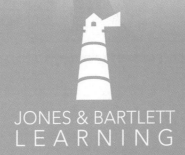

JONES & BARTLETT
LEARNING

Pharmacology for Nurses

The Pedagogy

Pharmacology for Nurses drives comprehension through various strategies that meet the learning needs of students while also generating enthusiasm about the topic. This interactive approach addresses different learning styles, making this the ideal text to ensure mastery of key concepts. The pedagogical aids that appear in most chapters include the following:

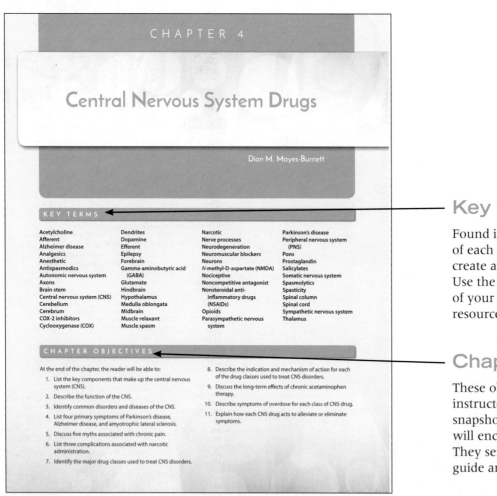

Key Terms

Found in a list at the beginning of each chapter, these items will create an expanded vocabulary. Use the access code at the front of your book to find additional resources online.

Chapter Objectives

These objectives provide instructors and students with a snapshot of key information they will encounter in each chapter. They serve as a checklist to help guide and focus study.

TABLE 4-1	Most Common Opioids			
Generic	Trade Name	Administration Routes	Natural/Other	Agonist/Antagonist
Morphine	MS Contin	Subcut./IM/IV/PO	Natural	Agonist
Codeine	Lodine	PO/IM/Subcut.	Natural	Agonist
Hydromorphone	Dilaudid	Subcut./IM/IV/PO/REC	Semi-synthetic	Agonist
Meperidine	Demerol	Subcut./IM/IV/PO/REC	Synthetic	Agonist
Fentanyl	Duragesic	IV/IM/lozenge/buccal tab/transdermal patch	Synthetic	Agonist
Methadone	Dolophine	Subcut./IM/IV/PO	Synthetic	Agonist
Tramadol	Ultram	PO	Synthetic	Agonist
Naloxone	Narcan	Subcut./IM/IV	Semi-synthetic	Antagonist

Best Practices

Key concept notes reinforce correct methods and techniques and provide information on matters in day-to-day practice.

Best Practices

Selecting an appropriate analgesic is achieved with consideration of the risks and benefits to the patient, the type and severity of pain the patient may be suffering, and the risk of adverse effects.

Best Practices

Analgesics should be dosed routinely to ensure constant blood levels of analgesic so that pain relief is uninterrupted.

Best Practices

The risk of side effects with long-term use of NSAIDs means treatment of chronic pain requires a combination of drugs, lifestyle modifications, and other treatment modalities.

a response; agonists mimic the actions of endogenous opioid ligands. The best-known drugs with *mixed* agonist–antagonist activity are the opioids. For example morphine is an agonist of opioid receptors, while naloxone is an antagonist to morphine and other opiate drugs (and therefore a receptor *antagonist*). The drugs buprenorphine and pentazocine have both agonist and antagonist effects (TABLE 4-1).

Among the class of NSAIDs are COX-2 inhibitors. These drugs are selective in that they directly target COX-2, an enzyme responsible for inflammation and pain, yet have a less severe impact on the gastrointestinal (GI) tract than traditional NSAIDs such as salicylates (aspirin). The more benign GI effects of COX-2 inhibitors reduce the risk of peptic ulceration associated with the traditional NSAIDs (Chan et al., 2017; Whittle, 2000), although overall gastrointestinal toxicity of selective COX-2 inhibitors has been questioned (Hima & Venkat, 2016). Celecoxib is an example of a COX-2 inhibitor.

Analgesics provide *symptomatic* pain relief but do not alleviate the cause of that pain. The NSAIDs, due to their dual activity, may be beneficial in both regards, as we shall see later in this chapter.

Acute Versus Chronic Pain

One person's pain perception may be very different from another person's, but the one commonality is that a sensory pathway spans from the affected organ to the brain. Analgesics work at the level of the nerves, either by blocking the signal from the PNS or by distorting the perception by the CNS. Selecting an appropriate analgesic is achieved with consideration of the risks and benefits to the patient, the type and severity of pain the patient may be suffering, and the risk of adverse effects. The healthcare provider would also want to examine whether the type of pain the patient is experiencing would be categorized as acute or chronic.

Acute pain is self-limiting in duration and includes postoperative pain or pain due to an injury or infection. Given that pain of this type is expected to be short term (usually less than 12 weeks' duration), the long-term side effects of analgesic therapy may be ignored. These patients may be treated with narcotics without concern of possible addiction. One important consideration with patients in severe pain is that they should not be subject to the return of pain. Analgesics should be dosed routinely to ensure constant blood levels of analgesic, rather than waiting to provide patients with appropriate medications until

---

effects. When the procedure is over, remind the patient not to arise too quickly to avoid possible dizziness due to orthostatic hypotension. Remind patients to call immediately if they experience side effects or notice areas of irritation or increased bleeding, warmth, or swelling at area of injection.

CHAPTER SUMMARY

This chapter has explored the CNS, touched briefly on the PNS, and discussed key conditions affecting the CNS as well as the drug classes most commonly used as treatments for specific CNS diseases and disorders. If there is one all-encompassing theme to this chapter, it is the principal necessity to support patients' ability to maintain physiological function and a sense of "normalcy" as they cope with the neurologic disorders for which they are being treated. Whether the problem is pain centered or focused on loss of memory (as in Alzheimer disease), physical capability (as in Parkinson's or ALS disease), or simply a matter of suppressing seizures, the therapeutic goal is the same: manage the condition with the goal of restoring normalcy to the extent possible. Where disease and/or symptom progression is inevitable, the goal becomes maintenance of high function and independence for as long as possible. In such cases (and, indeed, in any CNS disorder), medication is rarely used alone; it is most often supported with multiple adjunct therapies (or sometimes is better regarded as an adjunct to other modalities).

Key concepts include the importance of neurotransmitters such as *dopamine* and *acetylcholine* in brain-centered progressive disorders such as Alzheimer and Parkinson's disease, the function of glutamate and NDMA in memory and cognition, and the central role that prostaglandins play in inflammatory conditions. Management of pain is a challenging objective for the clinician because it is so often performed ineffectively. However, maintaining physiological function and supporting patients' ability to cope with various diseases and symptoms is as important as pain control.

Critical Thinking Questions

Analyze and evaluate content from each chapter using these end-of-chapter questions.

Critical Thinking Questions

1. What are the advantages and disadvantages of NSAID analgesia versus opioid analgesia?

2. What distinguishes epilepsy from non-epileptic seizures? Why would therapy for each type of seizure disorder be different?

3. Name three common myths surrounding pain medications. How do these medications potentially affect therapy and clinical response to the patient?

4. In Alzheimer disease, the key diagnostic symptom is dementia; in Parkinson's disease, the most frequent identifying symptom is tremor and changes in gait. How do these differences alter the therapeutic approach to patients with these diseases?

5. What is the principal function of glutamate?

6. What are the roles of prostaglandins in inflammatory diseases? How do NSAIDs affect prostaglandin production?

7. Which of the following medications is most appropriate for a patient with a spinal cord injury who has a history of benzodiazepine addiction: cyclobenzaprine, diazepam, aspirin, or dantrolene?

8. ALS is a progressive neurodegenerative disease with varied etiology. What are typically the first symptoms seen in the progression of this disease?

9. What are the key symptoms or lab findings that would indicate toxicity in a patient on long-term acetaminophen therapy?

CASE STUDIES

Case Scenario 1

Ms. Smith, a 78-year-old woman with a history of gastric ulcers and stroke, comes into the clinic following an accident where her car was rear-ended. She is complaining of headache and pain in her neck and shoulders. The nurse takes the patient's vital signs: B/P, 123/68; P, 88; R, 18; T, 98.9. Ms. Smith states that she has allergies to **penicillin** and **codeine**, and has been taking Coumadin since her stroke three years ago. After a brief examination, the physician's assistant tells Ms. Smith that he believes she has whiplash and prescribes her **cyclobenzaprine** and **aspirin**.

Case Question

1. Is aspirin the best or most appropriate medication that should have been ordered?
   a. Yes, because it acts both as an anti-inflammatory and a pain medication.
   b. No, the patient would do better taking ibuprofen because it is less upsetting to the stomach.
   c. No, the patient should take acetaminophen because she has both a history of peptic ulcers and is currently taking warfarin.
   d. None of the above.

   Answer: The answer is c. Because Ms. Smith has a history of ulcers and is receiving anticoagulant therapy post stroke, aspirin should be avoided because it would both increase the anticoagulant effects of the warfarin and increase her risk of gastric ulcers.

CASE STUDIES

Case Scenario 2

Nathaniel, an EMT and girls' soccer coach in Connecticut, was flying home to Tulsa for a visit. When his father, Louis, picked him up at the airport, Nathaniel noticed that Louis seemed different. He didn't think much of it at the time, but as the week progressed, he noticed that his father was frequently confused, had difficulty organizing and planning, and was quite moody when normally he was always laughing and telling jokes. He had always loved making flies for his favorite hobby, fly-fishing, but Nathaniel's mother reported that he no longer made the flies or even went into his workshop anymore. She also stated that she noticed when they watched TV, Louis had difficulty following the plot of any of the shows they were watching.

Nathaniel felt that his father might have some mild dementia, which concerned him because his father was only 58. He made an appointment for his father with his doctor; following examination and testing, Louis was diagnosed with early-stage Alzheimer disease.

Case Questions

1. Because Louis is relatively young, and has been diagnosed with early-stage Alzheimer disease with what appear to be only mild symptoms, which medication would be *best* to start him on?

Case Studies

Scenarios encourage active learning and promote critical thinking skills. Students can read about real-life scenarios and analyze each situation presented.

SECOND EDITION

Pharmacology for Nurses

Blaine Templar Smith, RPh, PhD

Pharmacy Consultant
Editor and Author

Former Chair
Department of Pharmaceutical Sciences, Saint
   Joseph College School of Pharmacy

Former Assistant Professor
Massachusetts College of Pharmacy and Health
   Sciences - Worcester
College of Pharmacy, University of Oklahoma

Diane F. Pacitti, RPh, PhD

Pharmacy Educator
Editor and Author

Adjunct Pharmacology Faculty
Manchester Community College
Capitol Community College

Former Chair
Holyoke Community College

Former Assistant Professor
Department of Pharmaceutical Sciences, Saint
   Joseph College School of Pharmacy Department
   of Pharmacology, Springfield College
Massachusetts College of Pharmacy and
   Health Sciences - Worcester

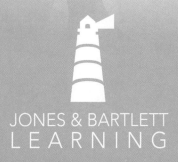

JONES & BARTLETT
LEARNING

World Headquarters
Jones & Bartlett Learning
5 Wall Street
Burlington, MA 01803
978-443-5000
info@jblearning.com
www.jblearning.com

Jones & Bartlett Learning books and products are available through most bookstores and online booksellers. To contact Jones & Bartlett Learning directly, call 800-832-0034, fax 978-443-8000, or visit our website, www.jblearning.com.

Substantial discounts on bulk quantities of Jones & Bartlett Learning publications are available to corporations, professional associations, and other qualified organizations. For details and specific discount information, contact the special sales department at Jones & Bartlett Learning via the above contact information or send an email to specialsales@jblearning.com.

14734-6

Production Credits
VP, Product Management: Amanda Martin
Director of Product Management: Matthew Kane
Product Specialist: Christina Freitas
Project Specialist: Alex Schab
Senior Marketing Manager: Jennifer Scherzay
Production Services Manager: Colleen Lamy
Product Fulfillment Manager: Wendy Kilborn
Composition: S4Carlisle Publishing Services

Cover Design: Michael O'Donnell
Text Design: Michael O'Donnell
Rights & Media Specialist: John Rusk
Media Development Editor: Troy Liston
Cover Image (Title Page, Part Opener, Chapter Opener):
  © Foxie/Shutterstock
Printing and Binding: LSC Communications
Cover Printing: LSC Communications

Library of Congress Cataloging-in-Publication Data
Names: Smith, Blaine T., editor.
Title: Pharmacology for nurses / [edited by] Blaine Templar Smith.
Description: Second edition. | Burlington, Massachusetts : Jones & Bartlett
  Learning, [2019] | Includes bibliographical references.
Identifiers: LCCN 2018023083 | ISBN 9781284141986 (hardcover)
Subjects: | MESH: Pharmacological Phenomena | Drug Therapy | Nurses'
  Instruction
Classification: LCC RM301.28 | NLM QV 37 | DDC 615.1--dc23
LC record available at https://lccn.loc.gov/2018023083

6048

Printed in the United States of America
22 21 20 19 18   10 9 8 7 6 5 4 3 2 1

Dedication

This book is dedicated to the memory of my mother,
Joan (Joanna) Lou Templar Smith, PhD (1927–2013),
my life-long editor and editorial advisor. – Blaine T. Smith

Dedicated to my mother as well: the single strongest, most faithful,
and resilient person I have ever known. – Diane F. Pacitti

Contents

    Diane F. Pacitti, RPh, PhD, and Blaine Templar Smith, RPh, PhD

Amy Rex Smith, DNSc, RN, ACNS, BC, and Blaine Templar Smith, RPh, PhD

Introduction

Pharmacology for Nurses is an earnest attempt to provide a fundamentally solid yet quickly learnable foundation from which to teach nursing pharmacology courses. It was created to provide an alternative pharmacology textbook for nurses to those previously available. There is a tendency for nursing pharmacology textbooks to be either overly complex or overly simplified for the needs of nursing students. This is not to say comprehensive pharmacology textbooks are not of value. It is a simple fact of the education paradigm that pharmacology must be a component of nursing education, but there is insufficient time to delve into the details of each topic during the regular curriculum. Therefore, the authors recognized a need for a "core" pharmacology textbook that not only provides a solid foundation for nurses but also is compatible with the realities of course constraints encountered in any curriculum.

The textbook is divided into three major sections. The first section provides the general information needed to make the student comfortable with both how pharmacology fits into professional nursing and the mathematical foundation on which later sections are based. The second section is intended to provide basic pharmacology and is arranged by organ or physiologic system. The reader's previous understanding of physiology is usually assumed, so physiology review is minimized in order to more directly address common systems of drug receptors utilized for medical interventions. The third section is dedicated to the physiologic systems that, though regularly encountered in practice, are not considered primary systems.

After reading this textbook, presumably in association with pharmacology courses offered, it is hoped the essentials for capable professional nursing practice will be afforded, while offering a nonintimidating presentation of the topic. It is our hope that this instills a true interest in pursuing more in-depth pharmacology education as situations inevitably present themselves in everyday professional nursing practice.

About the Editor

Blaine Templar Smith, RPh, PhD, earned bachelor degrees in chemistry and pharmacy and a PhD in pharmaceutical sciences (with emphasis in nuclear pharmacy and immunology) at the University of Oklahoma. Dr. Smith is a registered pharmacist in both Oklahoma and Massachusetts, practicing in a very wide spectrum of settings, including hospital in-patient, long-term care centers, independent and chain retail pharmacies, and Indian Health Service clinics and hospitals. He completed a postdoctoral fellowship at the University of Oklahoma Genome Sequencing Center, participating in the Human Genome Project.

Dr. Smith has been a faculty member at the University of Oklahoma College of Pharmacy and the Massachusetts College of Pharmacy and Health Sciences, Worcester; faculty member and Chair of the Department of Pharmaceutical Sciences at the Saint Joseph University School of Pharmacy; and Visiting Fellow at the University of Massachusetts Medical School.

He has written, edited, and published reference books and textbooks related to the fields of medicine, pharmacy, pharmaceutics, physical pharmacy, nuclear pharmacy, immunology, molecular biology, diagnostic imaging, and nursing. Additionally, he provides online education (both live and asynchronous) and continuing health profession education for healthcare professionals' licensure requirements.

Contributors

Dwayne Accardo, DNP, CRNA, APN
Assistant Professor, Program Director for DNP Nurse
  Anesthesia
University of Tennessee Health Science Center
Memphis, Tennessee

Catherine Bodine, RN, BSN
Clinical Research Communication Specialist
Duke Clinical Research Institute
Durham, North Carolina

Jacqueline Rosenjack Burchum, DNSc, FNP-BC, CNE
University of Tennessee Health Science Center
Memphis, Tennessee

Hoi Sing Chung, PhD, RN
Assistant Professor
University of Memphis
Memphis, Tennessee

Karen Crowley, DNP, APRN-BC, WHNP, ANP
Assistant Professor and Associate Dean of Online
  Nursing
Regis College
Weston, Massachusetts

William Mark Enlow, DNP, ACNP, CRNA, DCC
Assistant Professor of Nursing
Columbia University
New York, New York

Christopher Footit, RN, CS
Footit and Associates
Hadley, Massachusetts

Sue Greenfield, PhD, RN
Associate Professor
School of Nursing
Columbia University
New York, New York

Tara Kavanaugh, RN, MSN, MPH, ANP-BC, FNP-BC,
WHNP-BC
Holyoke Community College
Holyoke, Massachusetts

Dion M. Mayes-Burnett, RN
Manager of Alzheimer, Dementia, and PTSD
Norman Veterans Center
Norman, Oklahoma

Sarah Nadarajah, RN, BSN
Nurse Coordinator, Reproductive Medicine
Reproductive Science Center
Lexington, Massachusetts

Jean Nicholas, MSN
Spencer, Massachusetts

Diane F. Pacitti, PhD, RPh
Pharmacology
Manchester Community College Pharmacy Technician
  Training Program
Manchester, Connecticut

Ashley Pratt, MSN, WHNP-BC
Coastal Women's Healthcare
Scarborough, Maine

Cliff Roberson, DNP, CRNA, APRN
Assistant Program Director
Assistant Professor of Nursing
Graduate Program in Nurse Anesthesia
School of Nursing
Columbia University
New York, New York

Amy Rex Smith, DNSc, RN, ACNS, BC
Associate Professor, Department of Nursing
Graduate Program Director MS in Nursing Program
College of Nursing and Health Sciences
University of Massachusetts Boston
Boston, Massachusetts

Blaine Templar Smith, PhD, RPh
Pharmacy Consultant
Editor and Author
Former Chair, Department of Pharmaceutical Sciences,
  Saint Joseph School of Pharmacy
Former Assistant Professor, College of Pharmacy,
  University of Oklahoma

Linda Tenofsky, PhD, ANP-BC
Professor
Division of Nursing
Curry College
Milton, Massachusetts

Diana M. Webber, DNP, APRN-CNP
College of Nursing
University of Oklahoma
Oklahoma City, Oklahoma

Reviewers

Bruce Addison, DO, TAMUCC
Adjunct Professor
Assistant Clinical Professor Family Medicine TAMU
  HSC
Adjunct Clinical Professor
Family Medicine North Texas State University, HSC
Fort Worth, Texas

Karen J. Anderson, PhD, RN, CNE
School of Nursing & Health Professions
Oakwood University
Huntsville, Alabama

Mindy Barna, MSN, RN
Director of Practical Nursing
College of Saint Mary
Omaha, Nebraska

Patricia J. Bartzak, DNP, RN, CMSRN
Assistant Professor of Nursing
Anna Maria College
Paxton, Massachusetts

Christine M. Berte, APRN-BC
Professor
Western Connecticut State University
Danbury, Connecticut

Karen P. Black, MSN, APRN, PMHNP-BC
Assistant Professor
University of Louisville
Louisville, Kentucky

Sonya Blevins, DNP, RN, CMSRN, CNE
Assistant Professor of Nursing
University of South Carolina, Upstate
Simpsonville, South Carolina

Susan Braud, RN, MSN, CCRN
Assistant Professor of Nursing
Lynchburg College
Lynchburg, Virginia

Robin Webb Corbett, RN, BSN, MSN, PhD
Associate Professor
East Carolina State University
Greenville, North Carolina

Celeste S. Dunnington, RN, MSN
Dean, Associate Professor
Rielin & Salmen School of Nursing
Truett McConnell University
Cleveland, Georgia

Bruce E. Fugate, MSN, RN, CNE
Assistant Professor, Nursing
Southern State Community College
Hillsboro, Ohio

Laurie Gelardi, RNC, DNP, CCNS, CPNP, NNP
Assistant Professor
California State University Northridge
Northridge, California

Sheila Grossman, PhD, APRN, FNP-BC, FAAN
Professor, Family Nurse Practitioner Coordinator,
  Director of Faculty Scholarship & Mentoring
Egan School of Nursing & Health Studies
Fairfield University
Fairfield, CT

Tony Guerra, PharmD
Professor of Pharmacology
Des Moines Area Community College
Des Moines, Iowa

Katherine S. Herlache, MSN
Professor
School of Nursing and Health Professions
Marian University
Fond du Lac, Wisconsin

Jan Herren, MSN, RNC
Assistant Professor
Southern Arkansas University
Magnolia, Arkansas

Tara M. Howry, RN, MSN
Instructor
Craven Community College
New Bern, North Carolina

Jennifer C. Johnson, MSN, RN
Assistant Professor
Baldwin Wallace University Accelerated Bachelor
 of Science in Nursing Program
Berea, Ohio

Lynn A. Kelso, MSN, APRN, FCCM, FAANP
Assistant Professor of Nursing
University of Kentucky College of Nursing
Lexington, Kentucky

Josef Kren, PhD, ScD
Professor
Bryan College of Health Sciences
Lincoln, Nebraska

Nancy Kupper, RN, MSN
Associate Professor of Nursing
Tarrant County College
Fort Worth, Texas

Deborah L. Mahoney, RN, MSN, CCM
Nursing Instructor
College of St. Elizabeth and Union County College
Plainfield, New Jersey

Gerald Newberry, RN, MSN
Assistant Professor of Nursing
Eastern Michigan University
Ypsilanti, Michigan

Katharine O'Dell, PhD, RN-NP
Associate Professor of OB/GYN, Division
 of Urogynecology
UMass Memorial Medical Center
Worcester, Massachusetts

Patti Parker, PhDc, APRN, CNS, ANP, GNP
Assistant Clinical Professor
University of Texas at Arlington
College of Nursing Graduate School
Arlington, Texas

Amanda M. Passint, DNP, RN, CPNP-PC
Assistant Professor
Wisconsin Lutheran College
Milwaukee, Wisconsin

Pamela Preston-Safarz, DNP, RN
Instructor
Saint Anselm College
Manchester, New Hampshire

Edilberto A. Raynes, MD, PhD
Instructor
Grand Canyon University
Brentwood, Tennessee

Kathleen S. Sampson, MSN, RN, CCRN
Nursing Faculty
Carroll University
Waukesha, Wisconsin

Diana Shenefield, PhD, MSN, RN
Director of Nursing
Huntington University
Huntington, Indiana

Mary J. Sletten, DM(c), MSN, RN
Associate Professor
Doña Ana Community College
Las Cruces, New Mexico

Jane L. Smith, PhD, RN
Assistant Professor of Nursing, School of Nursing
New Mexico State University
Las Cruces, New Mexico

Beryl Stetson, RNBC, MSN, CNE, LCCE, CLC
Professor of Nursing, Chairperson for the Health
 Science Education Department
Raritan Valley Community College
Branchburg, New Jersey

Rebecca Swartzman, DNP, RN
Professor
Simpson University
Redding, California

Amy E. Tingle, PharmD
Clinical Pharmacist
Texas Tech University Health Sciences Center School
 of Pharmacy
Austin, Texas

Elizabeth A. Tinnon, PhD, RN, CNE
Assistant Professor
University of Southern Mississippi
Hattiesburg, Mississippi

Theresa Turick-Gibson, EdD (c), MA, PPCNP-BC, RN-BC
Professor
Hartwick College
Oneonta, New York

Sherry Vickers, RN, MSN, CNE
Associate Professor of Nursing
Jackson State Community College
Jackson, Tennessee

Michael H. Walls, MSN, PhD, RN
Assistant Professor, Manager, Medical-Surgical Nursing
Malek School of Health Professions
Marymount University
Arlington, Virginia

Cynthia Watson, DNP, APRN, FNP-BC
Assistant Professor
University of Louisiana at Lafayette College of Nursing
 and Allied Health Professions
Lafayette, Louisiana

Sue Winn, RN, MSN
Nursing Instructor
City College, MSU Billings
Billings, Montana

Lisa D. Wright, DNP, ANP-C, CPHQ
Adjunct Faculty
Jefferson College of Health Sciences
Carilion Clinic
Roanoke, Virginia

Maureen E. Yoder, MSN, RN
Assistant Clinical Professor
Northern Arizona University
Flagstaff, Arizona

Pharmacology for Nurses: Basic Principles

Introduction to Pharmacology

Jean Nicholas

KEY TERMS

Assessment
Controlled substances
Drug classification

Drug name
Goals
Medication errors

Nursing diagnoses
Nursing process
Pharmacology

Prescription drugs

CHAPTER OBJECTIVES

At the end of the chapter, the reader will be able to:

1. Discuss how drugs are classified.
2. Differentiate between *brand* versus *generic* drug names.
3. List the five steps of the nursing process.
4. Identify categories of controlled substances.
5. Name two sources for obtaining drug information.
6. Discuss legal and ethical responsibilities of the nurse when administering medication.
7. Define *medication error*.

Introduction

In modern health care, there is an increasing reliance on medication therapy to manage illness and disease, to slow progression of disease, and to improve patient outcomes. Medications offer a variety of potential benefits to the patient: relief of symptoms, support for necessary physiological processes, and destruction of toxic substances or organisms that cause disease, to name a few. Yet medications also have the potential to do harm, even when administered properly—and the harm is likely to be exacerbated if medications are administered incorrectly. The administration of drugs introduces opportunity to affect either remedy or harm.

As the persons most often charged with administering medications to patients, nurses can minimize any harm associated with medications by carrying out this task with few, if any, errors (Institute of Medicine [IOM], 2007). A 2007 IOM (now the National Academy of Science) report on medication safety, titled *Preventing Medication Errors*, emphasized the urgency of reducing medication errors, improving communication with patients, continually monitoring for medication errors, providing clinicians with decision-support and information tools, and improving and standardizing medication labeling and drug-related information (IOM, 2007).

If one of nursing's primary roles is the safe administration of medications, it is important to realize that this requires knowing not only how to correctly administer medications to patients, but also how to determine whether the intended effects are achieved and whether any adverse, or unintended, effects have occurred. Without adequate understanding of drugs and their effects on the body, nurses are unable to meet their professional and legal responsibilities to their patients. This text will provide the reader with that knowledge.

Nursing and Pharmacology

Pharmacology is the study of the actions of drugs, incorporating knowledge from other interrelated sciences, such as pharmacokinetics (how the body absorbs, distributes, metabolizes, and excretes a drug) and pharmacodynamics (a drug's mechanism of action and effect on an organism). Knowledge of the various drug classes enables the nurse to understand how drugs work in the body, to achieve the therapeutic (intended) effects, and to anticipate and recognize the potential side effects (unintended or unavoidable) or toxicities. To understand the pharmacology of drugs, and related information, such as drug interactions and side effects, it is important to understand drugs' mechanisms of action, at the *molecular* level. Rather than merely understanding a drug's actions, interactions, side effects and dosage requirements, the nurse should strive to understand the process behind these elements of drug administration. This requires at least a fundamental understanding of drug–drug receptor interactions, even if at an elementary "lock and key" level. Only then will drug effects, interactions, and side effects, and the logic behind dosing regimens, reveal a complete picture. Chapter 2 continues this discussion in depth.

The value of this knowledge in nursing cannot be overemphasized. The nurse's role as caretaker puts the nurse in the position of being closest to the patient and best able to assess both the patient's condition prior to use of a medication as well as the patient's response to the medication—two key components of appropriate medical therapy. Clearly, under these circumstances, it is ideal for the nurse to have a solid, in-depth understanding of when, how, and for whom medications are best used, and what the expected response is when specific pharmaceutical therapies are implemented.

At the most basic level, nurses must learn the various diagnostic and therapeutic classes of medications; recognize individual drug names, both trade and generic; know about the applications and availability of prescription and nonprescription medications, a particularly the restrictions regarding controlled substances; and be familiar with sources, both printed and online, where the nurse may obtain specific information about

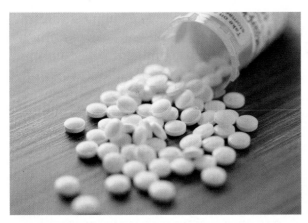

© Hero Images/Getty Images

particular drugs, including dosage, interactions, and contraindications.

Drug Classifications

Drugs are classified by how they affect certain body systems, such as the use of *bronchodilators* for respiratory conditions; by their therapeutic use, such as *antinausea*; or based on their chemical characteristics, such as *beta-blockers*. Many may fit into more than one drug classification due to the various effects that they exert in the body. Because drugs in the same *class* have many features in common, categorizing them in these ways helps nurses become familiar with many of the drugs they are administering. For example, although there are many types of angiotensin-converting-enzyme inhibitors, they have many common side effects.

Drug Names

Nurses must know both the *trade* name of a drug, which is assigned by the pharmaceutical company that manufactures the drug, and the *generic* name, which is the official drug name and is not protected by trademark. When a manufacturer receives a patent for a new drug, this means that no other company can produce the drug until the patent expires. Once this patent has expired, other companies may manufacture the drug with a different trade name but equivalent chemical makeup. Some companies choose to use the generic name only—for example, lisinopril is now manufactured by many different drug companies. Generic names are not capitalized.

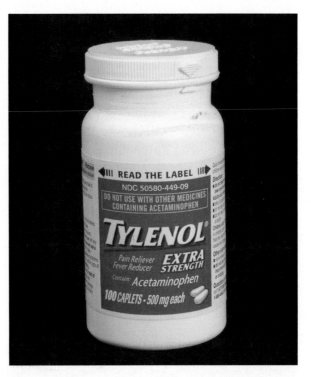

Drugs may be prescribed and dispensed by either trade name or generic name, as generic drugs are considered equivalent in most cases. Generic drugs are typically less expensive than trade-name drugs.

Prescription and Nonprescription Drugs

In the United States, consumers have two ways to legally access drugs. One is to obtain a *prescription* for the drug from a licensed provider, such as a physician, dentist, or nurse practitioner; the other is to purchase drugs that do *not* require a prescription on an *over-the-counter (OTC)* basis. Some drugs previously available only by prescription have now become available OTC. Thus, it is essential for the nurse to gather information about the patient's use of both prescription drugs and OTC medications, as some combinations of different types of drugs can affect the actions and toxicities of either. Various drug laws regulate these ways of acquiring drugs.

Controlled Substances

The Comprehensive Drug Abuse Prevention and Control Act was passed in 1970 and

> **Best Practices**
>
> Nurses are required to keep controlled substances in secure, locked locations, administering them only to patients with valid prescriptions or physician's orders.

regulates the manufacturing and distribution of substances with a potential for abuse—examples include narcotics, hallucinogens, stimulants, depressants, and anabolic steroids. These controlled substances are categorized by schedule (Schedules I–V), based on their therapeutic use and potential for abuse (TABLE 1-1). The Drug Enforcement Agency (DEA) enforces the law and requires all individuals and companies that handle controlled substances to provide storage security, keep accurate records, and include the provider number assigned by the DEA on all prescriptions for controlled substances. Schedule I drugs have a high potential for abuse and the potential to create severe psychological and/

or physical dependence; and in most cases, Schedule I drugs are illegal substances. Therefore, Schedule I drugs are not dispensed, except in rare instances of specific scientific or medical research. No refills can be ordered on Schedule II drugs; instead, providers must write a new prescription.

Nurses are required to keep controlled substances locked in a secure room or cabinet, administering them only to patients with valid prescriptions or physician's orders. Nurses must maintain accurate records of each dose given and the amount of each controlled substance on hand, and must report any discrepancies to the proper authorities.

Sources of Drug Information

With Internet access readily available for personal as well as professional use, obtaining drug information is easy. For the beginning student, however, access to a pharmacology textbook is helpful for learning and understanding the therapeutic uses of drugs. Drug reference guides are helpful when looking up a specific drug and the nursing implications of administering that agent. Drug information can be obtained through authoritative sources such as *American Hospital Formulary Service*, published by the American Society of Health-System Pharmacists (www.

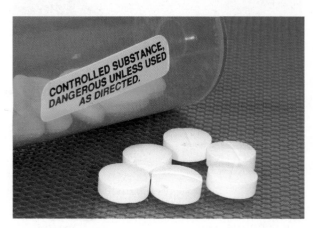

© Scott Rothstein/iStock/Thinkstock.

TABLE 1-1	Controlled Substances Categories Designated by the U.S. Government	
Schedule	Dispensing Requirements	Examples
I	Drugs not approved for medical use, except specific protocols: high abuse potential.	LSD, marijuana, heroin, gamma-hydroxybutyrate (Ecstasy)
II	Drugs approved for medical use: high abuse potential. Must be kept in locked safe. No refills without a new prescription.	Opioid analgesics (e.g., codeine, morphine, hydromorphone, methadone, oxycodone), central nervous system stimulants (e.g., cocaine, amphetamine), depressants (e.g., barbiturates—pentobarbital)
III	Less potential for abuse than Schedule I or II drugs but may lead to psychological or physical dependence. Prescription expires in 6 months.	Anabolic steroids; mixtures containing small amounts of controlled substances, such as codeine
IV	Some potential for abuse. Prescription expires in 6 months.	Benzodiazepines (e.g., diazepam, lorazepam), other sedatives (e.g., phenobarbital), some prescription appetite suppressants (e.g., mazindol)
V	Written prescription requirements vary with state law.	Antidiarrheal drugs containing small amounts of controlled substances (e.g., Lomotil)

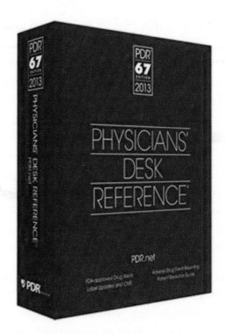

ahfsdruginformation.com); *Tarascon Pharmacopoeia*, published by Jones & Bartlett Learning; or *Drug Facts and Comparisons*, published by Lippincott Williams & Wilkins/Wolters Kluwer. These resources are updated periodically. *The Physicians' Desk Reference* is published yearly and includes pharmaceutical manufacturers' package inserts for specific drugs. Nurses can also obtain package inserts from the dispensing pharmacy—this is helpful when a drug is relatively new and information is not readily available from other resources.

Online resources and mobile applications include Micromedex and Lexicomp, both of which are searchable databases offering drug information, drug interactions, drug identification tools, medical calculators, and patient counseling information.

Continuing education about drug therapy is an essential part of professional nursing. Reading current peer-reviewed journal articles, which often include information about drug therapy for specific conditions, should be part of every nurse's professional development.

QSEN Competencies

The Quality and Safety Education for Nurses (QSEN) project, developed by the American Association of Colleges of Nursing, identified six competencies to prepare nurses with the knowledge, skills, and attitude needed to improve workplace quality and safety within healthcare systems. These competencies are as follows:

- Patient-centered care
- Teamwork and collaboration
- Evidence-based practice
- Quality improvement
- Safety
- Informatics

Overview of the Nursing Process

The **nursing process** is a systematic, rational, and continuous method of planning, providing, and evaluating individualized nursing care to optimize the administration of medications. The nursing process involves critical thinking throughout each of its five steps: assessment, nursing diagnosis, planning and establishing goals or outcomes, intervention, and evaluation. Administering medications involves much more than the psychomotor skill of preparing and giving medications; the nurse must use cognitive skills throughout the nursing process to ensure patient safety during drug therapy. The QSEN competencies, especially safety and patient-centered care, are woven into the framework of the nursing process.

> **Best Practices**
>
> Continuing education about drug therapy is an essential part of professional nursing.

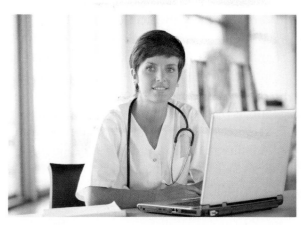

© goodluz/Shutterstock.

Assessment

Assessment involves collecting subjective and objective data from the patient, significant others, medical records (including laboratory and diagnostic tests) and others involved in the patient's care. These data may affect whether a medication should be given as ordered, or whether a provider's order should be questioned and confirmed. In addition, in the assessment step the nurse gathers data about the drug(s) that he or she is responsible for administering and monitoring. Assessment is ongoing throughout the entire nursing process, as patients' conditions may change. Nurses must continually monitor drug effects, both therapeutic and unintended. A complete medication history and nursing physical assessment are parts of the assessment step.

Nursing Diagnosis

The second step of the nursing process involves clustering the data gathered during the assessment, analyzing it for patterns, and making inferences about the patient's potential or actual problems. Nursing diagnoses, as developed by the North American Nursing Diagnosis Association (NANDA), are statements of patient problems, potential problems, or needs. This text will address nursing diagnoses that pertain more specifically to drug therapy. Some examples of selected diagnoses follow:

- Patient has a knowledge deficit related to drug therapy and reasons for use; need for follow-up tests and office visits
- Patient is at risk for injury related to adverse effects of medication
- Patient is at risk for falls related to various anticipated or unanticipated side effects of medications
- Diarrhea (or constipation) related to side effects of medications
- Ineffective health maintenance related to inability to make appropriate judgments or to lack of resources

Planning

Once the data have been analyzed and nursing diagnoses identified, the planning phase begins. During this phase, goals and outcome criteria are formulated. Nurses will prioritize identified needs, keeping patient comfort and safety as top priorities. The planning step incorporates the QSEN competency of patient-centered care. Patients are seen as full partners in the planning process and the goals recognize the patient's preferences and values. In *patient* terms, the goals and outcome criteria identify the expected behaviors or results of drug therapy. For example, the patient may be expected to and agree to do the following:

- List the steps for correctly drawing up his or her insulin dosage
- Demonstrate the correct technique for self-administration of a medication patch
- Verbalize the most common side effects of a medication
- Report pain relief of at least 3 on a scale of 10 within 30 minutes

Goals are usually broad statements for achievement of more specific outcome criteria. A timeline is often included so that there can be realistic achievement of goals. During the planning phase, the nurse must familiarize himself or herself with any special information or equipment needed to administer a medication. If knowledge attainment by the patient is the goal, appropriate patient teaching materials must be obtained. Because many medications are administered by the patient himself or herself (or the family), teaching is an important part of the nursing process for drug therapy.

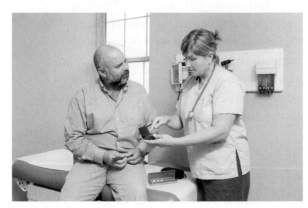

© Fertnig/iStockphoto.

Intervention

The intervention (or implementation) phase of the nursing process involves carrying out the planned activities, being mindful that ongoing assessment of the patient is needed before every intervention. For example, perhaps a patient has a laxative ordered daily but has been having loose stools all night. The nurse will need to assess this patient's current condition (i.e., complaint of loose stools) and decide how to proceed with the intervention (e.g., withhold the medication and notify the prescriber). Here, the nurse will value the patient as expert on his or her own health and symptoms, in conjunction with objective assessment. As this example illustrates, interventions for drug therapy involve not only the actual administration of medications, but also observation of the effects of the medications, as well as provision of additional measures to optimize the effects of certain medications, such as increased fluid intake to promote bowel elimination or reduce fever.

During the intervention process, the nurse encounters a variety of points at which he or she is required to make assessments and decisions about whether to proceed. Certain medications, such as antihypertensive or cardiac drugs, will require specific actions at the time of administration, such as measuring blood pressure or heart rate. If the identified parameters for these vital signs are not met, the medication may not be given.

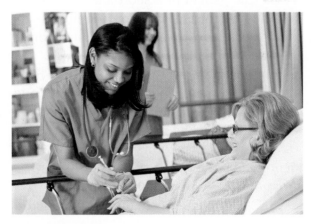

© asiseeit/iStockphoto.

Clearly, nurses require specific skills related to the intervention decision-making process. While these skills will not be enumerated in detail in this chapter, in general they include the following elements:

- Knowing and following correct procedures for confirming whether the medication is appropriate for the patient
- Knowing and following correct procedures for administering medications via different routes (oral, injection, intravenous, and so forth)
- Having the ability to identify and avoid factors that contribute to errors

Evaluation

The evaluation phase of the nursing process is a continuous process of determining progress toward identified goals. For some medications, the response can be identified quickly—for example, relief of pain following administration of an analgesic, again, utilizing patient-centered care as an approach to the evaluation. For other medications, the response is slower and must be monitored on an ongoing basis. A newly prescribed antihypertensive medication, for example, may require follow-up visits to the clinician's office for blood pressure checks and assessment of side effects. Evaluation may involve reviewing pertinent laboratory and other diagnostic tests, observing patient performance of a learned procedure, or interviewing patients and significant others about the effects of their medications.

Documentation is an essential component of all phases of the nursing process. Specific guidelines for documentation of medication administration and related teaching are prescribed by state nursing practice statutes and The Joint Commission (formerly the Joint Commission on Accreditation of Healthcare Organizations).

Patient- and drug-specific variables affect the nursing process as it relates to drug therapy. Factors such as the patient's age, physical condition (e.g., renal or liver impairment), psychological/mental ability to self-administer medication, and educational level are integral parts of the nurse's knowledge base for safe medication administration.

The nursing process is a dynamic tool used to enhance the quality of patient care. Each step involves critical thinking to provide individualized, safe, effective, and thoughtful patient care. Use of this process enables nurses to incorporate safe administration and monitoring of drug therapy into the overall plan of care for each patient, whatever the setting.

Cultural Aspects of Drug Therapy

As the United States becomes increasingly culturally diverse, nurses administering and monitoring medications must be aware of how various cultural beliefs and practices affect health care, particularly the use of medications. In addition, physical differences may affect how certain cultural or ethnic groups respond to specific medications. For many years, research on drugs was carried out using only white male subjects. Thus, the medications' effects on females or nonwhite males could not be accurately predicted, but rather were determined only by observing patient outcomes. Response to drug therapy is highly individualized, and nurses must be careful not to assume an eventual successful or failed

> **Best Practices**
>
> A careful nursing assessment will include cultural beliefs and practices that may impact drug therapy.

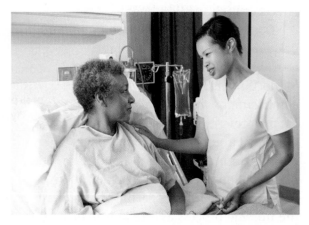

© monkeybusinessimages/iStockphoto.

response just because a patient appears to belong to a certain ethnic or cultural group.

Examples of cultural considerations affecting nursing care in drug therapy include pain response, belief in traditional "healers" versus belief in the medication's effectiveness for restoring health, use of herbal remedies, ability to communicate effectively with healthcare providers, and compliance with long-term drug therapy. A careful nursing assessment will include cultural beliefs and practices that may impact drug therapy. Nurses are encouraged to learn about cultural and ethnic groups commonly encountered in the healthcare settings of their practices.

Legal-Ethical Aspects of Drug Therapy

The legal responsibilities of nurses for medication administration are defined in state nurse practice acts and healthcare organization policies and procedures. The Eight Rights of Medication Administration, discussed in detail in Chapter Three, form the basis of safe drug therapy (Bonsall, 2011). These eight rights, briefly, ensure that (1) the right drug is given to (2) the right patient at (3) the right dose via (4) the right route at (5) the right time, for (6) the right reasons, with (7) the right documentation, to obtain (8) the right response. Some clinicians and institutions include two additional rights: right education (correctly educating the patient in therapeutic effects of the drug as well as expected side effects) and right to refuse (the patient or responsible party has the right to refuse medication administration). Most medication errors result from the failure to follow one of these "rights." Beyond maintaining awareness of these Eight Rights, nurses must possess the cognitive and psychomotor skills required to safely administer medication and monitor the effects.

Ethical aspects of nursing care were identified by the American Nurses Association (ANA) in the 2001 *Code of Ethics* (ANA, 2001). These guidelines provided ethical principles to be adhered to by every professional nurse. The Code included principles recommending that nurses (1) respect the dignity of all patients, regardless of ethnicity, socioeconomic status, or specific health problem; (2) participate in activities to support maintenance of their professional competence; (3) protect patients' privacy and confidentiality; and (4) make a commitment to providing quality patient care in every setting.

Since the original *Code of Ethics* was released, the ANA has added more provisions, along with interpretive statements. The 2015 *Code of Ethics for Nurses with Interpretive Statements* comprised nine provisions (ANA, 2015):

1. Respect for human dignity
2. Primacy of patient interests
3. Protection of patient privacy and confidentiality
4. Authority, accountability, and responsibility for nursing practice
5. Duty to self and others
6. Maintaining an ethical environment
7. Contributions through research and scholarly inquiry
8. Health as a universal right
9. Articulation and assertion of nursing values

Medication Errors

Medication errors are a daily occurrence in many healthcare facilities, sometimes resulting in serious—even fatal—consequences. It should be the goal of every healthcare professional to be aware of the potential for errors and to strive for prevention of these problems. Errors can occur during the prescribing, dispensing, administration, or documentation phases of medication administration. Thus, the error may be detected by the pharmacist, physician, nurse, or other staff, such as the person transcribing the order to the patient's medication administration record (MAR). The ECRI Institute noted in their Top 10 Patient Safety Concerns for 2017 list that information management in electronic health records, unrecognized patient deterioration,

and implementation and use of clinical decision support were the top three causes for medical errors. Opioid administration and management of new oral anticoagulants were medication-specific concerns on the list (ECRI Institute, 2017).

How Often Do Medication Errors Occur?

Medication errors have the potential to occur at numerous times during the complex delivery process, but their actual incidence is difficult to quantify. The reason the frequency of medication administration errors is difficult to calculate is because error rates vary depending on the method of measurement used to assess the errors (McBride-Henry & Foureur, 2006). The most accurate way to measure the occurrence of medication administration errors is through direct observation of practice (Barker, Flynn, & Pepper, 2002; Barker, Flynn, Pepper, Bates, & Mikel, 2002; Keers, Williams, Cooke, & Ashcroft, 2013b; Thomas & Peterson, 2003); self-reported data underrepresents true error rates (Nanji, Patel, Shaikh, Seger, & Bates, 2016). Two observational studies discovered that medication administration error rates in acute care settings varied between 14.9% (Tissot et al., 2003) and 32.4% (Schneider, Cotting, & Pannatier, 1998), with medication error rates for intravenous medications being significantly higher during the preparation (26%) and administration (34%) stages (McBride-Henry & Foureur, 2006; Keers, Williams, Cooke, & Ashcroft, 2013b; Wirtz, Taxis, & Barber, 2003). Observed medication administration demonstrated errors in nearly one out of every five doses (Barker, Flynn, Pepper, et al., 2002). Of note, studies primarily target inpatient care; thus, medication errors occurring in nursing homes or ambulatory surgery centers (and other outpatient care facilities) are not captured in the data (Makary & Daniel, 2016).

How Can Medication Errors Be Prevented?

In 2003, the Institute for Safe Medication Practices (ISMP) identified several key areas

Many medication errors occur during times of a patient transfer—for example, when a patient is being transferred from intensive care to a patient unit, from an inpatient unit to an outpatient facility or home, or from the care of one provider to another.

of focus for error prevention. Many errors occur during patient transfer—for example, when a patient is being transferred from intensive care to a patient unit, from an inpatient unit to an outpatient facility or home, or from the care of one provider to another. Medication reconciliation forms are now being used in many facilities to prevent medications from being omitted during transfers and to prompt physicians to review existing medication orders when transferring care. Bedside rounds, in which the nurse coming onto the succeeding shift accompanies the nurse going off-shift, are another helpful means of communicating medication changes. Nurses must be vigilant to ensure that these tools are utilized properly if they are to be effective in preventing errors.

Another area of focus is patient identification. Recent technological advances have been developed to reduce medication error rates by better associating patient and medication identities. Special patient wrist bracelets with bar-coding that require nurses to scan the bracelet before administering a medication are now being used, which facilitates matching the "right drug" to the "right patient." Every nurse should develop the habit of verifying patients' identities by asking each to state his or her name and date of birth. Photo identification can be used for nonverbal patients.

Environmental factors may also contribute to errors. Increased workload, working with acutely ill patients, distractions while preparing and administering medications, problems with medicine supply and storage, and nurse/staff fatigue have all been noted to lead to a higher number of errors (Anderson & Townsend, 2010; Keers, Williams, Cooke, & Ashcroft, 2013a).

The ISMP continues to identify areas of best practice. They released the 2016–2017 Targeted Medication Safety Best Practices for Hospitals, which consists of 11 medication-specific practices for

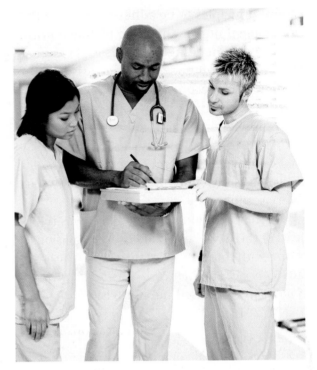

© Photos.com.

hospital-based and other healthcare settings, targeting areas in which there continue to be harmful and fatal errors (ISMP, 2016). Nurses should be active on committees and in professional organizations that are looking at these practice issues.

Hospitals and other providers have worked with pharmaceutical companies to reduce errors caused by similarly named drugs. Nurses should assess the patient and know why a patient is receiving a particular medication. They must carefully read medication labels, compare the labels to the prescribed order, and follow guidelines for proper use. For example, a medication label may say, "Do not crush."

Finally, all nurses must be responsible for maintaining and updating their knowledge of the medications they administer and the equipment they use. Patient teaching is also a key to preventing errors. An informed patient will question his or her nurse if the medication looks different from the usual "pill." In some cases, a generic version of a drug could have been substituted; in other cases, an error might be prevented.

Conclusion: Pharmacology in Nursing Practice

Given the central role of medical therapy in modern health care, the need for nurses to have a solid foundation in pharmacology is profound. Understanding how a drug acts in the body, how the body acts on the drug, and anticipating potential positive and adverse effects of drugs is tantamount if nurses are to knowledgeably administer drugs to patients. Recognizing drug actions based on knowledge of pharmacology enables the nurse to anticipate whether changes in patient symptoms indicate drugs are having its intended or adverse effects, whether medications are acting as drugs or poisons—"pharmacons." The act of administering medications is where the theory of medicine is put into practice. It is also where the general understanding of human biochemistry manifests in the reality that all people are different. Nurses are tasked with identifying how these differences may affect the use of a medical therapy in a patient and with determining the actions necessary to ensure the therapy's success. By learning about pharmacology, nurses can equip themselves to make sure that the tools of medicine are used appropriately to heal illness and relieve distress in their patients.

CHAPTER SUMMARY

- Pharmacology is the study of the actions of drugs, incorporating knowledge from other sciences.
- Drugs are classified based on their action or effect on the body or by their chemical characteristics.
- Nurses must be familiar with both generic and trade names of drugs.
- Controlled substances are categorized based on their potential for abuse and their prescribed uses.
- Drug information is available from many sources; nurses should familiarize themselves with reliable tools to gain knowledge of drug therapy.
- The five steps of the nursing process—assessment, nursing diagnosis, planning and goal setting, intervention, and evaluation—are a key part of safe drug administration.
- The success of drug therapy may vary because of cultural beliefs or ethnic differences.
- Nurses must follow legal and ethical guidelines for drug administration.
- Nurses must be aware of the potential for medication errors, working to provide a safe environment for drug therapy.

Critical Thinking Questions

1. What is pharmacology?
2. List three characteristics of a medicine used as a basis for drug classification.
3. Discuss the rationale for nurses knowing both generic and trade names of drugs.
4. What is an example of a Schedule II drug? What are the prescriptive limitations placed on such a drug?
5. Describe the five steps of the nursing process.
6. Identify at least three factors that can contribute to medication errors.

REFERENCES

American Nurses Association (ANA). (2001). *Code of ethics.* Retrieved from http://www.nursingworld.org/codeofethics

American Nurses Association (ANA). (2015). *Code of ethics for nurses with interpretive statements.* Retrieved from http://nursingworld.org/DocumentVault/Ethics-1/Code-of-Ethics-for-Nurses.html

Anderson, P., & Townsend, T. (2010). Medication errors: Don't let them happen to you. *American Nurse Today, 5*(3), 23–27.

Barker, K., Flynn, E., & Pepper, G. (2002). Observation method of detecting medication errors. *American Journal of Health-System Pharmacy, 59,* 2314–2316.

Barker, K., Flynn, E., Pepper, G., Bates, D., & Mikel, R. (2002). Medication errors observed in 36 health care facilities. *Archives of Internal Medicine, 162*(16), 1897–1904.

Bonsall, L. (2011). *8 rights of medication administration.* Retrieved from http://www.nursingcenter.com/Blog/post/2011/05/27/8-rights-of-medication-administration.aspx

ECRI Institute. (2017). *ECRI Institute names top 10 patient safety concerns for 2017.* Retrieved from https://www.ecri.org/press/Pages/Top-10-Patient-Safety-Concerns-for-2017.aspx

Institute of Medicine (IOM). (2007). *Preventing medication errors.* Retrieved from http://nationalacademies.org/HMD/Reports/2006/Preventing-Medication-Errors-Quality-Chasm-Series.aspx

Institute for Safe Medication Practices (ISMP). (2003, September 4). *Cultural diversity and medication safety.*

Retrieved from https://www.ismp.org/newsletters /acutecare/articles/20030904.asp

Institute for Safe Medication Practices (ISMP). (2016). *2016–2017 targeted medication safety best practices for hospitals*. Retrieved from http://www.ismp.org/Tools /BestPractices/TMSBP-for-Hospitals.pdf

Keers, R.N., Williams, S.D., Cooke, J., & Ashcroft, D.M. (2013a). Causes of medication administration errors in hospitals: A systematic review of quantitative and qualitative evidence. *Drug Safety*, 36(11), 1045–1067.

Keers, R.N., Williams, S.D., Cooke, J., & Ashcroft, D.M. (2013b). Prevalence and nature of medication administration errors in health care settings: A systematic review of direct observational evidence. *Annals of Pharmacotherapy*, 47(2), 237–256.

Makary, M., & Daniel, M. (2016). Medical error—the third leading cause of death in the US. *BMJ, 2016*, 353. doi: 10.1136/bmj.i2139

McBride-Henry, K., & Foureur, M. (2006). Medication administration errors: Understanding the issues. *Australian Journal of Advanced Nursing*, 23(3), 33–41.

Nanji, K.C., Patel, A., Shaikh, S., Seger, D.L., & Bates, D.W. (2016). Evaluation of perioperative medication errors and adverse drug events. *Anesthesiology, 124*(1), 25–34.

Schneider, M., Cotting, J., & Pannatier, A. (1998). Evaluation: Nurses' errors associated with the preparation and administration of medications in a pediatric intensive care unit. *Pharmacy World Science*, 20(4), 178–182.

Thomas, E. J., & Peterson, L. A. (2003). Measuring errors and adverse events in health care. *Journal of General Internal Medicine*, 18(1), 61–67.

Tissot, E., Cornette, C., Limat, S., Mourand, J., Becker, M., Etievent, J., . . . Woronoff-Lemsi, M. (2003). Observational study of potential risk factors of medication administration errors. *Pharmacy World Science*, 25(6), 264–268.

Wirtz, V., Taxis, K., & Barber, N. (2003). An observational study of intravenous medication errors in the United Kingdom and in Germany. *Pharmacy World Science*, 25(3), 104–111.

CHAPTER 2

Introduction to Drug Action: The Interplay of Pharmacodynamics and Pharmacokinetics

Diane F. Pacitti

KEY TERMS

Absorption
Active ingredient
Active metabolite
ADME
Adverse effect
Adverse event
Affinity
Affinity constant (k_A)
Agonist
Antagonist
Area under the curve (AUC)
Bile
Bioavailability
Biopharmaceutics
Biotransformation
Blockers
Brand name
Central compartment
Chemical name
Clearance
Clinical pharmacology

Compartmental model theory
Competitive antagonist
Distribution
Dose
Dose-response curve
Dosing interval
Dosing regimen
Drug
Drug action
Drug-activity profile
Duration of action
Efficacy
Elimination
Elimination rate constant (k_e)
Endogenous
Enterohepatic circulation
Exogenous
First-order
First-pass effect
Half-life ($t_{1/2}$)
Inactive metabolite

Inhibitors
Irreversible receptor antagonists
Lag-time
Ligand
Margin of safety
Mechanism of action
Metabolism
Metabolite
Minimum effective concentration (MEC)
Minimum toxic concentration (MTC)
Noncompetitive antagonist
One-compartment model
Onset time
Pharmaceutical
Pharmacodynamics
Pharmacokinetics
Pharmacologic activity
Plasma-level time curve
Plasma proteins

Potency
Presystemic elimination
Pro-drug
Rate process
Receptor
Renal clearance
Saturable-binding kinetics
Second-messengers
Side effects
Signal transduction
Steady-state drug levels
Therapeutic drug monitoring (TDM)
Therapeutic index
Therapeutic response
Therapeutic window
Toxicity
Toxicology
Volume of distribution (V_D)
Zero-order

CHAPTER OBJECTIVES

At the end of the chapter, the reader will be able to:

1. Define key terms.

2. Explain how a drug "knows" where to go following administration to a patient.

3. Explain what is meant by drug action, describing the events required for a drug to elicit a therapeutic response.

4. Differentiate the meaning of "drug action", using pharmacokinetic and pharmacodynamic parameters.

5. Explain why a specific dose of drug is required to achieve a therapeutic response.

6. Describe the difference between an agonist and antagonist.

7. Discuss the factors that can affect the pharmacodynamic parameters, such as time of drug onset, duration of action, minimum therapeutic dose, and receptor-drug binding.

8. List the factors that affect the bioavailability of a drug.

9. Explain how different routes of drug administration affect the therapeutic drug response.

10. Explain the physiological factors that influence the pharmacokinetic parameters, such as the rate and extent of drug absorption, distribution, metabolism, and excretion (drug action).

11. Describe how a dosing regimen is developed for a medication, in pharmacokinetic terms.

12. Discuss the factors that can affect optimal therapeutic response, drug therapy, and clinical patient care.

Introduction

The effective use of drugs in clinical practice requires a thorough understanding of both the foundational principles of pharmacology *and* the specific pharmacological characteristics of the major drug classes currently used in healthcare practice. The molecular basis of drug action—for all drugs—is based upon similar principles of pharmacology. To fully understand the molecular basis of drug action, the complex interactions between a drug and the body must be examined, including the consequences these interactions have on the drug's therapeutic or desired effects. This chapter provides the foundational principles and concepts necessary for learning how drugs are used in prevention and treatment of disease.

What Happens After a Drug Is Administered?

The question of how a drug works on the molecular level to produce a desired, therapeutic drug response underpins the study of pharmacology.

A drug is administered to a patient for a reason: to achieve a desired beneficial, or clinically observable, therapeutic effect. For this to occur, the drug itself must ultimately be delivered to a specific place in the body, called the drug's "site of action," to produce its desired effect, known as the **"therapeutic response."** To fully understand how the drug acts on the body, one must consider the fate of the drug following its administration to a patient. **FIGURE 2-1** illustrates the different sites inside the body where the drug can interact before it produces a physiological response.

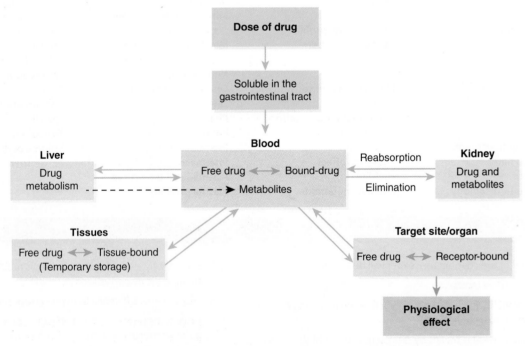

FIGURE 2-1 Pathways of a drug movement within the body (following oral administration). Note the number of sites/variables with which the drug can interact before producing a physiological effect.

Courtesy of Diane Pacitti. © 2017

Of note is the *lack* of a definitive path upon which the drug follows after it enters into the body to produce a response.

Drug action can be illustrated by following the movement of the drug molecule throughout the body, starting from the time the initial dose of drug enters the patient's body, to its interaction with its target site, until finally, the drug has completely moved out (**elimination**) of the body. Imagine that a drug could be tagged with a visible marker, thus enabling an observer to visualize and follow the drug as it moved through the body. The observer would be able to identify the precise macromolecules with which the drug interacted that result in an alteration of a specific biochemical or physiological process(es).

A number of questions arise from this scenario:

- *How* does the drug know where to go? *Does* it know where to go?
- *Why* would the medicine be administered in one manner and not another? *When* would a specific route of administration (ROA) be chosen?
- What happens *to the body* after the drug is administered? Where *else* does the drug "go" as it moves throughout the body?
- *After* the drug is administered, *how long* does it take the drug to work?
- *How* does the drug get to its intended site of action? Once there, *how* does it work?
- *How much* of the drug is needed to affect an observable change in the patient's symptoms?
- What dose of drug is "too much," and what happens if *too much* drug is given?
- *How often* does the medication need to be given to the patient, and how long should the therapy regimen continue? What if a dose is missed?
- Which patient parameters should be monitored while the patient is taking this medication?
- How does the body *eliminate* the drug?
- *How long* will it take for the drug to be completely removed from the body?

To safely administer medications, a nurse must know the answers to a range of potential questions about his or her patients' medication therapy. These questions are easily answered after grasping the basic principles and concepts necessary for understanding drug action, including the major determinants that influence the therapeutic response of a drug, in a clinical setting. The approach to understanding how these questions are addressed is the objective of this chapter.

Making the Connection: Pharmacology in Clinical Nursing Practice

Pharmacology (derived from the Greek word *pharmakon*, which translates into *poison* in classic Greek and *drug* in modern Greek, and *-logia*, meaning "the knowledge gained through study"), is the branch of medicine and biology concerned with the study of drug action—or, "how a drug works". In its broadest sense, pharmacology studies how chemical substances affect living organisms. More specifically, it is the study of the interactions between a living organism and a chemical substance that result in *a visible change* to the organism's normal or abnormal biochemical (or physiological) function(s). The resultant change is called a **drug action**. *Note:* The term "drug action" *alone* does not characterize *the outcome* of the change as beneficial, therapeutic, or toxic to the organism. Drug action simply means that an alteration in a physiological or biochemical process takes place *because* of the drug's interaction with a specific site within the body. If such chemical substances have *medicinal properties*—meaning they work in such a way as to correct an abnormal biochemical or pathophysiological function (including restoration of biochemical functions that are absent, intermittent, or subnormal)—they are said to be *pharmacologically active* and are considered **pharmaceuticals**. The field of pharmacology encompasses a broad range of scientific disciplines including biochemistry, physiology, pathophysiology, and chemistry, in addition to the study of the chemical structure of drugs, their chemical properties, toxicology, therapy, and medical applications.

Pharmacokinetics Versus Pharmacodynamics

The two major underpinnings of pharmacological study are *pharmacodynamics* and *pharmacokinetics*. The core principles of *both* (pharmacodynamics and pharmacokinetics) must be examined to characterize drug action, and are discussed later in this chapter. **Pharmacodynamics** is the study of "*what the drug does to the body*." More specifically, it describes the molecular interactions of a drug with specific biological molecules that lead to a desired therapeutic response. The study of **pharmacokinetics** is referred to as "*what the body does to the drug*" and quantifies the rate of drug movement in the body. Specifically, pharmacokinetic studies characterize the speed of drug **absorption**, **distribution**, **metabolism**, and drug elimination (excretion). The interaction between a drug and its target site is essential for understanding the molecular basis of drug action (*pharmacodynamics*); equally as critical is characterization of the rate and extent of the drug's movement in the body (*pharmacokinetics*). The **efficacy** of drug therapy (meaning, how *well* the drug works) is evaluated using components of *both* pharmacodynamics and pharmacokinetics. (*The term efficacy will have a more specific meaning, later in this chapter.)

The safe administration of medication is critical to providing optimal nursing care. A thorough review of the different ways medication is administered in the clinical setting, emphasizing the safe nursing practices associated with each, is given elsewhere in this text (Chapter 3). However, even if a drug is *administered* safely, a lack of understanding about *how* and *why* the drug works imperils the goals of medication therapy. Much of importance occurs within the span of initial drug administration and the action(s) of the drug, which ultimately produce a clinically beneficial response. It is *paramount* that the actions occurring between these two points are fully understood by the nurse. This chapter links drug action within the body at the molecular level to the patient's therapeutic drug response in the clinical setting, considering the host of variables that influence drug action. Knowing which pharmacodynamic and pharmacokinetic factors influence drug action equips the practitioner to better predict the therapeutic response of a medication, and tailor drug therapy to individual patients. Understanding "*the whole story,*" from proper administration to expected responses, enables the nurse to anticipate the timing of drug effects, the actions of drugs, and potential adverse effects and interactions.

The Relationship Between the Drug and the Body

To understand the molecular basis of pharmacology, the complex interrelationships between the drug and the body must be considered, *as well as* the consequences these interactions have on the drug's therapeutic or desired effects. The *molecular basis of drug action*, for *all* drugs discussed in this text, is based upon these *same concepts and principles* of pharmacology.

What Is a Drug?

Before examining drug action on a molecular level, it is necessary to first clarify what is meant by the terms *medication* and *drug*.

A **drug** is a substance or chemical capable of altering a biochemical or physiological process(es) in the body; these responses may be desirable (therapeutic) or undesirable (adverse). Drugs do not change the basic nature of these functions, or create new functions. This is a *vital* tenet of pharmacology: drugs do not confer any new functions on a tissue or organ in the body; *they simply modify existing functions*. For example, drugs can only affect the *rate* at which existing biologic functions proceed: they can speed up or slow down the biochemical reactions that cause muscles to contract, kidney cells to regulate the volume of water and salts retained or eliminated by the body, glands to secrete substances (such as mucus, stomach acid, or insulin), and nerves to transmit messages. Within the Federal Food, Drug, and Cosmetic Act (FD&C), the United States Food and Drug Administration (FDA) defines a drug* as:

1. A substance recognized by an official pharmacopoeia or formulary.
2. A substance intended for use in the diagnosis, cure, mitigation, treatment, or prevention of disease.
3. A substance (other than food) intended to affect the structure or any function of the body.
4. A substance intended for use as a component of a medicine but not a device or a component, part or accessory of a device.

Biological products (including *therapeutic biological products*, defined as proteins derived from living material, such as cells or tissues) used to treat or cure disease are included within this definition and are generally covered by the same laws and regulations, but differences exist regarding their manufacturing processes (chemical process versus biological process).
(Food and Drug Administration [FDA], n.d.)

Therefore, chemical substances such as water (H_2O), caffeine, metals (e.g., titanium, copper), illicit street drugs (e.g., heroin, crack cocaine), and mosquito-repellant (insecticide) spray *all* qualify as "drugs" (and rightly so). It quickly becomes evident that not all drugs are therapeutically beneficial, or even legal to use, in the United States. In contrast, a **medication** is defined as a drug that is used for the purpose of restoring a dysfunctional or pathologic process in the body to its desired function or process; conventionally termed a "medicine". The terms *drug* and *medication* are synonymous with what the FDA defines as an **active ingredient**. An active ingredient is any component that provides pharmacological activity or other direct effect in the diagnosis, cure, mitigation, treatment, or prevention of disease, or to affect the structure or any function of the body of man or animals (FDA, n.d.). Throughout this text, the words drug, medication, and active ingredient are used interchangeably.

Advances in New Drug Development: Personalized Medicine

The goal of **medication therapy** is to restore a dysfunctional or pathological biochemical or physiological process. Unfortunately, drugs cannot restore structures or functions *already damaged beyond repair* by the body. This fundamental limitation of drug action underlies much of the frustration when trying to treat tissue-destroying or degenerative diseases such as heart failure, arthritis, muscular dystrophy, multiple sclerosis, and Alzheimer disease (Arrowsmith, 2012). Yet, the completion of the human genome sequencing project along with rapid developments in genomics has dramatically transformed pharmacotherapeutic treatment approaches for many diseases, some with no previous drug choices. The National Research Council outlined the development toward a more individualized, gene-based pharmacotherapeutic treatment of human disease—termed *precision-based medicine* (Desmond-Hellmann et. al, 2011). There are a growing number of research initiatives to accelerate progress toward what drug development companies are calling "a new era of precision-medicine" (Kambhampati, 2014; Abrams, Conley & Mooney, 2014; Carter et. al, 2017). Personalized medicine promises to increase benefits and reduce risks for patients by improving both the safety and efficacy of medical products (Kambhampati, 2014; Food and Drug Administration [FDA], n.d.).

Drug Nomenclature

Every drug has (at least) three names: (1) a chemical name, (2) a generic name, and (3) a brand name (there can be one or more proprietary or trade names).

1. The **chemical** name is designated according to rules of nomenclature of chemical compounds (IUPAC—International Union of Pure and Applied Chemistry).

2. The **generic** name refers to a common established name regardless of its manufacturer. There is only one generic name for a drug.
3. The **brand** name is selected by the manufacturer and is *always* capitalized.

Chemical Name

The **chemical name** is a precise description of the chemical composition and molecular structure (see **FIGURE 2-2**) of a compound. In the early stages of drug research and development (commonly referred to as "R and D", for Research and Development), a chemical substance with potential pharmacological activity (i.e., a new drug candidate) is identified by its "chemical name"; that is, its molecular, atomic, or chemical structure. In most cases, the chemical name is too complex and cumbersome for general use; researchers may assign the compound a code name, a reference number, an acronym, or abbreviate the chemical name.

Generic Name

The generic name is the "official name" of the drug; there is only *one* generic name for any drug or medication. Although the FDA must approve *both* the generic *and* the brand name of a new drug, the FDA does *not* assign the new drug its generic name. In the United States, the generic name of a

medication is assigned by the United States Adopted Names (USAN) Council, an official body formed precisely for this purpose. Many generic names are a shorthand version of the drug's chemical name, structure, or formula (American Medical Association [AMA], n.d.). According to the USAN, the council strives to assign generic drug names that are useful and meaningful for their primary users: health professionals. (Physicians, for example, are *not* interested in knowing the chemical structure of drug molecule). "Consideration of the needs of health professionals has led to a system in which distinctive nonproprietary names are given that indicate relationships that exist between the new entity and older drugs. Conversely, misleading names that might suggest nonexistent relationships are avoided" (Wells, 2017).

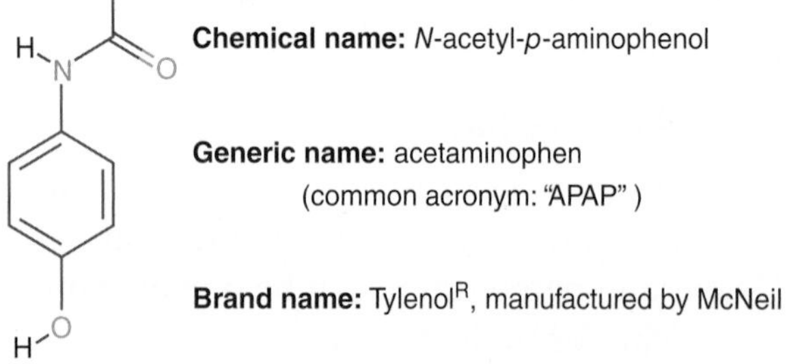

Brand Name

The **brand name** (also known as the "trade name" or "proprietary name") is created by the company requesting initial FDA approval for the drug and identifies it as the exclusive property of that company. While a drug is under patent protection*, the company markets it under its brand name. When the drug is no longer protected by the patent (the patent has expired), the original company may market the drug under *either* the generic name *or* its brand name. Other companies that file for approval to market the off-patent drug must use the same generic name but can create their own unique brand name. As a result, the same generic drug may be sold under either its generic name or one of many brand names. Therefore, one drug may have at least three different names: one chemical name, one generic name, and *one or more* brand names.

*A Note about Patent Protection - **Patent Protection for Drugs**

In the United States, a company that develops a new drug can be granted a patent for the drug itself, for the way the drug is made, for the way the drug is to be used, and

Chemical name: *N*-acetyl-*p*-aminophenol

Generic name: acetaminophen
       (common acronym: "APAP")

Brand name: Tylenol^R, manufactured by McNeil

FIGURE 2-2 The complexity of drug nomenclature. Chemical name: *N*-acetyl-p-aminophenol. (Molecular structure of $C_8H_9NO_2$). Different names for the same drug molecule (medication). Note the degree of complexity among the three different names. These three names are interchangeable, and all refer to the same drug!

Reproduced from the Open Chemistry Database. Retrieved from https://pubchem.ncbi.nlm.nih.gov/compound/acetaminophen#section=To.

even for the method of delivering and releasing the drug into the bloodstream. Patents grant the company exclusive rights to a drug for 20 years; although additional patents can be filed in an attempt to extend the patent life. Usually, it takes about 10 years between the time a drug is discovered, the company files a New Drug Application (NDA) with the FDA (petition for approval, when the patent is obtained), and the FDA grants approval of the drug. The company may have only half of the patent "time" left to exclusively market a new drug (and profit from its use). Companies that manufacture generic drugs typically sell their product at a lower price than the original brand-name drug because the generic manufacturer does not have to recover the original costs of drug development and spends less on marketing. (Smith Marsh, 2017)

Key Notes on Drug Naming

- When a new drug is approved by the FDA, it is given a **generic** (official) name and a **brand** (proprietary or trademark or trade) name.
- **Generic** and **brand** names *must* be unique to prevent one drug from being mistaken for another when drugs are prescribed and prescriptions are dispensed. To prevent this possible confusion, the FDA must agree to every proposed brand and generic name.
- **Generic names** are usually more complicated and harder to remember than **brand names**.
- In the clinical practice of medicine, prescribers tend *not* to be interested in the drug's **chemical name** or physiochemical properties when prescribing drug therapy for their patients. Hence, the *chemical* name of a drug tends *not* to be used outside of the fields of pharmaceutical science, research, and/or drug development.
- It is common practice for government officials, researchers, and others who write

about the new compound, to use the drug's **generic name** because it refers to the drug itself, not to a company's brand of the drug or a specific product.
- Prescribers often use the **brand name** on prescriptions, because it is easier to remember *and* because they are introduced to new drugs by the *brand name* (by pharmaceutical sales representatives).
- **Brand names** are typically "catchy," often related to the drug's intended use, and relatively easy to remember, so that doctors will prescribe the drug and consumers easily recognize the name (most commonly from advertising).

Source: Smith Marsh, 2017.

The Liver: Anatomical First Stop for Orally Administered Drugs

In order to ensure the safety of compounds introduced into the body, the FDA categorizes and distinguishes compounds used for drug therapy through an approval process that assigns them as either prescription, or over-the-counter (OTC medications). However, the human body cannot distinguish between a prescription medication and a poisonous toxin: both are **exogenous** chemicals (meaning, chemical substances *produced outside of the body*). Fortunately, inherent physiologic processes serve to protect the body from potentially toxic compounds. Every compound that enters the human body is subjected to these same physiologic and biochemical processes.

As an example, a food or any other substance ingested by mouth is subjected to the rigors of the gastrointestinal (GI) system tract and its digestive processes. Food is broken down by enzymatic processes into smaller particles and transported to the duodenal region of the small intestine. Digestive processes continue until food breakdown is complete, releasing vitamins, nutrients, and other essential compounds in the duodenum, where the absorption of most soluble chemical substances takes place. Compounds

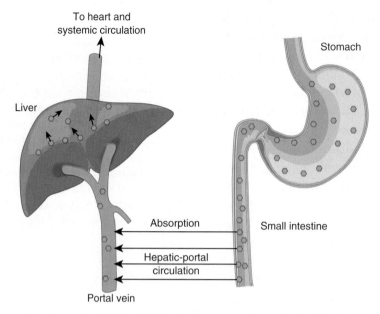

FIGURE 2-3 Physiologic protection of systemic circulation. The blue circles represent drug molecules. Following drug administration, the drug in the small intestine is absorbed into the hepatic portal vein, where it passes through the liver before it is "delivered" to the systemic circulation (the entire body).

absorbed from this region of the GI tract do *not* immediately enter the systemic circulation (bloodstream); they *first* enter into the hepatic portal vein, which shunts all orally absorbed substances to the *liver* (**FIGURE 2-3**). The liver serves as the "filter" through which compounds are "screened" by inherent (built-in) metabolic and enzymatic processes; pathways in the liver *may* (or *may not*) remove *or* chemically inactivate drugs, nutrients, or potential toxins (by metabolic breakdown processes, discussed in further detail later in this chapter). As a consequence, drugs that pass through the digestive tract may *not* attain the same concentration in the bloodstream as was present in the GI tract, before the absorption process.

The human body does not "know" if the administered drug compound is a nutrient, a poison, a vitamin, or a medication—*it does not discriminate*. The liver serves *only* as an *anatomical first stop* for chemical substances absorbed from the duodenal region of the small intestine—*before* they can reach the systemic circulation. Following passage through the liver, the vena cava carries blood from the liver to the bloodstream (*systemic circulation*; i.e., circulation throughout the entire body). This is illustrated in Figure 2-3.

The chemical changes a drug undergoes as it passes through the liver *may* affect the drug's ability to interact with its target site of action; it depends *how* the chemical changes affect the drug's molecular (i.e., chemical) structure. A structurally-changed drug (**metabolite**) may not retain the chemical properties required to elicit a therapeutic response. If the drug's metabolite *can* elicit the same therapeutic response as the "parent drug" (chemical structure of the intact drug), it *retains its pharmacological activity,* and is termed an **active metabolite**. Conversely, if the chemical changes render the drug *unable* to elicit a therapeutic response, the metabolite is deemed *pharmacologically inactive*, and termed an **inactive metabolite**. For this reason, the amount of drug surviving these liver processes, and thus the resulting therapeutic drug response, may be less than anticipated when the drug was originally administered orally; this is called the **first-pass effect** (metabolism, metabolites, and *the first-pass effect* are discussed later in this chapter).

It is important to note that *not* every drug, chemical substance, or even poisonous compound is subjected to the metabolic processes present in the liver (many compounds are *not* affected by the metabolic pathways).

Key Notes

- The anatomical shunting of orally ingested chemical substances to the liver, *before* it circulates throughout the entire body, is just *one* of the body's built-in (inherent) physiologic protective mechanisms.
- Although the liver is the primary site of chemical detoxification and protection, *it is not the only site* where metabolic processes take place.
- Medications can be broken down into inactive forms by enzymatic processes located *within the gastrointestinal tract*, thereby preventing the drug from ever reaching the bloodstream.

Nursing Considerations

The amount of medication (or any chemical substance) that the liver can metabolize depends on the overall health of the liver. Consider a medication that must be chemically changed (metabolized) in order to be eliminated from the body; the drug is *completely dependent* upon an enzymatic (metabolic) pathway in the liver to change its chemical structure into a form that can then exit the body (i.e., if it is not metabolized by the liver, it will not be eliminated [removed] from the body). A patient with a history of hepatitis or cirrhosis is likely to have impaired liver function due to direct damage caused by disease. A patient with impaired liver function will not have the same metabolic capacity as a healthy patient. Thus, a patient with hepatic dysfunction who is given a drug that relies on the liver to be eliminated may experience toxicity from the "regular" dose of this medication. In other words, the dose of the drug may need to be lowered, to prevent drug toxicity.

Drug Meet Patient; Patient Meet Drug

The introduction of a drug into a patient, presuming that the drug does, in fact produce a clinically beneficial effect, can result in several clinical outcomes. The *optimal* outcome a drug can produce is a therapeutic response (beneficial effect) without causing any ill effects for the patient. However, because the drug travels throughout the body via the bloodstream to reach its intended target, a number of alternative outcomes can occur. These include: (1) no therapeutic response in a patient (although this is very rare); (2) a side effect (common); or (3) an adverse event (uncommon). The occurrence of side effects does not necessarily preclude the use of a drug. A **therapeutic response** means that the medication produces a beneficial effect for the patient. Understanding "response" requires knowing *how* and *where* in the body a drug produces it. Ideally, a drug administered to a patient would move only (and specifically) to its site of action, where it would produce its intended therapeutic response without affecting other sites in the body, where its effects are neither required nor wanted. This selectivity is called the "magic bullet" and describes the *ideal* medication—one that every pharmaceutical company and research pharmacologist strives to create. However, very rarely (if ever) does this occur with the medications currently in use. The assumption that all drugs act *selectively*, leading to only the desired results, is flawed because most drugs *lack* selectivity; that is, a drug may also produce unintended and often unpredictable effects on the body. Because the drug travels via the bloodstream to reach its intended target, inevitably, unintended sites within the body are exposed to the drug, potentially causing unpredictable (and unwanted) physiological or biochemical responses. Thus, when drugs do not act "ideally," it is important to understand why and perhaps even to anticipate deviations from ideal behavior.

As mentioned, the most common unintended therapeutic drug responses are side effects. **Side effects** are *responses in tissues* where *the drug's effects are neither needed nor wanted*, causing problematic, but not harmful, symptoms such as nausea, fatigue, headache, and similar uncomfortable responses. Drug side effects result from the drug's "accidental" interaction, or interference, with of one or more of the body's (healthy) physiologic systems, while the drug's therapeutic effects help to repair the intended dysfunctional system. Side effects range in severity from mild (barely noticeable), to nuisances (somewhat bothersome), to—at worst—severe. In severe cases, an unintended drug effect causes such a significant impact on the patient's daily functioning that the patient may choose to stop taking the medication as a result. An example of a particularly troublesome side effect (but one that is not harmful or toxic to the patient) that may lead to the discontinuance of drug therapy is nausea. Although nausea is extremely uncomfortable, the drug itself is not causing harm or damaging the biological function of body systems (except if nutritional intake is adversely affected).

In some cases, drug therapy produces the desired therapeutic drug response but at the same time produces *harmful* effects; some of these effects are severe enough to be life-threatening. When an unintended drug effect causes harm to the functioning of a body system, it is termed an **adverse effect** (also referred to as an **adverse event**) and usually requires the patient to discontinue that medication. For example, a widely prescribed class of medications used to treat high cholesterol levels (statins) is associated with development of *rhabdomyolysis*, a rare but life-threatening disorder in which skeletal muscle tissue is damaged. Should a patient experience muscle pain not attributable to other causes following the initiation of statin drug therapy, the patient would alert their prescriber immediately, as the muscle pain could be an early sign of this adverse effect (Lopez-Jimenez, et. al. 2014).

Although steroids ("glucocorticoids") are highly effective anti-inflammatory medications, long-term use of these medications in the treatment of chronic inflammatory disease is associated with several serious adverse reactions. Glucocorticoid use causes hyperglycemia (abnormally high blood sugar levels), which, if left untreated, may lead to diabetes. Acceleration of bone loss, which can lead to osteoporosis (Ferris & Kahn, 2012), is another potential adverse effect associated with long-term glucocorticoid use. For this reason, steroid medications are frequently used only on a short-term basis, to "kick-start" healing, without allowing sufficient time for the side effects to do long-term damage.

Toxicology

Toxicology is the study and characterization of the adverse effects caused by excessively high concentrations of drug in the body and the harmful, potentially fatal results that may result. Most drugs used for their medicinal effect have the potential to become **toxic** (i.e., capable of causing harm or death; to produce toxic effects); it all depends upon the **dose**, or *amount of the drug* that is administered to the patient. The first recorded toxicologist, Paracelsus (circa 1500) was quoted as saying, "All substances are poisons; there is none which is not a poison. The right dose differentiates a poison and a remedy." Most often, this is simply paraphrased: "*the dose makes the poison.*"

Thus, both in this text and others, the reader is reminded of the root word of pharmacology, *pharmakon*, and its *two* meanings—drug and poison—with good reason. Medications do not affect all individuals in the same way. In fact, they do not always affect the same individual in the same way, each time they are used. The same drug that is therapeutic for one patient can produce harmful, even toxic effects, when administered to another. Unfortunately, there are a limited number of signs alerting the practitioner to which patients should or should not use a given medication. Therefore, it is important to weigh each drug's potential for harm against the anticipated benefits in each patient accordingly. *All drugs* must be treated as potential "toxins." Toxic effects, or **toxicity** implies drug poisoning, the consequences of which can be extremely harmful and may become life-threatening. In such situations, the drug should be stopped immediately and supportive therapy to treat the harmful effects may be required.

Nursing Considerations

Toxic effects should not be confused with *adverse* or *side effects. Side effects* (and adverse effects) occur when drug concentrations are within therapeutic levels, as a result of that drug's interaction with sites *other* than the drug's target site, producing unwanted, but not fatal, effects. **Toxicity** is a result of *"too much drug" in the body,* when the amount of drug present in the body exceeds the "dose"; hence the derivation of the term *overdose.*

What, Then, Is the Right Dose?

One must consider the relationship between drugs and the body to answer this question. Thus far, the mechanism of drug action has been described in terms of the interaction between the drug and a functionally important structure within the body. This *alone* is not sufficient to determine the "right dose" of medication for any given patient. Not only does the drug interact with the body,

the body interacts with the drug molecule. This may be likened to the "pharmacology coin": Up until this point, the focus has been on only one side of the coin. There is a flipside, however, and *its* characteristics must be examined thoroughly as well, to determine the coin's value. In pharmacological terms, knowledge of "where" and "how" drug action occurs does not provide enough information to determine "how much drug" (right dose of medication) is required to produce a therapeutic drug response. To determine the optimal dose of a drug, one must examine factors that affect *the fate* of the drug as it moves throughout the body *as well as the rate* (speed) at which the drug movement occurs. In other words, one must examine what the drug does to the body *and* what the body does to the drug.

The Interplay of Pharmacokinetics and Pharmacodynamics

What happens when drug and patient meet is a complex, challenging interplay of the two sides of the pharmacology coin: pharmacodynamics and pharmacokinetics. **FIGURE 2-4** illustrates that

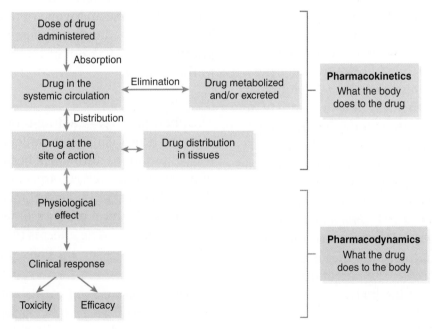

FIGURE 2-4 The interplay of pharmacokinetics and pharmacodynamics: The components, text boxes and all shapes that are colored in purple are pharmacokinetic parameters. Those same items that are colored in blue are pharmacodynamic parameters. Note the *interdependence* of the pharmacological response on the drug concentration at the site of action. This is only *one* of the components involved in the complex interplay of the drug-body interactions.

Courtesy of Diane Pacitti. © 2017

both pharmacokinetic and pharmacodynamic parameters influence the ability of a drug to produce a therapeutic response following the introduction of a drug into the body.

Pharmacodynamics

Pharmacodynamics describes qualitatively the therapeutic activity of a drug once it is in the bloodstream, and characterizes the interaction of the drug with its target site, known as the **mechanism of action (MOA)**. The MOA identifies the target molecule with which the drug interacts and describes *how* the interaction produces a therapeutic drug response. This allows one to calculate how a given amount of a drug will get from point A (the place where the drug enters the body) to point B (the place in the body where the drug's activity is wanted). Pharmacodynamic studies delineate factors such as dose, onset of drug action, and drug response. These will be discussed later in this chapter.

Pharmacokinetics

Pharmacokinetics is the quantitative (numerical) study of the rate of drug movement throughout the body, focusing on the biological processes by which substances move in the body as a function of time. The study of pharmacokinetics can be summarized as the study of how fast the drug reaches the bloodstream (*absorption* process), how fast the drug gets to its site of action (*distribution*), how long the drug stays in its chemically active form (is the drug metabolized—yes or no), how long the drug stays inside the body before being eliminated, how fast the drug is eliminated from the body (processes of *elimination*), and how often the drug needs to be dosed (dosing interval). Pharmacokinetics uses mathematical equations to predict the rate of drug movement throughout the body.

Biopharmaceutics

The third key area of pharmacological study is known as **biopharmaceutics**. It is the study of the design and development of drug dosage forms that will (1) deliver the chemically active form of the drug in sufficient amount (dose); (2) withstand physiologic conditions inside the patient's body; (3) release the active drug at a tolerable therapeutic rate (i.e., neither too slowly nor too quickly); and (4) determine the route of administration to achieve the optimal therapeutic outcome without causing physiologic adverse effects for the patient. The chemical properties of the drug molecule govern the drug's formulation into what is termed its "dosage form" (e.g., capsule, tablet, solution, transdermal patch). These same chemical properties, in turn, determine which route of administration (ROA) would be the best way to deliver the drug so that it gets where it is needed in an appropriate concentration, without causing physiologic adverse effects for the patient.

An excellent and thorough review of the different routes of drug administration encountered in the clinical setting is given in Chapter 3 of this text. Not only does it build on the foundational principles introduced in this chapter, the emphasis placed upon the safe practices throughout the nursing process while administering medication strengthens the discourse and scope of this discussion. The study of medication dosage forms (biopharmaceutics) will not be addressed in detail in this chapter.

Nursing Considerations

The pharmacology of a drug is often confused with the drug's clinical, therapeutic response. It is important to distinguish between *actions* of drugs and their *effects*. *Actions* of drugs are the biochemical physiological mechanisms by which the chemical produces a response in living organisms. The effect is the observable, clinical outcome—or, the consequence of a drug action.

- The *pharmacology* of a drug defines the *mechanism of drug action*; the mechanism of action explains *how* and where in the body the drug *works*, and identifies the biological molecule to which the drug binds at the drug's target site of action.

- The *therapeutic response* of a drug is the desired effect, or clinical outcome of drug therapy, and explains the desired end result of drug therapy.

Consider the following scenario: A patient is diagnosed with strep throat and prescribed an antibiotic—penicillin—to treat the infection. *"How* does the drug work, to treat strep throat?"

- The HOW is the pharmacology and explains *the mechanism of action* of penicillin; The mechanism of action explains how penicillin works to kill and/or remove the Gram-positive-bacteria (*Streptococcus*) that is the *cause* of the infection.
  - Penicillin interferes with the structure and synthesis of the bacterial cell wall; bacterial cell walls "break," causing the bacterial cell contents to spill out. This kills the bacterium.
- The clinical response of penicillin is relief of any sore throat pain or possible fever. That is, improvement in patient symptoms due to eradication of the bacteria—the cause of the strep throat.

Clinical Pharmacology

The interplay of the research areas—pharmacodynamics and pharmacokinetics—answers many of the key clinical questions that come with the decision to prescribe a medication and initiate a patient on a drug treatment regimen. **Clinical pharmacology** is the *application* of the concepts and principles of pharmacology to enable the practitioner to properly evaluate and manage drug therapy for patients in the clinical care setting. In pharmacology, the key questions about the clinical use of medication are:

1. *For what reason* is the medication being given—that is, *what condition* is being treated, and what are the intended effects? (In other words, *Why?*)
2. *What is the dose* of the medication that must be given to achieve therapeutic effects without causing harm? (*How much?*)

3. When should this dose be repeated to maintain those effects? (*How often?*)
4. By which method is the medication best administered for this patient? (*Where?*)

The key difference between pharmacology and clinical pharmacology is that simply knowing the chemical properties of the drug is not enough to predict the therapeutic drug response in the clinical setting; the practitioner must also evaluate and individualize medication therapy for each patient. Every drug has a dose required to produce a therapeutic response (known as the **therapeutic dose**). However, drug *action is different in every patient*, even though the same medication is administered under identical conditions. This introduces once again a critical consideration—one which the nursing professional frequently encounters in the clinical setting: What, then, is the "right" dose? Clinical pharmacology applies these basic pharmacological principles to determine what the right dose is, for optimal patient care.

The reliance of pharmacokinetic effects upon drug concentration at the target site provides the *key link* between pharmacokinetics and pharmacodynamics. Given that the goal of medication therapy is to achieve a therapeutic effect:

- Drug action occurs only when there is a sufficient concentration of drug present at the site of action; *and*
- The rate and extent of drug distribution determines the amount of drug to reach the site of action.

Which side of the coin should be studied first? Pharmacokinetics *or* pharmacodynamics? It literally becomes a "toss-up"; *both sides* must be examined, to accurately characterize the patient's therapeutic response and the outcome of the medication therapy. FIGURE 2-5 illustrates the interdependence between pharmacodynamic and pharmacokinetic parameters. The mechanism of *how* a drug interacts with its receptor site to produce a beneficial drug response is addressed first. Consideration of pharmacokinetics, or the rate processes of drug movement throughout the body, will follow.

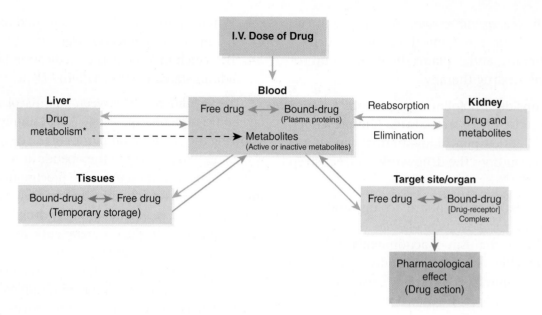

FIGURE 2-5 Pathways of drug movement after entering the bloodstream.
Courtesy of Diane Pacitti. © 2017

Pharmacodynamics

Pharmacodynamics is the study of the mechanism of drug action. The mechanism of drug action describes both *where* the interaction (drug's target site) takes place and *how* the change (therapeutic response) occurs. In other words, it considers both *drug action*, which refers to the initial consequence of a drug-receptor interaction, and *drug effect*, which refers to the subsequent effects. The *drug action* of **digoxin**, for example, is via inhibition of membrane Na^+/K^+-ATPase pump on cardiac tissue; the *drug effect* is augmentation of cardiac contractility (Chapter 6).

What the Drug Does to the Body

A medication, or "drug", is administered to a patient for a reason. It does not matter what the reason is. It does not matter what the drug is. It also does not matter who the patient is. What matters is what happens *after* the drug is administered to the patient. *Does the drug produce the therapeutic effect, for which it was prescribed*? To answer this, one must address drug action—*at the molecular level*—that leads to a drug's therapeutic response.

It was originally thought that the drug itself "knew" where "to go" in the body. All the drug molecule had to do, after reaching the bloodstream, was travel directly to the "spot" in the body that needed "to be fixed," and once there, fix the problem for which it was given and the drug would exit the body. Another dose of drug would only be necessary *if* the "problem" occurred again. For example, consider an adult with a sore throat, who has taken a single oral dose of an over-the-counter analgesic, to relieve the sore throat pain. The patient asks, "How does the medication get rid of this pain in my throat?" It was believed that the medication "knew" just where the pain source was located and moved directly to that site in the body, where it would work to alleviate the pain. It is *now* known that drugs ingested by the oral route must not only survive the rigors of the gastrointestinal digestive processes, but also then travel to the liver, before they even enter the bloodstream! But what about the throat pain? The over-the-counter analgesic moved right past it, after it was swallowed; yet in most cases it does prove effective, and temporarily relieves the mild to moderate throat pain for which it was taken. But the question remains unanswered: How *does* the drug know where to go?

The Mechanism of Drug Action

The key to answering the question of *how* the drug relieves sore throat pain hinges upon the overarching principle of pharmacology: Drugs do not produce "new" responses in the body; they merely interact with a structure in the body, resulting in alterations of physiologic or biochemical processes that *already exist*. While it is widely accepted that the effect of most drugs results from interactions with **receptor** molecules, the concept of a "molecular drug target" inside the body with which the drug interacted was not widely accepted until the middle of the twentieth century. It was originally thought that drugs exerted their effect on the body based upon the chemical properties of the drug molecule itself. Later theories of drug action proposed that there was a structure inside the body, complementary in shape and specificity to the structure of the drug molecule, to which the drug bound. However, *the existence* of such "drug-specific molecules" could only be inferred from the chemical structures of the drugs. In 1907, Paul Ehrlich developed his own theory, which included the binding of drugs to molecular drug targets receptors that he called chemoreceptors (Ehrlich, 1913). However, it was not until the first "receptor" molecule (the beta-receptor) was isolated and its receptor interactions characterized, that the "receptor theory" was accepted by the scientific community. With the discovery of the "receptor" molecule came theories regarding the *mechanism* of the drug-receptor interaction. Originally, the belief was that a drug "fit" into the receptor molecule in the same manner in which *a key* fits *into a lock* to open a door; this model was aptly named the "lock and key" model. Simply put, the receptor is a "lock" with a specific keyhole, and the drug is the "key" that fits (into the lock), to open the door. (**FIGURE 2-6**. In pharmacology, if the "right" drug finds the right "receptor", it produced the drug's therapeutic response. Unfortunately, the mechanism of drug action is not this simplistic.

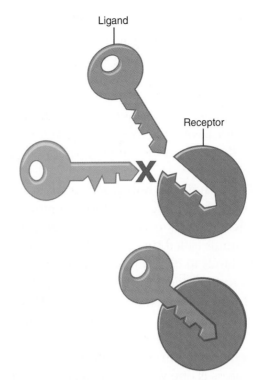

FIGURE 2-6 Cartoon illustration of the degree of ligand-receptor binding specificity between the drug and the binding site(s) on a target receptor molecule.

Courtesy of Hana Tisserand. http://tisserandinstitute.org/cleaning-receptors-myth/

The Receptor Molecule

The "functionally important" molecule in the body with which the drug interacts (to produce its therapeutic response) is known as the "drug target". For most drugs, this *target molecule* is a macromolecular protein called a *receptor*. **Receptors** are large protein molecules located either outside the target cell called *extracellular* receptors, or inside the cell, called *intracellular* receptors. The receptor types are discussed in further detail later in this chapter.

It is of import to note, however, that the actual drug-target may not even *be* a receptor molecule. Although the term "receptor" is ubiquitously used to describe the target molecule with which the drug interacts, *not all drugs exert their pharmacologic actions via receptor-mediated mechanisms*. There are other mechanisms by which a drug produces its effect. For instance, the mechanism of action for a number of drugs (discussed throughout this textbook) is attributed to the *physicochemical properties of the drug molecule*. Examples include osmotic diuretics, purgatives, antiseptics, antacids, chelating agents, and urinary acidifying and alkalinizing agents. Certain cancer and antiviral chemotherapeutic agents are structural analogs of pyrimidine and purine bases; these drugs serve as suicide substrates for DNA or RNA synthesis, and elicit their effects when they are incorporated into nucleic acids.

For most drugs, however, the target *is*, in fact, a receptor molecule. Most receptors have specific, naturally-occurring (**endogenous**) compounds called **ligands**. When the proper ligand binds to its receptor, it causes a stimulation (or *activation*) of the receptor molecule, which leads to a biological response. This response manifests as a change in an existing physiological or biochemical process within the body. Quite often, the affected physiological process is one which plays a critical role in maintaining optimal health. For almost all receptors that have been identified to date, endogenous ligands specific for each receptor

have been identified and characterized. A ligand has a specific three-dimensional shape that "fits" into its binding site on the receptor molecule. The receptor binding site is highly discretionary and will only bind compounds (ligands) with specific chemical structures. Therefore, the ligand must "fit" and bind to the receptor (three dimensionally) in a very precise manner. Even a slight change to the chemical structure of the molecule can render it unable to properly fit into the receptor's binding site (**FIGURE 2-7**). The degree to which the ligand is able to elicit a therapeutic response is dependent upon the interaction between the ligand-binding site and the receptor, the specifics of which are addressed in the following section.

The Nature of Ligand-Receptor Interactions: Chemical Bonding Interactions/Forces

The target site on the receptor molecule has a high degree of binding-specificity as well. Like any other chemical-bonding interaction, the

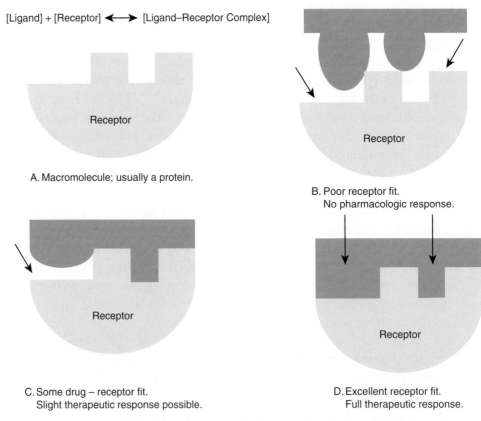

[Ligand] + [Receptor] ⟷ [Ligand–Receptor Complex]

Receptor

A. Macromolecule; usually a protein.

Receptor

B. Poor receptor fit.
No pharmacologic response.

Receptor

C. Some drug – receptor fit.
Slight therapeutic response possible.

Receptor

D. Excellent receptor fit.
Full therapeutic response.

FIGURE 2-7 Ligand-Receptor Complex: If the body lacks the ligand, either from a disease-state or congenital disorder, a drug (medication) may serve to bind the receptor as the "ligand" itself would, (replacing the natural compound), thus resulting in the desired physiological (pharmacological) response. When the drug binds to its receptor site, it produces the intended pharmacological response.

Courtesy of Diane Pacitti. © 2017

binding of a ligand (or drug) to a receptor is determined by chemical bonding forces that allow interaction(s) between functional groups on the ligand and complementary binding surfaces in the receptor (**FIGURE 2-8**). Ligands bind to their target site on the protein molecule "using" chemical bonds, non-covalent in nature (meaning "reversible"); Bonds include the following "intermolecular forces":

1. *Hydrogen bonds* result from electrostatic attraction between an electronegative atom (oxygen or nitrogen) and a hydrogen atom that is bonded covalently to a second electronegative atom. They result from electrostatic attraction between an electronegative atom (oxygen "O"; or nitrogen, "N") and a hydrogen (H) atom that is bonded covalently to a second electronegative atom. Example: N-H ----- O=C- -O-H----- O=C-

2. *Ionic bonding* is a very important bonding mechanism between a drug and receptor, as many drugs are weak acids or bases. These drugs become "ions," meaning they have either a positive or a negative charge (positive and negative charges interact) when in the physiological environment of the body (pH averages 7.4). The nature of the ionic chemical bond is a basic attraction between net positive (+) and negative (–) charges.

3. *Van der Waals forces* are the weakest bonds between a drug molecule and its receptor-binding site. They are short range, weak hydrophobic attraction forces caused by slight charge displacements that occur only when chemical groups come into close contact with one another. The bond occurs when a drug is within close contact to its receptor site, and this close proximity can cause non-polar groups such as hydrocarbon chains to associate with each other in the aqueous physiological environment.

4. *Covalent bonds* are strong, irreversible chemical bonds (sharing of electrons) that form when a drug's chemical group shares electrons with a chemical group on the receptor. This bond is irreversible; thus, the drug-receptor complex will never dissociate. Compounds that are bound by covalent bonds are usually toxins or poisons to the human body.

Nursing Considerations

The effects of most drugs used in clinical practice are temporary, because the interaction of the drug with the target site is *reversible*. Consider the effects of a drug that entered the body, and bound covalently to its target site - that drug would permanently remain in the body. An example of one of the *few* drugs that *does* utilizes covalent bonding is **aspirin (ASA)**. This medication irreversibly acetylates platelets, thereby suppressing the production of prostaglandins and thromboxanes (due to its *irreversible* inactivation of the cyclooxygenase [COX] enzyme).

The Drug-Receptor Complex

If the body lacks the ligand, either from a disease-state or congenital disorder, a drug (medication) may serve to bind the receptor as the "ligand" itself would (replacing the natural compound). Therefore, the drug must be a close structural mimic of the endogenous compound, (to "fit" the target site on the receptor).

Note: Knowing the exact structure of the endogenous ligand allows synthetic chemists to design structural mimics of the ligand molecule. This knowledge greatly expands the pharmaceutical industry's arsenal of potential new drugs.

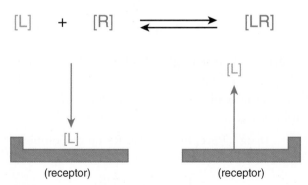

FIGURE 2-8 The extent to which a ligand will bind to its receptor molecule & form a [ligand-receptor] complex is dependent upon the degree of chemical attraction between the two molecules, expressed by the affinity constant, k_A (see text).

drug's *"association rate"*, or, *"on"* rate

$$[\text{Drug}] + [\text{Receptor}] \underset{k_{-1}}{\overset{k_{+1}}{\rightleftharpoons}} [\text{Drug-Receptor Complex}]$$

drug's *"association rate"*, or, *"off"* rate

FIGURE 2-9 A drug molecule will bind to a receptor molecule if there is a sufficient degree of chemical attraction between the two molecules. The *strength* of the bond between two molecules is based solely upon chemical bonding; that is, the degree of "chemical attraction" between the two. The complex formation occurs at a speed known as the drug's *association rate*, also referred to as the *drug's on rate* (meaning, how quickly the drug associates, or binds to, the receptor). The rate of complex formations is represented by the rate constant k_{+1}. The bond between the drug and its receptor, forming the drug-receptor complex, is reversible (meaning the drug eventually disassociates or "falls off" the receptor). The amount of time the drug remains bound to the receptor is based upon the degree of chemical bonding attraction (and also the basis of the duration of a drug's action). The drug-receptor complex breakdown occurs at a speed known as the drug's *dissociation rate*, or *off rate*, and is represented by the rate constant. k_{-1}.

Courtesy of Diane Pacitti. © 2017

What are the chances that a that any molecule, such as a ligand (or drug), will bind to a receptor-binding site? It depends on the *degree of chemical attraction* (i.e., the strength of the "chemical bonding forces) between the two molecules (covalent bonds are the strongest; Van der Waals are the weakest). The equation in **FIGURE 2-9** shows the interaction that is reversible. The drug binds to the receptor, and then "falls off."

The *strength* of the drug-receptor complex is measured in terms of **affinity**; that is, *how much the drug is attracted to the receptor* (or target). *Affinity* is the measure of the strength of the bonds, or tightness, of the drug-receptor complex. The strength of the binding complex is represented by an **affinity constant**, referred to as k_A (**FIGURE 2-10**). This term is widely used to describe drug-receptor binding. The *magnitude* of k_A indicates the degree of attraction with which a drug (or ligand) binds to a receptor. The stronger the affinity, the longer the drug–receptor complex will exist before the drug is released from the site.

The length of time the drug remains bound to its receptor [between a drug and a receptor] is also the basis of the *duration of action* for a medication (the duration of drug action in addressed in further detail later in this

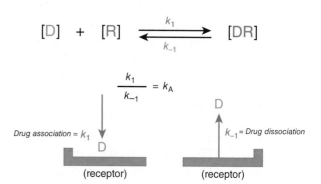

FIGURE 2-10 Drug is abbreviated as "D"; receptor is "R". The brackets represent the "molar concentration". Note that the binding constant k has "A" as its subscript. This indicates that the bonding constant is expressed in terms of the "association" of the drug with the receptor molecule [DR]. The rate of drug binding to the receptor is represented by "k_1", and rate which the drug "leaves" or "falls off" (dissociates) the receptor is represented by "k_{-1}". The association constant k_A is calculated from the ratio of the molar concentration of reactants [D] and [R], and the molar concentration of the product [DR]. Drug binding to its receptor ("on") and the dissociation ("off") of the drug from the receptor. (One could also characterize the drug-receptor binding interaction in terms of the parameter "k_D", known as the "dissociation complex". The ratio of the "on" and "off" rates would simply be inverted to calculate the dissociation complex.)

Courtesy of Diane Pacitti. © 2017

chapter). The strength of a bond between a drug and a receptor protein can be expressed mathematically, as well. Consider that the following:

Drug + Receptor ↔ Drug-Receptor Complex

Or

(D) + (R) ↔ (DR)

This equation assumes one binding site per receptor molecule:

$$k_A = \frac{[DR]}{[D][R]}$$

Where [DR] = bound drug-receptor complex and [D] and [R] = free, or the receptor molecule and drug separate from one another. An association constant, k_A, can be expressed as the ratio of the molar concentration of the products and the molar concentration of the reactants.

The Drug-Receptor Interaction and Therapeutic Response

If a drug binds to a receptor molecule to form a receptor-bound complex (drug-receptor complex [DR]), one can expect the bound complex to induce that receptor's therapeutic response. The assumption that must be made is this: when the drug binds to the target binding site on the receptor molecule, it will produce the intended therapeutic response.

This is known as the *receptor occupancy theory*, and is illustrated in FIGURE 2-11. The equation illustrates that the formation of a drug–receptor complex is responsible for a desired pharmacologic effect. What about the *extent* of the drug response? The degree to which a drug is able to produce a therapeutic drug response is based upon both the affinity of the drug for the receptor, and the efficacy. *Efficacy* is pharmacodynamic measure of the therapeutic response, and is related to the number

of receptor-drug complexes which can form *at* the drug's target site of drug action. Efficacy is discussed in further detail later in this chapter.

Types of Receptors

Most receptors are one of three types of large protein molecules: (1) those located outside the target cell, called cell-surface receptors or *extracellular receptors*; (2) *transmembrane receptors*, which cross, or span, the cell membrane— these receptor-types have binding sites located on both the outside and inside of the cell; or (3) those located inside the cell, called *intracellular receptors*. (The best-characterized receptor molecules are regulatory proteins, enzymes, transport proteins, and structural proteins. [Note: for the purpose of understanding the molecular mechanism of drug action, it is not necessary to know what pharmacological response each of these receptor-types produces]).

Transmembrane Receptor Activation and Response

The transmembrane receptor has a specific ligand binding site on the outside surface of the cell. For example, four *different* transmembrane receptors are illustrated in FIGURE 2-12; in this figure, note that each of the receptors has a specific ligand-binding (receptor) site located on the outside of the cell and "connections", or "responders" of some type located on the inside of the cell. When the cell-surface-receptor site is "occupied" (ligand binds), the transmembrane receptor undergoes a transformational change in shape (conformational change), which then "signals" a "messenger" inside the cell, to amplify the signal. One receptor binds one ligand – and triggers a chain of biochemical events ("amplification") to take place inside the cell.

Signal Transduction

The ligand-receptor complex formation initiates a complex set of reactions inside the cell via a process known as **signal transduction**.

Receptor occupancy theory

The general theory of drug receptor interaction can be expressed by the equation:

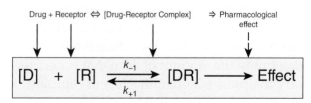

Drug + Receptor ⇔ [Drug-Receptor Complex] ⇒ Pharmacological effect

$$[D] \; + \; [R] \; \underset{k_{+1}}{\overset{k_{-1}}{\rightleftarrows}} \; [DR] \longrightarrow \text{Effect}$$

FIGURE 2-11 Receptor Occupancy Theory
Courtesy of Diane Pacitti. © 2017

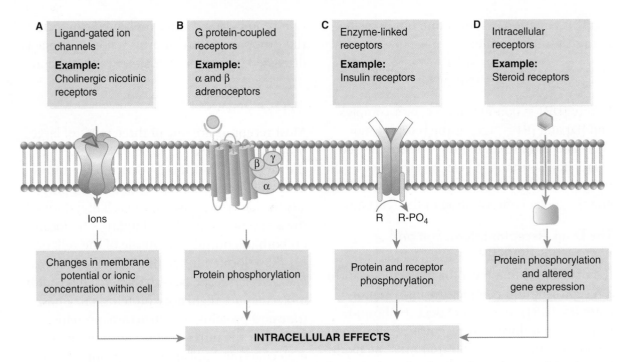

FIGURE 2-12 Types of receptors. Each of the four different receptor types illustrated utilizes cell-surface signaling pathways to affect a change within the cell.

Courtesy of Diane Pacitti. © 2017

The signal is amplified by activating what is known as a **"second-messenger system"** inside the cell. **Second messengers** are systems that are activated upon stimulation of the receptor. Although only one molecule can stimulate one receptor (at any one time), the stimulated receptor can produce multiple second messengers, each of which can stimulate other molecules within the cell. *One molecule* (ligand, drug, etc.) *can therefore cause a large effect.*

Key Points

When the ligand binds to its receptor site, the receptor complex undergoes a "conformational change" (meaning the shape of the entire receptor changes); this change then initiates a complex set of biochemical reactions *within* the cell, called signal transduction. In effect, one ligand binds to one receptor site, and converts an extracellular signal into an intracellular signal—which then signals the "messenger" inside the cell *to amplify the signal*. These interactions and the resulting conformational changes in the receptor initiate biochemical and physiological changes that characterize the drug's response.

The Dose-Response Relationship

In previous discussions in this chapter, it was said that a drug can only exert its desired (therapeutic) affect when enough of the drug molecule is present at the active site to produce a physiological response. The concentration of drug that is reached at site of action depends on the dose and dosage form in which the drug was administered and the physiochemical properties of the drug itself, as well as physiological processes of the body. An amount of drug is administered to a patient and the desired therapeutic drug response occurs. *How much* drug is required to produce a therapeutic drug response? The amount is known as the **dose** of a drug.

Pharmacodynamic studies are performed to characterize *how much drug is required to produce a therapeutic response*. Specifically, to determine the amount of drug that is necessary to produce a quantifiable and clinically observable response, defined (increasing) amounts of drug are administered to healthy volunteers and the therapeutic response is measured. The data is known as the *dose-response curve*. The "dose-response curve" is obtained graphically: the amount of drug is plotted on the X-axis, and its corresponding therapeutic response on the Y-axis. **Dose-response curves** are used to present data describing *the ability of a drug to produce a given physiological effect.*

A plot of the log of [D], (in which [D] is the concentration of drug), versus the pharmacological effect results is a sigmoidal-shaped curve, and is the most common "graphical" presentation of the "dose-response data"; depicted in FIGURE 2-13. It is *the way the data is graphed* which yields the shape of the curve—the *X-axis is the log dose).* The resulting sigmoidal curve is depicted in the following graph:

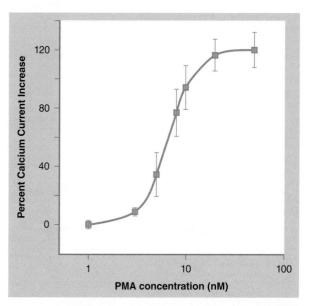

FIGURE 2-13 The sigmoidal-shaped curve is the most recognizable "dose-response" graph when speaking of a drug- receptor binding.

Data from U.S. Occupational Safety and Health

In FIGURE 2-14, the graph in 2-14a illustrates the raw drug concentration plotted on the X-axis. A graph of the amount of drug versus the therapeutic drug effect produces a rectangular curve that plateaus when the maximal therapeutic response is reached. This is a cumbersome graph because drug concentrations often vary over 100- to 1,000-fold, necessitating a long X-axis. To overcome this problem, the log of the drug concentration is plotted on the X-axis; the same data is graphed and the resultant curve is illustrated in Figure 2-14b (log of [D]) of the drug concentration on the X-axis. Note the difference in the shapes of the curves.

Pharmacodynamic Parameters Obtained from the Dose-Response Curve

The graphs in Figures 2-14a and 2-14b depict and characterize the relationship between the dose of a drug and the amount of drug required to produce the maximum physiological (therapeutic) effect. Graphs such as these are often used to compare the effectiveness of two drugs or characterize the degree of drug responses.

Efficacy

Efficacy is a measure of the *maximal therapeutic response that a drug is able to produce* and is dependent on the number of drug-receptor complexes formed. When all the receptors are

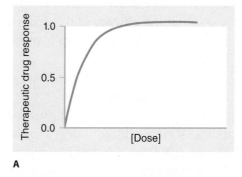

A

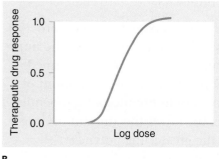

B

FIGURE 2-14 a: The dose-response curve. For example, a clinical study examines the effect of increasing amounts of an analgesic on pain threshold. To present the data, the concentration of the drug is plotted on the X-axis and the effect on pain threshold is plotted on the Y-axis. The resultant "dose-response curves" are shown in Figure 2-14b; both graphs depict the therapeutic effect of the drug on the Y-axis, but *the difference between the two graphs is the way in which the dose is plotted on the X-axis.*

occupied at a drug's site of action, the maximum therapeutic response is achieved.

On a log dose-response curve, the efficacy of a drug can be readily observed by looking at the *height of the sigmoidal curve*, and reading over to the Y-axis to determine the percentage of the maximal response.

Potency

Potency is a measure of *how much drug is required to elicit a therapeutic response*. The lower the dose required to achieve the *maximal therapeutic response*, the *more potent the drug*. By convention, in the field of pharmacology, potency is expressed as "the dose of drug that gives 50% of the maximal response," known as the ED_{50}. In this way, two or more drugs may be compared by examining the values of the ED_{50}, in the absence of graphical data (log-dose response curve).

On a log-dose response curve (sigmoidal curve), *the potency* of a drug can be readily observed by looking at the placement of the sigmoidal curve on the X-axis; its position on the X-axis quickly indicates that the farther to the left that the curve begins on the X-axis, *the more potent* the drug. That is, it takes *less drug* to produce a therapeutic response.

Potency vs. Efficacy: A Source of Confusion

The difference between potency and efficacy can be evaluated quickly by looking at a comparison between two drugs on a log-dose response curve. *The amount of drug* it takes to elicit the maximum therapeutic response of the drug is a measure of the drug's *potency*; a separate and distinctive parameter, easily confused with efficacy.

- **Efficacy** is the maximal response produced by a drug and depends on the number of drug-receptor complexes formed.
- **Potency** is a measure of the amount of drug necessary to produce a therapeutic response; the lower the amount of drug needed, the greater the potency.

FIGURE 2-15 compares three drugs that produce the same degree of therapeutic activity (i.e., all three drugs have the *same efficacy*) but

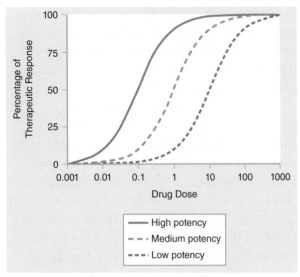

FIGURE 2-15 Dose-response graph comparing three different drugs. This dose-response graph compares the pharmacological response/activity of three different drugs that produce the *same therapeutic response*. (Pharmacological response is plotted on the Y-axis; the log of the drug dose amount is plotted on the X-axis; 100% is the maximum pharmacological response - % therapeutic response.) All three drugs produce the same degree of the desired response; that is, all three have the same efficacy (biological response). The *dose* required to produce a percent of therapeutic response is different among these three drugs–a shift of the curve to the right means it takes more drug to produce the same degree of drug response; therefore, it is said that the drug has a lower potency when compared to the others.
Courtesy of Diane Pacitti. © 2017

have three *different potencies*. Note, in this graph, the sigmoidal curve the farthest to the left represents the drug with the highest potency.

Nursing Considerations

A patient has an attack of gouty arthritis, and the prescriber would like the patient to receive a short course of a nonsteroidal anti-inflammatory drug (NSAID) medication. The prescriber has two choices: **ibuprofen**, 600 mg or **piroxicam**, 20 mg. Both drugs produce the same degree of pain relief; therefore, it is said that the efficacy of the drugs is the same.

Which of the two drugs is more potent? Why?

Which of the two drugs has a greater affinity for the receptor? Why?

The efficacy of the two drugs is the same, as a dose of either drug produces the same degree of pain relief. Yet, it takes 600 mg of **ibuprofen** and 20 mg of **piroxicam** to achieve that same degree of pain relief. **Piroxicam** is clearly the more potent of these two drugs, as it requires a lower dose to achieve the same effect. This does not mean **piroxicam** is "better" than **ibuprofen**; simply that it takes less of the drug to produce the same effect.

Affinity cannot be determined from the data given in the question as there is no mention of the binding strength of either drug to the receptor. Recall that affinity measures the degree of binding strength between two molecules and predicts the likelihood of two molecules forming a bonded complex.

Limitations of a Dose-Response Curve

The dose-response graph yields information that accounts for the amount of drug that produces the maximal therapeutic drug response. However, it does not give *any* information about the effect of the drug on the patient, the duration of action of the drug, the optimal dose, or the resultant effect on the patient: it does not include TIME. It is a graph simply showing the amount of drug required to produce the maximal therapeutic drug response. This by no means is meant to minimize the information gained from the dose-response relationship. The studies are essential for analysis of the drug's pharmacological properties.

The Drug Activity Profile

A fundamental principle of pharmacology is the amount of time it takes to produce a drug action, or alternatively, to produce a therapeutic, clinically observable effect. While a dose-response curve provides an instant view of the efficacy of a drug, it lacks the amount of time it takes to achieve a therapeutic drug response. For *this* information, one must look to the **drug activity profile**: a graphical representation of the concentration of drug in the body over a given period of time, using the information gleaned from the dose-response curve. (This graph is synonymous with a **concentration-response graph**.) A dose of drug is administered to a patient; the concentration of drug in the body is measured at periodic time intervals. The concentration of drug is plotted on the Y-axis, and the corresponding time of the blood draw is noted on the X-axis. The resultant graph represents the relationship between the amount of drug and the time the drug produces a therapeutic drug response; either its beneficial or toxic action (**FIGURE 2-16**).

The drug-activity profile is a measure of the amount of drug in the bloodstream at

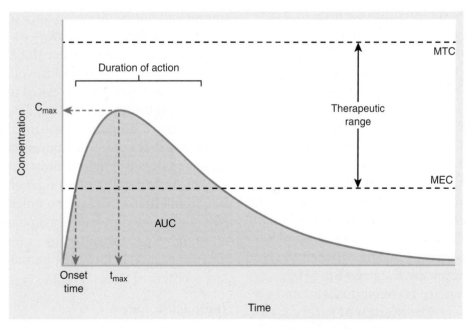

FIGURE 2-16 "Drug activity profile" (also known as the *concentration-response graph*). The drug-plasma level time curve indicates a number of pharmacodynamic parameters: the onset of action, duration of action, the therapeutic index, the minimum toxic concentration (MTC), and minimum effective concentration (MEC) for a given drug.

periodic time intervals; this information is used to determine the amount of drug required to be in the body to produce a therapeutic effect.

Pharmacodynamic Parameters Obtained from the Drug Activity Profile

Figure 2-16 illustrates a drug activity profile from which the following pharmacodynamic parameters can be determined: the *onset* of drug action, the *duration* of drug action, the minimum effective concentration (MEC), and the minimum toxic concentration (MTC). Each of these will be discussed in greater detail.

The amount of drug it takes to produce the intended pharmacological response of the drug is termed the drug's **minimum effective concentration (MEC)**. The drug must be present in a concentration at least as large as the MEC; thus, the MEC is used to determine **the dose** (or amount) of drug *that is given to the patient*. The drug's dose may be considerably more than the amount of drug required to achieve the MEC at the target site, but it must not be so large that it delivers too much drug to the site of action (or to unrelated locations) and produces toxic effects. The maximum dose of a drug that may be given to a patient without producing toxic effects is termed the *maximum effective concentration* (i.e., the maximum amount of drug that produces a therapeutic response, without signs of toxicity), and defines the uppermost dosage limits, or the maximum dose of drug that can be safely administered. The drug dose that no longer produces the intended therapeutic response but produces the first signs of drug toxicity is known as the **minimum toxic concentration (MTC)** and delineates the toxic dose for that drug. (Note that there is a very fine line between the *maximum effective concentration* and the MTC.)

The difference between the MEC and the MTC represents the **margin of safety** for a medication and is defined as the **therapeutic window**, also known are the **therapeutic index**. The dose of a drug that is required to deliver the optimal concentration at the active site depends on the pharmacokinetic and biopharmaceutical parameters of the drug, as well as physiological processes in the body that affect the drug as it moves throughout the body. The therapeutic window will be discussed further in this chapter.

Duration of Action

The **duration of action** is defined as *the length of time a drug exhibits a therapeutic effect* after the drug is administered, or the duration of the pharmacologic effect. This is determined by measuring the amount of time that the drug concentration is at or above the minimum effective concentration (MEC). In an earlier discussion it was said the duration of drug action is related to the affinity (degree of attraction) between the drug and the receptor molecule. In fact, the longer that the drug is bound to its receptor (drug-receptor complex), the more likely it is that the blood levels of drug will stay above the minimum effective concentration.

Onset of Action

The **onset of action** is the *time it takes for the drug to reach the MEC*. A measurable response will not be observed until the drug *exceeds the minimal concentration*—at its site of action—necessary to produce the desired response. Factors which effect the onset time for a drug are more likely related to the route of drug administration and the dosage form of the drug. A drug that is absorbed quickly will reach that minimum concentration more rapidly than a drug that is slowly absorbed. When comparing the onset time of drug action, recall that a drug with a quicker onset will require *less* time to exert a pharmacologic effect. *Increasing* the onset time means *more* time is required before the pharmacologic effect is observed.

Therapeutic Index

Drugs produce both desired and undesired (adverse) effects. The ratio of the minimum concentration of drug that produces toxic effects (*MTC*) and the minimum concentration that produces the desired effect (*MEC*) is termed the **therapeutic index**. The term *therapeutic window* is also used to refer to the span of concentration between the MEC and MTC. *The larger the therapeutic window for a drug, the "safer" it is to use that drug without causing unwanted toxicity in patients.* Another way of assessing the therapeutic index, also known as the margin of safety, is to use the ratio between two factors: the lethal dose 50 (LD_{50}), the dose of drug lethal in 50% of the laboratory animals tested, and the effectiveness dose (ED_{50}), the dose that produces the therapeutic effect in 50% of a similar population. The closer the ratio is to "1," the greater the danger in administering the drug to humans. Some drugs have a small therapeutic range and the difference between the effective dose and the toxic dose is small. **Digoxin**, **lithium**, and **warfarin** are examples of drugs with a *narrow* therapeutic index. During the course of drug therapy with these medications, particularly with **warfarin**, blood levels are drawn on a regular basis (e.g., weekly) to ensure that the drug concentration levels remain within therapeutic limits. This close monitoring of drug plasma levels is also known as **therapeutic drug monitoring (TDM)**. In contrast, **naloxone** is an example of a drug with a *wide* margin of safety.

Classes of Medications

After *any* drug binds to the ligand-binding site on a receptor, the drug may *either initiate a response* or *prevent a response from occurring*.

An **agonist** is a drug that produces a stimulation-type (*activates the receptor*) response. The agonist is a very close mimic to the ligand (endogenous compound) that normally stimulates that receptor; it therefore "fits" with the receptor site and is able to *initiate a response*. In contrast, an **antagonist** is a drug that binds to the receptor site and *blocks* or *depresses the biological response*

for that receptor. Because the *antagonist* binds to the *same site as the agonist* for that receptor, it also prevents the agonist or the receptor's ligand from binding to the receptor site. This type of antagonist is known as a **competitive antagonist**, because it "competes" with the agonist for the same binding site on the receptor. An antagonist that binds to a site *other* than the ligand-binding site, and blocks receptor-activation is known as a **non-competitive antagonist**. Since a non-competitive antagonist does *not* bind with the ligand-binding site, it blocks receptor activation in the presence of endogenous ligand. This is an important distinction which must be made; each is discussed in further detail.

Agonist Drugs
Mimic Ligand-Receptor Activation Responses

An agonist is a drug that binds at the exact same place on the receptor as the ligand. Thus, it is capable of producing a stimulation-type response. Agonist binding induces a conformational change in the receptor such that cellular signaling pathways are activated; these activated pathways trigger a series of biochemical events that ultimately lead to an alteration in cellular function, producing the *same effect as the endogenous ligand itself*. However, not all agonist drugs are capable of initiating the maximal response that the naturally occurring ligand is able to produce. Therefore, agonists can be further divided into *full* and *partial agonists*. Full agonists are compounds able to elicit a maximal response following receptor occupation and activation; partial agonists are compounds that *can* activate receptors but are unable to elicit the maximal response of the receptor system.

Antagonist Drugs
Block the Receptor's Activation Response

While it seems intuitive that inducing a therapeutic response would be an important part of therapy, *disrupting* (or "blocking") *such responses is equally*, if not more, important—particularly in situations in which the typical physiological response has become abnormal or compromised. An antagonist is a drug that binds to the receptor molecule and *prevents the receptor's biological or functional* activation process. Once bound, the drug may be unable to effectively alter the receptor in a manner that can initiate a change in cellular function. Antagonist molecules often bind at the same place on the receptor that the agonist binds (and therefore, where the ligand binds); occupation of the receptor by a "competitive" antagonist molecule prevents the binding and actions of agonists; this is discussed further in the next section.

Different Types of Antagonists

Antagonists can be reversible or irreversible. The most common type of antagonist drug-receptor interaction is known as the **competitive antagonist** (see above). This type of antagonist is known as *competitive,* because it (the drug) "competes" for the endogenous ligand-binding site on the receptor. Antagonists are also referred to as **blockers**, or **inhibitors.** (There are many examples of drugs that bind the active binding site on the receptor *intentionally to block* its activity—these appear throughout this text). Competitive antagonists block the ligand site, preventing the normal ligand from interacting with the receptor site. Competitive antagonists reversibly bind to the ligand-binding site binding to the receptor; blockade of the ligand-binding site can be overcome by increasing the agonist concentration. (The presence of the antagonist does *not decrease the maximal response* of the agonist) (see FIGURE 2-17).

In contrast, a **noncompetitive antagonist** binds to a site *different from the endogenous ligand's binding site* (responsible for activation of the receptor response) but it is still able to block the receptor's "normal" physiological response. The noncompetitive antagonist binds to a site—other than the ligand-bind site—on the receptor (and therefore, does *not* compete with the endogenous ligand (hence

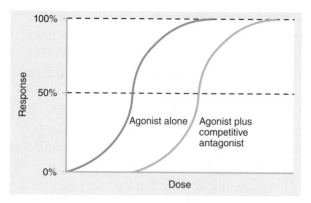

FIGURE 2-17 Hallmark log-dose response curve illustrating a competitive antagonist (discussed in text): Receptor blockade can be overcome by increasing the agonist concentration; the sigmoidal curve "shifts to the right"; meaning that the dose of the drug can be increased to overcome the presence of the competitive antagonist.

the name *"non-competitive antagonist"*). *Its* inhibitory action *cannot* be overcome by increasing the ligand or agonist concentration, nor can the presence of the ligand or agonist affect (diminish) the inhibitory action of the non-competitive antagonist.

Irreversible receptor antagonists are *chemically reactive compounds*. The antagonist covalently binds to the receptor. Because the bond is covalent, this compound can *not* disassociate from the receptor; the physiological response is completely blocked and cannot be undone. This is not a desired interaction, in most cases, as the receptor loses its functionality completely.

Nursing Considerations

Many "agonists" drug classes have been developed to bind to an endogenous ligand's binding site and stimulate its ligand-receptor's response. Many "antagonists" drug classes have been designed to interrupt, or block a particular process that contributes to disease, as well. For example, the enzyme aromatase converts testosterone to estradiol, an estrogen—a normal and necessary part of the female hormonal cycle. However, certain estrogen-dependent cancers affecting breast and ovarian tissue in women grow more rapidly in the presence of estrogen. Thus, a class of medications called aromatase inhibitors was developed to suppress the activity of the aromatase enzyme, effectively decreasing the body's synthesis of estradiol, and reducing the amount of estrogen available to promote tumor growth.

Variability in Pharmacodynamics

There is remarkable variability in drug responses from one individual to the next. Two patients can be given the same dose of the same medication and have completely different responses; the pharmacologic response to a drug is different in every human body. Therefore, one patient might take 500 mg of acetaminophen and have a completely different response than another patient. What causes this variability in drug response?

Some of the variability stems from the differences *the differences between individual persons*. These individual-level factors include the following:

- Body size and body mass (volume of distribution)
- Gender
- Chronological age
- Genetics/pharmacogenetics

- General health of the person
- Psychological aspects (e.g., placebo effect)

Other sources of variability occur due to the administration *of the drug itself* to that individual:

- Dosage
- Potency of the drug
- How the drug is formulated (e.g., liquid, capsule, tablet, sustained release)
- Route of medication administration (e.g., IV, oral, inhalation)
- Single dose (acute) versus maintenance (chronic) versus steady state
- Physiological tolerance of the drug (i.e., drug allergy, drug resistance)
- Interaction with other drugs and other substances that may be present in the body

Pharmacokinetics

How the Body Affects the Drug

Pharmacokinetic studies investigate and characterize the *rate* of *drug* movement throughout the body (see **FIGURE 2-18**)—specifically, the physiological processes of drug **absorption**, **distribution**, **metabolism**, and **elimination**; often

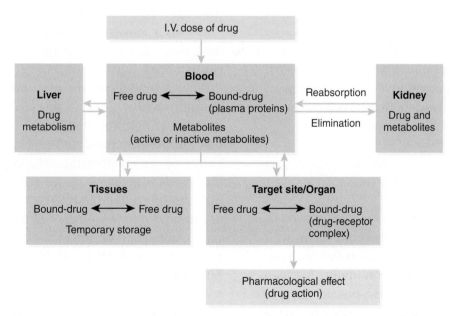

FIGURE 2-18 What the body does to the drug. What happens to a drug following an intravenous (IV) bolus dose of drug that is administered to a patient?

Courtesy of Diane Pacitti. © 2017

referred to by the acronym **ADME** (pronounced "add-mee").

- **A**bsorption: The process of drug movement, from the site of administration, into the systemic circulation.
- **D**istribution: The process of drug movement, from the systemic circulation, to the site of drug action.
- **M**etabolism: Chemical alteration(s) to the structure of the drug molecule.
- **E**limination: Process(es) of irreversible drug removal from the body.

Each drug moves throughout the body at a particular rate, depending on the physiochemical characteristics of the drug, the manner in which it is administered, and its interaction with the patient's body. *Pharmacokinetic studies* characterize the rate of drug movement throughout the body by measuring the amount of drug in the body over a given period of time. *Pharmacokinetic models* are developed to predict the patterns of drug movement when the drug is administered to the general population. The mechanism and rates of the absorption of drugs into the body, their distribution to various body sites, their metabolism into inactive (or active) compounds, and their routes of elimination are essential to understand how a drug works (drug action). The relationship of the amount of drug in the body at any time is used to determine pharmacokinetic parameters of half-life, steady-state drug levels, rates of drug clearance and bioavailability.

Overview of the Pharmacokinetic Processes, ADME

Absorption

Absorption is the process of drug movement *from* its site of administration *into* the systemic circulation; this definition implicitly means that the drug must cross a physiological barrier to reach, or enter, the systemic circulation. The *rate* of drug absorption is dependent on the *route* of drug administration (ROA). Consider a drug administered orally: It must "survive" (remain pharmacologically intact) the physiological conditions of the upper gastrointestinal (GI) tract (mouth, esophagus, stomach, and duodenum) as well as passage through the liver, before the drug reaches the bloodstream. Recall from discussion earlier in this chapter the variables along this route of administration which may (or may not) affect *the amount of the drug dose* that enters into the systemic circulation (the amount of the dose may be significantly decreased from the amount of drug present in the dosage form). Contrast this with a drug administered intravenously (IV): The drug is "placed" directly into the bloodstream (vein), in the form and concentration selected by the clinician. The onset of drug action is immediate, and the amount of drug needed to achieve a therapeutic effect may be smaller than with an orally administered drug.

Distribution

The process of drug **distribution** is *the movement of the drug from, or "out of," the systemic circulation to its target site of action*. The drug may distribute out of the bloodstream into organs or tissues, or simply stay within the systemic circulation. The physiochemical characteristics of the drug itself dictate where the drug "goes" as it moves throughout the body. The drug may diffuse into a particular tissue, because it "has affinity" for those tissues. The drug may bind to plasma proteins, such as albumin, within the systemic circulation itself. The amount of time a drug "stays" in the body is highly dependent upon the rate and extent of drug distribution. If a drug is *highly distributed*, it means that the drug *partitions*, or diffuses, out of the bloodstream into tissues/organs and *remains* (outside of the systemic circulation) for a period of time, before it returns to the bloodstream to be eliminated. Little or no "distribution" means the drug spends much less time in the body; it enters the bloodstream, interacts with its site of action, and is eliminated quickly. Drug distribution is discussed later in this chapter, as well.

Metabolism

Drug **metabolism** is any alteration or change to the chemical structure of the drug molecule by the body. Metabolic processes dictate how/if the chemical structure of the medication is "changed" or structurally altered, and may create secondary pharmacologically active drug products, called **metabolites**, which may or may not be therapeutically active. The different metabolic processes are addressed later in this chapter.

Elimination

Drug elimination (the term *excretion* is often used in place of elimination, although they are not the same) is the *irreversible drug removal from the body*. It is worth noting that the term *elimination* does not identify the mechanism or site of the drug removal processes. Drug elimination processes are complex and can involve multiple organ systems. *Pharmacokinetic rate processes* used to characterize the drug elimination rate constant, k_e, represent the fraction of drug eliminated, by all mechanisms, from the body. Drug elimination is discussed later in this chapter.

Nursing Considerations

Pharmacokinetic studies are performed with one goal—to obtain the rate constant for elimination, which means: How fast is the drug being eliminated in terms of time?

1. Why does the nurse need a working knowledge of the elimination rate constant?
   Because it is used to determine the *half-life* for that drug.
2. Why is the half-life important?
   The half-life determines how long the drug will stay in the body, *and* is used to design drug-dosing regimens.

Also, it is frequently necessary to predict how a *drug concentration* in the plasma (or other body fluid) *will change over time*. Although "pharmacokinetic studies" seem particularly daunting, this chapter aims to present material in a manner that is relatable *and* useful to the clinical practice of nursing.

Overview of Pharmacokinetic Terminology

The Pharmacokinetic Parameters Used to Characterize the Rate of Drug Movement

Each drug moves throughout the body at a particular rate, or speed, that is dependent on properties of the drug molecules and its interaction with the body. The rate of the drug's movement is represented, in pharmacological terms, by its rate constant, k (a lower-case k in italics); a subscript indicates which ADME process is being discussed—that is, the rate constant for drug absorption is k_a, for distribution it is k_d, and for elimination, k_e. The rate constant for a drug is determined from data obtained from pharmacokinetic drug studies plotted on a graph, called the drug's **plasma-level time curve**. The plasma level time curve is also used to characterize the **rate process** of drug movement (zero- or first-order). The rate constant of elimination, k_e, is used to calculate the most important pharmacokinetic parameter: the drug's **half-life**, known as $t_{1/2}$. Each will be discussed in turn.

Nursing Considerations

Kinetic parameters for all drugs approved for by the FDA are readily found on the drug's package insert, which contains the full prescribing information of each drug product.

Pharmacokinetic Studies and Determination of Kinetic Parameters

The Plasma Level-Time Curve

Similar to the pharmacodynamic dose-response curve discussed earlier, a plasma level-time curve is a highly useful tool used to determine characteristic properties of drug behavior after it enters the body.

A pharmacokinetic drug study is conducted in the following manner: A patient is given a specific dose, or amount, of drug, represented as "D", by intravenous (IV) bolus injection (bolus means "all at once"). The route of administration *must* be IV bolus to determine the rate constant for elimination (k_e) in pharmacokinetic studies, as *only one* kinetic process—elimination—is occurring. Blood draws are taken at specified time intervals, and the amount of drug in each blood sample is measured. The concentration of drug in the plasma is represented by C_p: "**C**" represents *the concentration* of drug; the subscript "**p**" means that the drug being sampled was drawn from the plasma (bloodstream). The amount of drug in the body determined at the time of each blood draw is plotted at the corresponding *time point* of the blood draw, **t**, on the X-axis on graph paper. The units on the Y-axis (C_p) represent the drug concentration, which is usually expressed as "mg/ml" or "ng/ml" (amount of drug/blood volume); on the X-axis, units are measurements of time (t), most commonly measured in hours. The resultant graph is known as the *plasma-level time curve*. The time of drug administration by IV bolus injection is called "time zero," or "t_0". Immediately following the administration of an IV bolus drug dose, the drug is in the bloodstream, and the process of drug elimination begins. The highest plasma drug concentration (C_p^{max}) occurs at the time of the IV bolus dose (at t^0) and is known as the "initial plasma drug concentration," or $C_p^{\,0}$. To find the rate constant k_e, one must calculate the slope of the "line of best fit" resulting from a plot of the drug concentration C_p versus time t (the slope IS the rate constant.) A plasma-level time curve is shown in **FIGURE 2-19**.

Rate Processes of Pharmacokinetics

Drugs generally exhibit either a **zero-order** or **first-order** rate process.

Zero-Order Rate Process

Drugs characterized as following a zero-order rate process (for any of the ADME processes) have a *rate* of drug elimination that is *constant*; that is, the drug is eliminated from the body at a *fixed rate* and independent of the amount of drug that is in the body. The *amount of drug eliminated from the body per time does not change.*

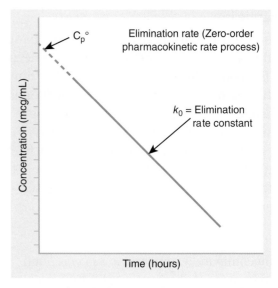

FIGURE 2-19 Plasma level-time curve illustrates a zero-order process of drug elimination following a single IV bolus dose of drug. The data is graphed using regular (rectangular) graph paper to obtain a straight line. The elimination rate constant is the slope of the straight line obtained from the resultant graph.

Courtesy of Diane Pacitti. © 2017

If a straight line can be drawn through the data after it is plotted on regular rectangular graph paper, it immediately reveals that the rate process for that drug follows a zero-order rate process for elimination. Figure 2-19 illustrates a plasma level-time curve typical for a drug that exhibits a zero-order rate process of elimination. The rate constant, k_0, is obtained from the slope of the straight line on the plasma-level time curve.

Key Points

Note: The *rate process* for drug elimination (i.e., irreversible removal of drug from the body) does not identify *how* the drug is being moved out the body (e.g., urine, feces).

Nursing Considerations

There are very few drugs that are eliminated at a fixed rate; the best-known drug that follows a zero-order rate process for elimination is alcohol. No matter what alcohol dose is "administered," the rate of alcohol elimination out of the body does not change. This is due to the elimination mechanism of alcohol—enzymes in the liver metabolize alcohol into a pharmacologically inactive form, and this is constant. The elimination rate will not change—approximately 10 mL of ethanol are eliminated per hour. (However, the rate *can* differ among the general population due to genetics, alcohol overuse, and other factors.) Contrary to popular belief, caffeine (coffee) *does not speed up* the elimination of alcohol from the body. **Caffeine** itself is a drug; its drug action is stimulation of the sympathetic nervous system (Chapter 5) .

The First-Order Rate Process

For a drug that exhibits (or follows) a first-order kinetic rate process (any ADME process), the rate of drug elimination is dependent upon *the amount of drug that remains in the body*; the rate of elimination is *not* constant. Unlike drugs that follow a zero-order rate process of elimination (which eliminates drugs at a constant rate no matter how much drug is in the body) the rate of elimination for drugs that follow first-order kinetics *does* change. Thus, for a patient with a high concentration of drug in his or her body, drug elimination occurs at a faster rate. As the amount of drug in the patient's body decreases (because it is being eliminated), the rate of drug elimination slows (decreases) proportionally. The rate constant (k_e), represents the fraction of drug eliminated from the body—and *this* is constant (**FIGURE 2-20**).

The same data as seen in Figure 2-20 is also plotted in **FIGURE 2-21**, but this time the data is graphed using semi-logarithmic graph paper. The Y-axis is rectangular (i.e., normal), and the X-axis is in log units. The graph is *transformed into a straight line when the data is plotted on semi-log graph paper*. A straight line is obtained for a drug that exhibits first-order kinetics, and a curved line for a drug that follows zero-order kinetics (to be clear, a zero-order rate process of elimination on semi-log graph paper results in a curved line—not a straight line).

Further Explanation of Rate Constants in Pharmacokinetics

As mentioned, rate constants are represented by the lowercase letter "*k*," in italics. But

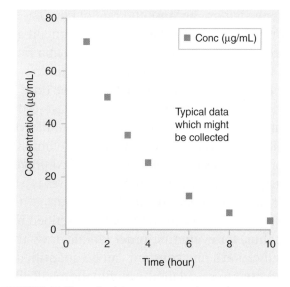

FIGURE 2-20 Plasma-level time curve on regular graph paper illustrates a drug that follows a first-order rate process of elimination. Note that there is not a straight line.

Courtesy of Diane Pacitti. © 2017

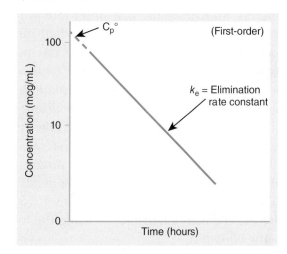

FIGURE 2-21 Plasma level-time curve for a first-order rate process on semi-logarithmic graph paper.

Courtesy of Diane Pacitti. © 2017

what, exactly, *is* the rate constant? And how can there be a "constant" if, as has been discussed, the elimination rate for drugs that follow a first-order kinetic rate process *slows down over time*? To answer this question, understand that there are two different rates being considered when looking at the rate of elimination for drugs that follow a first-order kinetic rate process. The first is the fairly straightforward concept of the rate at which the drug leaves the body, or *the elimination rate*. The second is the rate at which *the elimination rate changes over time*. For a drug that follows a zero-order rate process, this rate of change is zero, because the rate of elimination is constant (unchanging) over time; if a zero-order kinetic drug is eliminated at a rate of 1 mg/100 ml per hour, it will be eliminated at that rate from the moment the dose is administered until the moment the last of the drug leaves the body. For a drug that follows a first-order rate process, the rate of elimination decreases over time as mentioned previously, but the rate at which it decreases is a constant that is specific to the given drug. It is this second, constant rate that is described by k_e; thus, for every first-order kinetic drug, the medication's rate constant can be quantified and used to calculate the elimination half-life.

Half-Life in Pharmacokinetics

The most valuable of the pharmacokinetic parameters, aside from the first-order rate process for elimination, k_e, is the drug's half-life, $t_{1/2}$. For drugs that follow a first-order rate process for elimination, because the *rate constant* does not change, one can easily calculate the half-life for any drug; it, too, *does not change*. This value identifies how long it will take the body to eliminate one-half of the total amount of drug administered. For a drug that follows a first-order rate process, one needs to know *only* the elimination rate constant, k_e, to calculate the drug's half-life, by using the following equation:

$$t_{1/2} = \frac{0.693}{k_e}$$

For example, a 500mg dose (*D*) of a drug is administered to a patient; the half-life is the amount of time it takes for the dose of drug to decrease by 50%. Alternatively, it is the time it takes for the amount of drug remaining in the body to be one-half of the original dose, which in this case, is 250 mg. How long does it take? If the value of k_e is known (or looked up in a reference), one simply uses the simple equation given above to calculate the half-life. The half-life can then be used to determine the amount of a drug that remains in the body at *any* given time, using the first-order elimination rate constant, k_e.

(Conversely, if one knows the drug's half-life, the equation above can be used to calculate the rate constant for elimination.)

For a drug that follows a first-order kinetic rate process, at $1t_{1/2}$, one-half of the initial dose is gone from the body. At $2t_{1/2}$, three-fourths of the initial dose is gone from the body. At $3t_{1/2}$, seven-eighths of the initial dose is gone from the body, and so on up to $10_{t_{1/2}}$, when virtually all of the drug is "cleared (*out* of the body)"—meaning whatever remains is such a small amount it is undetectable. Ten half-lives are considered the completion of the drug elimination process (although it theoretically takes an infinite amount of time to completely eliminate the drug due to the rate equation).

Nursing Considerations

In clinical practice, when a patient asks, "How long will it take for this drug to be gone from my system?" the standard answer is *five half-lives*, which is the amount of time is takes for approximately 95% of the drug to be eliminated.

A patient may state: "This medication is giving me terrible headaches, and I am going to stop taking it. How long will it take for this drug to get out of my system?" The simplest way to answer this question is to use the numerical value of the drug's half life and multiply it by 5 to estimate the amount of 95% drug eliminated by the body (only about 5% of drug remains in the body). The answer, for a drug that follows first-order kinetics, can also be calculated if the clinician only has access to the k_e; $t_{1/2}$ is found using the first-order rate equation for half-life.

To obtain the *precise* half-life value, clinicians commonly rely on the package insert for the medication, in the "pharmacokinetics" section, or another source of drug information, such as Lexicomp (Chapter 1).

Drug Absorption: The "A" in ADME

- The movement of all drug molecules from the site of administration to the systemic circulation.

- The rate and extent of drug absorption depends on the drug's ability to cross a cellular membrane, along with a number of other factors.
- Passage of drug across a cell membrane depends upon the physiochemical nature of both the drug and the cell membrane.

Absorption is the process of drug movement (drug molecule) from the site of administration into the systemic circulation. A key point to understand is that with most routes of drug administration, the drug must cross a physiological barrier to reach the systemic circulation. Thus, a drug that has not passed through all the barriers between its original point of entry (i.e., site of drug administration) and the circulation system *cannot* be said to have been absorbed. Therefore, *there is a delay* in the time it takes for the drug to become "absorbed"—that is, to actually reach the bloodstream and begin to circulate throughout the body. (The exception to this is drugs that are designed for topical use that are never meant to enter the systemic circulation; to do so may even prove harmful. This topic—routes of administration—is discussed in further detail in Chapter 3.)

The more complex the physiological barrier, the longer it takes for the drug to cross into the systemic circulation. One exception to this rule occurs with IV bolus drug administration. When a drug is administered intravenously, there *is* no absorption process; there *is no barrier* the drug needs to cross; the drug is injected directly *into* the systemic circulation. Immediately following an IV bolus drug dose, the drug is detected in the systemic circulation. This route of drug administration *is the fastest way to get a drug* into a patient's body. For all *other* routes of drug administration, there is a delay from the time of administration to the time the drug enters the systemic circulation.

The Pharmacokinetics of Oral Absorption

After an oral dose of drug is administered, *two* pharmacokinetic processes are occurring simultaneously – the processes of both drug

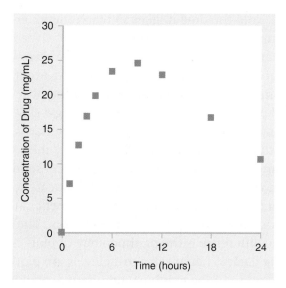

FIGURE 2-22 Plasma-level time curve: Plasma drug levels obtained following administration of a single oral dose of drug. Note that the data is plotted on rectangular graph paper.
Courtesy of Diane Pacitti. © 2017

absorption *and* drug elimination. **FIGURE 2-22** illustrates data points on a plasma level time curve following administration of a single oral dose of drug. Contrast this with the graph obtained following a single IV dose of drug, in Figure 2-19, where there is no absorption process.

When a drug is administered by the oral route, the drug can *not* immediately enter into the bloodstream; the drug must pass through the GI tract and the liver before it can enter the bloodstream. The time it takes for the drug to enter the bloodstream is known as the **lag-time**; it takes even longer for the drug to reach peak plasma drug levels. Contrast this with a drug administered intravenously; the moment the drug dose is administered, it is present in the bloodstream. In fact, the time of IV drug administration is the same as when (the time) the drug is at its highest plasma levels!

Inherent in the definition of absorption is the *barrier* between the drug and the bloodstream. The amount of time it takes the drug to reach the systemic circulation directly corresponds with the complexity of the barrier between the drug at its administration site and the bloodstream.

Note the time it takes to reach the maximum drug concentration levels – t^{max}. Two pharmacokinetic rate processes are taking place—first-order absorption and first-order elimination. Figure 2-22 illustrates a typical plasma level-time curve following a single oral dose of a drug, plotted on regular rectangular graph paper. In FIGURE 2-23, the same plasma drug levels are plotted on semi-log graph paper, for purposes of delineating the two concurrent pharmacokinetic rate processes—absorption *and* elimination. The key difference is the methodology of plotting data: When plasma drug levels are plotted on semi-log graph paper, pharmacokinetic parameters can be obtained from the resultant plasma-level time curve, much in the same manner as the rate constant for elimination was determined following a single IV bolus drug dose. The first-order rate constant for elimination, k_e, is determined from the slope of the straight line obtained on semi-log graph paper. The plasma-level time curve in Figure 2-23 can be used to determine k_e, but, the data points used to determine an accurate k_e occur only at the tail end of this plasma level time curve. Why? One must be absolutely certain that the drug absorption process is complete, and the data used to determine

the k_e represents ONLY the first-order *elimination* rate process. When the rate of elimination is the *only* kinetic process occurring, the tail-end of the straight line on the plasma-level time curve can be extrapolated and used to determine k_e.

Key Points

As the last pharmacokinetic process, the rate of elimination appears on a plasma-level time curve at the tail end of the semi-log graph of the data C_p versus t. The plot of these data becomes a straight line on semi-log graph paper when only the rate process of elimination is occurring, and the slope of the line, which represents the rate constant for elimination, can be readily determined. (The first-order rate constant for absorption k_a can also be determined using the same plasma-level time curve on semi-log graph paper; the methodology is beyond the scope of this text.)

Bioavailability

Bioavailability is defined as the total amount of drug (as a fraction of the total amount of drug in the administered dose) that reaches the systemic circulation in its pharmacologically active form, capable of producing a therapeutic drug response. Bioavailability is a measure of *the extent* of absorption and is generally determined by calculating the **area under the curve (AUC)**. (The "curve" is the resultant plasma-level time curve following a single dose of a drug.) The AUC represents the total amount of drug that entered the bloodstream; its value is numerically determined by adding all of the data points *on* the plasma level-time curve: from the time the drug entered the bloodstream until the drug was completely out of the bloodstream. It is, quite literally, an accounting of *how much drug* entered the bloodstream following a single dose of a medication. A quick estimate of a drug's bioavailability can be more easily observed by looking at the plasma-level time curve. Literally, everything under the plasma-level time curve represents the total amount of drug

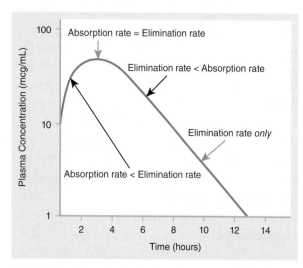

FIGURE 2-23 Plasma-level time curve plotted on semi-log graph paper; data obtained following a single oral dose of drug. Comparison between the rate of absorption and rate of elimination is indicated on the plasma level-time curve.

Courtesy of Diane Pacitti. © 2017

that entered the bloodstream. Drugs administered intravenously are 100% bioavailable—the entire amount of the drug dose enters into the bloodstream. With all other routes of drug administration, the entire dose of the drug may or *may not* reach the bloodstream, meaning one cannot be assured that 100% of the dose will be absorbed. The *rate* of absorption is determined by calculation of t^{max}, or the time required to reach the peak drug blood concentration (C^{max}). Regardless of the shape of the AUC (i.e., fast or slow t^{max}, low or high C^{max}), if the AUCs are the same, the same amount of drug was absorbed.

Many factors affect bioavailability. As discussed earlier in this chapter, an oral dose of drug must pass through the gastrointestinal tract before reaching the systemic circulation. Recall that the drug must first disintegrate and then dissolve in gastric or enteric juices, and survive the digestive enzymes. Food slows down gastric transit time from the stomach into the intestines, slowing the rate of absorption, as well.

The plasma-level time curve in **FIGURE 2-24** illustrates the dramatic differences between both the rate and extent of drug absorption (bioavailability) when a single dose of the same drug is given in three different dosage forms. Biopharmaceutics and drug formulation affects the bioavailability; you can see that the same drug product in three different formulations results in three different AUCs.

Factors Affecting the Rate and Extent of Absorption

The rate and extent of absorption depends on a number of factors, including the following:

- The route of drug administration
- Degree of complexity of the membrane
- Physiochemical properties of the drug
- Surface area at the site of absorption
- Dosage form of the drug
- Physiology of the patient (i.e., motility of the GI tract)

FIGURE 2-25 illustrates the vast difference in both the rate and extent of drug absorption following a single dose of the same drug. Both the dosage form and route of drug administration differ; note the overall effect the

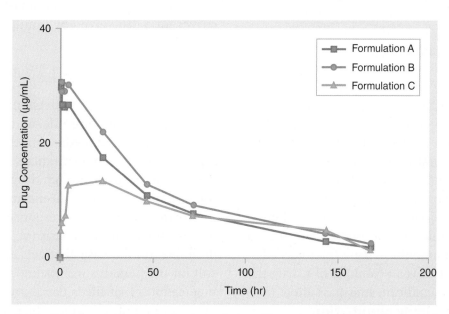

FIGURE 2-24 Bioavailability differs dramatically when the drug is given in three different dosage forms, depending on the dosage form of a drug plasma-level time curve.

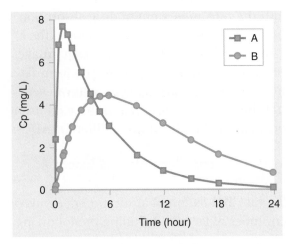

FIGURE 2-25 Plasma-level time curve indicates the amount of drug that reaches the bloodstream for the same dose of drug administered by two different routes of administration: the blue line represents the amount of drug in the body following administration via the rectal route (suppository), and the red line, following oral dosage form. Note the extensive *decrease* in the amount of drug that reaches the bloodstream when the drug is given orally.

Courtesy of Diane Pacitti. © 2017

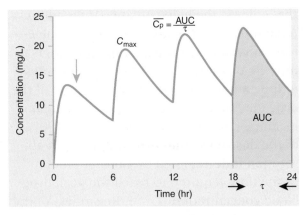

FIGURE 2-26 Plasma-level time curve: multiple oral dosing.

Courtesy of Diane Pacitti. © 2017

different ROAs have on the bioavailability, time to reach C^{max}, the level of C^{max} achieved, and the duration of action.

Impact of First-Pass Effect on Bioavailability

Recall that an orally administered drug is shunted to the liver before it enters the bloodstream for the first time. If a drug is extensively metabolized into an inactive metabolite by the liver, each pass through the liver will only serve to further decrease the amount of pharmacologically active drug; that is, decrease the amount of active drug that enters the systemic circulation. The greater the extent of drug metabolized by the liver (rendering it inactive), the greater the impact on the bioavailability of the drug. Consider an orally administered drug that is 80% metabolized in the liver, rendering it pharmacologically inactive. Only 20% of the pharmacologically active drug will enter the systemic circulation the first time—a *much smaller* amount of drug than was administered. This is an example of a drug that undergoes a significant first-pass effect (also called **presystemic elimination**).

For drugs that are highly metabolized by the liver, the oral route of administration may

be preferred, but the clinician may select an alternative ROA that bypasses the liver. For example, drugs administered parenterally, transdermally, or by inhalation are examples of ROAs in which the drugs are absorbed into the systemic circulation, without first passing through the gastrointestinal tract, thus avoiding the first-pass effect. Drugs may also be metabolized by *the intestinal mucosal cells* into a pharmacologically inactive form; these drugs demonstrate poor systemic bioavailability when given orally. It is therefore advantageous to select an alternative ROA that will bypass the first pass through the liver. The effect of bypassing the liver can be seen quite clearly by examining the plasma-level time curves for a drug given by multiple ROAs. See **FIGURE 2-26**.

Steady-State Drug Levels

The clinician needs to understand a drug's half-life, elimination profile, and affinities because the goal of medication therapy is to maintain plasma concentrations of the drug at a level that ensures enough drug is present, at the minimal effective concentration (MEC), to provide a therapeutic response on a more-or-less continual basis (or, if that is not desirable, on the basis that gets an optimal result for the patient's well-being). Recall that a medication's half-life is the amount of time it takes for half of the drug to be excreted from the body. Of course, half-life applies only to an individual dose—so what happens when a second dose is given before the first dose is fully excreted? The result of repeat dosing depends on *when* the second dose is given in relation to the first (i.e., the dosing interval, τ) and how much of the drug the second dose contains. Ideally, the new (second) dose would be calculated so that it supplies enough drug to keep the therapeutic effects going without introducing any potential toxicity (i.e., keep blood levels above MEC and below MTC; further discussion of this point appears in the section on pharmacodynamics, earlier in this chapter). If a second dose is given before the first drug dose is completely eliminated from the body, the second drug dose results in a higher maximum plasma drug concentration (C^{max}). With each consecutive dose, drug continues to *accumulate* in the body until the maximum drug concentration plateaus (shown in Figure 2-26). This is known as **steady-state drug levels**, in which the concentration of drug entering the body equals the amount of drug being eliminated. This in–out balance is represented as C_p^{ss}. In general, medications reach steady-state drug levels between five and six half-lives (note that this is the same amount of time that a drug is said to be eliminated from the body, as well). Those with short half-lives reach steady state relatively quickly, and those with long half-lives require longer to reach steady state.

Nursing Considerations

A drug administered by continuous IV infusion achieves desired steady-state drug levels immediately. One must calculate the desired amount of drug to be delivered at a given flow rate, set on the IV infusion pump, to deliver a the steady-state drug level.

Distribution: The "D" in ADME

Distribution is the process of drug movement *from the bloodstream to its target site of action.* After a drug moves from its site of administration into the bloodstream, it then moves throughout body, via the bloodstream, to its site of drug action. The movement of the drug throughout the body, and hence its "ability to distribute," reflects various physiological factors as well as the physiochemical properties of the drug. To understand how a drug is distributed, the clinician needs to identify or understand the following:

- The process by which drugs are carried throughout the body and delivered to targets of action
- The blood/blood flow at the absorption site and throughout the rest of the body
- The capacity for passage across a cell membrane, which depends on the physiochemical nature of both the drug and the cell membrane
- The affinity of the drug for a tissue or organ; that is, the partitioning and accumulation of the drug in the tissue

Drug concentration in untargeted sites may cause side effects. Once the drug is absorbed into the bloodstream, the drug molecules move freely throughout the body via the systemic circulation. The drug may distribute, or move, out of the systemic circulation into organs or tissues, bind with plasma proteins within the systemic circulation, or simply stay within the systemic circulation. Ideally, the drug would move throughout the body directly to its site of drug action, leave its site of action, and be eliminated (exit) from the body directly (recall the "magic bullet theory of drug action" described earlier in this chapter).

Pharmacokinetics: Rate of Drug Distribution

Drug movement is dependent upon the physiochemical characteristics of the drug molecule *and* its interactions with the anatomical and physiological surroundings following its administration. Once a drug enters the systemic circulation, the chemical composition of the drug molecule governs its ability to diffuse out of the bloodstream and into tissues, organs, or other areas.

The *rate of drug movement* to its site of action is derived in the same manner as the rate

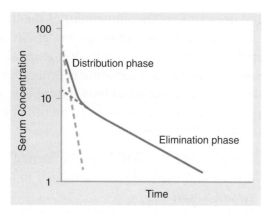

FIGURE 2-27 Plasma-level time curve: Data is plotted on semi-log graph paper, following a single intravenous dose of drug. This drug exhibits first-order rate processes of drug distribution *and* drug elimination. This drug distributes into two compartments; therefore, has a first-order rate constant for both distribution *and* rate constant for elimination. Two pharmacokinetic rate processes occur simultaneously, and account for the shape of the plasma-level time curve.

Courtesy of Diane Pacitti. © 2017

constant for elimination—by using the drug plasma level versus time curve. This rate is mathematically derived from the slope of the line obtained using a semi-logarithmic graph paper (assuming a first-order rate process). The *rate* of drug movement from the bloodstream to various tissues/organs/sites is represented by the rate constant for distribution, or k_d (**FIGURE 2-27**).

Pharmacokinetic Models: Compartmental Model Theory

Mathematical pharmacokinetic models are developed to describe the movement of a drug in the body after it has entered the bloodstream. The **compartmental model theory** of drug distribution defines specific areas within the body as "compartments" — that is, groups of tissues with similar blood flow and drug affinity. For some drugs, only one compartment matters—the circulatory system, the **central compartment**—because they stay in the blood and do not move into other tissues. These drugs are said to follow a **one-compartment model**. For other drugs, a two- or three-compartment model is more appropriate. The mathematical equations developed by modeling are used to predict the amount of drug in the body as the drug becomes distributed, moving from the bloodstream to tissues and back to the bloodstream

prior to elimination. Compartmental models are used to visualize and represent where a drug moves as it travels throughout the body once it has reached the bloodstream; compartments illustrate the distribution patterns for a particular drug. For example, if a drug moves out of the bloodstream (central compartment) into tissues (second compartment) and/or other distinct areas outside of the bloodstream to reach its target site(s), it is said to exhibit a two-compartment (or possibly more) model for drug distribution.

There is a rate constant for drug distribution into each distinct compartment to account for the movement of drug throughout the body. In the mathematical model of pharmacokinetics, one important question is this: What is the rate of drug movement? That is, how long does it take for the drug to move from the place where it enters the body to its site of action? As previously stated, the rate of drug movement is derived by plotting the plasma drug concentration (C_p) against time and then calculating the distribution rate constant, or k_d.

One-Compartment Model

In a one-compartment pharmacokinetic model, there is no rate constant for distribution because drugs *do not move out of the bloodstream* and into other tissues—that is, they stay within the central compartment, and have only a rate constant for elimination (k_e). Qualitatively speaking, once such a drug enters the bloodstream, the rate of drug movement is completely dependent the elimination rate; i.e., upon the amount of drug remaining in the body at any time (i.e., a first-order rate process). Because the drug remains in the central compartment (bloodstream), and does not leave, no actual distribution takes place. Thus, when dealing with a drug that follows the one-compartment model, the rate of drug movement is due to the elimination rate process only.

FIGURE 2-28 illustrates the simplest model of drug distribution, made even simpler due to the route of drug administration—IV—such

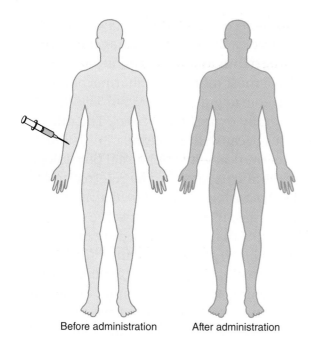

Before administration   After administration

FIGURE 2-28 One-compartment model.

that there is no "absorption" process for which to account.

The drugs that follow this simplest model of drug distribution are characterized by the following traits:

- The drug stays within the bloodstream and has no affinity for tissues outside the compartment of the central circulation.

- There is *no* rate constant for drug distribution(k_d)—because *there is no* distribution.
- As soon as the drug enters the bloodstream, the process of elimination begins.

Multicompartment Model

Once a drug enters the systemic circulation, a pattern of distribution becomes evident.

- One-compartment model: Into the body (bloodstream), circulation in the bloodstream, out of the body.
- Two-compartment model: Into the body (bloodstream), circulation in the bloodstream, distribution from bloodstream to tissue or other compartment, back to the bloodstream, out of the body (**FIGURE 2-29**).
- Distribution of the drug out into tissues—the second compartment—is often referred to as the "peripheral" compartment.
- This compartment(s) includes(s) physiological spaces that are less well-perfused, such as adipose tissue and skeletal muscle, and therefore the administered drug will equilibrate more slowly in those regions ("compartments"). The duration of the

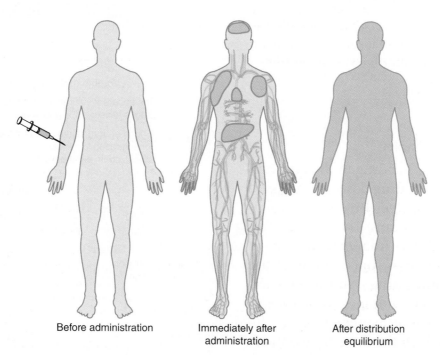

Before administration   Immediately after administration   After distribution equilibrium

FIGURE 2-29 Multicompartment model.

drug effect at the target tissue will often be affected by the *redistribution* from one compartment to another.

- If more than two compartments are involved, pharmacologic modeling becomes more challenging, because it is necessary to assess how fast the drug moves among multiple compartments. The elimination rate of a drug is much simpler to determine using a plasma-level time curve when there are more than at least two different rates of distribution on the graph. The total amount of time the drug spends in the body, moving into and out of the systemic circulation, can be determined if the time of drug administration and the elimination rate constant are known. This will be a finite amount of time, which can be calculated.

Key Points

What *cannot* be determined is the amount of time a drug spends in any given compartment, interacting with its site of action, before returning to the circulation to be cleared. Nor is it known how many compartments the drug passes through when it leaves the circulation and goes out to the tissues. Drugs that follow multicompartment models become distributed into different compartments at different rates, and determining not only the path the drug travels but also the speeds at which it travels through different sections of the path is extremely challenging.

Volume of Distribution

The amount of the drug in the body, or the amount of a drug dose, is expressed in units of mass (weight)—grams, milligrams, or micrograms. The *amount of drug* in the body differs from *the concentration of drug* in the body, as concentration represents how much drug is in the body as a solution (weight/volume), which means there must be a measurement of the fluid volume in which the drug is "dissolved," or contained. The amount of fluid neces-

sary to account for the concentration of drug in the body is known as the **volume of distribution (VD)** and is perhaps one of the most difficult of pharmacokinetic concepts to grasp (FIGURE 2-30). The V_D is generally expressed in liters. The difficulty arises because the volume of distribution is theoretical—it is not a real physiological volume. It may also be referred to as the *apparent volume of distribution*, for this same reason. However, it serves as an indicator of the extent of drug distribution in the body, and for this and other reasons is an invaluable pharmacokinetic value.

If a drug tends to stay within the systemic circulation, it will appear to have a volume of distribution equal to that of the volume of the bloodstream (5 L), or less (the total volume of the "central compartment"). However, if a drug has an affinity for a distant compartment, meaning that the drug travels out of the bloodstream and into tissues, organs, or other sites beyond the central circulation, the time it takes for the drug to reach its site of action (or final destination) becomes much longer. Not only does this affect the amount of time the drug stays in the body, but it also effectively "hides" the drug in a compartment outside the bloodstream, vastly increasing

Volume of distribution

- The apparent volume in which the dose of drug is "dissolved", or distributed.

- A dose of drug is injected, and the plasma concentration is measured. The dose is "dissolved" in an apparent volume.

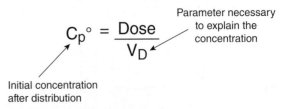

$$C_p^{\circ} = \frac{Dose}{V_D}$$

Initial concentration after distribution

Parameter necessary to explain the concentration

FIGURE 2-30 The volume of distribution serves as an indicator of the *extent* of drug distribution, that is, a measure of how long it stayed outside the bloodstream, effectively hiding. For example, drugs that must travel to difficult-to-reach "compartments" such as bone, joint fluid, the prostate gland, and others to reach their target sites of action, typically have a very "large" volume of distribution.

the apparent volume of distribution. Consequently, the half-life of this drug will be much greater, as the rate of elimination is much slower.

Once the drug exits the systemic circulation and enters two, three, or four (or more) different compartments, it must eventually return to the systemic circulation to be eliminated from the body. The mechanism of elimination does not affect the distribution of the drug, nor does the extent of distribution affect where the drug is distributed as it moves throughout the body.

A few generalizations can be made regarding volume distribution. First, if V_D for a drug is 5 L or less, it can be inferred, just from the V_D value, that the drug most likely remains within the central compartment (the bloodstream), has a shorter half-life (than a drug with a higher V_D), spends less time in the body, is eliminated more rapidly, and has a shorter dosing interval, meaning it must be dosed more frequently. In contrast, if V_D for a drug is much larger than the physiological volume of the compartment (or is a volume that is anatomically possible), such as 250 L, it is deduced that the drug does not stay within the central compartment, but rather distributes in the body into a second, third, or even more distant compartment, where it travels based upon its chemical characteristics. This drug will be eliminated much more slowly from the body in comparison to drugs that follow a one-compartment model. The elimination rate for such a drug, along with its half-life, will be much longer. The dosing interval for a drug with a large volume of distribution, therefore, is less frequent than that for a drug with a volume of distribution of 5 L.

Drug Binding to Plasma Proteins

Drugs can, and very often do, bind to plasma proteins (usually albumin). While the binding of drugs is reversible, drugs have differing affinity for binding to these proteins. If two or more drugs are present in the bloodstream simultaneously, both having a high affinity

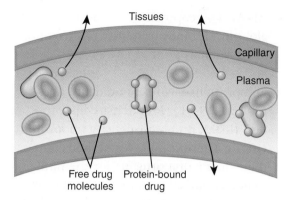

FIGURE 2-31 Schematic representation of protein binding.

for binding to the same plasma protein, there will be a drug "competition" for binding sites on that particular plasma protein. Only unbound forms of a drug (otherwise known as the "free" form of the drug) move out of the bloodstream and reach target sites in the tissues to cause a pharmacologically relevant effect (**FIGURE 2-31**). Conversely, bound drugs are unable to diffuse out of the bloodstream and into the tissue (or to their target site of action) due to their large size when bound in a drug–protein complex.

Of import in the assessment of a drug's binding capacity is the fact that a drug may bind to various macromolecular components in the bloodstream as it enters the systemic circulation, where there are numerous proteins in the blood. This drug–protein complex literally becomes trapped within the systemic circulation. However, most drugs' binding processes are reversible, such that the drug–protein complexes will (eventually) dissociate.

The following proteins most commonly bind to drug molecules:

- Albumin—a protein synthesized by the liver. It is the major component of plasma proteins responsible for reversible drug binding. Many weakly acidic (anionic) drugs bind to albumin by electrostatic and hydrophobic bonds (the same intermolecular bonding forces previously discussed, in the pharmacodynamics section). Weakly acidic drugs such as salicylates, phenylbutazone, and penicillins are highly-bound to albumin.

- α1-Acid glycoprotein (orosomucoid)—a globulin. It binds primarily basic (cationic) drugs such as **propranolol, imipramine,** and **lidocaine**.
- Lipoproteins—very-low-density lipoprotein (VLDL), low-density lipoprotein (LDL), and high-density lipoprotein (HDL). These complexes of lipids and proteins may be responsible for the binding of drugs if the albumin sites become saturated.
- Erythrocytes (red blood cells)—may bind both endogenous and exogenous compounds.

The bonding interaction between a drug and plasma protein is reversible and varies in strength, depending on the affinity that the drug has for the plasma protein. Recall the discussion earlier the chapter describing the nature of drug-receptor interactions; the extent which a drug binds to its receptor is dependent upon the degree of "chemical binding attraction" between the two molecules. The very same kinetic principles apply to characterize the interaction between drugs and plasma proteins: identifying how strong the bond will be between the drug and protein, and how long the bond lasts. The extent to which a drug binds to a plasma protein is dependent upon the affinity of the drug-protein complex. The attraction may be strong because a protein has multiple binding sites to which the drug molecule can attach, or it may be strong because the molecular configuration of the site forms a strong chemical bond with the drug molecule. Drugs have different affinities for plasma proteins; some have no affinity at all.

The extent of the drug's capacity to bind to plasma proteins has an impact upon the therapeutic response of the drug, in part, due to the "availability" of the drug to reach its molecular site of action. Only "free" or unbound drug is able to diffuse out of the bloodstream, distribute to the drug's target tissues, and produce the desired therapeutic response. The extent of drug–protein binding in the plasma or tissue will affect the V_D, as well. The formation of a drug-protein complex essentially confines the bound drug to the bloodstream until it dissociates from the plasma protein molecule. This binding appears as a measurable decrease of the drug in the central compartment and makes the volume of distribution much greater. The strength of a bond between a drug and a protein can be expressed mathematically, as was discussed previously in the pharmacodynamics section, for the drug-receptor binding interaction. Given:

$$\text{Protein} + \text{drug} \leftrightarrow \text{protein–drug complex}$$
$$\text{Or}$$
$$(P) + (D) \leftrightarrow (PD)$$

The magnitude of K_A is indicative of the degree of protein–drug binding. Drugs strongly bound to proteins have a very large K_A and exist mostly as the protein–drug complex. Thus, large doses of such a drug may be needed to obtain a reasonable therapeutic concentration of free drug.

Competition for Binding Sites

Earlier, a brief mention was made regarding the fact that drugs sometimes compete for binding sites. In the competition for protein-binding sites, someone always loses the battle and is not able to compete with the strength of its opponent. In this case, the "strength" in question is the binding attraction of the drug for the plasma protein molecule itself. The drug with the stronger affinity will push aside the drug with the weaker affinity and bind to the protein; this process, called displacement, has potentially significant consequences for the patient.

Displacement of drugs from plasma proteins (for example, by other drugs taken at the same time) can affect the pharmacokinetics of a drug in several ways:

- Directly increase the free (unbound) drug concentration as a result of reduced binding in the blood

- Increase the free drug concentration that reaches the receptor site directly, causing a more intense pharmacodynamic response
- Increase the free drug concentration, causing a transient increase in V_D, which then decreases (partly) this free plasma drug concentration
- Increase the free drug concentration, resulting in more drug diffusion into tissues of eliminating organs, particularly the liver and kidney, resulting in a transient increase in drug elimination

Ramifications of Protein Binding on Therapy

The effects of protein-binding competition among drugs can have direct significance for patient outcomes. For example, consider a scenario in which a patient has been prescribed Drug A. This patient is taking Drug B, which has a higher affinity for binding plasma proteins than Drug A. The patient neglects to inform his doctor that he uses Drug B on occasion. Drug B competes with Drug A for protein-binding sites and, due to its greater affinity, successfully displaces Drug A about 75% of the time. This decreases Drug A's protein binding significantly. As a result, the concentration of free Drug A increases, distributed into all tissues. More of Drug A will then be available to interact at receptor sites, which produces a more intense pharmacologic effect. The plasma levels of Drug A may even become too high, causing potential harm to the patient as well. In addition, the elimination half-life of Drug A may be decreased, as binding to plasma proteins typically lengthens the half-life of a drug. Collectively, as a result of its displacement from the plasma proteins when Drug B is present, the clinical effects of Drug A become unpredictable.

Metabolism: The "M" in ADME

Metabolism is defined as *the chemical change of the structure of a drug molecule* by an enzymatic reaction in the body; also called **biotransformation**.

The liver produces enzymes that are capable of chemically reacting with and changing the chemical structure of a drug molecule, often rendering that changed drug molecule into a *pharmacologically inactive* compound. However, not *all* drugs are metabolized, and not all drug biotransformation reactions occur in the liver; there are metabolic enzymes present in other tissues throughout the body as well.

Some drugs are eliminated chemically unchanged from the body into the urine, by the kidneys. For other drug molecules, their chemical structure is such that the drug must be chemically changed in order for it to be eliminated by one of the elimination pathways in the body. For example, enzymes in the liver can change the chemical structure of drugs suitable for excretion in the kidneys (usually by making them more hydrophilic, or water soluble). The liver serves as a hub for numerous metabolic and enzymatic reactions, with drug biotransformation being just one of those reactions. The majority of drugs that require a metabolic chemical transformation are acted upon by enzymes present in the liver. The family of enzymes most notable and responsible for chemically changing the structure of drug molecules is known as the cytochrome P-450 (CYP-450 family of enzymes) enzymes.

For a drug that cannot be eliminated from the body unless the chemical structure of that molecule is changed, biotransformation reactions convert drug molecules into more water-soluble compounds that can be eliminated from the body. Most biotransformation reactions occur in the liver, although there are other body tissues (such as intestinal wall, kidney, skin, blood) in which enzymatic transformation takes place. The discussion that follows focuses on those enzymes present in the liver. Drug molecules travel into the liver via one of two routes: (1) the hepatic portal vein, which provides 75% of the liver's blood flow and transports the venous blood returning from the small intestine, stomach, pancreas, and spleen, and (2) arterial blood from the hepatic artery.

Enzyme Reactions in the Liver

Hepatic biotransformation enzymes are responsible for the inactivation and subsequent elimination of drugs that are not easily cleared through the kidney. For these drugs, there is a direct relationship between the rate of drug metabolism (biotransformation) and the elimination half-life for the drug.

Some drugs, such as ethanol, undergo Michaelis-Menten pharmacokinetics, referred to as **saturable-binding kinetics**. When drug concentration is low relative to enzyme concentration, there is plenty of enzyme available to metabolize, or biotransform, the drug molecules. The presence of abundant enzymes to catalyze the reaction means that the metabolism is a first-order process. However, when the drug concentration is high, enzymes soon become saturated and can no longer metabolize the drug. In this scenario, the reaction rate is at a maximum, and the rate process becomes zero-order (discussed earlier in this chapter).

What does this mean for the patient? Two key issues are involved. First, what concentration of the drug reaches the liver? If it is a high concentration, as is true for drugs that are subject to first-pass effects, more enzymes are needed to metabolize the high drug concentration than for a drug that bypasses the liver. If it is a lower concentration, as is true for drugs that pass through the systemic circulation prior to reaching the liver, the quantity of enzymes needed may be smaller. This brings us to the second issue: Is the liver capable of producing enough enzymes to metabolize the drug completely—or, more to the point, at what level of concentration can the liver not metabolize all of the drug?

Most drugs are eliminated after being processed by the kidneys, but the molecules must be water soluble. A lipid-soluble drug would be easily reabsorbed by the renal tubular cells and, therefore, would tend to remain in the body. In this circumstance, the chemical

composition of the drug—specifically, its polarity—makes a difference. Many drugs start out as lipid-soluble, less-polar molecules. The biotransformation process usually (but not always) creates a metabolite of the drug that is generally more polar than the parent compound; polar metabolites are unable to diffuse out of the systemic circulation, and therefore, are not pharmacologically active. Instead, they are filtered through the glomerulus and are more rapidly excreted (the process of renal excretion is described later). This allows the drug to be eliminated faster than if it remained lipid soluble.

Many drugs, despite undergoing a chemical or structural change by a metabolic process, remain pharmacologically active. These compounds are called **active metabolites**; despite being structurally different than their "parent drug", active metabolites can still bind to the drug's target site and produce a drug action. Because they are capable of binding to the receptor site resulting in drug action, active metabolites effectively prolong the pharmacological activity of the drug, before being eliminated.

In rare cases, a drug is intentionally formulated as an *inactive* compound called a prodrug. A prodrug has no pharmacological activity before it enters the body. After the drug is administered to the patient, it *requires* a metabolic enzyme process or biotransformation reaction *inside the body* to chemically change its structure into its pharmacologically active form. A prodrug can be designed to improve drug stability, to increase systemic drug absorption, or to prolong the duration of the drug's activity.

Metabolism and Liver Blood Flow

Blood flow to the liver plays an important role in the extent of drug metabolized after oral administration. Changes in blood flow to the liver may substantially alter the proportion of drug metabolized and, therefore, the proportion of bioavailable drug. The quantity of enzymes involved in metabolizing drugs is not uniform throughout the liver. Some enzymes are produced only when blood flow travels from a given direction. Because of this, changes in blood flow can greatly affect the fraction of drug metabolized. This factor explains why the presence of hepatic disease—which can cause tissue fibrosis, necrosis, and hepatic shunt, all of which change blood flow—can have a significant effect on the bioavailability of drugs administered to a particular individual. Also, there is genetic variability in drug-metabolizing enzymes from individual to individual (pharmacogenomics).

Drug Interactions Involving Drug Metabolism

Enzymes involved in the metabolism of drugs may be altered by diet and by the administration of other drugs and chemicals. Enzyme induction is a drug- or chemical-stimulated increase in enzyme activity, usually due to an increase in the amount of enzyme present. Enzyme induction usually involves some onset time for increased protein (enzyme) production. Enzyme inhibition may occur due to substrate competition or due to direct inhibition of the drug-metabolizing enzymes (particularly one of the cytochrome P-450 enzymes). For example, grapefruit juice, which contains a bioflavonoid called naringin, is at least partly responsible for inhibition of the enzyme cytochrome P-4503A4, which is present in the liver and intestinal wall. This inhibitory effect can lead to an increased concentration of drug in the body, possibly leading to toxic levels of the drug. A nutrient may mimic, enhance, or suppress the effects of certain drugs in the body, resulting in unintended toxic effects.

A well-documented example of such an interaction occurs between the prescription drug warfarin, which is used to decrease the risk of blood clots, and vitamin K, found in dark-green, leafy vegetables. Vitamin K promotes the clotting cascade, and warfarin acts by inhibiting the body's ability to recycle this vitamin. If a patient normally eats a lot of leafy greens prior to being prescribed warfarin, and then reduces or eliminates greens from his or her diet, this change

can exacerbate the drug's effects and leave the patient prone to excessive bleeding and poor wound healing. Conversely, a patient on warfarin who does not normally include leafy greens in his or her diet but who begins to eat more of them (perhaps to improve his or her health) may inadvertently decrease the drug's action and become vulnerable to a blood clot.

Nursing Considerations

Such diet–drug interactions need to be explained to the patient prior to beginning medication therapy. While a nurse may not want to discourage a patient from eating healthy foods, it may be necessary to adjust the patient's medication dose and monitor his or her plasma drug levels more closely until the effects of the dietary change are ascertained. (A valuable resource for obtaining such information is the National Institutes of Health's patient education pages on drug–nutrient interactions; for example, the page on the vitamin K/warfarin interaction, found at http://www.cc.nih.gov/ccc/patient_education /drug_nutrient/coumadin1.pdf, contains a helpful list of foods high in vitamin K.)

It is important for nurses to be aware that dietary factors can and do alter how patients metabolize certain drugs. Such knowledge can help the patient avoid unintended drug–food interactions, and potentially adverse events.

Elimination: The "E" in ADME

Drugs may be eliminated from the body through a variety of processes. However, the key components are the biliary system in the liver—the mechanism by which toxins extracted from the detoxification channels are removed to the excretory system—and the renal system.

Biliary Excretion of Drugs

The biliary system of the liver is an important mechanism for the excretion of drugs. Bile appears to be an active secretion process by hepatic cells and is made up of mainly water, bile salts, bile pigments, electrolytes, and, to a lesser extent, cholesterol and fatty acids. A drug or its metabolite is secreted into bile and, on contraction of the gallbladder, is then excreted into the duodenum via the common bile duct. At this point, the drug or its metabolite may be excreted into the feces or, alternatively, the drug may be reabsorbed and become systemically available and therefore pharmacologically active. The cycle in which the drug is absorbed, excreted into the bile, and reabsorbed is known as enterohepatic circulation. The biliary secretion process may become saturated in some cases, however.

The following are general rules:

- Drugs with molecular weights (MW) in excess of 500 are mainly excreted in the bile.
- Drugs with MW between 300 and 500 are excreted in both the urine and the bile.
- Drugs with MW less than 300 are almost exclusively excreted via the kidneys into urine.

To be excreted into bile, drugs must usually have a strong polar group in addition to a high MW. Many drugs excreted into bile are glucuronide metabolites (glucuronide conjugation increases the MW by 200).

Drug Clearance

Clearance is a pharmacokinetic term used to describe drug elimination from the body without identifying the elimination process. It differs from elimination in that clearance can include drugs that break-down without being excreted. The simplest concept of **clearance** is defined as *the fixed volume of fluid (containing the drug) cleared of drug per unit of time*. Often, the fluid in this definition is plasma. Thus, clearance may also be defined as the rate of drug elimination divided by the plasma drug concentration or, in pharmacokinetic terms,

$$Cl_t = kV_D$$

where Cl_t is the sum total of all the clearance processes in the body, including clearance through the kidney, lung, and liver.

Because V_D and k are both constant, clearance will remain constant as long as elimination is a first-order process. An important note with respect to Cl_t is that clearance values are often normalized on a per-kilogram body weight basis; thus, the patient's body weight will change the volume of distribution.

Drugs are typically excreted by one of three processes: (1) glomerular filtration; (2) active renal secretion in the proximal tubules of the kidney; or (3) tubular reabsorption in the distal tubules (lipid-soluble drugs). Renal clearance is defined as the volume of plasma that is cleared of drug per unit time through the kidneys. It can be expressed as the constant fraction of V_D in which the drug is contained that is excreted by the kidney per unit of time.

Glomerular Filtration

Drug molecules generally are eliminated through the first process, glomerular filtration—a unidirectional process that occurs for most small molecules (MW < 500), including undissociated (non-ionized) and dissociated (ionized) drugs. The major driving force for glomerular filtration is hydrostatic pressure within the glomerular capillaries (FIGURE 2-32). When clinicians want to measure a patient's glomerular filtration rate, they do so using a drug that is known to be eliminated by filtration only (inulin, or creatinine, is most often used).

Glomerular filtration of drugs is directly related to the free or non-protein-bound drug concentration in the plasma. Protein-bound drugs generally are not eliminated by glomerular filtration in the kidneys because the molecules tend to be too large; instead, such bound drugs are usually excreted by active secretion, following capacity-limited kinetics. As the amount of free drug in the plasma increases, the glomerular filtration for the drug will increase proportionately, thereby increasing the renal drug clearance.

Active Renal Secretion

Active renal secretion is an active transport process that occurs in the proximal tubule.

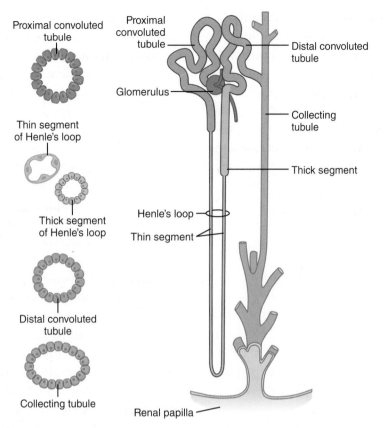

FIGURE 2-32 The structure of the renal tubule, illustrating its relationship to the glomerulus and the collecting tubule.

In the following way: The filtrate leaving the glomerulus passes through the tubules to allow key nutrients contained in it—including water, as the kidneys are also responsible for maintaining blood volume—to be reabsorbed. Unwanted molecules, which include protein-bound drug molecules that could not be filtered out by the glomerulus, are not reabsorbed, but rather are "carried" out of the plasma by a variety of transporter molecules, including P-glycoproteins (PGPs), organic anion transporters (oats), and organic cation transporters (cots), among others. (This process is called active transport because it requires an energy input; the molecules that transport the drug must work against a concentration gradient, so the active tubular secretion rate is dependent on renal plasma flow.)

Most of these transporters are not specific to a particular substance, meaning that any transporter molecule can attach to any substance present in the filtrate. As a consequence, the process can become saturated if the amount of drug molecules needing transport surpasses the availability of transporter molecules. Drugs with similar structures can compete for the same carrier system.

Tubular Reabsorption

Tubular reabsorption is a passive transport mechanism in which drug molecules are reabsorbed from the plasma rather than being excreted into the urine. This process occurs after a drug is filtered through the glomerulus and is often influenced by the differences in pH between the filtrate and the urine. Urine that is highly concentrated (i.e., more acidic) tends to promote more reabsorption of drugs that are acids or weak bases, though this process is influenced by the pH of the fluid in the renal tubule (i.e., urine pH) and the pKa of the drug. Non-ionized drugs are easily reabsorbed from the renal tubule back into the body, but the ionized forms of such drugs are less readily reabsorbed and, therefore, will be excreted faster. The rate of urine flow also influences the amount of filtered drug that is reabsorbed. Specifically, drugs that increase urine flow (e.g., diuretics) will decrease the time for drug reabsorption and promote their excretion.

Case Study: Making the Connection to Clinical Nursing

Considerations Affecting Drug Delivery: Dosing Frequency, Timing, and Route

Consider the following situation a nurse may encounter in clinical practice. A 13-year-old male patient, newly diagnosed with type 1 diabetes, is being taught how to use insulin to treat his condition. He asks the nurse the following questions:

- Why do I have to keep taking insulin over and over again? Wouldn't it make more sense to just take one big dose, instead of a lot of smaller ones?
- Why does insulin have to be given using a needle? I don't want to stick myself with a needle, what, five times a day?! If insulin needs to be given more than once a day, can't I take a pill or a liquid of some kind, something I can swallow?
- Why do I have to take two different forms of insulin? Why can't I just take one?

Now consider the true questions being asked by the patient. He wants to know, in essence, two things: (1) why one dose of the medication (in this case, insulin) will not cure, correct, or fix the underlying *cause* of his illness in a permanent way and (2) why he is being asked to take the medication by a specific ROA, according to a specific dosing regimen.

To answer his first question, the term *cure* must first be clarified, because a common (and erroneous) assumption that many patients, and indeed many healthcare providers, make is that the end result of medication therapy is curing disease. If we define cure as "ending the disease process and restoring normal function," then we must acknowledge that most drugs *do not actually cure disease*. Antibiotic agents, antiviral agents, and some biological anticancer medications are exceptions, because they actively attack disease-causing organisms or cells. That is not true of most medications (and even with most "cures," the medications tend to act in concert with the patient's physiology, although there are a few exceptions). Most medications' actions simply support or suppress existing body processes to interrupt either the dysfunction itself or, more often, the symptoms caused by the dysfunction that are unpleasant for the patient to experience. *Interrupting*, however, is not the same as *ending*—for a patient to be "cured" of a disease, the disease process must actually end. Most of the time, it is the body's own healing capacity that determines whether a disease or injury ultimately resolves itself or continues, albeit in a controlled state. In many situations, medication therapy is capable of restoring "normalcy" to body systems in *biochemical* terms, but not *functional* terms. For example, a person with low thyroid function can take **levothyroxine** to increase the thyroid hormone level to "normal"—but he or she must continue taking the drug to maintain that state, because the drug only *replaces* a missing component *without actually fixing the dysfunctional thyroid*.

That brings us back to the patient's first question: Why must a drug (almost always) be given more than once to achieve a therapeutic result? In general terms, the answer to this question is that body systems are dynamic, not static. When dysfunction occurs, it will generally continue occurring unless or until something happens to restore normal function. Sometimes the body lacks sufficient resources (for whatever reason) to resolve an injury or infection.

The portion of the original dose of the drug that enters the body does not permanently remain in the body (because drugs do not irreversibly "bind" to their sites of action). Recall from earlier in this chapter the manner in which the drug interacts with its target and then *dissociates*. Dissociated drug molecules leave the site of action, return to the systemic circulation (bloodstream), and are eliminated by the body. Each dose of drug "works" only for a specific period of time before it is eliminated. The dose must be repeated for the duration of the symptoms or dysfunction; each dose of drug works at its site of action to alleviate the symptoms or dysfunction. Drugs are designed to reach a specific site of action in the body where the pathology is located and "work" to alleviate the problem—*temporarily*. How long a drug takes to be eliminated depends in a manner consistent with the chemical properties of the compound; that is, the pharmacokinetic parameter drug half-life ($t_{1/2}$). Some drugs last 4 hours, some 12 hours, others a full day. This is the basis for the design of the dosage regimen, and explains why *multiple* doses of medication may be needed to achieve the desired response.

Chronic Medication Use: Long-Term Dosing Regimens

The situation faced by the patient with newly diagnosed type 1 diabetes is somewhat more complicated. This patient has a chronic condition for which correcting the disease process is not currently possible. Therefore, the patient must use chronic medication therapy—which raises many considerations not pertinent to short-term medication regimens.

In short-term, acute conditions, medication supports or suppresses a normal body function to promote healing. In chronic conditions, however, medication often replaces or restores a physiological function or factor that has gone so seriously awry that it cannot be brought back to normal, or that has stopped working entirely. What is the malfunctioning or missing piece of the physiological system? Which physiological or biochemical process is affected in this pathophysiological state, and what is the normal condition? In type 1 diabetes, the biochemical process that has become dysfunctional is the patient's ability to produce the hormone known as insulin.

The solution sounds simple, but in clinical practice, effective insulin therapy is difficult to achieve, as the levels of insulin are not at a constant level in the body under normal physiological conditions. *Emulating normal fluctuations of insulin concentrations is daunting.* A patient attempting to replace the missing insulin relies on what amounts to a system of "informed guesswork." The patient must measure blood sugar and carbohydrate intake and use these parameters to calculate a dose of insulin that can counterbalance from food, all without supplying too much insulin that blood glucose levels fall too low (causing fatigue, shakiness, seizures, loss of consciousness, or even, in extreme cases, death).

To answer the patient's second question about why two types of insulin are needed, the nurse must explain to the patient that normally the pancreas releases insulin in the healthy body in two different ways. Unfortunately, this requires the patient to use two types of insulin, to mimic "healthy" physiological responsive actions of the pancreas. In addition to maintaining a baseline insulin level, "bursts" of insulin are required to effectively deal with increases in blood glucose after meals. Therefore, the standard drug therapy regimen for type 1 diabetes is insulin replacement for both the baseline levels and the spikes and, therefore, two different insulins: *(1)* a long-acting form of insulin that is injected once daily and *ensures baseline insulin levels* and *(2)* a short-acting form of insulin that is injected *with meals to replace the insulin spike* that accompanies rising postprandial glucose levels.

The patient's question about why insulin must be injected, rather than taken

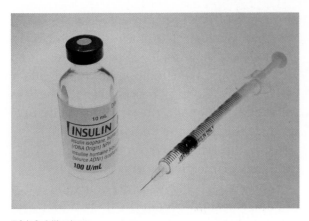

© Carlos Davila/Alamy Images

by mouth, is simpler to answer. Insulin is a protein molecule (a biological drug)—if ingested orally, it is rapidly degraded and completely destroyed by enzymes present in the gastrointestinal tract. Subcutaneous injection, by comparison, delivers the insulin into the bloodstream rapidly, circumventing gastrointestinal metabolism, so that drug response can be seen within 15 to 30 minutes. At the present time, there is no other bioavailable dosage form of insulin (aside from the parenteral routes of administration).

Such considerations are fundamental to identifying which drug to use, at which dose, at which frequency, and by which manner of delivery. In pathologies where physiological and biochemical systems are challenged but remain fundamentally intact, medication can reduce symptoms or speed the healing response so that the body can fend off the disease and return to a healthy state. In contrast, when the body's underlying functions are compromised, as in autoimmune disorders, metabolic disorders, cardiovascular disease, and so forth, often the best drug therapy can do is to restore a semblance of normal function or relieve symptoms, without fixing the actual problem. What this means for the patient is that the drug may need to be taken indefinitely. The drug used to treat type 1 diabetes, insulin, is essentially a *synthetically identical* hormone produced in

the pancreas, albeit one altered to extend its life in the body.

CHAPTER SUMMARY

Medication therapy requires knowledge of both physiology (how the body works) and biochemistry (how chemicals work upon the body). Fortunately for the clinician, much of the biochemistry is worked out before drugs are approved for use, so there is guidance available. Even so, it is up to the clinician to keep the pharmacokinetic and pharmacodynamic parameters in mind and apply them to each specific situation when choosing a drug for treatment and, especially, when deciding how to administer the drug. It would take decades of study to identify the properties of each and every drug—and even then, given that new drugs are continually entering clinical trials, the clinician would never be able to keep up. Moreover, the "old standbys" of therapy often are found to be problematic in some respects when used in different regimens, for long-term therapy, or for new indications. Thus, practitioners must keep abreast of the various sources of information and learn to identify clinical situations that favor the use of one medication over another.

The nature of this text is such that it focuses on general principles; the specific details of pharmacodynamics and pharmacokinetics for individual drugs, or even individual drug classes, cannot be given here due to space constraints. However, there are abundant resources for obtaining this information. Following are a series of resources (websites) that can offer more specific guidance when it comes to identifying these parameters for particular medications.

1. Interactive Clinical Pharmacology: http://www.icp.org.nz/
2. First Key: Pharmacodynamics for Nurses: https://nursekey.com/pharmacodynamics/
3. A First Course in Pharmacokinetics and Biopharmaceutics by David Bourne: https://www.boomer.org/c/p4/index.php?Loc=OUHSC33
4. Basic Principles and Pharmacodynamics: https://clinicalgate.com/basic-principles-and-pharmacodynamics/
5. Pharmacokinetics and Biopharmaceutics: Advanced Course by David Bourne: https://www.boomer.org/c/p4/?Loc=Advance
6. An online course in Basic Pharmacokinetics by Makoid, Vuchetich, and Banakar: http://klinikfarmakoloji.com/files/PKINBOOK.PDF
7. Pharmacology Corner: http://pharmacologycorner.com/
8. USC Laboratory of Applied Pharmacokinetics: http://www.lapk.org/
9. MoDRN: ADME and Toxicology: https://modrn.yale.edu/education/undergraduate-curriculum/modrn-u-modules/adme-and-toxicology
10. Pharmacology for Nurses: https://pharmafactz.com/pharmacology-for-nurses-rapid-revision-of-drugs/

1. Define the process of absorption.

2. List factors that may affect the rate of drug absorption; explain the reason(s) for each. (Hint: Recall the "definition" of absorption.)

3. Which factors may affect the extent of drug absorption? Explain the reason(s) for each.

4. Identify the physiological barrier(s) for each of the following routes of drug administration. How does the barrier affect the rate of drug absorption for each?
   a. IV bolus injection
   b. Oral tablet
   c. Transdermal patch
   d. Intramuscular injection
   e. Rectal suppository

5. Place the predicted rates of drug absorption (for the routes of administration (ROAs) listed in Question 4) in order from the fastest rate to the slowest rate (based on the physiological barrier).

6. What is meant by the "first-pass effect," with respect to drug absorption?

7. Identify the route(s) of administration that bypass the "first-pass effect" following drug administration. Explain your answer considering the site of drug absorption.

8. Which route of elimination is most subject to the "first-pass effect"? Why?

9. Explain what is meant by "steady-state" plasma drug levels.

10. Will a drug given as an oral solution be 100% systemically available (bioavailable)? Why or why not?

11. Describe, in words, the meaning of $t_{1/2}$ for a drug.

12. A medication has a short half-life (approximately 3 hours). Discuss how the (elimination) half-life ($t_{1/2}$) for a medication affects its dosing interval and, consequently, the design of the dosing regimen.

13. How long will it take to eliminate 75% of a drug, if the drug's $t_{1/2}$ is 6 hours?

14. Explain why a healthy, adult patient would need to take 600 mg of ibuprofen, but only 10 mg of piroxicam, to obtain the same degree of pain relief.

15. Explain "volume of distribution." Why is this kinetic parameter necessary? What information does it give about the overall distribution for a medication?

16. What information does the V_D value give about the overall half-life of a drug? Which predictions can be made about the extent of distribution and the rate of elimination for such a drug?

17. Mrs. S. Takes Drug A at the same time as she takes Drug B. Both drugs bind to albumin (one of the plasma proteins) and compete for the same binding sites on this plasma protein in the bloodstream. Drug A has a much higher affinity for the plasma protein than Drug B. Which Drug (A or B) will be more likely "inactivated"?

For Questions 18–20, choose the correct answer. More than one answer may be correct.

18. Which factor(s) affect(s) the distribution of a drug in the body following systemic administration?
   a. Extent of drug binding to plasma proteins
   b. Lipophilicity of the drug molecule
   c. MW of the drug molecule
   d. Affinity of the drug for peripheral tissues

19. What assumption(s) might you make if a drug has a large volume of distribution (i.e., 250 L)?
   a. The drug is highly bound to plasma proteins.
   b. The drug exhibits one-compartment model kinetics.
   c. The drug distributes extensively in tissues.
   d. The drug is excreted exclusively by the kidney.

20. Which of the following factors may explain a long half-life for a drug?
   a. The rate of elimination is very fast for that drug.
   b. The volume of distribution is 3 L.
   c. The drug distributes into a peripheral tissue compartment.
   d. All of these factors will result in an increased drug half-life.

REFERENCES

Abrams, J., Conley, B., Mooney, M., Zwiebel, J., Chen, A., Welch, J.J....Doroshow, J. (2014). National Cancer Institute's Precision Initiatives for the new National Clinical Trials Network. In *American Society of Clinical Oncology educational book* (pp 71–76). Alexandria, VA: American Society of Clinical Oncology.

American Medical Association (AMA). (n.d.). USAN council. Retrieved from https://www.ama-assn.org/about/usan-council

Arrowsmit, J. (2012). A decade of change. Nature Reviews Drug Discovery, 11, 17–18.

Boundless. (2016). Types of receptors. Boundless Biology Boundless. Retrieved from https://www.boundless.com/biology/textbooks/boundless-biology-textbook/cell-communication-9/signaling-molecules-and-cellular-receptors-83/types-of-receptors-381-11607/

Brater D.C., Daly W.J. (2000). Clinical pharmacology in the Middle Ages: principles that presage the 21st century. *Clinical Pharmacology and Therapeutics, 67*(5), 447–450.

Carter, A., Chang, H., Church, G., Dombkowski, A., Ecker, J., Elad., D.. . .Wong, W. (2017). Challenges and recommendations for epigenomics in precision health. *Nature Biotechnology* 35, 1128–1132. DOI: 10.1056/NEJMp1500523.

Collins, F. & Varmus, H. (2015) Perspective: A new initiative on precision medicine. *New England Journal of Medicine, 372*, 793–795.

Desmond-Hellmann, S., Sawyers, C.L., Cox, D.R., Fraser-Liggett, C., Galli, S.J., Goldstein, D., ... Morrison, S.J. (2011). Toward precision medicine: Building a knowledge network for biomedical research and a new taxonomy of disease". *Washington DC: National Academy of Sciences*. Retrieved from http://www.nap.edu/catalog/13284/toward-precision-medicine-building-a-knowledge-network-for-biomedical-research.

Ehrlich, P. (1913). Chemotherapeutics: Science, principles, methods and results. *Lancet, ii*, 445–451.

Ferris, C.H., & Kahn R. (2012). New mechanisms of glucocorticoid-induced insulin resistance: Make no bones about it. *The Journal of Clinical Investigation, 122*(11), 3854–3857. https://doi.org/10.1172/JCI66180.

Food and Drug Administration (FDA). (n.d.). Drugs @ FDA Glossary. Retrieved from https://www.accessdata.fda.gov/scripts/cder/daf/index.cfm?event=glossary.page

Hollinger, M.A. (2003). *Introduction to pharmacology* (p. 4). Boca Raton, FL: CRC Press.

Kambhampati, D. (2014). FDA – Paving the way for personalized medicine. *Health & Medicine*. Retrieved from https://www.slideshare.net/devkambhampati/dr-dev-kambhampati-fda.

Krsiak, M. (1991). Ethnopharmacology: A historical perspective. *Neuroscience and Biobehavioral Reviews, 15*(4), 439–445.

Lopez-Jimenez, F., Simha V., Thomas, R., Allison, T., Basu, A., Fernandes, R., . . .Wright, R.S. (2014). A summary and critical assessment of the 2013 ACC/AHA Guideline on the Treatment of Blood Cholesterol to Reduce Atherosclerotic Cardiovascular Disease Risk in Adults: Filling the Gaps. *Mayo Clinic Proceedings, 89*(9), 1257–1278. Retrieved from https://www.mayoclinicproceedings.org/article/S0025-6196(14)00570-9/abstract

Maehle, A.H., Prüll, C.R., & Halliwell, R.F. (2002). The emergence of the drug receptor theory. *Nature Reviews Drug Discovery, 1*(8), 637s–641.

Rahman, S.Z. & Khan, R.A. (2006). Environmental pharmacology: A new discipline. *Indian J Pharmacol.* 38(4): 229–30.

Rang, H.P. (2006). The receptor concept: Pharmacology's big idea. *British Journal of Pharmacology, 147*(Supplement 1), S9–S16.

Rang, H.P., Ritter, J.M., Flower, R.J., & Henderson, G. (2007). *Rang & Dale's pharmacology (6th edition)*. London: Churchill Livingstone.

Ruhoy, I., & Daughton, C. (2008). Beyond the medicine cabinet: An analysis of where and why medications accumulate. *Environment International, 34*(8), 1157–1169.

Smith Marsh, D.E. (2017). Overview of generic drugs and drug naming. *Merck Manual*. Retrieved from http://www.merckmanuals.com/home/drugs/brand-name-and-generic-drugs/overview-of-generic-drugs-and-drug-naming.

Spear, B.B., Heath-Chiozzi, M., & Huff, J. (2001). Clinical application of pharmacogenetics. *Trends in Molecular Medicine, 7*(5), 201–204.

U.S. Food and Drug Administration. (2013). *Paving the way for personalized medicince: FDA's role in a new era of medical product development*. Washington, DC: U.S. Department of Health and Human Services. Retrieved from https://www.fdanews.com/ext/resources/files/10/10-28-13-Personalized-Medicine.pdf

Wells, B. (2017). Philosophy of USAN program. *USAN Insider, 8*(2), 1.

EXTERNAL LINKS

American Society fr Pharmacology and Experimental Therapeutics: https://www.aspet.org/

British Pharmacological Society: https://www.bps.ac.uk/

Pharmaceutical company profiles at NNDB: http://www.nndb.com/lists/623/000098329/

International Conference on Harmonisation: http://www.ich.org/home.html

US Pharmacopeia: http://www.usp.org/

International Union of Basic and Clinical Pharmacology: http://www.iuphar.org/

IUPHAR Committee on Receptor Nomenclature and Drug Classification: http://www.guidetopharmacology.org/

https://clinicalgate.com/basic-principles-and-pharmacodynamics/

CHAPTER 3

Medication Administration

Tara Kavanaugh

KEY TERMS

Buccal	Intraosseous	Medication administration	Subcutaneous
Depot preparations	Intrathecal	error	Sublingual
Injectable pen	Intravenous	Medication error	Transdermal
Intramuscular		Oral	Transmucosal

CHAPTER OBJECTIVES

At the end of the chapter, the student will be able to:

1. Define key terms.

2. Discuss the nurse's role in medication administration.

3. Identify the Eight Rights of Medication Administration and three patient checks.

4. Identify the steps in administering medications using different delivery methods.

5. Discuss current trends in medication administration.

6. Identify methods to help reduce medication errors.

Introduction

Medication is transferred into the body's tissues in one of three ways (as mentioned in Chapter 2): (1) by ingestion and absorption in the digestive tract; (2) by passive transfer through porous tissues, such as the skin, the alveoli of the lungs, and the mucous membranes; or (3) by insertion directly into the interior tissues via subcutaneous, intramuscular, or intrathecal injection or intravenous/intraosseous infusion. The central goal of nursing pharmacology is to enable nurses to provide medications to patients safely and appropriately using the route best suited for the administration. Within that seemingly simple statement is held a complex set of information defining the nurse's relationship with his or her patients.

To safely administer medications, a nurse must know the answers to a range of potential questions about his or her patients and their medications: who, what, when, how, and why (TABLE 3-1).

Medication errors are no small matter in nursing practice. The Institute of Medicine's (IOM) first Quality Chasm report, *To Err Is Human: Building a Safer Health System*, noted that medication-related errors contribute to significant morbidity and mortality; errors accounted "for one out of every 131 *outpatient* deaths and one out of every 854 *inpatient* deaths in the United States" (IOM, 1999, p. 27; see also Hughes & Blegen, 2008). Furthermore, according to the IOM (1999), medication errors accounted for more than 7,000 deaths annually in the United States.

TABLE 3-1	Key Questions When Administering Medications	
General Questions	What Nurses Need to Know Is…	Goal
Who	Who is the patient? This means: What is the patient's age, sex, and mental and physical health status? Are there any factors that could contraindicate this medication being administered? Is this *patient* the same individual for whom the medication was ordered?	Ensure that the medication is appropriate for the patient's needs, keeping in mind factors such as physiological issues (e.g., ability to absorb oral medications), biochemical issues (e.g., other medications the patient takes), and social factors (e.g., the patient's known religious or cultural preferences) that may affect whether an ordered medication is appropriate for a given patient. Avoid administering the ordered medication to the *wrong patient*.
What	What *medication* is to be delivered to this patient? What *dose* was requested on the medication order?	Ensure that the *correct medication* is administered in accordance with the prescription or orders of the prescriber. Ensure that the dose administered is in accordance with the orders of the prescriber and cross-check that the dose ordered is appropriate for patient needs.
When	What is the appropriate *time* to administer this medication? When did this patient last have a dose of this (or any) medication?	Avoid administering medication too frequently, too infrequently, at inappropriate times of day, or in inappropriate combination with another medication. Avoid delivering a medication for a longer or shorter *duration* than was ordered by the prescriber. Avoid overmedication or potential interactions between medications.
How	*In what manner* is this medication *typically* administered? Which *route* of delivery was ordered for this patient? Do any factors contraindicate the ordered delivery route in this patient?	Avoid selection of inappropriate delivery *procedures* (e.g., intramuscular injection for a medication intended for intravenous delivery). Ensure that the medication is delivered via the route ordered by the prescriber. Avoid using inappropriate methods of medication delivery.
Why	*What condition* is the medication intended to treat? What is the response that is expected from the use of this medication?	Avoid using medications that are not indicated for a particular condition. Ensure that unexpected or unintended actions (e.g., medication allergy) are noted and treated as necessary in a timely fashion.

Note: If any of these questions is overlooked before medication is administered, the potential for a medication error increases.

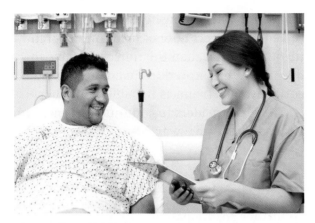

© Jupiterimages/Photos.com/Thinkstock.

More recently, the Department of Health and Human Services (DHHS) estimated that one in seven Medicare patients experienced an adverse event during a hospital stay and 31% of those were due to medication error (DHHS, 2010). Contemplating these facts makes it

clear that nurses must take an approach toward medicating patients that focuses on ensuring the *right* amount of the *right* medication gets to the *right* patient at the *right* time—always.

Before Administering Medications: The Eight Medication "Rights"

A variety of protocols have been instituted to help avoid medication errors. For example, many hospitals and practices use an eight-point checklist (TABLE 3-2) that includes identifying the correct patient (*who*) by cross-checking the names on the medication order and on the patient's identification bracelet; using two documented patient identifiers, such as name and date of birth; and asking the patient to verbally identify himself or herself, if able to do so. Additionally, using technology, such as a bar-code system when

TABLE 3-2	The Eight Rights of Medication Administration
Patient Right	**Nursing Interventions**
Delivered to the RIGHT patient	Confirm the patient's identity by cross-checking the medication order and the patient's ID If the patient is awake/conscious ask them to state their name and their date of birth
The RIGHT medication	Check the medication label against the medication order
Given for the RIGHT reason	Does it make sense to give this medication to this patient? What is the patient's medical history?
The RIGHT dose	Check the medication order for correct dosage. Verify against available drug references. Verbally confirm with another nurse.
Via the RIGHT route	Confirm the correct route of administration through drug references and by reviewing the medication order.
At the RIGHT time	Check the medication order for correct timing of medication administration. Review patient chart for time of previous medication administration.
With the RIGHT response	What are the expected outcomes for how this patient should respond to the medication? Verify against manufacturer guidelines and available drug references. Ensure the drug leads to the desired effect. Monitor the patient and document the monitoring process as well as any nursing interventions performed
The RIGHT documentation	Review the medication order for the correct frequency of medication administration, as well as correct site for administration. Document administration of medication after it has been given. Note patient vital signs and pertinent lab values.

it is available, can decrease medication errors. Checking the medication label against the medication order can ensure that the correct medication is being prepared for the patient (*what*). Checking the medication order for the correct dosage and verifying its appropriateness by comparing information with drug references, as well as double-checking with another nurse, can also reduce dosing errors. Determining the route of the medication that should be given (*how*) can be verified via a drug reference book, and confirming the order can reduce errors associated with the wrong route of administration. Furthermore, knowing the appropriate time when a given dose should be administered by checking the prescribed or ordered frequency of the medication dosing, as well as knowing when the previous dose of a medication was given, can eliminate timing errors (*when*). After a medication is administered, it is important to document that the drug was administered both in a timely fashion and in a correct manner to avoid duplicate dosing and prevent missed doses, note pertinent information such as lab values and vital signs, and review documentation regarding the sites used for previous medication administration. Finally, knowing the reason (*why*) a medication is ordered or prescribed, as well as the expected outcomes, will allow the nurse to provide optimal care for his or her patients.

All of these procedures must precede *any* delivery of medication. A nurse who fails to perform them has made a medication error

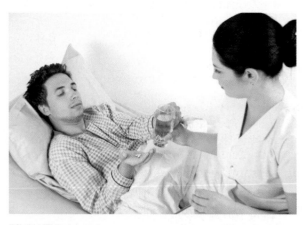

© Blaj Gabriel/Shutterstock.

regardless of whether the patient actually received the correct dose of medication—if for no other reason than the nurse is unable to document that procedures were performed correctly, which affects the ability of other healthcare providers to continue treatment in a safe and effective way.

Procedures for Administering Medications

To further ensure patient safety, each route of administration (TABLE 3-3) has procedures that should be followed. These procedures shall be delineated individually below. However, before describing how medications are administered, it is important to review the obstacles that can interfere with performing this task.

Which Factors Hamper Safe Medication Administration?

The goal of any healthcare provider is to administer medication in accordance with correct procedure. However, *any* procedure can be derailed by the following factors that commonly contribute to human error (Reason, 2000; Southwick, 2012):

- *Fatigue*. Tiredness reduces attentiveness to details, making it more likely that a step in a procedure will be missed or performed incorrectly.
- *Interruption*. Stopping midway through a task or being interrupted during a task increases the likelihood that steps will be missed or improperly performed.
- *Multitasking*. Attempting to juggle multiple tasks at the same time usually results in one or more of those tasks being performed poorly.
- *Emotional stress*. An individual who is under emotional stress—whether the source is personal (e.g., marital difficulties, a sick relative) or professional (e.g., fear of layoffs, workplace conflicts)—is more prone to making errors.

Such factors are not always in the nurse's control. If a facility is short-staffed, due to illness for instance, it may not be possible to

TABLE 3-3	Routes of Administration	
Route of Administration	Route Meaning	Example of Medication*
Sublingual (SL)	Under the tongue	Nitroglycerin
Inhalation	Into the lungs	Albuterol
Intranasal	Within the nose	Midazolam
Intravenous (IV)	Into the vein	Furosemide
Intramuscular (IM)	Within the muscle	Glucagon
Subcutaneous (SC/SQ)	Between the dermis and muscle layer	Insulin
Endotracheal (ET)	Via an ET tube	Atropine
Oral	By mouth	Fluoxetine
Buccal	Between the cheek and gum	Glucose
Rectal (PR)	Rectum, urethra, or vagina	Diazepam
Transdermal (TD)	Applied topically to the skin as in a patch	Lidocaine
Aural	Ear	Levofloxacin
Intradermal (ID)	Within the dermal layer of the skin	PPD (purified protein derivative; Mantoux tuberculosis [TB] test)
Ocular	Drops in the eye	Betaxolol ophthalmic
Gastric	Via a gastric tube	Activated charcoal
Intraosseous (IO)	Into the marrow cavity of the bone when quick IV access is not practical	Furosemide
Intrathecal route[†]	Lumbar puncture	Baclofen

*Note that many drugs are available in forms for administration via multiple routes.
[†]Intrathecal medications are generally not administered by nursing staff due to the specialized nature of lumbar puncture procedures. Most such medications are administered by anesthesiologists or other specialist technicians. However, nurses need to maintain awareness of the effects of medications given by this route.

avoid working long or multiple shifts, leading to fatigue and emotional stress. However, maintaining awareness of susceptibility to these factors can help the nurse avoid the errors these factors tend to encourage.

Systemic Factors in Medication Errors

It is likewise important to realize that errors do not occur simply because of factors specific to an individual; often, systemic or cultural factors in institutions also create an environment that is error-promoting. For example, studies have found that the transition between shifts—that is, when a new team of providers assumes care for patients after the previous team members finish their working day—is a key period during which errors may develop due to ineffective communication of patients' status (Carayon & Wood, 2010). Thus, having

systemic institutional processes in place designed to limit errors and foster a safety culture (Singer & Vogus, 2013), such as implementing a handoff program (Starmer et al., 2014) and mitigating interruption-related errors (Prakash et al., 2014), is crucial to reduce such errors and ensure correct administration of medications (Reason, 2000).

The procedures we describe in the following sections include protocols to help avoid conditions that contribute to medication errors. Most institutions will have specific checklists or processes that must be followed, some of which are specific to particular medications that are prone to be confused (e.g., medications with similar-sounding names), that are similar in function but have critical differences in timing (e.g., short-acting versus long-acting insulins), or that may have

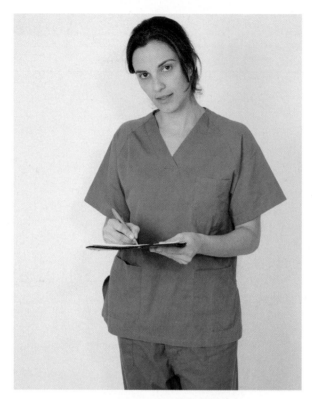

© Adam Gregor/Shutterstock.

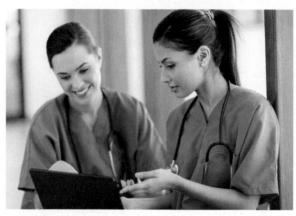

© michaeljung/Shutterstock.

medication record or patient chart, (3) clean dispensing containers, and (4) drug reference books or approved apps. It is important to gather your supplies prior to the procedure to decrease interruptions. Handwashing should be performed prior to and after all of the necessary steps in the medication administration procedure. All legitimate prescriptions should, at a minimum, include the name of the drug (usually the generic name, but the trade name can be written), the dose of the medication to be given, the *intended* administration time, the *actual* time of administration, and the route of administration. If the prescription is handwritten, it should be legible, unambiguous, and contain complete information (e.g., correct dose, route of administration) (Albarrak, Al Rashidi, Fatani, Al Ageel, & Mohammed, 2014; Brits et al., 2017; Cerio, Mallare, & Tolentino, 2015; Walker, 2016). Additionally, the medical chart should contain the patient's name, date of birth, and medical record number affixed via a nonremovable label on the chart, and it should clearly state whether the patient has any known allergies to any substances, especially medications (Ferguson, 2005). An

profound effects if dosed incorrectly (e.g., anticoagulant or antiarrhythmic agents).

Proper Procedure for Administering All Medications

No matter which delivery route is used, certain steps should be followed when giving any form of medication. First, the equipment necessary to administer a medication should be gathered prior to the procedure. This equipment includes (1) any necessary keys for opening the medication-dispensing devices, (2) the

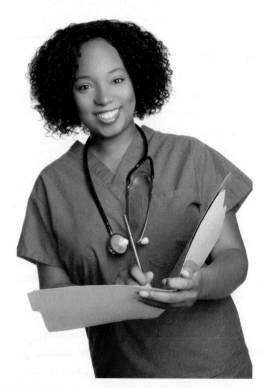

© Hero Images/Getty Images

updated weight should be documented in the patient chart and recorded on the medication administration record flow sheet; this should be checked for discrepancies for any weight-dependent medication dosages, especially for pediatric patients (Ferguson, 2005).

Facility-based policies will exist regarding the number of providers necessary to check the appropriateness of medication prescriptions. Adherence to such policies is especially important when administering controlled substances, pediatric doses of medications, and high-alert medications, which include such drugs as **insulin** and **heparin**. Pediatric dosing and administration of controlled substances require that two nurses check preparations prior to administration of the medications. For all medication administration, at a minimum, the nurse should check the name of the medication (both the generic and trade names), the dose required, time for proper administration, and the previous time the drug was given (or the most recent time that the drug was taken by the patient). In addition, the legibility of the prescription, the provider's signature, the date when the order or prescription was written by the prescriber, any known patient allergies, and the expiration date of the drug should be included on the order or patient chart (Ferguson, 2005). Any discrepancies between the ordered medication and the medication the nurse has to administer should be verified with the prescriber, or, if that prescriber is not available, with another qualified prescriber familiar with the patient.

Before administering the medication, the nurse must verify that the patient receiving the medication is the patient for whom the medication is prescribed. One way to do this is to check the patient identification band on the patient's wrist, or ask the patient to state his or her name and to match it with the name in the medical record (Ferguson, 2005). Additionally, a second identifier is necessary to verify the patient's identity; this may include the patient's date of birth for easy verification. Some facilities use bar-coded or radio-frequency identification labels on wristbands for patient identification (Probst, Wolf, Bollini, & Xiao,

2016; Strudwick, Clark, McBride, Sakal, & Kalia, 2017), although crinkles, food spills, and barcode blurring due to bathing may cause errors (Sandler, Langeberg, Carty, & Dohnalek, 2006). Informed consent should be obtained prior to administering any medication, to determine the patient's understanding of the medication and its side effects, as well as the option for the patient to refuse any medications (Ferguson, 2005). Any refusal of medication should be appropriately documented in the patient record and reported to the prescribing provider.

Administering Oral Medications

Oral medications in this context are those given by mouth and swallowed (**FIGURE 3-1**). It is important to note that some other medications are ostensibly delivered orally (e.g., sublingual medications) but are not swallowed; the key difference is that oral medications are designed to pass through the digestive tract, while the other types of delivery bypass the digestion process. Rationale for either type was discussed in Chapter 2.

Oral medications should be administered using an appropriate delivery system. Solid medications such as tablets and capsules should be given in clean, dry, disposable

Best Practices

It is important to gather your supplies prior to the procedure to decrease interruptions and their potential negative consequences.

Best Practices

Before administering the medication, the nurse must verify that the patient receiving the medication is the patient for whom the medication is prescribed. Matching the patient's name and birth date to the name and birth date on the order is the easiest way to do this.

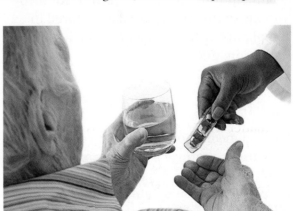

FIGURE 3-1 Proper oral medication administration.
© JPC-PROD/Shutterstock.

subcutaneous = under the skin (handwritten)

containers, whereas oral liquid medications, and those requiring oral syringes, should be measured in syringes designed specifically for the medication-dispensing purpose (Ferguson, 2005). Patients should be placed into a comfortable position and assisted if necessary. It is important to note that medications *should not* be left out for a patient to take at his or her convenience. If the patient is not present when the medication is due, or if the patient does not wish to take it at the prescribed time, then the nurse should return to administer the dose later (documenting the reason for the discrepancy in timing). Additionally, consideration should be given to the patient's ability to swallow oral medications; all medications should be given in the manner prescribed, and crushed only if ordered to do so by the prescriber, and if it is appropriate to crush the specific dosage form of the medication (Morris, 2005). Pharmacy / pharmacists can be valuable sources for these questions.

When dispensing oral medications, the nurse should sign the prescription or medical record to verify that the medication has been administered as ordered, and should do so *only after the patient has taken the medication*—not when the medication is placed into the dispensing containers (Ferguson, 2005). The nurse should also note the effectiveness of the medication given and document it in the patient record. All medications should be replaced and stored in compliance with the policy of the institution (Ferguson, 2005).

Injecting Medications Safely

Injected medications are delivered into the body using a syringe by one of six routes (Table 3-3). These are intradermal, subcutaneous, intramuscular, intravenous, intraosseous, and **intrathecal**. The most common of these are subcutaneous, intramuscular, and intravenous. **Subcutaneous** medication

intramuscular = into muscle (handwritten, vertical)

is delivered "under the skin" (*sub* = "under", *cutis* = "skin") by a syringe placed within the fatty layer of tissue just below the dermis (National Institutes of Health [NIH], 2012). The subcutaneous route is sometimes selected because there is little blood flow to the fatty tissue, and the injected medication is therefore absorbed slowly, sometimes taking as long as 24 hours to be absorbed. Examples of medications that are injected subcutaneously include **heparin**, growth hormone, **insulin**, and **epinephrine** (NIH, 2012). **Intramuscular** injections, as the name implies, are administered directly into muscle tissue. Intramuscular injections are utilized as a medication delivery method because there are no significant barriers to drug absorption and are designed such that they may be absorbed rapidly or slowly (Lehne, 2013).

A variety of considerations affect safety when delivering medications by injection. First, the nurse needs to ascertain which type of injection is required: Is the medication intended for subcutaneous delivery or intramuscular delivery? Second, the nurse should consider the needs of the patient receiving the injection: Is this a pediatric patient who may be unwilling or unable to sit still for an injection? If so, the nurse may need to get an assistant or request a parent's help in holding the child still while delivering the injection. Third, the patient's physical presentation may affect safe and appropriate medication delivery; for example, in a particularly slender patient, the layer of subcutaneous fat may be narrow enough that a syringe inserted at too great an angle (more than 45°) might inadvertently inject the medication into muscle instead fat, while in an obese patient, the opposite problem might impede an intramuscular injection. Note that the nurse's own safety is important as well when it comes to medication injection, as improperly handled syringes can cause needle-stick injuries.

Giving Subcutaneous Injections

Before giving a subcutaneous injection, the nurse should wash his or her hands thoroughly

The Parts of the Syringe

A syringe has three major parts: the needle, the barrel, and the plunger (FIGURE 3-2). The needle goes into the skin to enable medication transfer from the barrel. The barrel holds the medicine, and the plunger is used to force the medication out of the syringe. The syringe has marks on the side of the barrel (like a ruler) to indicate the number of cubic centimeters (cc) or milliliters (mL) that can be contained in the syringe, and increments thereof.

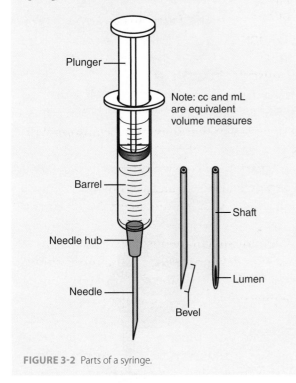

Plunger

Note: cc and mL are equivalent volume measures

Barrel

Shaft

Needle hub

Lumen

Needle

Bevel

FIGURE 3-2 Parts of a syringe.

for at least 20 seconds, and assemble the equipment necessary, including the following:

- Medication in either a multidose vial of liquid or a vial of powder requiring reconstitution, as directed by the manufacturer
- Syringe or pen and needle, appropriate for the size of the adult or child: 0.5 cc, 1 cc, or 2 cc with 27-gauge ⅝-inch needle; 3 cc Luer-Lock syringe if the solution is more than 1 cc; 25- to 27-gauge ⅝-inch needle or 0.3 mL insulin syringes with 31-gauge – 1/4 to -1/2 inch needle in special circumstances
- Container for syringe disposal
- Sterile 2×2-inch gauze pad
- Alcohol pads

Preparing the Medication for a Subcutaneous Injection

- Check the label to verify the correct medication and remove the soft metal or plastic cap protecting the rubber stopper of the vial.
- If the medication is in a multidose vial, record the date and time the vial was first opened on the label.
- Clean the exposed rubber stopper with an isopropyl alcohol wipe, remove the syringe from the plastic or paper cover, and attach the needle securely to the syringe, if it is indicated.
- Next, pull back and forth on the plunger by grasping the plunger *handle*, so that contamination of the sterile plunger shaft will be prevented.
- With the needle capped, pull back on the plunger to fill the syringe with air equal in volume to the amount of medication to be administered.

Remove the cap covering the needle and set it on its side to prevent contamination, also taking care not to touch the sterile needle. The inside of the cap and the needle are sterile, and the cap will be used to cover the needle until the time of medication administration. With the vial upright, push the needle through the cleansed rubber stopper on the vial (FIGURE 3-3).

Inject the air (if appropriate) in the syringe into the vial to prevent a vacuum from forming. If too little air or no air is injected, it is difficult to withdraw the medication. If too much air is injected, the plunger may be forced out of the barrel, causing the medication to spill. Remember that there are a few injectable medications for which you want to prevent positive pressure from causing the medication to spill on the nurse or the patient.

Turn the needle and vial upside down with the needle remaining in the vial, making

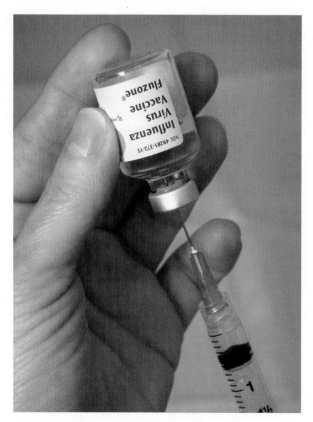

FIGURE 3-3 Dispensing medication into a syringe.
Courtesy of Jim Gathany/CDC

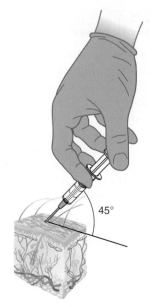

FIGURE 3-4 Image of administering a subcutaneous injection (45° angle).

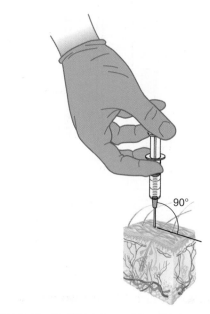

FIGURE 3-5 Image of injection at a 90° angle.

sure that the needle is pointed upward. Ensure that the tip of the needle is completely covered by the medication to make it easier to draw up the medication without any air. Pull back on the plunger to fill the syringe with the correct volume of the medication. Keep the vial upside down with the needle in the vial, continuing to point them upward. Tap the syringe with the fingertips to remove any air bubbles in the syringe. Once the bubbles are at the top of the syringe, gently push on the plunger to force the bubbles out of the syringe and back into the vial. Alternatively, if the bubbles cannot be removed from the syringe by tapping with the fingertips, push all of the medication slowly back into the vial and repeat the previous steps if necessary. It is important to remove the air from the syringe because air takes up the needed space for the medication and because such bubbles can cause pain or discomfort or air emboli if they are injected. After removing the bubbles, check the volume of the medication in the syringe to verify that the *volume* (and therefore the *dose*) is the correct.

Push the needle into the subcutaneous tissue at a 45° or 90° angle, being careful not to bend the needle (**FIGURE 3-4**, **FIGURE 3-5**, and **FIGURE 3-6**).

Injectable Pens

For some medications, a pen-like device, which delivers premeasured dosing, is available. If the nurse is using such an **injectable pen**, the following steps will be employed.

Comparison of angles of injection.

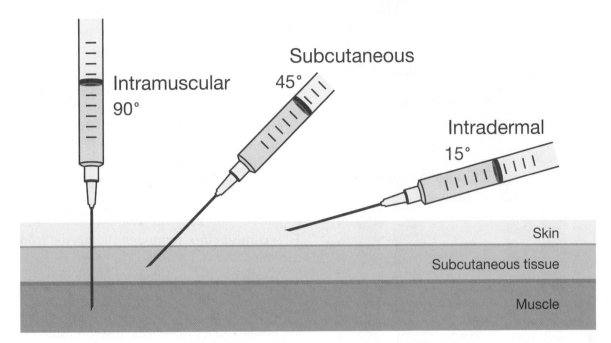

FIGURE 3-6 Subcutaneous injection administration.
© solar22/Shutterstock

First, attach the needle to the pen by cleaning the top of the pen with an alcohol wipe and screw the needle onto the injectable pen. Next, use the dial on the pen to set the appropriate dose volume. If priming of the injectable pen is required, this step should be performed before setting the dose. Many injectable pens are manufactured so that a "priming volume" may be set with a dial. To prime, the pen needle should be pointed up and the injection button depressed completely. The nurse should see a drop or stream of liquid. If a stream of liquid is not visible, the priming steps should be repeated until this occurs. Dial in the prescribed volume of medication. After the medication is correctly prepared, carefully replace the needle cap to prevent contamination, being careful not to stick any fingers with the needle (NIH, 2012).

Rotating Injection Sites for Subcutaneous Injections

It is important to rotate the injection sites to keep the skin healthy and to prevent scarring and hardening of the fatty tissue. Scarring and hardening of the skin may prevent absorption of the medication. Each injection site should be at least one inch away from the previous injection site. A series of injections should be started at the highest physical point possible on the patient (such as the upper arms) (FIGURE 3-7); the sites should then move to the furthest point from the initial injection site on the body part, such as the upper thighs. It is preferable to use all of the sites available on one body part before moving to another body part, although this may need to be altered for patient comfort. Injections should not be administered in red, inflamed, burned, swollen, or damaged skin (NIH, 2012).

General Guidelines for Subcutaneous Injections

Cleanse the skin thoroughly in a back-and-forth motion with an alcohol swab to eliminate microbes at the injection site. Allow the alcohol to dry completely. Take the cover off the needle, being careful not to

Best Practices

Before injections, remove the air from the syringe because air takes up space that should be filled with medication. In addition, bubbles can cause pain or discomfort or air emboli if they are injected.

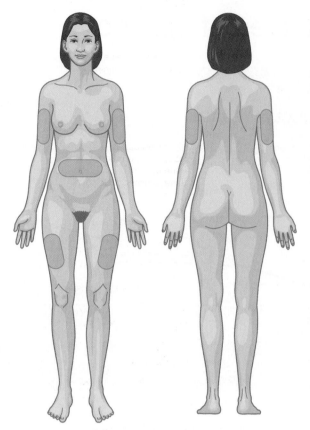

FIGURE 3-7 Example of injection site rotation choices.

contaminate the needle. Place the cover on its side. The nurse who is administering the dose should hold the syringe in one hand like a pencil or dart, grasp the patient's skin between his or her thumb and index finger with his or her other hand, and pinch the skin in an upward fashion. The needle should then be quickly thrust all the way into the skin. Avoid pushing the needle into the skin slowly or thrusting the needle in with great force. A common mistake is pressing down on the top of the plunger while piercing the skin; this can result in the medication being released before the needle is in position, resulting in deposition of medication on the skin surface, or within the skin layers, rather than under the skin; for this reason, it is important to keep one's thumb or finger off the plunger until the needle is completely inserted.

Insert the needle at a 90° right angle into the skin (see Figure 3-5). This angle is important to ensure that the medication will be injected into the fatty tissue. If the patient receiving the injection is a small child or has very little subcutaneous fat or thin skin, a 45° angle is used (see Figure 3-4). If using a pen needle, insert the pen needle at a 90° angle.

After the needle is completely inserted into the skin, release the grasped skin and press down on the plunger to inject all of the medication into the subcutaneous layer at a slow and steady rate. If using a pen, press the injection button completely until it "clicks," and keep the pen in position for 10 seconds before removing the needle from the skin.

As the needle is pulled out of the skin where it was inserted, gently press a 2×2-inch gauze pad onto the needle insertion site. Keeping pressure over the needle insertion site prevents the skin from retracting while removing the needle, causing less pain. The gauze also helps to seal the punctured tissue, preventing any leakage of medication. If indicated, press or rub the injection sites. Not all medications should be massaged into the skin, so the medication manufacturer's information should be consulted. If any fluid or blood is noted at the injection site, press another 2×2-inch gauze pad onto the injection site.

If using a pen, untwist the needle on the pen and safely dispose of the needle. Replace the pen cap and store as instructed (NIH, 2012).

Intramuscular Injections

Some medications, as noted earlier, are injected directly into muscle tissue (**FIGURE 3-8**). The primary reasons for using intramuscular injections of medications are (1) administration of poorly soluble drugs and (2) administration of **depot preparations**, which are preparations of medications that are absorbed slowly over an extended period of time (Lehne, 2013). The rate of absorption is determined by two factors: the water solubility of the drug and the blood flow to the injection site. Drugs that are highly soluble

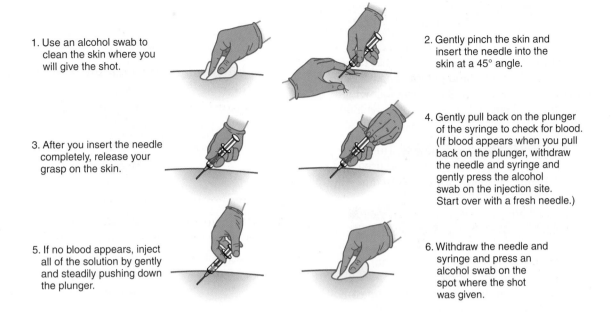

1. Use an alcohol swab to clean the skin where you will give the shot.

2. Gently pinch the skin and insert the needle into the skin at a 45° angle.

3. After you insert the needle completely, release your grasp on the skin.

4. Gently pull back on the plunger of the syringe to check for blood. (If blood appears when you pull back on the plunger, withdraw the needle and syringe and gently press the alcohol swab on the injection site. Start over with a fresh needle.)

5. If no blood appears, inject all of the solution by gently and steadily pushing down the plunger.

6. Withdraw the needle and syringe and press an alcohol swab on the spot where the shot was given.

FIGURE 3-8 How to give an intramuscular injection.

in water will be rapidly absorbed, within 10 to 30 minutes, whereas drugs that are poorly soluble will be absorbed at a rate greater than 30 minutes (Lehne, 2013, p. 34).

Anatomic Locations for Administering Intramuscular Injections

The muscle chosen for the injection must be able to be exposed completely and easy to access (Beyea & Nicoll, 1995). However, the patient's circumstances must also be considered. Muscles change with age and cannot always be used successfully for every type of intramuscular injection. The dorsogluteal muscle, for example, is never used for children younger than age three because it has not developed completely. The deltoid cannot be used if the area is very thin or fragile with no muscle mass or is underused, such as in a frail older adult or infant. It is generally considered good practice to avoid giving an injection in the dominant arm because any pain or swelling in the injection site might hamper the patient's ability to function using that arm.

The following sites are most commonly used for intramuscular injections.

Vastus Lateralis Muscle (Thigh)

The thigh is used most often for children younger than age three but can also be used for adults. There is some evidence of reduced infant distress during medication administration at this site (Taddio et al., 2015). Another advantage to this location is that it is easy to view the thigh if the patient needs to administer his or her own injectable medication. In infants and children, the site for injection lies below the greater trochanter of the femur and within the upper lateral quadrant of the thigh. For adults, the site is four inches below the greater trochanter and four inches above the knee, lateral to the middle third of the vastus lateralis muscle. This may be visualized as dividing a patient's thigh from the knee to the hip into three equal parts. The middle third is where an injection should be administered (**FIGURE 3-9** and **FIGURE 3-10**) (Beyea & Nicoll, 1995; Winslow, 1996).

Ventrogluteal Muscle (Hip)

The ventrogluteal muscle is a good location for adults and children aged seven months and older. This site's utility is due to the ease with which bony landmarks may be

Safe Needle Disposal

After any injection, it is important to dispose of needles properly to avoid injuries or the possibility of needle reuse (and potential contamination or infection transmission). The following guidelines will ensure such errors are avoided (NIH, 2012):

- Do *not* recap needles after use. Doing so increases the likelihood that the used needle will be mistaken for an unused needle and inadvertently reused.
- Immediately after use, place the needle, with or without the syringe, in a hard plastic or metal container with a tightly secured lid. Keep the container out of reach of children or pets.
- If used in a home setting, when the container is full, take it to an appropriate facility for proper disposal.

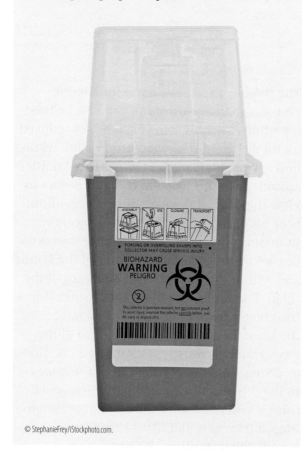

© StephanieFrey/iStockphoto.com.

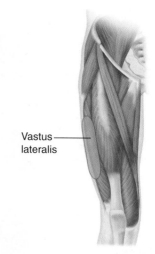

Vastus lateralis

FIGURE 3-9 Administering a vastus lateralis injection.

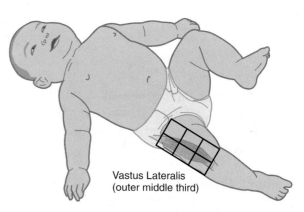

Vastus Lateralis
(outer middle third)

FIGURE 3-10 Proper visualization of thigh.

& Nicoll, 1995; Winslow, 1996). To find the correct location to give a ventrogluteal injection (in the hip), place the palm of the hand against the greater trochanter and place the index finger on the anterior superior iliac spine. Extend the middle finger along the iliac crest toward the iliac tubercle (right hand to left hip and left hand to right hip; see **FIGURE 3-11**).

Deltoid Muscle (Upper Arm Muscle)

The patient receiving a deltoid intramuscular injection can be lying down, sitting, or standing. The entire upper arm and shoulder area should be exposed to correctly identify the landmarks. The correct location to give the injection is 1–2 inches (2.5–5 cm) below

identified, and there is little danger of inadvertently piercing blood vessels or nerves. The patient should lie on his or her side when receiving a ventrogluteal injection (Beyea

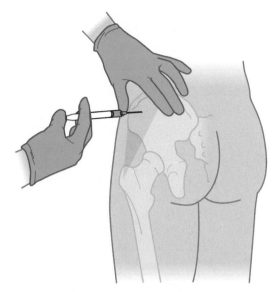

FIGURE 3-11 Administering a ventrogluteal injection.

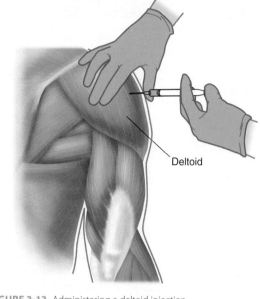

FIGURE 3-13 Administering a deltoid injection.

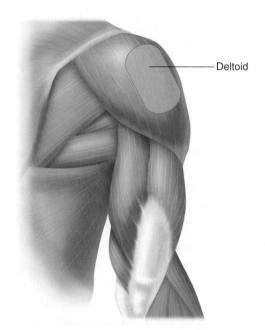

FIGURE 3-12 Location for administering a deltoid injection.

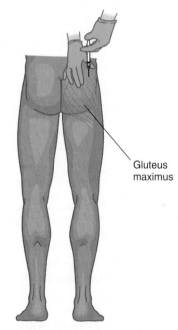

FIGURE 3-14 Administering a dorsogluteal injection.

the bottom of the acromion process
(**FIGURE 3-12** and **FIGURE 3-13**) (Beyea & Nicoll,
1995; Winslow, 1996).

Dorsogluteal Muscle (Buttocks)

Expose one buttock cheek completely. Draw an
imaginary line between the superior iliac spine
and the greater trochanter. Give the injection
in an area above this imaginary line (**FIGURE 3-14**)
(Beyea & Nicoll, 1995; Winslow, 1996).

Supplies Needed for Administering Intramuscular Injections

- Individually wrapped alcohol wipes, or
  the equivalent.
- Sterile 2×2-inch gauze.
- The vial or ampule of medication being
  administered.
- The correct-size needle and **sy**ringe
  (1 cc, 3 cc, 5 cc, 10 cc, 20 cc, 30 cc, or
  60 cc syringes; ½-inch, 5/8-inch, 1-inch,

TABLE 3-4	Needle Lengths and Injection Sites for Intramuscular Injections	
Birth–18 Years		
Age	Needle Length	Injection Site
Newborn*	5/8" (16 mm)†	Anterolateral thigh
Infant 1–12 months	1" (25 mm)	Anterolateral thigh
Toddler 1–2 years	1"–1¼" (25–32 mm) 5/8"†–1" (16–25 mm)	Anterolateral thigh§ Deltoid muscle of the arm
Child/adolescent 3–18 years	5/8"†–1" (16–25 mm) 1"–1¼" (25–32 mm)	Deltoid muscle of the arm§ Anterolateral thigh
Aged ≥19 Years		
Sex/Weight	Needle Length	Injection Site
Male and female <60 kg (130 lbs)	1" (25 mm)¶	Deltoid muscle of the arm
Female 60–90 kg (130–200 lbs) Male 60–118 kg (130–260 lbs)	1"–1½" (25–38 mm)	
Female >90 kg (200 lbs) Male >118 kg (260 lbs)	1½" (38 mm)	

*Newborn = first 28 days of life.
†If skin stretched tight, subcutaneous tissues not bunched.
§Preferred site.
¶Certain experts recommend a 5/8" (16-mm) needle for patients who weigh <60 kg (130 lbs)
Data from Poland, et al. (1997). JAMA 1997 June; 277(21):1709-1711.

or 1.5-inch needle, ranging from 15- to 33-gauge needle diameter). The needle length and injection site for intramuscular injections appear in **TABLE 3-4**.

- Gloves for the protection of the patient and person providing the intramuscular injection.
- A sharps container to dispose of the used syringe and needle.

General Procedure for Administering Intramuscular Injections

As with other procedures, the supplies required (see the preceding list) should be assembled and checked prior to the procedure. The location of the injection should likewise be determined in advance, considering the patient's needs and circumstances. The nurse should wash his or her hands with soap and water for at least 20 seconds and pat them completely dry.

Next, the nurse should put on gloves and open one of the packages of alcohol wipes. The nurse should take the cover off the needle by holding the syringe with his or her writing hand and pulling on the cover with the other hand. This can be thought of as similar to taking a cap off of a pen. The nurse should hold the syringe in his or her dominant hand, then place the syringe under his or her thumb and first finger. The nurse should let the barrel of the syringe rest on the second finger of his or her hand, as is typically done when writing with a pen or pencil.

Wipe the area with the alcohol wipes where the needle will be inserted, and let the area dry completely. Depress and pull the skin a little with the free hand. The nurse should continue to hold the skin a little to the side of where he or she plans to insert the needle. Next, the nurse should use his or her wrist to insert the needle at a 90° angle (i.e., straight into the muscle). The nurse should think of this action similar to that of throwing a dart (**FIGURE 3-15**).

Avoid trying to forcefully push the needle into the patient's muscle, because doing so will cause bruising. The needle is sharp and

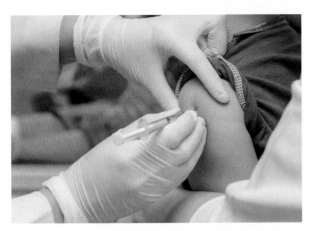

FIGURE 3-15 Administering an intramuscular injection.
© weerayut ranmai/Shutterstock.

will go through the skin easily if the wrist action is correct. Remember to let go of the skin to prevent the needle from jerking sideways. Push down on the plunger and inject the medicine. Do not force the medicine through the syringe by pushing too hard on the plunger, because some medications will burn or hurt if they are administered too quickly.

After all of the medicine is injected, pull the needle out quickly at the same angle that it was inserted. Finally, use the 2×2-inch dry sterile gauze to press gently on the location where the needle entered, and apply a bandage as necessary (Higgins, 2005).

Examples of medications that are given as an intramuscular injection include **epinephrine** pens, antibiotics, pain medications such as **morphine** and nonsteroidal anti-inflammatory drugs (NSAIDs), vitamin B_{12}, and vaccinations. Intramuscular injections should not be administered into broken or damaged skin.

Intravenous and Intraosseous Medications

When speed of delivery is important, medications may be delivered directly into the bloodstream by one of two means: intravenous or intraosseous.

Intravenous medications are delivered via a device that punctures a vein and infuses medication directly into the bloodstream at a specific rate and concentration.

Medications can be administered via a peripheral line, a saline IV lock, a direct IV line, or a central venous catheter. In addition, medications can be delivered by rapid injection (called a "push" or "IV push"), infused continuously over a specified time period, or given intermittently by mixing them into IV solutions (usually normal saline) at predetermined times. Over 90% of hospitalized patients receive IV therapy of some form during their hospital stay (Institute for Safe Medicine Practices [ISMP], 2015).

Intraosseous access is similar in nature except that the puncture goes into bone marrow of a long bone in the arm or leg rather than a vein. The long bones' marrow contains a network of blood vessels that feed into the central venous canal, so intraosseous access is just as effective as intravenous access for delivering medicines. This route of administration is generally used when intravenous access is difficult or impossible to achieve—for example, in small children with circulatory collapse or adult individuals experiencing vasoconstriction due to shock.

IV Medication Safety Issues

In its guide to standardization of high-risk IV medications, the San Diego Patient Safety Consortium (2006) lays out a compelling argument for being especially careful when administering IV medications. It notes that IV medications are associated with the highest risk of harm, with 61% of serious and/or life-threatening adverse drug events occurring with these medications. Equally important is the fact that many of the medications given via IV are high-risk drugs in and of themselves, including drugs such as **insulin**, **heparin**, **morphine**, and **propofol**. Certain of these drugs have been designated "high-alert medications" by the Institute for Safe Medicine Practice (ISMP) due to the drugs' propensity toward serious harm. These drugs have a narrow therapeutic index and there is a higher risk of patient injury or death associated with the drugs (ISMP, 2015). A complete list of high-alert medications can be found at

www.ismp.org/tools/highalertmedicationlists
.asp. Given that a very common form of
administration error in IV medications is
incorrect dosing, it is essential that nurses
administering intravenous/intraosseous
medications pay special attention to the Eight
Rights, and particularly to ensuring the right
dose. A key point to remember is that for IV
delivery, the dose means the *rate* of delivery
as well as the *amount* of medication delivered.

Matters of Key Concern When Administering IV Medications

Some of the most important issues to be
considered during IV medication administration include the potential for allergic
reaction, synergistic or antagonistic effects
between medications, and complications of
the procedure.

Patient's Allergy History

A medication delivered via IV goes directly
into the circulation. Allergic reactions to medications delivered by IV therefore tend to be
considerably more severe than allergic reactions to those medications delivered by other
routes. If the patient has a history of allergy
to the prescribed, or similar, medications, the
drug should not be used so that severe allergic responses can be at least partly avoided.
Be aware that just because there is no *known*
history of allergy does not mean the patient
will not have an allergic response. At the
medication's first use, any reactions (e.g.,
hives, difficulty breathing) should be considered a potential allergic response, treated appropriately, and documented.

Synergistic or Antagonistic Effects

Medications given in close proximity in time
and location may alter each other's activity. For example, **heparin's** anticoagulant
effect increases in the presence of
penicillin. Thus, when giving an
IV medication to a patient who has
already received another medication by this or any other route, it
is important to double-check for
potential drug interactions.

Best Practices

In intravenous deliv-
ery, the dose means
the *rate* of delivery as
well as the *amount* of
medication delivered.

Complications

Potential complications related to cannula
insertion or use of IV medications include
hematoma; infiltration; extravasation; phlebitis; thrombosis; venous spasm; puncture of
artery, nerve, tendon, or ligament; septicemia; and fluid overload. Some medications, if
infused too rapidly, can cause life-threatening
reactions as well. If a central venous catheter
is used, pneumothorax is another concern.
Nurses should be alert to the specific symptoms of these complications.

Administering an IV Medication

After undertaking the necessary checks
for correct patient, medication, and dose,
collect the supplies needed to administer
the medication:

- Medication to be administered
- Alcohol swabs
- Tape or occlusive dressing
- Syringe with needle
- Sterile saline or water (diluent)
- Sodium chloride flush syringe
- Heparin flush (if central venous catheter is indicated)
- Surgical gloves
- Tourniquet

Ensure that the patient is comfortable and
warm; this prevents vasoconstriction. Keeping
in mind that gaining intravenous access may
be frightening to some patients, the nurse
should project a reassuring, confident manner. Turn on and position any supplemental
light as needed before beginning. If the patient is supine in a mobile bed or gurney, the
nurse should raise the bed sufficiently high
so that he or she can work without bending
over, as comfort for the nurse will assist in accuracy of performing the puncture. A patient
who is seated should place the arm to be used
on a flat surface so that the nurse can have
unimpeded access to it.

Identifying a Site

The veins most commonly used for intravenous access are located in the hand or arm.

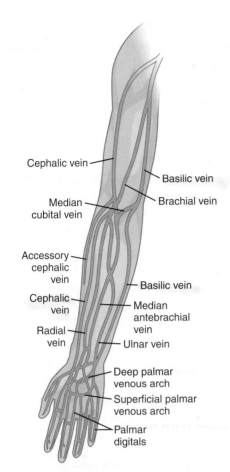

FIGURE 3-16 Veins used for intravenous access.

Cephalic vein

Basilic vein

Median cubital vein

Brachial vein

Accessory cephalic vein

Basilic vein

Cephalic vein

Median antebrachial vein

Radial vein

Ulnar vein

Deep palmar venous arch

Superficial palmar venous arch

Palmar digitals

They include the dorsal digital and metacarpal veins, the cephalic vein, and the basilic vein (**FIGURE 3-16**).

Examine the arm or appendage to spot large or prominent veins, tapping if necessary to promote greater blood flow. Allow the patient's arm to hang down so that gravity can further promote blood flow. If these strategies do not identify any obvious veins, apply a tourniquet. If the patient (or chart) reports prior IV medication administration, ask the patient where the "best veins" have been for previous administrations, as patients usually know. Bear in mind that if the patient has had prior venous access in recent weeks, it may not be possible to reuse a vein that has already been accessed; look for evidence that a vein may have been recently used, and, if possible avoid any veins that show signs of bruising or new healing. If avoidance is not possible, choose the site that seems to have had the least recent use.

Once the patient and environment are ready and an appropriate site has been identified, the nurse should wash his or her hands for 20 seconds, pat them dry, and put on gloves. If indicated, apply the tourniquet 4–6 inches above the site. Sitting or standing in a comfortable, stable position, the nurse rests the heel of the dominant hand on the patient's arm (or other appendage) into which the access is to be inserted. The nurse then grasps the cannula controls between his or her thumb and index finger and lowers them so that they just touch the insertion point. The bevel of the needle should be facing up, and the angle of entry should be shallow, 20–30° at most. The nurse presses the tip first gently, then firmly, against the skin, informing the patient what is happening as it occurs, in order to avoid surprising the patient (which can lead to jerking or jumping). The tip should be allowed to rest a few seconds on the skin surface, then gently and quickly pressed through the skin. The hub of the cannula should be held stable as the needle is withdrawn. If a tourniquet is in place, it should be removed *immediately* once the cannula is in place to avoid loss of access and bleeding from the site.

For a more in-depth discussion regarding cannula placement, a nursing practice handbook should be consulted.

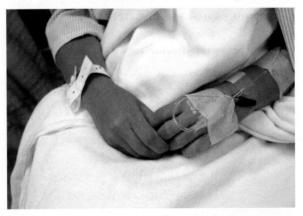

© Elena Ray/Shutterstock, Inc.

With access established, the next step is to begin infusing the medication.

Inhaled Medications

Medicine delivery via inhalation is primarily used to treat respiratory disorders for obvious reasons: Inhalation offers the most direct pathway into the lungs and sinuses. Inhalation is also used for some anesthesia drugs. Although *therapeutic* inhalation delivery may eventually include medications for nonrespiratory diseases (for example, diabetes researchers are exploring the potential for an inhaled form of insulin), for the purposes of this text, it is assumed that the medications are intended as therapy for a respiratory disorder, such as asthma, chronic obstructive pulmonary disease (COPD), sinus congestion, or bronchitis; are inhaled forms of vaccines; or are inhalation anesthesia drugs.

There are three principal methods for inhaled medication delivery: (1) an inhaler device, (2) a nasal spray, or (3) a nebulizer. This section describes each method in turn.

Proper Procedure for Using a Metered-Dose Inhaler or Dry-Powder Inhaler

Metered-dose inhalers (MDI, "puffers") are most frequently used to administer medications for chronic respiratory illnesses such as COPD or asthma. These hand-held devices deliver the medication in aerosol form by means of a propellant in the medication canister so that it can be inhaled directly into the lungs (FIGURE 3-17). A similar device called a dry-powder inhaler (DPI) does not use a propellant; instead, the medication is simply inhaled from the device in the form of a fine, dry powder—much like breathing in dust or pollen. The inhaler used by the patient depends on the medication; only those medications that are produced in dry-powder form can be delivered with a DPI.

The greatest obstacle to delivery of medication via either type of inhaler is improper patient technique. The correct method needed to deliver the full dose accurately is neither self-evident nor easy to learn, although the use of *spacers* with metered-dose inhalers (MDIs) can improve delivery (Figure 3-18c). Because most of these medications are intended to be self-administered, it is important that a nurse assist the patient in learning how to use the device properly to maximize the benefits the patient gets from the medication (Melani, 2007).

It is also important that the inhaler be kept clean. Buildup of debris can clog the inhaler's exit hole, preventing medication from being released and potentially reducing the dose of medication the patient receives. When working with a patient who uses an inhaler, particularly if the inhaler is not used frequently, examine the hole where the medicine comes out of the inhaler. If any powder or debris is noted in or around the opening, the inhaler should be cleaned. To do so, remove the canister from the L-shaped plastic mouthpiece. Rinse the cap and the plastic mouthpiece in warm water. Let the components air-dry thoroughly (overnight if necessary). When the mouthpiece is completely dry, put the canister back inside the mouthpiece and replace the cap. Do not rinse the other parts. The unit *may* need to be primed again (see following paragraphs) to restore proper function.

Delivering Medication with an Inhaler

Assemble the necessary components, including the medication, the inhaler, and the spacer (if used), and perform the standard checks to ensure the medication, dose, and patient are correct. Take off the cap and shake

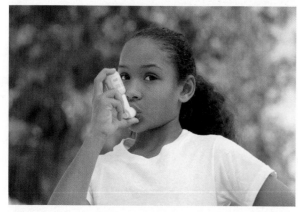

FIGURE 3-17 Use of a metered-dose inhaler (MDI) or dry-powder inhaler (DPI).

© bikeriderlondon/Shutterstock.

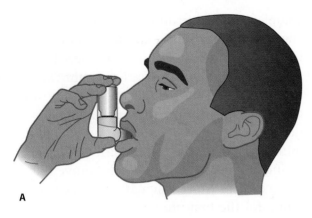

A

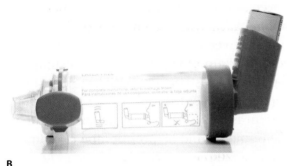

B

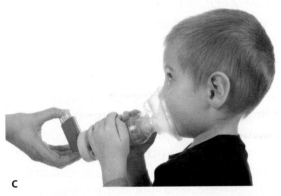

C

FIGURE 3-18 (A) Proper use of metered-dose inhaler (MDI).
(B) Inhaler spacer. (C) Use of a spacer to assist with proper inhaler use.
© Rob Byron/Shutterstock.
© LSOphoto/iStockphoto

insert the inhaler into the round end of the spacer and put the spacer's flat mouthpiece completely inside his or her mouth (it should not simply be pressed against the lips). If the spacer has a mask, fit the mask over the nose and mouth.

Instruct the patient to breathe in slowly through the mouth while pressing down on the inhaler once (**FIGURE 3-19**). If a spacer is being used, press down on the inhaler unit before inhaling slowly. Instruct the patient to begin to breathe in slowly through the spacer within five seconds of inhaler actuation. Remind the patient to keep breathing in slowly and as deeply as he or she can.

With or without a spacer, after inhalation, instruct the patient to hold his or her breath while counting to 10 slowly, if the patient is able to hold the breath that long. If the patient is unable to hold his or her breath for 10 seconds, the patient should be instructed to hold the breath for as long as possible, albeit less than 10 seconds. Inform the patient that holding his or her breath for as long as possible allows the medicine to better penetrate into the lungs.

the inhaler hard. If the patient has not used the inhaler before or has not used it in a while, the device may need to be primed to prepare it for administration of the aerosolized spray (**FIGURE 3-18**). (The patient will need to look at the instructions that came with the inhaler to learn how to do this properly.)

Instruct the patient to breathe out or exhale completely. Next, instruct the patient to hold the inhaler about one inch in front of his or her mouth (about the width of two fingers away). If using a spacer, the patient should

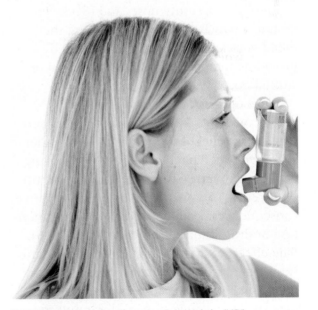

FIGURE 3-19 Actuation of a metered-dose inhaler (MDI).
© Stockbyte/Thinkstock.

If the patient is using inhaled *rescue* medicine (beta-agonists), wait at least five minutes before taking the next puff of the medication. Subsequent inhalations or "puffs" should be spaced one to five minutes apart and not exceed the prescribed dose. Remind patients that they should wait at least five minutes between inhalations or "puffs" of other medicines.

Finally, after they have finished using their inhaler, patients should rinse their mouths with water, gargle, and spit, especially if the medicine contains a steroid. This will help reduce unwanted side effects.

The procedure for DPI administration is the same as for MDIs, except that DPIs do not employ a spacer as an option for administration.

Proper Procedure for Administering a Nasal Spray

Nasal sprays are generally used for conditions affecting the nose or sinuses, such as congestion related to colds or allergies. The medications are usually one of three types: (1) steroids, which work by decreasing inflammation within the nasal passages; (2) anticholinergics, which work by decreasing secretions from the glands lining the nasal passages, thereby diminishing the symptoms of a runny nose; and (3) decongestants, which work by constricting the blood vessels in the nasal lining, thereby providing temporary relief for a clogged or stuffed nose (Wade, 2016).

Decongestant nasal sprays are available as over-the-counter products. They provide quick relief of symptoms, but the relief is limited, often having the result of causing patients to overuse them in search of continuous relief. This overuse usually has negative consequences, leading to rhinitis medicamentosa or drug-induced rhinitis (Wade, 2016). Side effects of overuse of nasal decongestant sprays can include increased risk for sinus infections, headaches, coughing, nasal passage swelling, congestion, and, rarely, septal perforation (Wade, 2016). A patient who complains of congestion should be questioned about over-the-counter decongestant use before a prescription nasal spray is offered.

As with inhalers, there is a "right way" and a "wrong way" to use a nasal spray, and patients who will be using such a medication at home should be taught how to administer it correctly. Instruct the patient to shake the bottle gently and remove the dust cover or cap. If the patient is using the pump for the first time or has not used it for a week or more, he or she must prime the pump by holding the pump with the applicator between the forefinger and middle finger and the bottom of the bottle resting on the thumb. Instruct the patient to point the applicator away from his or her face. If the patient is using the pump for the first time, the pump should be pressed down and released six times to prime it. If the patient has used the pump before, but not within the past week, the pump should be pressed down and released until he or she sees a fine spray (FIGURE 3-20A). Next, instruct the patient to blow his or her nose until the nostrils are clear (FIGURE 3-20B). Have the patient hold one nostril closed with his or her finger; next, tilt the head slightly forward and carefully put the nasal applicator into the other nostril, being sure to keep the bottle upright. The patient should hold the pump with the applicator between his or her forefinger and middle finger, with the bottom resting on the thumb. The patient should be instructed to begin to breathe in through the nose. While breathing in, the patient should use the forefinger and middle finger to press firmly down on the applicator and release the spray (FIGURE 3-20C). Instruct the patient to breathe gently in through the nostril and breathe out through the mouth. If the patient's healthcare provider told him or her to use two sprays, the same process should be repeated using the same nostril, with the patient then switching sides to the other nostril. Finally, wipe the applicator with a clean tissue and cover it with the dust cover or cap.

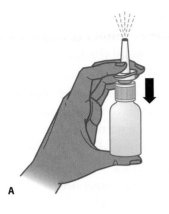

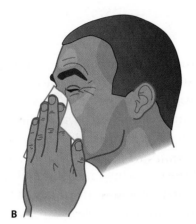

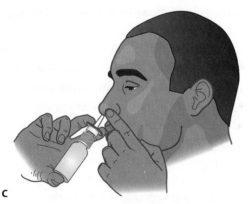

FIGURE 3-20 Procedure for nasal spray administration. (A) Priming. (B) Clearing nostrils. (C) Administration.

Using a Nebulizer

A nebulizer delivers medication by producing a mist that is inhaled by the patient. This method of delivery is preferred for patients who lack the ability to exert conscious control over their inhalation and exhalation. Examples of these types of patients include young children, older adults with chronic conditions

that affect their lung function and voluntary muscle control, and those patients who are cognitively impaired (Dhand et al., 2012)—or for a few medications for which hand-held inhalers are not appropriate or available for delivery of the required drug. When used correctly, nebulizers are just as effective as MDI/DPI devices, and in some patients they may be more effective, as the use of a nebulizer mask or mouthpiece reduces the likelihood of underdosing due to the errors in delivery technique often seen with inhalers. If a nebulizer is to be used in the home setting, the patient or the patient's caretaker must be given instruction on its proper use.

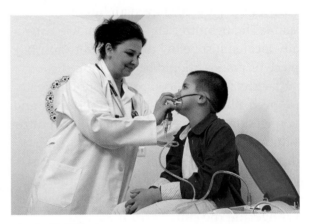

© LeventKonuk/iStock/Thinkstock.

Preparing for Nebulizer Therapy

The nebulizer device usually consists of a compressor machine attached with tubing to a mouthpiece or mask (**FIGURE 3-21**). A mouthpiece is inserted into the patient's mouth between the teeth such that the lips surround the mouthpiece and form a seal. A mask is fitted over the mouth and nose and is often secured with an elastic strap (if no strap is present, it must be held securely, but not tightly, to the face).

To use the nebulizer, the compressor should be placed on a table or solid surface next to the chair or bed where the patient will sit or lie; the compressor's on-off switch should be within easy reach of the patient if the medication is self-dispensed. The tubing

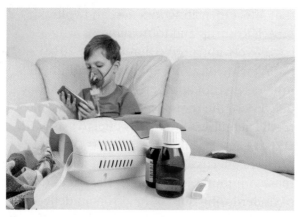

FIGURE 3-21 Nebulizer.
© Gerain0812/Shutterstock

should be free of tangling or kinks, and sufficiently long that the mask or mouthpiece reaches the patient's face with length to spare. The nebulizer cup—a receptacle usually located just below the nebulizer mouthpiece or mask—should be placed on the surface as well. The compressor should be properly plugged into an electrical outlet, and verification should be made that the nebulizer is functioning properly; a clean measuring dropper or syringe should be readily accessible. The patient or care provider should wash and dry his or her hands before handling the syringe and the cup.

Using the Nebulizer

Remove the top of the nebulizer cup. The dose of medicine to be placed in the cup should be confirmed and measured into a syringe or dropper, then dispensed into the bottom of the cup. It is best to place the tip of the measuring device into the cup, rather than letting the medication drip down from above the cup, to avoid spillage. Replace the top of the nebulizer cup, attach the cup to the mouthpiece or mask, and make sure that the tubing is connected to both the cup and the compressor. Switch the compressor on; the mist should be visible through the tubing at the compressor end. If the patient is sitting, he or she should sit up straight, breathing slowly and deeply through the mouth. If possible, the patient should hold his or her breath for 2 or 3 seconds before exhaling, to improve the

penetration of the medication into the airways. Continue the treatment for 7 to 10 minutes to ensure that all of the medication is delivered. When the treatment time is finished, the mouthpiece/mask should be removed and the patient instructed to take several deep breaths and cough into a tissue to remove any secretions. The compressor may be turned off and the tissue discarded. Remember to properly clean the nebulizer after use.

Medication Transfer Across Permeable Tissues

While injected medications are inserted *into* tissues, other delivery forms place the medication *onto or against* a tissue. These methods take advantage of tissue permeability to transfer medication into the body. They can be classified broadly into two groups: **transdermal** methods, in which medication is spread or placed upon the skin and allowed to enter and/or cross the skin barrier, and **transmucosal** delivery systems, which introduce medication into areas of mucous membranes so that the medication can pass through the membrane into the bloodstream. *Transdermal* delivery systems include medicated patches and topical creams, gels, ointments, and lotions. *Transmucosal* delivery makes use of sublingual (under the tongue), buccal (between cheek and gums), vaginal, and anal mucosa, as appropriate.

Administering a Transdermal Patch

Use of transdermal patches has become increasingly common in recent years. Most people have become aware of this delivery option through widely marketed nicotine-replacement patches used to aid in smoking cessation, but other medications (e.g., pain medications or hormone therapies) are now being provided in this manner, due to its convenience, the different timing of drug activity (Prausnitz & Langer, 2008), and, in some instances, the ability to bypass the liver's detoxification channels, which can cause oral or injected medications to be eliminated before

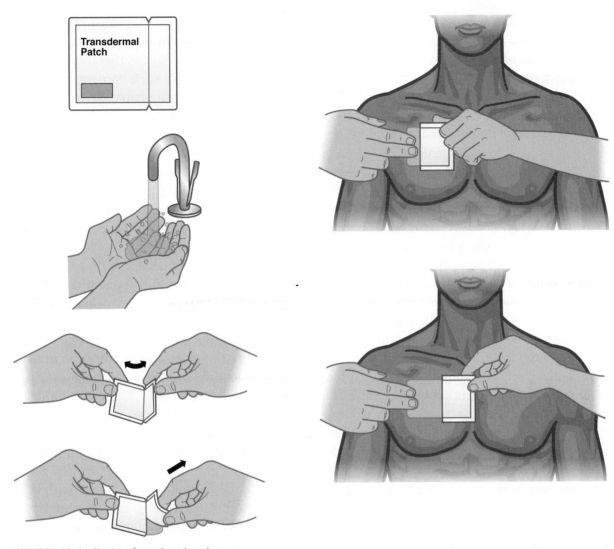

FIGURE 3-22 Application of transdermal patches.

they reach their destinations (Morrow, 2004), as discussed in Chapter 2.

To properly apply a transdermal patch, the patient or nurse should wash his or her hands thoroughly with soap and water for at least 20 seconds (FIGURE 3-22A). Nurses should don appropriate gloves for their protection from absorbed medication. Each patch is individually sealed in a protective package. Open the package at the tear mark if there is one present, or cut the package with scissors if not, taking care not to cut the patch inside. Carefully remove the patch. The patch is attached to a pre-labeled adhesive liner (FIGURE 3-22B). The liner has a slit that divides the backing into two strips. Hold the patch with the adhesive pointed away. For easier application of the

patch, the slit should never be facing toward the patient, to ensure that it will not stick to other areas of the body. Rotate the patch as necessary to place the slit in a vertical position. Bend both sides of the adhesive liner away at the slit (FIGURE 3-22C) and slowly peel off only one of the strips of the liner. Do not touch the exposed sticky side of the patch. Use the remaining strip as a "handle" to apply the sticky side of the patch to the skin (FIGURE 3-22D). Press the sticky side on the chosen skin site and smooth it down. Fold back the unattached side of the patch. Grasp the remaining strip and remove it while applying the remainder of the patch to the skin (FIGURE 3-22E). Press the patch on the skin and smooth it down with the palm of a hand. Once the patch is in place, *do not* test the adhesion by pulling on it. After applying the patch, instruct the patient to wash his or her hands to remove any drug. At the time recommended by the prescribing provider, and verified via a literature check, remove and discard the old patch. Place a new patch on a different skin site according to the healthcare provider's instructions.

The patch should be applied to clean, dry, hairless skin. If hair is likely to interfere with the adhesion of the patch, the hair can be clipped or shaved, being careful not to break the skin. Do not apply a transdermal patch to any areas with broken or irritated skin, or immediately after bathing or showering, so the patch will be able to properly adhere to the skin. It is best to wait until the skin is completely dry. It is important to rotate the sites used for patch application so that the medication can properly absorb into the skin, and to prevent irritation or breakdown of the skin.

Consult the manufacturer's prescribing information to determine if the medication patch can be cut. Certain topical medication patches cannot be cut because doing so will alter the absorption of the medication. Also, with some medications—particularly hormonal therapies such as testosterone—great care should be taken to avoid the medication coming in contact with the skin of individuals other than the patient. For example, one precaution that patients or caregivers applying any transdermal medication should take when washing after application is to place a tissue in their hand before opening doors or turning on a faucet, so that any medication on the hands prior to washing is not transferred to the door or faucet handle.

Applying Topical Preparations

Topical preparations include ointments, creams, gels, and lotions that are applied to the skin, usually on or above an area affected by an injury, an allergic response, or an infection. Most people have had experience using some form of topical preparation,

even if it is merely a soothing aloe gel to treat a sunburn, or lotion for dry skin. What they may not realize, however, is that the majority of people do not apply such preparations properly. For example, most people fail to wash their hands first unless they are visibly dirty, and often (unless an open wound is involved) they will not wash or dry the skin to which the medication is applied. Yet doing so is the key first step to ensuring that the medication is applied in such a way as to maximize its effects while minimizing possible contamination.

In the correct approach to applying a topical preparation, the person who is applying the medicine (be it nurse or patient) must wash his or her hands with soap and water for at least 20 seconds. It is *especially* important that handwashing precede application in cases where the medication is intended to treat wounded, abraded, inflamed, or healing skin, to reduce the possibility of microbial contamination. Gloves should be worn by nurses applying medications on patients. The skin itself should also be washed and patted (not rubbed) dry—again, a particularly important step when the skin *is* the treatment target. Be sure that the skin in the affected area is completely dry before applying any topical preparation.

Apply a thin layer or film of medication to the entire area of the skin that is affected, using either a gloved finger or cotton-tipped applicator. Rub the medication into the skin completely and gently, unless otherwise indicated by the manufacturer's directions. After the topical medication has been applied, wash the hands with soap and water to remove any remaining medication. Treated areas may be covered with normal clothing, but bandages, dressings, or wraps should not be placed over the area unless indicated by the prescribing healthcare provider. Remind the patient to be careful not to wash or wipe off medication from the affected areas of the skin to prevent loss of the medication. Instruct the patient not to swim, bathe, or shower immediately after applying medication because these activities will prevent the medication from properly absorbing into the skin.

Best Practices

To avoid accidentally transferring topical medications to other people, put a tissue in your hand when turning the faucet on to wash up after application. Always wear gloves to avoid inadvertent medication absorption.

As with transdermal patches, it is important to prevent cross-contamination of other people by ensuring that topical medication is not spilled or wiped on surfaces, clothing, towels, and so forth that might be touched by someone else. The nurse or patient applying the topical medication should use only disposable cloths or tissues to wipe medication off hands, and should put a tissue in the hand to grasp door handles or faucet fixtures if he or she must touch them before washing up.

Vaginal Rings

Vaginal rings are a form of transmembrane delivery that is generally utilized to provide hormonal medications, specifically sex steroids. These devices are used for delivery of contraceptives and of hormones for relief of menopausal symptoms. They are flexible rings that are inserted into the vagina and left in place for up to three weeks of continuous contraception, or up to three months of continuous hormone therapy to replace loss of estrogen during menopause. Vaginal estrogen is used to treat vaginal dryness, itching and burning, painful or difficult urination, and incontinence in perimenopausal or postmenopausal women (NIH, 2010a). It is also used to treat "hot flashes" in women who are experiencing menopause (NIH, 2010b).

Administering Vaginal Rings

After performing the Eight Rights checks, the nurse should wash his or her hands for at least 20 seconds and dry them thoroughly. Remove the vaginal ring from the pouch and save the foil wrapper to properly dispose of the previously used hormonal ring after it is removed. Ask the patient to either lie down on her back with her knees bent or have her squat or stand with one leg up on a chair, step, toilet, or other elevated object; it is best to allow the patient to choose the position that is most comfortable for her so that the nurse can insert the vaginal ring. The nurse should hold the ring between his or her thumb and index finger and press the opposite sides of the ring together to form a figure-eight shape (FIGURE 3-23).

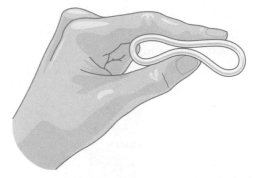

FIGURE 3-23 Hold the vaginal ring between thumb and index finger, pressing the opposite sides of the ring together to form a figure-eight shape.

The nurse can either hold open the labial folds of the patient's vagina or have the patient hold open her own folds of skin around her vagina with her hand. Place one side of the figure-eight tip of the ring into her vagina and then use an index finger to gently insert the ring into her vagina.

The vaginal ring does not need to be positioned a certain way inside the patient's vagina but it will be more comfortable and less likely to fall out if it is placed as far back in the vagina as possible (FIGURE 3-24). Inform the patient that the ring cannot go past her cervix so it will not "go too far" in her vagina or "get lost" when it is inserted. If she feels discomfort when the ring is inserted, the nurse should use his or her index finger to insert it farther back into the woman's vagina. The nurse should inform the patient that the ring may fall out if it is not inserted deeply into the vagina, if the vaginal muscles are weak, or if the woman is straining during a bowel movement. If the ring falls out, it should be washed with warm water and reinserted into the vagina following the steps outlined previously. If the ring falls out and is lost, insert a new ring and leave the new ring in place for the manufacturer's intended duration. If it falls out often, the patient should consult her healthcare provider.

The nurse should remind the patient that the vaginal ring can be left in place during sexual intercourse. If the patient chooses to remove it, or if it falls out, the ring should be washed with warm water and replaced in the vagina as soon as possible.

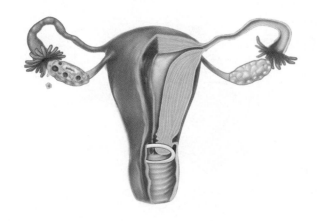

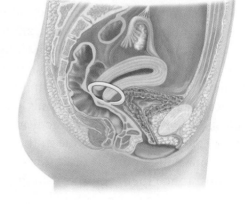

FIGURE 3-24 Proper location for vaginal ring placement.

When it is time to remove the ring from the patient's vagina, instruct the patient to find a position that is most comfortable for her. The nurse should hook his or her index finger under the front rim of the ring or hold the rim between the index and middle fingers to then pull it out from its resting location. The nurse should gently pull downward and forward to remove the ring from the patient's vagina. The used ring should be discarded in a sealed trash can out of reach of children and pets. Do not flush the used ring down the toilet. Finally, insert a new ring into the patient's vagina as directed according to the prescribing provider's instructions (NIH, 2010a, 2010b).

Administering Rectal Suppositories

To administer a rectal suppository, after performing the Eight Rights checks, the nurse should wash his or her hands thoroughly with soap and water for at least 20 seconds and dry them completely. If the suppository is soft, hold it under cool water or place it in the refrigerator for a few minutes to harden it before removing the wrapper. Remove any wrapper that is present. If half of the suppository is indicated for use, cut the suppository lengthwise with a clean, single-edged razor blade. Consult the manufacturer's directions about suppositories that can be safely cut in half without affecting the efficacy of the drug. The nurse should put on disposable gloves to administer the suppository.

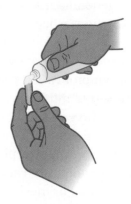

FIGURE 3-25 Lubrication of rectal suppository prior to administration.

Lubricate the suppository tip with an appropriate lubricant (**FIGURE 3-25**). The use of an improper lubricant (such as an aqueous-based lubricant used with a water-soluble suppository base) may compromise the integrity of the delivery system. The manufacturer's literature for individual suppositories should be consulted for advice regarding suggested appropriate lubricants. If there is no lubricant available, the nurse should moisten the patient's rectal area with cool tap water. The nurse should instruct the patient to lie on his or her side with the lower leg straightened out and the upper leg bent forward at the knee toward the stomach (**FIGURE 3-26**).

Lift the upper buttock to expose the rectal area and insert the suppository with the finger, pointed end first, until it passes the muscular sphincter of the rectum, about a half to one inch in infants, and one inch in adults

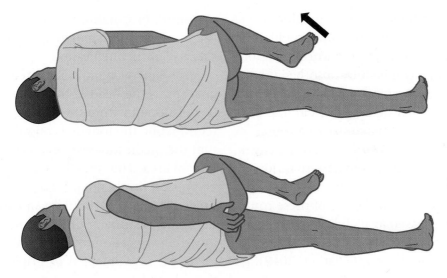

FIGURE 3-26 Proper positioning of the patient for rectal suppository administration.

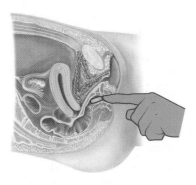

FIGURE 3-27 Proper positioning of a rectal suppository.

(FIGURE 3-27). (If the suppository is not inserted past the sphincter, the suppository may not remain in place.) Have the patient hold his or her buttocks together for a few seconds and remain lying down for five minutes to avoid dislodging the suppository (FIGURE 3-28).

The nurse should discard any used materials such as gloves and wrappers, and wash his or her hands thoroughly.

Buccal and Sublingual Administration

The membranes of the mouth offer certain advantages for administering medications. Key among them is the speed with which such medications are transferred into the bloodstream. The permeability of the oral membranes is considerably greater than that of the skin, although the extent of this permeability depends on where in the mouth the medication is placed, as membrane thickness varies in different parts of the mouth. **Sublingual** (below the tongue) placement results in very rapid absorption due to the thinness of the membranes in this location, which is why rescue medications such as

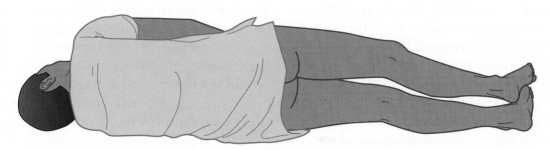

FIGURE 3-28 Temporary patient positioning after rectal suppository administration.

nitroglycerin for angina relief, and glucose gel for hypoglycemia in diabetes, are provided for sublingual use. This approach works well for medications that can be fully absorbed if held in place for a short time, but not quite as well for medications that need to be held in place over a longer time to maximize absorption. In the latter case, **buccal** (between the cheek and gum) placement is used despite its lower absorption rate.

Recent advances in the use of these routes have led to increased availability of drugs delivered by buccal and sublingual systems (Senel, Rathbone, Cansiz, & Pather, 2012). A variety of medications is currently available, including fast-dissolving tablets, films/strips, or sprays. Some are available in this form as over-the-counter products.

Aside from the rapidity of absorption, an advantage of sublingual and buccal delivery is that this route bypasses the digestive tract and the liver, delivering the drug directly into the bloodstream. This can allow for lower quantities of drug to be highly effective (Lam, Xu, Worsley, & Wong, 2014), resulting in fewer side effects (Narang & Sharma, 2011) (refer to Chapter 2). A disadvantage of this delivery system is that it cannot be used in unconscious or combative patients.

Administering a Sublingual or Buccal Medication

Sublingual Medications

Patients should be advised to refrain from smoking for an hour prior to use of the medication, as smoking causes vasoconstriction that will impede sublingual absorption. Likewise, the patient should be advised to neither eat nor drink while taking the medication to avoid swallowing it, which may reduce or obviate its absorption as well. The patient should remain seated and upright while the medication is in place, to avoid accidental swallowing or aspiration of the medication. After performing the Eight Rights checks and prior to administration, the patient should be asked about or inspected for sores, cuts, abrasions, or irritation to the oral mucosa, as the presence of such damage may contraindicate use of the medication.

If the medication is delivered via sublingual spray, the head of the spray bottle should be positioned within the mouth, behind the teeth, while the tongue is raised to ensure that the medication is delivered into the sublingual area. The spray bottle's button should be pressed firmly the prescribed number of times. The patient should wait about 10 minutes before eating or drinking anything to allow the medication to be fully absorbed.

In the case of tablets or strips, the patient should rinse his or her mouth with water prior to placing a tablet or strip under the tongue. The tongue is then raised and the strip or tablet placed underneath it; the tongue may be lowered once the medication is in place, and if possible the patient should tilt his or her head forward to reduce the chance of swallowing it. The patient should avoid standing, moving, talking, opening the mouth, eating, or drinking for at least 10 minutes to ensure the medication is fully absorbed and to minimize the chance of swallowing or dislodging the tablet or strip. Some medications may cause a tingling sensation while in place, but they should not be moved to another location unless strictly necessary for the patient's comfort. (This sensation *may* also be an indication the medication is working correctly.) Most of the time, patients can place tablets or strips into their own mouths without difficulty, but for those patients who cannot, the nurse should be certain to take standard precautions (gloves) prior to placing the medication.

Buccal Medications

The procedure for administering buccal medications is similar to that of sublingual medications, except that the tablet or strip is placed between the cheek and gum line as far back toward the back molars as possible. After the medication is in place, the mouth should be kept closed for up to 10 minutes to allow for complete absorption.

Medication Errors

Earlier in this chapter, the need to avoid medication errors was discussed briefly. That discussion is expanded upon here to emphasize the magnitude and gravity of this problem. It is important for nurses, as the people most commonly charged with delivering medications to patients, to have a strong awareness of the root causes of medication errors, and to understand the steps and systems that can be put in place to reduce their incidence.

Administering medication is where the "rubber meets the road" in medical therapy—it is not only the point at which the therapeutic decisions are put into action, but is also the last point at which errors in the preceding decision-making process (prescribing and dispensing) can be identified prior to causing harm. Nurses should strive to avoid medication errors in their daily practice; thus, not only must they know how to administer medications properly but also they must be alert enough to identify errors made in previous therapeutic stages.

What are Medication Administration Errors?

A **medication error** is defined as follows:

> ...any preventable event that may cause or lead to inappropriate medication use or patient harm while the medication is in the control of the health care professional, patient or consumer. Such events may be related to professional practice, health care products, procedures and systems, including prescribing, order communication, product labeling, packaging, and nomenclature, compounding dispensing, distribution, administration, education, monitoring, and use. (National Coordinating Council for Medication Error Reporting and Prevention, 2018)

Note that a medication error can occur at any point in the pathway from prescription onward. Indeed, many such errors have been found to occur at the point at which the prescription is actually *written*—which means that the nurse's checks are a key means of restoring accuracy to the treatment process. In this context, however, the concern centers on errors in *administration* of medication—that is, the ways in which implementation of the therapeutic plan can go wrong.

The definition given by physicians in the literature for a **medication administration error** is a deviation from the physician's medication order as written on the patient's chart (Headford, McGowan, & Clifford, 2001; Mark & Burleson, 1995). Interestingly, this definition of medication administration errors fails to consider that prescribing errors contribute to medication administration errors (Davydov, Caliendo, Mehl, & Smith, 2004; Headford et al., 2001; Wilson et al., 1998). A nurse who administers 10 mg of a drug to a patient in accordance with the physician's written instructions is, by this definition, not in error, even if the correct dosage for this patient should have been written as 10 mcg. Yet, an error has indeed been committed—a fairly serious one that, depending on the drug and whether the error is caught in time, could be life-threatening! The definition of "medication administration errors" that nurses use, and that is cited most often in the literature for nurses, is "mistakes associated with drugs and intravenous solutions that are made during the prescription, transcription, dispensing and administration phases of drug preparation and distribution" (Wolf, 1989, p. 8).

Wolf classifies the errors as either acts of commission or omission, either of which can now also include violations of the Eight Rights: administering the medication to the wrong patient; administering the patient the wrong drug; administering the patient the correct drug but at the wrong dose, via the wrong route, or with the wrong timing of drug administration; administering a contraindicated drug to the patient; injecting the drug at the wrong site; using the wrong drug form or the wrong infusion rate; using medication beyond its expiration date; or prescribing the wrong medication. Wolf (1989) further notes that errors can be classified as either occurring intentionally or unintentionally.

Medication administration errors are not always due to a mistake by the nurse, but the nurse may nonetheless help prevent them. A situation with high potential for error occurs when patients (or caretakers) are charged with administering their own (or someone in their care) medication but are given inadequate information for performing this task—or, having been given appropriate information, nonetheless fail to understand key points of how or when the medication is to be administered. At minimum, a nurse needs to ensure that the patient or caregiver knows each of the following pieces of information: the *name* of each medication that the patient is taking; *why* the patient is taking it; *how often or when* to take it; what the drug *looks* like; the appropriate *means of delivery* (e.g., ensure that medications designed to be delivered via buccal or sublingual delivery are not swallowed); the *dosage*; potential *adverse effects and interactions*; and *symptoms* to watch for (Anderson & Townsend, 2010).

Patients or caregivers who are under the significant stress of coping with an acute illness or injury may not fully grasp instructions given to them in a hospital setting. Thus, for patients being discharged following an acute illness or medical emergency, providing clear written instructions, in conjunction with a follow-up call by the nurse within the first few days after discharge, is very important to ensure that there is complete understanding of how to use medications.

Causes and Prevention of Medication Errors

Factors that contribute to medication errors can be divided into two subcategories: errors caused by the *system* (Keers, Williams, Cook, & Ashcroft, 2013) and errors caused by *individual healthcare professionals* (Kim & Bates, 2012; McBride-Henry & Foureur, 2006). Earlier, we noted some of the causal

factors for individual errors—fatigue, stress, multitasking, and interruption. In addition, medication administration errors can occur because of flaws in the institution's system and procedures, or the provider's equipment, procedures, operators, supplies, or environments (Anderson & Webster, 2001), and can occur anywhere in the system. Moreover, errors can occur because of the interface between the nurse and the system in which he or she works. For example, a nurse who undergoes inadequate training regarding the facility's procedures may learn what is taught, and may even recognize that the training is insufficient; if he or she has no opportunities to request or receive additional training, however, there is a systemic issue that affects individual performance.

Additionally, prescribing, preparing, and administering medications rely on numerous processes intended to ensure that the patient receives appropriate treatment, and problems can arise in any part of this system as well (McBride-Henry & Foureur, 2006). Finally, acuity levels or seriousness of illness, available nursing staff, access to medication, and policy documentation can affect medication administration error rates (McBride-Henry & Foureur, 2006).

Error avoidance must, therefore, be a priority not only for the individual nurse, but also for the facility for which the nurse works. Standardized procedures should be established and followed as a matter of daily routine, particularly in high-risk medication delivery systems such as intravenous medications. Tools such as procedural checklists can be valuable assets to assist in limiting errors, but only if the individual nurse commits to using them, and the facility culture promotes and reinforces their use. Communication among the various individuals working with a specific patient is a key component, yet systemic barriers to communication remain all too common. Such barriers may include lack of clear-cut processes, inadequate staffing (or the less-common problem of overstaffing, which means too many people are working on the same problem, thereby impairing communication and efficiency), poor staff training, cluttered or disorganized workspaces, inadequate lighting, or even something as simple as a failure to provide adequate office supplies such as pens, computers, printers, and so forth.

Conclusion: Medication Administration in Nursing Practice

Nurses are continually challenged to ensure that their patients are given the correct medication at the correct time. Obstacles such as inadequate nursing education about patient safety, excessive workloads, untrained staff, fatigue, illegible provider handwriting, flawed dispensing systems, and problems with the labeling of drugs are encountered by nurses on a daily basis. Moreover, harm from medications can arise from unintended sequelae, as well as from errors such as administering the wrong medication or administering the medication at the wrong time, at the wrong dose, via the wrong route, or to the wrong patient (Hughes & Blegen, 2008). Thus, nurses' understanding of pharmacology includes knowledge of not only how medications are administered, but also which factors can contribute to faulty administration of medications.

CHAPTER SUMMARY

- Medications are an essential therapeutic intervention, yet there are multiple challenges to administering them correctly.
- The Eight Rights of Medication Administration offer nurses a checklist for ensuring that the chance of errors is reduced.
- Medication delivery comes in a variety of forms, each with its unique administration procedures, challenges, advantages, and disadvantages.
- Understanding when and why a given delivery route is preferred for a specific drug is as important as knowing how to correctly administer the drug.
- Medication errors are not solely a matter of individuals making mistakes, however; nurses must also understand the potential for systemic problems that promote medication errors.

Critical Thinking Questions

1. What are the Eight Rights of Medication Administration? How can these be applied for patients who are noncommunicative, for any reason?

2. Why should nurses know the rationale for a prescription even if they are not the ones prescribing the medication?

3. Name the three basic ways medication can be transferred into the body's tissues/bloodstream, and provide two specific examples of delivery methods for each of the three forms of transfer.

4. Which modes of delivery may be used in an unconscious patient and which may not? If a route of administration is considered inappropriate for an unconscious patient, how can the nurse determine an alternative route to recommend to the prescriber?

5. The causes of medication errors occur at both an individual level and a systemic level. What is an example of a factor leading to an *individual* error? Which factors can be considered *systemic* factors leading to medication errors?

6. Which form of medication delivery has the highest error rate? At what point in the administration process do most of the errors occur and why?

SUGGESTED READINGS

American Society of Health-System Pharmacist. (n.d.). *How to use rectal suppositories properly*. Retrieved from http://www.safemedication.com/safemed/MedicationTipsTools/HowtoAdminister/HowtoUseRectalSuppositoriesProperly.aspx

Barker, K., Flynn, E., & Pepper, G. (2002). Observation method of detecting medication errors. *American Journal of Health-System Pharmacy, 59*, 2314–2316.

Barker, K., Flynn, E., Pepper, G., Bates, D., & Mikel, R. (2002). Medication errors observed in 36 health care facilities. *Archives of Internal Medicine, 162*(16), 1897–1904.

Bergogne-Bérézin, E., & Bryskie, A. (1999). The suppository form of antibiotic administration: Pharmacokinetics and clinical application. *Journal of Antimicrobial Chemotherapy, 43*(2), 177–185.

Bonsall, L. (2011). *8 rights of medication administration*. Retrieved from http://www.nursingcenter.com/Blog/post/2011/05/27/8-rights-of-medication-administration.aspx

Burstein, A.H., Fisher, K.M., McPherson, M.L., & Roby, C.A. (2000). Absorption of phenytoin from rectal suppositories formulated with a polyethylene glycol base. *Pharmacotherapy, 20*(5), 562–567.

DiPiro, J.T., Blouin, R.A., Pruemer, J.M., & Spruill, W.J. (1996). *Concepts in clinical pharmacokinetics* (2nd ed.). Bethesda, MD: American Society of Health-System Pharmacists.

Drugs.com. (2017). *How to give an intramuscular injection*. Retrieved from http://www.drugs.com/cg/how-to -give-an-intramuscular-injection.html

Flynn, E., Barker, K., Pepper, G., Bates, D., & Mikel, R. (2002). Comparison of methods for detecting medication errors in 36 hospitals and skilled-nursing facilities. *American Journal of Health-System Pharmacy, 59*, 436–446.

Institute of Medicine (IOM). (2007). *Preventing medication errors*. Washington, DC: National Academy Press.

Katzung, B.G. (1998). *Basic and clinical pharmacology* (7th ed.). Stamford, CT: Appleton & Lange.

MacDermott, B.L., & Deglin, J.H. (1994). *Understanding basic pharmacology: Practical approaches for effective application*. Philadelphia, PA: F. A. Davis.

Mylan Pharmaceuticals. (2006). *Nitroglycerin patch*. Retrieved from http://dailymed.nlm.nih.gov/dailymed /archives/fdaDrugInfo.cfm?archiveid=1448

National Institutes of Health (NIH)—Medline Plus. (2017). How to use a metered-dose inhaler. Retrieved from https://medlineplus.gov/ency/patient instructions/000042.htm.

Nursing and Midwifery Council. (2004). *Guidelines for the administration of medicines*. London, UK: Author.

Schneider, M., Cotting, J., & Pannatier, A. (1998). Evaluation nurses' errors associated with the preparation and administration of medications in a pediatric intensive care unit. *Pharmacy World Science, 20*(4), 178–182.

Stetina, P., Groves, M., & Pafford, L. (2005). Managing medication errors: A qualitative study. *Medsurg Nursing, 13*(3), 174–178.

Tissot, E., Cornette, C., Limat, S., Mourand, J., Becker, M., Etievent, J., … Woronoff-Lemsi, M. (2003). Observational study of potential risk factors of medication administration errors. *Pharmacy World Science, 25*(6), 264–268.

U.S. Department of Health and Human Services. (2007). *National Asthma Education and Prevention Program Expert Panel Report 3: Guidelines for the diagnosis and management of asthma*. Rockville, MD: National Heart, Lung and Blood Institute, U.S. Department of Health and Human Services.

Wakefield, D.S., Wakefield, B.J., Uden-Holman, T., & Blegen, M.A. (1996). Perceived barriers in reporting medication administration errors. *Best Practices and Benchmarking in Healthcare, 1*(4), 191–197.

WebMD. (2007). Steroid nasal sprays. Retrieved from http://www.webmd.com/allergies/guide/steroid _nasal_sprays

Wirtz, V., Taxis, K., & Barber, N. (2003). An observational study of intravenous medication errors in the United Kingdom and in Germany. *Pharmacy World Science, 25*(3), 104–111.

Wynne, A.L., Woo, T.M., & Millard, M. (2002). *Pharmacotherapeutics for nurse practitioner prescribers*. Philadelphia, PA: F. A. Davis.

REFERENCES

Albarrak, A.I., Al Rashidi, E.A., Fatani, R.K., Al Ageel, S.I., & Mohammed, R. (2014). Assessment of legibility and completeness of handwritten and electronic prescriptions. *Saudi Pharmaceutical Journal, 22*(6), 522–527.

Anderson, D., & Webster, C. (2001). A system approach to the reduction of medication error on the hospital ward. *Journal of Advanced Nursing, 35*(1), 34–41.

Anderson, P., & Townsend, T. (2010). Medication errors: Don't let them happen to you. *American Nurse Today, 5*(3), 23–27.

Beyea, S.C., & Nicoll, L.H. (1995). Administration of medications via the intramuscular route: An integrative review of the literature and research-based protocol for the procedure. *Applied Nursing Research, 8*(1), 22–33.

Brits, H., Botha, A., Niksch, L., Terblanché, R., Venter, K., & Joubert, G. (2017). Illegible handwriting and other prescription errors on prescriptions at National District Hospital, Bloemfontein. *South African Family Practice, 59*(1), 52–55. doi: 10.1080/20786190.2016.1254932

Carayon, P., & Wood, K.E. (2010). Patient safety: The role of human factors and systems engineering. *Studies in Health Technology and Informatics, 153*, 23–46.

Cerio, A.A.P., Mallare, N.A.L.B., & Tolentino, R.M.S. (2015). Assessment of the legibility of the handwriting in medical prescriptions of doctors from public and private hospitals in Quezon City, Philippines. *Procedia Manufacturing, 3*, 90–97.

Davydov, I., Caliendo, G., Mehl, B., & Smith, L. (2004). Investigation of correlation between house-staff work hours and prescribing errors. *American Journal of Health-System Pharmacy, 61*(1), 1130–1134.

Department of Health and Human Services, Office of Inspector General. (2010). *Adverse events in hospitals: National incidence among Medicare beneficiaries*. Retrieved from https://oig.hhs.gov/oei/reports/oei -06-09-00090.pdf

Dhand, R., Dolovich, M., Chipps, B., Myers, T.R., Restrepo, R., & Farrar, J.R. (2012). The role of nebulized therapy in the management of COPD: Evidence and recommendations. *COPD, 9*(1), 58–72.

Ferguson, A. (2005). Administration of oral medication. *Nursing Times, 101*(45), 24–25.

Headford, C., McGowan, S., & Clifford, R. (2001). Analysis of medication incidents and development of medication incident rate clinical indicator. *Collegian, 8*(3), 26–31.

Higgins, D. (2005). IM injection. *Nursing Times, 100*(45), 36–37.

Hughes, R.G., & Blegen, M.A. (Eds.). (2008). *Patient safety and quality: An evidence-based handbook for nurses*. Rockville, MD: Agency for Healthcare Research and Quality.

Institute for Safe Medicine Practices (ISMP). (2015). *ISMP safe practices guidelines for adult IV push medications*. Retrieved from http://www.ismp.org/Tools /guidelines/ivsummitpush/ivpushmedguidelines.pdf

Institute of Medicine (IOM). (1999). *To err is human: Building a safer health system*. Washington, DC: National Academy Press.

Keers, R.N., Williams, S D., Cook, J., & Ashcroft, D.M. (2013). Causes of medication administration errors in hospitals: A systematic review of quantitative and qualitative evidence. *Drug Safety, 36*(11), 1045–1067.

Kim, J. & Bates, D.W. (2012). Medication administration errors by nurses: Adherence to guidelines. *Journal of Clinical Nursing, 22*(3–4), 590–598.

Lam, J.K.W., Xu, Y., Worsley, A., & Wong, I.C.K. (2014). Oral transmucosal drug delivery for pediatric use. *Advanced Drug Reviews, 73*(30), 50–62.

Lehne, R.A. (2013). *Pharmacology for nursing care* (8th ed., pp. 33–34). St. Louis, MO: Elsevier Saunders.

Mark, B., & Burleson, D. (1995). Measurement of patient outcomes: Data availability and consistency across hospitals. *Journal of Nursing Administration, 25*(4), 52–59.

McBride-Henry, K., & Foureur, M. (2006). Medication administration errors: Understanding the issues. *Australian Journal of Advanced Nursing, 23*(3), 33–41.

Melani, A.S. (2007). Inhalatory therapy training: A priority challenge for physicians. *Acta Biomedica, 78*(3), 233–245.

Morris, H. (2005). Administering drugs to patients with swallowing difficulties. *Nursing Times, 101*(39), 28–29.

Morrow, T. (2004). Transdermal patches are more than skin deep. *Managed Care*. Retrieved from http://www.managedcaremag.com/archives/0404/0404.biotech.html

Narang, N., & Sharma, J. (2011). Sublingual mucosa as a route for systemic drug delivery. *International Journal of Pharmacy and Pharmaceutical Science, 3*(Suppl. 2), 18–22.

National Coordinating Council for Medication Error Reporting and Prevention. (2018). *What is a medication error?* Retrieved from http://www.nccmerp.org/about-medication-errors

National Institutes of Health (NIH). (2010a). *Estrogen vaginal*. Retrieved from http://www.nlm.nih.gov/medlineplus/druginfo/meds/a606005.html

National Institutes of Health (NIH). (2010b). *Ethinyl estradiol and ethonogestrel vaginal ring*. Retrieved from http://www.nlm.nih.gov/medlineplus/druginfo/meds/a604032.html

National Institutes of Health (NIH). (2012). *Patient education sheet: Giving a subcutaneous injection*. Retrieved from http://www.cc.nih.gov/ccc/patient_education/pepubs/subq.pdf

Nursing 2012 Drug Handbook. (2012). Philadelphia, PA: Lippincott Williams & Wilkins.

Poland, G.A., Borrd, A., Jacobson, R.M., McDermott, K., Wollan, P.C., Brakke, D., Charboneau, J.W. (1997). Determination of deltoid fat pad thickness: Implications for needle length in adult immunization. *JAMA, 277*(21), 1709–1711.

Prakash, V., Koczmara, C., Savage, P., Trip, K., Steward, J., McCurdie, T., … Trbovich, P. (2014). Mitigating errors caused by interruptions during medication verification and administration: interventions in a simulated ambulatory chemotherapy setting. *BMJ Quality & Safety, 23*, 884–892.

Prausnitz, M. R., & Langer, R. (2008). Transdermal drug delivery. *Nature Biotechnology, 26*, 1261–1268.

Probst, C.A., Wolf, L., Bollini, M., & Xiao, Y. (2016). Human factors engineering approaches to patient identification armband design. *Applied Ergonomics, 52*, 1–7.

Reason, J. (2000). Human error: Models and management. *British Medical Journal, 320*(7237), 768–770. Retrieved from http://www.ncbi.nlm.nih.gov/pmc/articles/PMC1117770/

San Diego Patient Safety Consortium. (2009). *Safe administration of high-risk IV medications. Intra- and inter-hospital standardization: Drug concentrations and dosage units* (Rev. ed.). Retrieved from https://www.hqinstitute.org/sites/main/files/file-attachments/sdpsc_safe_administration_of_high-risk_iv_medication.pdf

Sandler, S.G., Langeberg, A., Carty, K., & Dohnalek, L.J. (2006). Barcode and radio-frequency technologies can increase safety and efficiency of blood transfusions. *Laboratory Medicine, 3*(7), 436–439.

Senel, S., Rathbone, M.J., Cansız, M., & Pather, I. (2012). Recent developments in buccal and sublingual delivery systems. *Expert Opinion on Drug Delivery, 9*(6), 615–628.

Singer, S.J. & Vogus, T.J. (2013). Reducing hospital errors: Interventions that build safety culture. *Annual Review of Public Health, 34*(1), 373–396.

Southwick, F. (2012). *Six factors that lead to human error*. Retrieved from https://www.fiercehealthcare.com/hospitals/6-factors-lead-to-human-error

Starmer, A.J., Spector, N.D., Srivastava, R., West, D.C., Rosenbluth, G., Allen, A.D., … Landrigan, C.P., for the I-PASS Study Group. (2014). Changes in medical errors after implementation of a handoff program. *New England Journal of Medicine, 371*, 1803–1812. doi: 10.1056/NEJMsa1405556

Strudwick, G., Clark, C., McBride, B., Sakal, M., & Kalia, K. (2017). Thank you for asking: Exploring patient perceptions of barcode medication administration identification practices in inpatient mental health settings. *International Journal of Medical Informatics, 105*, 31–37.

Taddio, A., Shah, V., McMurtry, C.M., MacDonald, N.E., Ipp, M., Riddell, R.P., … Chambers, C. T. (2015). Procedural and physical interventions for vaccine injections: Systematic review of randomized controlled trials and quasi-randomized controlled trials. *The Clinical Journal of Pain, 31*(Suppl. 10), S20–S37. doi: 10.1097/AJP.0000000000000264

Wade, M. Reviewed by Ratini, M. (2016). *Can you overuse nasal spray?* Retrieved from http://www.webmd.com/allergies/features/nasal-spray-are-you-overdoing-it

Walker, E.E. (2016). Medication errors. *Imperial Journal of Interdisciplinary Research, 2*(5). Retrieved from http://www.imperialjournals.com/index.php/IJIR/article/view/439

Wilson, D., McArtney, R., Newcombe, R., McArtney, R., Gracie, J., Kirk, C., & Stuart, A.G. (1998). Medication errors in paediatric practice: Insights from a continuous quality improvement approach. *European Journal of Pediatrics, 157,* 769–774.

Winslow, E.H. (1996). The right site for IM injections. *American Journal of Nursing, 96*(4), 53. Retrieved from http://www.nursingcenter.com/journalarticle?Article_ID=102892

Wolf, Z. (1989). Medication errors and nursing responsibility. *Holistic Nursing Practice, 4*(1), 8–17.

Zuckerman, J.N. (2000). The importance of injecting vaccines into muscle: Different patients need different needle sizes. *BMJ, 321*(7271), 1237–1238.

SECTION II

The Pharmacology of Physiological Systems

CHAPTER 4

Central Nervous System Drugs

Dion M. Mayes-Burnett

KEY TERMS

Acetylcholine
Afferent
Alzheimer disease
Analgesics
Anesthetic
Antispasmodics
Autonomic nervous system
Axons
Brain stem
Central nervous system (CNS)
Cerebellum
Cerebrum
COX-2 inhibitors
Cyclooxygenase (COX)

Dendrites
Dopamine
Efferent
Epilepsy
Forebrain
Gamma-aminobutyric acid
  (GABA)
Glutamate
Hindbrain
Hypothalamus
Medulla oblongata
Midbrain
Muscle relaxant
Muscle spasm

Narcotic
Nerve processes
Neurodegeneration
Neuromuscular blockers
Neurons
N-methyl-D-aspartate (NMDA)
Nociceptive
Noncompetitive antagonist
Nonsteroidal anti-
  inflammatory drugs
  (NSAIDs)
Opioids
Parasympathetic nervous
  system

Parkinson's disease
Peripheral nervous system
  (PNS)
Pons
Prostaglandin
Salicylates
Somatic nervous system
Spasmolytics
Spasticity
Spinal column
Spinal cord
Sympathetic nervous system
Thalamus

CHAPTER OBJECTIVES

At the end of the chapter, the reader will be able to:

1. List the key components that make up the central nervous system (CNS).

2. Describe the function of the CNS.

3. Identify common disorders and diseases of the CNS.

4. List four primary symptoms of Parkinson's disease, Alzheimer disease, and amyotrophic lateral sclerosis.

5. Discuss five myths associated with chronic pain.

6. List three complications associated with narcotic administration.

7. Identify the major drug classes used to treat CNS disorders.

8. Describe the indication and mechanism of action for each of the drug classes used to treat CNS disorders.

9. Discuss the long-term effects of chronic acetaminophen therapy.

10. Describe symptoms of overdose for each class of CNS drug.

11. Explain how each CNS drug acts to alleviate or eliminate symptoms.

Nervous System Physiology

The nervous system has two major divisions: the **central nervous system (CNS)** and the **peripheral nervous system (PNS)**. The central nervous system is made up of the brain, brain stem, spinal cord, and an intricate network of neurons. The CNS (FIGURE 4-1) is responsible for sending, receiving, processing and interpreting sensory information from all areas of the body. It also receives information from and sends information to the peripheral nervous system (PNS). The PNS monitors and coordinates internal organ function and responds to changes in the external environment. Figure 4-1 illustrates how these two parts of the nervous system are divided, describing the paths they follow as well as the areas of the body they affect.

The brain is the control center of the body. It processes and interprets sensory input sent from the spinal cord. The brain consists of three structurally distinct components. The first, the **forebrain**, houses the **thalamus**, **hypothalamus**, and **cerebrum**. This area is responsible for functions such as receiving and processing sensory information, thinking, perceiving, producing and understanding language, and controlling motor function.

The **midbrain** and the **hindbrain** make up the **brain stem**. The midbrain connects the forebrain and the hindbrain, and is involved in auditory and visual responses as well as motor function. The midbrain also contains the **medulla oblongata**, which is responsible for autonomic functions such as breathing, heart rate, and digestion. The hindbrain extends from the spinal cord and

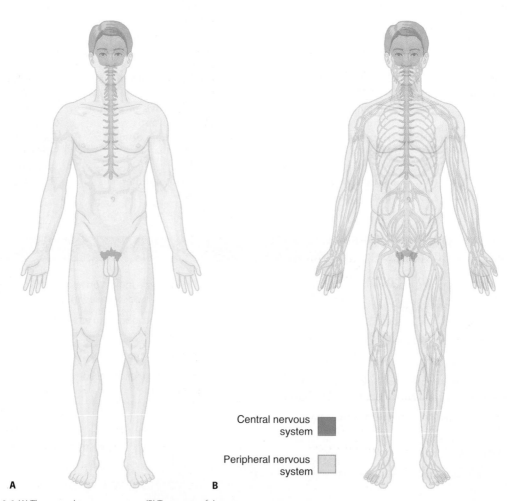

Central nervous system

Peripheral nervous system

A   B

FIGURE 4-1 (A) The central nervous system. (B) Two parts of the nervous system.

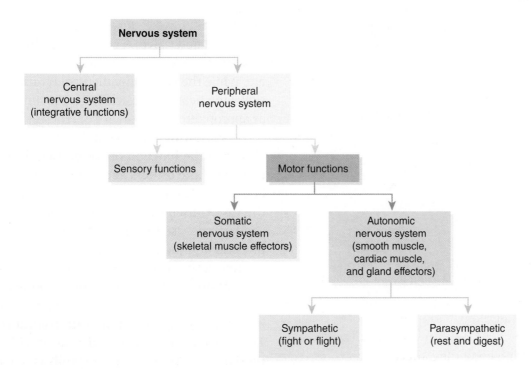

FIGURE 4-2 Major subdivisions of the nervous system.

contains the **pons** and **cerebellum**. This region assists in maintaining balance and equilibrium, as well as movement coordination and conduction of sensory information.

The **spinal cord** is a cylindrical bundle of nerves that is connected to the brain, running down the protective **spinal column**, extending from the neck to the lower back. Spinal cord nerves are responsible for transmitting information from body organs and external stimuli to the brain, and for sending information from the brain to other areas of the body.

Neurons are the basic units of the nervous system (FIGURE 4-2). All cells of the nervous system contain neurons, which in turn contain **nerve processes** ("fingerlike" projections) that consist of **axons** and **dendrites** (Figure 4-2). These cells work together to convey signals to different areas of the body.

The PNS consists of nerves outside the CNS. PNS nerves are classified by how they are connected to the CNS. Cranial nerves originate from or terminate in the brain, while spinal nerves originate or terminate in the spinal cord.

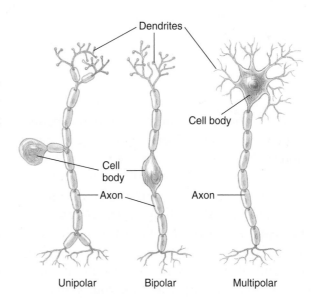

FIGURE 4-3 Cells of the nervous system.

The PNS (FIGURE 4-3, FIGURE 4-4) is divided into two major functional units, the sensory **(afferent)** and motor **(efferent)** functions; the motor (efferent) division is further subdivided into the **somatic nervous system** (voluntary nervous system) and the **autonomic nervous system** (involuntary nervous

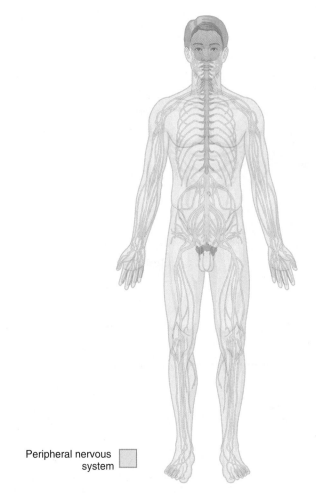

Peripheral nervous
system ☐

FIGURE 4-4 The peripheral nervous system.

system). The somatic nervous system consists of peripheral nerve fibers that send information to the CNS and motor nerve fibers that project to skeletal muscles. The autonomic nervous system can be further divided into the **sympathetic** and **parasympathetic nervous systems**. The sympathetic nervous system is responsible for generating the "fight-or-flight" response. When a person is afraid, the stimulated sympathetic nervous system prepares the body for action by increasing the heart rate, releasing glycogen from the liver into the blood, and other actions. The parasympathetic nervous system activates passive functions such as stimulating the secretion of saliva, or digestive enzymes into the stomach or small intestines ("rest and digest").

Generally, both the sympathetic and parasympathetic systems target the same organs,

but they often work antagonistically (discussed later in Chapter Five). For example, the sympathetic system causes the heart rate to accelerate, while the parasympathetic nervous system slows the heart rate. Each system is stimulated as appropriate to maintain homeostasis.

In reviewing the CNS and PNS, it becomes clear that the function of these systems to control all the centers and actions within the body. It is also simple to see how damage to the CNS caused by either disease or trauma can have devastating implications for both physical and mental health.

Recall that neurotransmission involves generation and propagation of action potentials along axons, which then trigger signaling across synapses, via neurotransmitters. These signals then cause reactions in either receiving neurons, or effector cells (such as muscle). The terminal actions may be either stimulating or inhibitory, depending on the type of receptors.

The major neurotransmitters in the CNS include gamma amino butyric acid (GABA), serotonin, acetylcholine, dopamine, norepinephrine, endogenous opioids (endorphins and enkephalins), and some amino acids, such as glutamic acid, aspartic acid, and histamine. There are other molecules understood to participate in neurotransmission, but this discussion will be limited to major neurotransmitters.

Drugs that affect these neurotransmitters in the central nervous system, their effects, and interactions with the immune system and inflammatory responses in relation to the central nervous system will be discussed in this chapter.

Conditions Affecting CNS Function

What causes these diseases or trauma to the CNS? The injuries and diseases that occur to the CNSs of thousands, even millions, of people worldwide have numerous causes. They can be attributed to viruses, toxins released from bacteria, toxic chemicals, congenital disorders, birth defects, lesions, tumors, autoimmune diseases, and trauma. These can affect the brain tissue, spinal cord, or major nerves directly, or they can impact specific components of the nervous system—individual nerves or even structures within nerves—resulting in effects that may be either localized or systemic. Examples of diseases, disorders, and trauma that affect the nervous system include encephalitis, meningitis, Huntington disease, Alzheimer disease, Parkinson's disease, Tourette syndrome, multiple sclerosis, epilepsy, fibromyalgia, accidents causing brain and spinal cord injuries, strokes, fractures, and torn ligaments, tendons, muscles, or nerve fibers.

Just as there are numerous diseases and causes of disease, the symptoms the patient might experience vary widely. Symptoms associated with a nerve disorder or injury may include persistent headaches, loss of sensation, memory loss, muscle weakness, tremors, nausea and vomiting, loss of bowel or urinary control, seizures, slurred speech, aphasia, dysphagia, intractable pain, paralysis, or blindness, to name a few. Symptoms may be barely noticeable, or they may be so significant as to impair the patient's ability to function. However, because the nervous system's functions are essential to movement, it is quite common for patients with CNS disorders or damage to complain of loss of function in an affected limb or system, as well as pain syndromes.

For many of these conditions, the therapy of choice is medication, perhaps in conjunction with physical therapy. Thus, it is important for the clinician to have a solid understanding of the types of medications available to treat CNS disorders and the effects that may be expected from their use.

Drugs Used for Conditions of the Central Nervous System

A wide range of therapies and medications is used to treat CNS diseases. This chapter focuses on drugs that treat CNS disorders including acute and chronic pain, the three most common neurodegenerative disorders, seizure disorders, and musculoskeletal dysfunction. The most commonly used medications for treating CNS issues will be discussed, including analgesics (both opioids and nonsteroidal anti-inflammatory drugs [NSAIDs]), local anesthetics, and muscle relaxants. Particular emphasis will be given to acute and chronic pain management, myths associated with pain, and the nursing process related to administration of CNS medications, as these are commonly seen in nursing practice and are of particular significance for patient care.

Classes of Medications for Treating CNS Disorders

CNS pharmacology will be addressed using the following system of categorization. These divisions are based on the groupings of the pharmacologic mechanisms of the drugs contained within each division.

1. Analgesics
   a. Opioids/narcotics
   b. NSAIDs (nonsteroidal anti-inflammatory drugs) and **acetaminophen**
2. Antiseizure/antiepileptic agents
3. Medications for neurodegenerative disorders
4. Muscle relaxants
5. Local anesthetics

Analgesics and Pain Management

Analgesics is a broad term used to describe medications that provide pain relief. The primary classes of analgesics are the *narcotics* or *opioids*, which include narcotic agonist–antagonist drugs; *NSAIDs*, including salicylates and COX-2 inhibitors. Other medications, such as **gabapentin**, an antiepileptic agent, are used to relieve pain (primarily neurologic pain), but these are not routinely classified as analgesics because pain relief is a useful coincidental effect of their activity.

In the narcotic drug class, medications are defined pharmacologically as agonists and antagonists. An agonist is a chemical (drug) that binds to a cellular receptor and activates

TABLE 4-1	Most Common Opioids			
Generic	Trade Name	Administration Routes	Natural/Other	Agonist/Antagonist
Morphine	MS Contin	Subcut./IM/IV/PO	Natural	Agonist
Codeine	Lodine	PO/IM/Subcut.	Natural	Agonist
Hydromorphone	Dilaudid	Subcut./IM/IV/PO/REC	Semi-synthetic	Agonist
Meperidine	Demerol	Subcut./IM/IV/PO/REC	Synthetic	Agonist
Fentanyl	Duragesic	IV/IM/lozenge/buccal tab/transdermal patch	Synthetic	Agonist
Methadone	Dolophine	Subcut./IM/IV/PO	Synthetic	Agonist
Tramadol	Ultram	PO	Synthetic	Agonist
Naloxone	Narcan	Subcut./IM/IV	Semi-synthetic	Antagonist

a response; agonists mimic the actions of endogenous opioid ligands. The best-known drugs with *mixed* agonist–antagonist activity are the opioids. For example morphine is an agonist of opioid receptors, while naloxone is an antagonist to morphine and other opiate drugs (and therefore a receptor *antagonist*). The drugs buprenorphine and pentazocine have both agonist and antagonist effects (TABLE 4-1).

Among the class of NSAIDs are COX-2 inhibitors. These drugs are selective in that they directly target COX-2, an enzyme responsible for inflammation and pain, yet have a less severe impact on the gastrointestinal (GI) tract than traditional NSAIDs such as salicylates (aspirin). The more benign GI effects of COX-2 inhibitors reduce the risk of peptic ulceration associated with the traditional NSAIDs (Chan et al., 2017; Whittle, 2000), although overall gastrointestinal toxicity of selective COX-2 inhibitors has been questioned (Hima & Venkat, 2016). Celecoxib is an example of a COX-2 inhibitor.

Analgesics provide *symptomatic* pain relief but do not alleviate the cause of that pain. The NSAIDs, due to their dual activity, may be beneficial in both regards, as we shall see later in this chapter.

Acute Versus Chronic Pain

One person's pain perception may be very different from another person's, but the one commonality is that a sensory pathway spans from the affected organ to the brain. Analgesics work at the level of the nerves, either by blocking the signal from the PNS or by distorting the perception by the CNS. Selecting an appropriate analgesic is achieved with consideration of the risks and benefits to the patient, the type and severity of pain the patient may be suffering, and the risk of adverse effects. The healthcare provider would also want to examine whether the type of pain the patient is experiencing would be categorized as acute or chronic.

Acute pain is self-limiting in duration and includes postoperative pain or pain due to an injury or infection. Given that pain of this type is expected to be short term (usually less than 12 weeks' duration), the long-term side effects of analgesic therapy may be ignored. These patients may be treated with narcotics without concern of possible addiction. One important consideration with patients in severe pain is that they should not be subject to the return of pain. Analgesics should be dosed routinely to ensure constant blood levels of analgesic, rather than waiting to provide patients with appropriate medications until

Best Practices

Selecting an appropriate analgesic is achieved with consideration of the risks and benefits to the patient, the type and severity of pain the patient may be suffering, and the risk of adverse effects.

Best Practices

Analgesics should be dosed routinely to ensure constant blood levels of analgesic so that pain relief is uninterrupted.

Best Practices

The risk of side effects with long-term use of NSAIDs means treatment of chronic pain requires a combination of drugs, lifestyle modifications, and other treatment modalities.

after the experience of pain returns. Often, it can take some time before the plasma concentration of analgesic drugs returns to effective levels, so waiting until pain recurs to administer analgesics may mean that the patient must then wait for an extended period of time for the medication to provide relief.

Chronic pain, classified as pain severe enough to impair function that lasts longer than three months, is much more difficult to treat, because the long-term use of medications makes the anticipated side effects more difficult to manage. With regard to narcotics, this may include the potential for tolerance and addiction, respiratory depression, or other side effects.

One of the more serious side effects of narcotic analgesics—respiratory depression—occurs when the medulla oblongata (moderator of unconscious crucial activities within the body, including respiration) detects variances in the levels of partial pressure of carbon dioxide (PCO_2) through specific chemoreceptors present in the carotid arteries. As PCO_2 increases, the medulla stimulates the respiratory muscles to breathe in a deeper, more rapid rhythm; this hastens the drop in PCO_2 as well as increases oxygenation of erythrocytes. In the presence of narcotics, the medulla is desensitized such that the brain remains unconscious of rising PCO_2 that normally leads the lung musculature to be understimulated, resulting in respiratory depression.

While some drugs, such as the selective COX-2 inhibitor celecoxib and the narcotic agonist–antagonist drugs **buprenorphine**, **nalbuphine**, and **pentazocine**, represent advances in the reduction of side effects, they are still not suitable for long-term management of severe pain. Although these classes of drug inhibit various isoforms of COX, thereby reducing the production of prostaglandins (a key component of the inflammatory reaction), it is precisely because of their inhibition of COX isoforms that NSAIDs may cause injury through their effects on various organ systems (Samad et al., 2001). The potential sequelae from organ damage include cardiovascular risk, acute renal failure, gastric ulceration and perforation, and decreased coagulation due to inhibition of platelet aggregation. For this reason, treatment of chronic pain requires a combination of drugs, lifestyle modifications, and other treatment modalities (Rosenquist, n.d.).

Chronic Pain Management: Myths and Facts

Pain is a normal part of people's daily lives. Pain occurs during childbirth, when scraping a knee while on the playground, postoperatively, or when getting whiplash in a fender-bender. Most of this pain is *acute*, meaning that it is of sudden onset, self-limiting, and usually of short duration, normally no longer than 12 weeks. In contrast, *chronic* pain, by definition, lasts longer than 3 months and may be severe enough to impair function and interfere with daily routines.

No one wants to be in pain. No one wants to be in a situation where they have discomfort so debilitating that they cannot work, rest, or simply enjoy life. Yet despite this, patients with chronic pain are occasionally branded with labels of being "lazy," "drug-seeking," or "whiny." They are often told—sometimes even by medical professionals!—that their pain is "all in your head," when in fact their pain is very real; very often, it may just be that the causes of the pain are not clearly defined or known. Ironically, while the patient's experience of pain is usually *not* a consequence of psychological issues, chronic pain syndromes can *cause* such issues, leading to depression, anxiety, and other disorders. Such issues often spring from patients' efforts to "just deal with it" and the difficulties associated with others' perceptions of what the patient should or should not feel. These issues can, in turn, affect the patients' ability to cope with chronic pain.

The following discussion illustrates some of the common myths and misconceptions associated with pain, including the medications used for chronic pain management, and presents the facts needed to exculpate these myths.

MYTH: "Chronic pain" is a psychological issue—it is mostly in the patient's head.

FACT: Chronic pain is a legitimate medical condition that can and should be treated. An exact cause cannot always be found; sometimes, clinicians lack the specialized training to recognize and treat common and unusual conditions that cause ongoing pain.

MYTH: Taking opioid painkillers leads to drug addiction.

FACT: Because people have often read sensational stories of numerous celebrities addicted to drugs, many people with chronic pain fear that taking opioids will lead to drug addiction. As a result, many people with terrible chronic pain refuse medication. When opioids are taken on a short-term basis and as directed, the risk of becoming addicted to this type of medication is very low. When used to treat chronic pain, *tolerance* to lower opioid doses can occur, and can be anticipated. This sometimes requires escalating the opioid dose, adding combinations of pain medications, and increased patient monitoring. Tolerance and addiction are not the same.

An interesting side point in regard to opioid painkillers is that they are all too often misused not by patients, but by prescribers. As detailed in both the literature (Chou et al., 2014; McNicol, Midbari, & Eisenberg, 2013) and a two-day FDA public conference on the subject of opioid abuse (Walker, 2012), little evidence supports the efficacy of long-term opioid use in chronic pain relief for conditions *unrelated* to cancer or acute injury due to accident or surgery; in the latter indications, however, evidence for their efficacy is abundant. Even so, the drugs are often prescribed for patients whose pain syndromes do not fall within those parameters and, therefore, who are unlikely to respond to the medications appropriately. Treating chronic pain with nothing more than a medication—and one that has little proven effect—contradicts current knowledge regarding the complex and multifaceted therapies required for relief.

MYTH: Addiction is the main risk to be concerned about when prescribing opioids.

FACT: Predicting which patients are at risk of addiction or aberrant behavior when using opioids is possible, given known risk factors

(Bolden et al., 2017). Thus, while addiction is a concern, the other risks associated with opioid use—risks that are more difficult to identify—are of considerably greater concern. These risks include respiratory depression and unintentional overdose death, serious fractures from falls, hypogonadism and other endocrine effects that cause a spectrum of adverse effects, increased pain sensitivity, sleep-disordered breathing, chronic constipation and serious fecal impaction, and chronic dry mouth, which can lead to tooth decay.

MYTH: Bed rest is usually the best cure for pain.

FACT: In the past, the medical advice for people with some types of chronic pain, such as back pain, was to rest in bed. But that is no longer the case. Now we know that for almost all types of chronic pain conditions, bed rest is almost never helpful, and in some cases it will actually worsen the problem. For most causes of pain, keeping up a normal schedule, including physical activity, will help the patient get better faster. Of course, there are situations where rest is important, especially for a day or two after acute injury, so the patient should be urged to follow a provider's advice.

MYTH: Increased pain is inevitable as we age.

FACT: Pain experts say that one particularly damaging myth about chronic pain is that pain is just a sign of aging and that not much can be done about it. They also suggest that too many doctors believe this myth as well. While it is true that the odds of developing painful conditions such as arthritis become higher as we age, those conditions can be treated and pain can be well controlled. *No matter what their age, no patient should have to settle for chronic pain.*

While there will always be myths and assumptions regarding pain, there will also always be answers to questions, and realistic facts to correct many of the myths associated with pain, and with pain medications and treatments. Always research your facts and discuss your concerns with your primary provider rather than suffer unnecessarily because of unfounded fears or lack of knowledge. As a nurse, researching drugs and medical conditions, and discussions with other healthcare professionals and specialists, should be routine practices.

Narcotics

Narcotics or opiates (**opioids**) comprise a variety of chemicals that owe their name to their derivation from the Asian poppy *Palaver somniferous*, also called the opium poppy. These drugs may be classified as natural, semi-synthetic, synthetic, or endogenous. *Natural opioids* such as morphine or codeine are created from opiate alkaloids extracted from the resin of the opium poppy. Semi-synthetic opioids are produced chemically by altering the natural opioids or morphine esters; examples of these drugs include **oxycodone** and **hydromorphone**. *Synthetic opioids* such as **meperidine**, **fentanyl**, and methadone are derived from non-opioid substances in laboratories, although they have similar mechanisms of action. *Endogenous opioids* are created naturally by the body and include substances called *endorphins*. The most common opioids are listed in Table 4-1.

Opioids work by "agonizing" *opioid receptors*, which are found in the brain, spinal cord, and gastrointestinal tract (**FIGURE 4-5**). This binding action blocks transmission of nerve impulses. **Morphine**, as well as other opioids, acts on an endogenous opioidergic system, which not only establishes the body's pain (**nociceptive**) threshold and controls nociceptive processing, but also participates in modulation

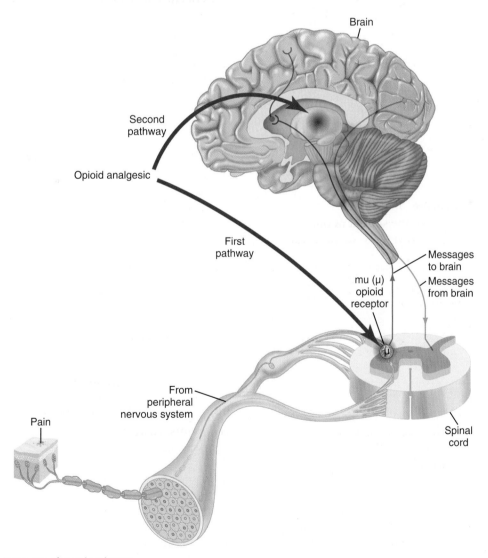

FIGURE 4-5 Action sites of opioid analgesics.

of gastrointestinal, endocrine, and autonomic function, as well as plays a possible role in cognition.

Opiate receptors are also responsible for some autonomic functions within the body. They may cause fluctuations in body temperature or alter heart rate and respiratory function. The endocrine system is also sensitive to changes in these receptors. Opiate receptors influence the neurotransmitters acetylcholine, dopamine, serotonin, and norepinephrine. These neurotransmitters cause the

sensations of well-being and euphoria that patients experience when medications such as morphine and hydrocodone bind to opiate receptors in the brain. A shortage or excess of these natural chemicals can drastically alter a person's emotional state.

Individually, the opioid receptors known as mu, kappa, delta, and nociceptin play antagonist and agonist roles within the body (TABLE 4-2). Mu receptors are necessary for the supraspinal analgesic effects from narcotics; they are also responsible for the feelings of

TABLE 4-2	Four Major Opioid Receptors

Receptor	Location	Function
Delta or DOP	**Brain:** • Pontine nuclei • Amygdala • Olfactory bulbs • Deep cortex • Peripheral sensory • Neurons	• Analgesia • Antidepressant effects • Convulsant effects • Physical dependence • Perhaps participate in mu-opioid
Kappa or KOP	**Brain:** • Hypothalamus • Periacqueductal gray • Claustrum	• Analgesia • Anticonvulsant effects • Dissociative and deliriant effects • Diuresis • Dysphoria • Miosis • Neuroprotection • Sedation
MU or MOP	**Brain:** • Cortex • Thalamus • Striosomes • Periacequductal gray • Rostral ventromedial • Medulla **Spinal cord:** • Substantia gelatinosa • Peripheral sensory • Neurons • Intestinal tract	**Mu1:** • Analgesia • Physical dependence **Mu2:** • Respiratory depression • Miosis • Euphoria • Reduced GI mobility • Physical dependence **Mu3:** • Possible vasodilation
Nociceptin receptor or NOP	**Brain:** • Cortex • Amygdala • Hippocampus • Septal nuclei • Habenula • Hypothalamus	• Anxiety • Depression • Appetite • Development of tolerance to Mu agonists

euphoria associated with opioid use, respiratory depression with overuse, and opioid dependence. Delta receptors are responsible for enabling the body to experience pain relief. They also permit the medication or natural neurotransmitters to exert an antidepressant effect and play a role in a person's physical addiction to opiates. Nociceptin receptors control appetite stimulation and are responsible for the formation of depressive conditions and anxiety disorders. When total sedation is required in anesthesia, it is the kappa receptors that are responsible. Epidural or spinal cord anesthesia would not provide pain relief without these receptors. Kappa receptors are also responsible for the pupil constriction (miosis) seen in patients taking opiates.

Narcotics dull the sense of pain and cause drowsiness or sleep. They are effective in relieving severe pain and are used preoperatively to reduce anxiety and induce anesthesia. They are used to suppress cough through direct action on the cough center in the medulla, and in severe cases of diarrhea, due to their direct actions on the intestines, in instances where these symptoms are not relieved by other medications. Caution should be exercised, however: In large doses, these medications can suppress the ability to breathe and cause coma and death.

Because narcotic drugs depress the CNS, they should not be taken with other drugs that depress the CNS, such as alcohol, barbiturates, and benzodiazepines. In addition, opioids are metabolized by the liver, so individuals with liver disease or damage may not metabolize and eliminate these medications as readily as healthy individuals, which can then potentially lead to accidental overdose. These drugs do not cure the source of the pain, but simply block the individual's perception of pain.

Side effects are essentially the same for all of the narcotics. They may include drowsiness, dizziness, confusion, sedation, euphoria, insomnia, seizures, heart palpitations, bradycardia, tachycardia, cardiac arrest, nausea, vomiting, constipation, urinary retention, rash, skin flushing, pruritus, respiratory depression, and apnea.

Among the many narcotics available, there are some with a few notable differences.

- **Hydrocodone** and **oxycodone** are often mixed with other non-opioid compounds such as **acetaminophen** and **ibuprofen** to achieve synergistic analgesic effects between the two compounds.
- **Tramadol** is a synthetic opioid analgesic that binds to mu opioid receptors and inhibits reuptake of norepinephrine and serotonin; consequently, it does not cause histamine release or affect heart rate like many opioids can. When metabolized, it becomes *O*-desmethyltramadol, a significantly more potent mu opioid antagonist. **Tramadol** and its metabolites are distinguished from more potent opioid agonists by their selectivity for mu opioid receptors.
- **Fentanyl**, besides the usual uses for opioids, is employed as an adjunct to general anesthesia, for conscious sedation, and for controlling breakthrough cancer pain. It is 100 times more potent than morphine. **Fentanyl** is a strong agonist at the mu opioid receptor sites. Although typically used for pain relief, it is often administered with a benzodiazepine for preoperative pain control and anesthesia. It is unique in that one of its administration routes is *transdermal* (i.e., via a patch applied to the skin). When the patch is used, it releases the drug across the skin, into body fats, so that it is slowly absorbed and distributed over 48 to 72 hours (which provides longer duration of action than typical of opioids).

Nursing Process

Assessment

When administering narcotics, the nurse or caretaker should regularly assess the patient regarding various

Best Practices

When using narcotic medications, be cautious about dosing because large doses of narcotic drugs can suppress respiration and other autonomic functions.

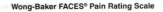
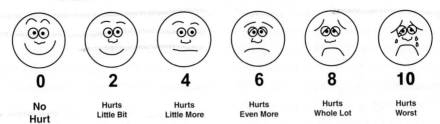

FIGURE 4-6 Wong-Baker FACES pain rating scale.

© 1983 Wong-Baker FACES Foundation. www.WongBakerFACES.org. Used with permission. Originally published in *Whaley and Wong's Nursing Care of Infants and Children.* © Elsevier.

aspects of pain, such as its location, type, and character, utilizing pain scoring methods such as having the patient rate the pain from "no pain" (0) to the "worst pain ever" (10). If the patient is unable to provide a rating, a facial scale that shows facial expressions ranging from comfort to excruciating pain can be used for this purpose (**FIGURE 4-6**).

The patient should not be required to wait too long between doses of analgesic medication. It is important to maintain adequate pain control. At the same time, watch for more frequent requests for pain medication, as that could indicate tolerance. Constipation is common with narcotic use, so provide stimulant laxatives as needed. Be sure to obtain baseline vital signs and monitor blood pressure, pulse, and respirations closely. Watch the patient's intake and outputs closely. Decreases in output could indicate urinary retention.

Regularly check the patient for signs of adverse reactions and CNS changes such as dizziness, hallucinations, euphoria, or pinpoint pupils. If the patient displays any of these signs or allergic or anaphylactic reactions such as rash, hives, or respiratory difficulty, contact the patient's primary provider immediately.

Administration

When administering any medication, it is important to know the ordered route and handling of the drug; to ensure the proper timing, dosage, and name of medication for the right patient; and to maintain thorough documentation. If the patient experiences nausea or vomiting, provide ordered antiemetic agents.

Follow all guidelines for the proper storage of each medication. Be sure to provide safety measures such as side rails, a night light, a clutter-free room, and a call bell and water within easy reach. Assist the patient with ambulation or other activities as needed. When the patient has been on a long-term regimen of narcotics, withdrawal of these drugs should be gradual to avoid adverse reactions.

Evaluate

Evaluation of a therapeutic response should include assessment for decreased or no pain, no facial grimacing, decreased cough, or decreased diarrhea.

Patient/Family Education

Teach patients to take the medication as prescribed and, if any CNS changes or allergic reactions occur, to contact the healthcare provider immediately. Instruct patients not to stop medications abruptly as symptoms of withdrawal could occur, including nausea, vomiting, cramps, fever, faintness, and anorexia. Advise patients that they should avoid alcohol or other CNS depressants unless prescribed by their primary provider and that physical dependence may occur with long-term therapy. Instruct patients to avoid hazardous activities

Best Practices

It is important to maintain adequate pain control, but watch for increased requests for pain medication as a possible sign of tolerance.

Best Practices

The antidote for overdose of narcotics is the antagonist **naloxone**.

such as driving if drowsiness or dizziness is present, and to change position or stand slowly, as orthostatic hypotension could occur. Female patients should not breastfeed their children while on narcotics, as these medications can pass through breastmilk.

Overdose

Serious symptoms of overdose may include decreased level of consciousness, pinpoint pupils, changes in heart rate, or decreased or absent respirations. Cyanotic lips and nails are caused by decreased oxygen in the blood as an indirect result of depressed respiratory rate. Other symptoms may include seizure activity, muscle spasms, or even death. The antidote for overdose of narcotics is **naloxone**, which reverses the adverse effects of the opiates due to its antagonistic actions.

Nonsteroidal Anti-Inflammatory Drugs

Nonsteroidal anti-inflammatory drugs (NSAIDs) reduce inflammation but are not related by structure or action to steroids (glucocorticoids), which also reduce inflammation. The NSAID class of drugs provides both analgesic and antipyretic effects. This large group of medications is available under an assortment of brand names, with the most recognizable members of this group being **aspirin, ibuprofen,** and **naproxen**, all of which are available as over-the-counter medications. Although all NSAIDs have a similar mechanism of action, individuals who do not respond to one may respond to another.

While these drugs are generally considered safe, some people may experience side effects with their use, though these unwanted effects are not the same as many of those seen with steroid use. NSAIDs are not narcotics, so they do not carry any risk of addiction.

NSAIDs work by reducing the production of **prostaglandins**. Prostaglandins are chemicals produced by the body that promote inflammation, pain, and fever. They also protect the lining of the stomach and intestines from the damaging effects of acid, and promote blood clotting by activating blood platelets. Prostaglandins also affect kidney function.

The enzymes that produce prostaglandins are called **cyclooxygenases (COX)**. Two types of COX enzymes are distinguished: *COX-1* and *COX-2*. Both enzymes produce prostaglandins that promote inflammation, pain, and fever; however, only COX-1 produces prostaglandins that activate platelets and protect the stomach and intestinal lining.

NSAIDs block COX enzymes and reduce production of prostaglandins. Therefore, inflammation, pain, and fever are reduced. Because the prostaglandins that protect the stomach and promote blood clotting also are reduced, NSAIDs, with the exception of COX-2 inhibitors, can cause ulcers in the stomach and intestines, and increase the risk of bleeding. TABLE 4-3 lists the most common NSAIDs, their administration routes, and their classifications.

NSAIDs are used for treating conditions that cause inflammation, mild to moderate

TABLE 4-3	Most Common NSAIDs		
Generic Name		Administration Route	Chemical Class
Acetylsalicylic Acid	Aspirin/ASA	PO/REC	Salicylate
Ibuprofen		PO/IV	Proprionic acid derivative
Naproxen		PO	Proprionic acid derivative
Ketrolac		PO/IV/IM	Acetic acid derivative
Celecoxib		PO	COX-2 inhibitor

pain, and fever. Examples include headaches, coughs and colds, physical injuries, gout, arthritis, menstrual cramps, and postoperative discomfort. These medications (especially aspirin) are also used for their antiplatelet effects. NSAIDs differ in potency and duration of action, as well as their tendency to cause GI ulcers and bleeding, because they differ in their relative inhibition of COX-1 and COX-2. As the individual drugs are addressed further in this section, more specific consideration of their actions and uses will be provided.

There are a few notable differences between NSAIDs. Celecoxib blocks COX-2 but has little effect on COX-1. Therefore, celecoxib is subclassified as a selective COX-2 inhibitor, which causes fewer instances of gastrointestinal bleeding or ulceration than other NSAIDs. This agent is used for the treatment of osteoarthritis, rheumatoid arthritis, acute pain, ankylosing spondylitis, and primary dysmenorrhea.

Ibuprofen is chemically similar to acetylsalicylic acid (ASA, or aspirin) and functions in a comparable way, minimizing the production of prostaglandins. In lower doses, it appears to irritate the esophageal and gastric linings less than the related NSAIDs, aspirin and naproxen. Ibuprofen is used for rheumatoid arthritis, osteoarthritis, primary dysmenorrhea, gout, dental pain, musculoskeletal disorders, fever, and migraine.

Aspirin is the only NSAID able to irreversibly inhibit COX-1; it is also indicated for inhibition of platelet aggregation because it inhibits the action of thromboxane A_2. This agent is useful in the management of arterial thrombus and prevention of adverse cardiovascular events.

Although naproxen is commonly used for headaches and menstrual pain, it is especially effective as an anti-inflammatory agent. For arthritis, sprains, and other inflammation-based pain, naproxen appears to be superior to ibuprofen in that it better targets muscle-tissue inflammation and has less of an anti-platelet effect than aspirin. Another difference between naproxen and the other NSAIDs is that the dosing interval for naproxen is longer (every 8–12 hours) than for other NSAIDs, which are usually dosed every 4–6 hours.

Ketorolac is a very potent NSAID that is used for short-term management of moderately severe, acute pain that would normally be treated with narcotics, such as kidney stone pain or postsurgical pain. It is more effective than other NSAIDs in reducing pain from both inflammatory and non-inflammatory causes. This agent acts by reducing the production of prostaglandins by binding to the COX-1 and COX-2 enzymes, thus reducing pain and inflammation as well as their signs and symptoms. Ketorolac is not to be used for more than five days due to adverse effects on the kidneys; it also causes ulcers more frequently than other NSAIDs.

Acetaminophen is an analgesic and antipyretic, but it is *not* an anti-inflammatory substance. As a result, it is relatively ineffective for treating arthritis, sprains, or other inflammatory conditions. Acetaminophen blocks pain impulses peripherally that occur in response to inhibition of prostaglandin synthesis, so it does not have anti-inflammatory properties. Its antipyretic action results from inhibition of prostaglandin synthesis in the CNS at the hypothalamic heat-regulating center. While acetaminophen has milder effects on the upper digestive tract than other over-the-counter pain relievers, it can have serious side effects in cases of overdose or long-term therapy such as renal failure and hepatic toxicity. This agent should be used with caution in patients who have renal or hepatic disease and should not be taken with alcohol. Acetaminophen does not decrease platelet aggregation and, therefore, is less likely to affect clotting capacity, which makes it a safer choice for hemophiliacs, patients taking "blood thinners," and for children. It is often used as a first-line medication in conditions such as headache, muscle aches, arthritis, backache, toothaches, colds, and fevers.

The most common side effects of NSAIDs are gastrointestinal symptoms, which are usually mild, but can be serious. Nausea, vomiting, indigestion, dyspepsia, stomach ulcers, and gastrointestinal bleeding are some adverse reactions that are seen. These symptoms result from NSAIDs' inhibition of prostaglandins, which, in addition to their pro-inflammatory functions, are responsible for producing the protective lining of the stomach and intestines.

Other side effects that can have serious consequences are the NSAIDs' effects on the cardiovascular system. It is believed that serious cardiovascular disease leading to heart attack and stroke is twice as likely in people using NSAIDs, even if there is no preexisting heart disease. The exception is low-dose aspirin, which is used for preventing strokes and heart attacks in individuals who are at high risk for such events. The reason aspirin works in this fashion is that it inhibits blood clotting for a prolonged period by irreversibly acetylating platelets, something none of the other NSAIDs do. Aspirin is therefore effective for preventing blood clots that cause clot-related cardiovascular conditions; however, if used in conjunction with another NSAID, aspirin negates at least some of the other drug's benefits, so a patient who takes aspirin for its cardiovascular benefits should not take a second NSAID drug for relief of pain for extended periods of time. Aside from aspirin, naproxen is considered the only other NSAID that possesses a low likelihood of causing cardiovascular disease.

NSAIDs affect the kidneys by reducing their efficiency in filtering and eliminating waste from the body—again due to their action on prostaglandins. Side effects can be compounded when NSAIDs are taken with other drugs that act on the kidneys, such as ACE inhibitors. Some common signs of adverse reaction on the kidneys are sodium or fluid retention and hypertension. More serious reactions could be pain or urinary retention. Hydration is very important for patients taking these medications. The effects of NSAIDs on both the kidneys and heart mean that they should be avoided in pregnant women, particularly late in pregnancy. They are also suspected to cause premature birth and miscarriage.

Mixing NSAIDs with other medications is something to be undertaken with caution. Some kidney and blood pressure medications' efficacy can be affected by NSAIDs. Moreover, antiplatelet effects can be experienced with NSAID use; this is especially true when aspirin is mixed with anticlotting medications such as heparin or warfarin. If mixed with alcohol, aspirin may increase the risk of gastrointestinal bleeding and ulceration.

Toxic effects are usually the result of overdose or chronic, long-term therapy. One of the first studies conducted on this issue (Singh, 1998) estimated that each year nearly 107,000 hospitalizations and 16,500 deaths in the United States are linked to NSAID-related complications. More recent studies have shown an overall decrease in NSAID-related mortality and morbidity (Gargallo, Sostres, & Lanas, 2014; Sostres, Gargallo, & Lanas, 2013). The severity of symptoms depends largely on the dosage taken and the timing of the medication. Multiple systems can be affected in NSAID-related toxicity; most notably, gastrointestinal and liver dysfunction can be manifested.

Gastrointestinal effects can be as serious as ulceration and bleeding. The possibility of liver toxicity increases in elderly individuals, in patients with history of liver failure, and with any alcohol consumption. Tenderness, jaundice, elevated liver enzymes, and liver failure can be seen in severe toxicity.

Other signs of toxicity in various body systems may include sodium and water retention, acute renal failure, and tissue death from renal necrosis associated with overdose. Overdose can also produce tachycardia and even cardiac or respiratory arrest; blood complications, though rare, can include decreased platelet counts, anemia, and reduced white blood cell count. Skin rashes can occur with minor acute toxicity, and in rare instances, a serious condition called Stevens-Johnson syndrome may occur, characterized by painful rash and blisters, with shedding of the epidural layer of the skin.

Significant toxicity can occur from interactions between NSAIDs and **lithium**, oral anticoagulants, oral hypoglycemic agents, **phenytoin**, **digoxin**, or aminoglycoside antibiotics.

Nursing Process

Assess

Due to the possibility of serious toxic reactions with overdose and chronic use of NSAIDs, the following parameters should be monitored: complete blood count (CBC), liver enzymes, and, in patients receiving diuretics, urine output and blood urea nitrogen (BUN)/serum creatinine. In patients with renal insufficiency, the provider should obtain a baseline of renal function, followed by repeat testing within two weeks to determine if renal function has deteriorated. It is important to monitor patient fluid intake and output closely, as changes in urine such as presence of blood or albumin could indicate nephritis and decreased output could pose the threat of renal failure. If changes in urine color, clay-colored stools, yellowing skin, or sclera is noted, the patient could be experiencing hepatotoxicity.

Request the patient to describe any pain, including its location, intensity, and duration, and identify whether anything worsens or improves the pain. Encourage use of numerical and facial scales as means to rate pain. If the patient shows signs of any of these symptoms, the primary provider should be contacted immediately, as the medication may have to be discontinued.

Administer

Most NSAIDs are given orally. Explain to the patient that many oral medications may be given crushed or whole and that chewable tablets may be chewed. However, consult with the pharmacy or manufacturer literature regarding the potential for modified dosage forms that should *not* be crushed.

Give medications with a full glass of water. Medications may be taken with milk or food as needed to decrease gastric symptoms. Oral suspensions should be shaken well before ingestion by the patient.

Perform/Provide

Make sure medications are stored at room temperature and out of the reach of children. Store suppositories at temperatures less than 80°F (27°C); some require storage at under 4°C.

Evaluate

Regularly evaluate the patient's therapeutic response to medications. Note whether there is an absence or diminished report of pain using pain scales such as a numerical scale of 0–10, where 0 is absence of pain and 10 is the worst pain possible; for children, mentally challenged patients, or patients who cannot verbalize their responses, a facial scale may be used for pain monitoring. Also monitor for a decrease in the patient's fever.

Patient/Family Education

Teach the patient to not exceed the recommended dosage of NSAIDs, as acute poisoning with liver damage may result. Tell parents to check products carefully and to avoid **aspirin** use in children, as this could potentially lead to Reye syndrome; also educate them that symptoms of acute toxicity include nausea, vomiting, and abdominal pain. Patients/parents should notify the prescriber immediately if these symptoms occur. Parents should be especially aware of the toxicity that may occur if NSAIDs are used with over-the-counter combination products that also contain NSAIDs.

Emphasize to the patient the importance of avoiding alcohol while taking NSAIDs, and of notifying the prescriber if the patient has liver dysfunction or a history of alcoholism to avoid hepatotoxicity. Instruct the patient about signs of chronic overdose, such as bleeding, bruising, malaise, fever, or sore throat. Diabetics may notice blood glucose monitoring changes due to drug interactions of hypoglycemic medications with NSAIDs, so encourage them to monitor their blood glucose regularly and report changes to the primary provider.

Seizure Disorders and Epilepsy

The brain is the center that controls and regulates voluntary and involuntary responses in the body. It is made up of trillions of cells that, through a sequence of events, transmit information by interacting with each other. In the normal brain, neuronal interchange occurs with few disruptions. When portions of the brain become overly stimulated, or when multiple cells break down at the same time in an abnormal fashion, however, a seizure may occur. If seizures recur or are prolonged over short periods of time, the potential for additional seizures increases as nerve cell death, scar tissue formation, and new axons accumulate.

After a nerve cell actuates, certain chemicals prevent a second firing of the neuron until the internal charge of the neuron returns to a resting state. One of the principal inhibiting chemicals in the brain is **gamma-aminobutyric acid (GABA)**. GABA causes chloride channels for negatively charged ions to open and flood into the excited neuron, which in turn decreases the internal charge and prevents the nerve cell from firing again. If there is a disruption in the cells that produce GABA or in the receptor sites for GABA, these channels may fail to open and moderate the excitability of the nerve cell.

Another chemical that plays a significant role in the pathophysiology of seizure activity is **glutamate**. A major excitatory mediator in the brain, glutamate binds to receptors that open channels for sodium, potassium, and calcium into the cell. Some genetic forms of seizures involve a predilection for excessively frequent or prolonged activation of glutamate receptors, which increases the excitability of the brain and the possibility of further seizure activity.

Seizure disorder is a broad term used to describe any condition in which a seizure may be a symptom. It is a term often used in place of *epilepsy*. The type of seizure a patient experiences depends on which part and how much of the brain is involved, as do the symptoms that the person has during a seizure. The cause of the seizure, including "unknown causes," also influences its manifestation. Two broad categories of seizures are distinguished: generalized seizures (absence, atonic, tonic–clonic, myoclonic) and partial seizures (simple and complex).

Non-epileptic seizures are essentially a symptom caused by either physiological or psychological conditions. When the seizure activity has a known cause, it is generally classified as a non-epileptic seizure. Such short, frequent events mimic epileptic seizures, but do not involve abnormal, rhythmic discharges of cortical neurons. Non-epileptic seizures are generally caused by illness, injury, or other issue that stimulates irregular brain activity. They may also be caused by infectious diseases such as HIV/AIDS, encephalitis, or meningitis. Other causes may include drug use, high fever (especially in children), abrupt cessation of certain medications, excessive alcohol consumption, traumatic brain injury, stroke, cardiovascular disorders, or even organ failure, such as of the liver or kidneys. If a seizure has no identifiable cause, it is considered an epileptic seizure.

Epileptic seizures are a symptom of **epilepsy**, a brain disorder in which clusters of neurons sometimes signal abnormally in the brain. When normal neuronal activity in the brain becomes disturbed, it may cause strange sensations, emotions, behaviors, convulsions, muscle spasms, or even loss of consciousness. This condition has many possible causes. Anything that disturbs the normal patterns of activity, such as brain damage, abnormal brain development, or illness, can cause seizure activity. Having a seizure, however, does not necessarily mean a person has epilepsy. Generally, a person is not considered to have epilepsy unless he or she has two or more episodes of seizure activity; even then, this diagnosis is only suspected until further testing is done to confirm its presence. Electroencephalography and brain scans are the diagnostic tests most commonly performed to definitively diagnose epilepsy.

Epilepsy is a relatively common condition, affecting 0.5% to 1% of the population. In the United States, approximately 2.5 million people have epilepsy, and about 10% of Americans will have at least one seizure in their lifetime (Epilepsy Foundation Michigan, 2011).

Once epilepsy is diagnosed, treatment should begin as soon as possible. A majority of patients have success with medications. When medications do not relieve seizure activity, surgery is sometimes an option.

Numerous medications are used to treat seizures and epilepsy. These medications are selected based on the type of seizure, age of the patient, side effects, and cost. There are three main goals of antiseizure/epileptic drug therapy: (1) to eliminate or reduce the frequency of seizure activity to the maximum degree possible; (2) to avoid the adverse effects associated with long-term treatment; and (3) to assist patients in maintaining or resuming their usual routines, psychosocial activities, and occupational activities so as to maintain as normal a lifestyle as possible.

Anticonvulsants

While the ideal antiseizure medication would prohibit seizures without resulting in any undesired adverse effects, most of the currently available drugs not only fail to adequately control seizure activity in some people, but also produce adverse effects that range in severity from minimal impairment of the CNS to hepatic failure. The healthcare practitioner must be careful to choose an appropriate combination of drugs that controls the seizures with a minimal degree of side effects. Some of the most commonly used anticonvulsants are described in TABLE 4-4.

Valproic Acid

Valproic acid is a carboxylic acid derivative. Valproate is the name given to valproic acid after it has converted to the active form in the body. Valproic acid is converted to valproate in the GI tract; thus, this medication must be delivered orally. It is used as an anticonvulsant as well as vascular headache suppressant. Valproic acid has also been used to treat manic episodes associated with bipolar disorder, as an adjunct in schizophrenia, to treat tardive dyskinesia, to minimize aggression in children with attention-deficit/hyperactivity disorder (ADHD), and for organic brain syndrome mania.

The mechanism of action by which valproate exerts its antiepileptic effects has not been established, but its action in epilepsy is believed to occur through increased GABA concentrations in the brain, which decreases seizure activity. Valproic acid (valproate) also blocks the voltage-gated sodium channels and T-type calcium channels. These mechanisms make valproic acid a broad-spectrum anticonvulsant drug.

Valproate is believed to affect the function of the neurotransmitter GABA in the human brain, making it an alternative to lithium salts in treatment of bipolar disorder. Its mechanism of action includes enhanced neurotransmission of GABA (by inhibiting GABA

TABLE 4-4	Anticonvulsants	
Generic	Administration	Chemical Class
Valproic acid	PO/IV/REC	Carboxylic Acid Derivative
Phenobarbital	Subc./PO/IV/IM	Barbituate
Levetiracetam	PO/IV	(-)-(S)-alpha-ethyl-2-oxo-1-pyrrolidine acetamide
Phenytoin	PO/IV	Hydantoin

transaminase, which breaks down GABA). However, several other mechanisms of action in neuropsychiatric disorders have been proposed for **valproic acid** in recent years (Rosenberg, 2007).

Phenobarbital

Phenobarbital is a barbiturate or barbituric acid derivative that acts as a nonselective CNS depressant. It is primarily used as a sedative hypnotic but also has application as an anticonvulsant. **Phenobarbital** enables binding to inhibitory GABA subtype receptors, and it alters chloride currents through receptor channels. It also restricts glutamate-induced depolarizations. In subhypnotic doses, it is used to treat all forms of epilepsy, status epilepticus, febrile seizures in children, sedation, and insomnia.

Phenobarbital agonizes GABA receptors, increasing synaptic inhibition. This has the effect of elevating the seizure threshold and reducing the spread of seizure activity from a seizure focus. Phenobarbital may also inhibit calcium channels, resulting in a decrease in stimulative transmitter release. The sedative–hypnotic effects of phenobarbital are likely the result of its effect on the polysynaptic midbrain reticular formation, which controls CNS arousal.

Levetiracetam

Levetiracetam is an anticonvulsant chemically unrelated to existing antiepileptic drugs. Its chemical class name is (–)-(S)alpha-ethyl-2-oxo-1-pyrrolidine acetamide. This agent is often used as monotherapy in partial seizures and as an adjunct to other medications in partial, primary generalized tonic–clonic, and myoclonic seizures. Like other anticonvulsants such as **gabapentin**, **levetiracetam** is also prescribed to treat neuropathic pain.

Electrical signals in the brain cause the release of neurotransmitters, which in turn assist in sending messages between neurons. If the release of these neurotransmitters occurs too often or is prolonged, an overload in the body's electrical signals can occur. This can then result in a seizure. Although the drug's mechanism of action is not entirely understood, it is believed that within the neurons in the brain, **levetiracetam** binds to a synaptic vesicle glycoprotein, SV2A. These molecules are found on the surfaces of tiny structures in the neurons called vesicles. It is this attachment of **levetiracetam** to the SV2A molecules that inhibits the abnormal spread of signals, which may otherwise lead to a seizure (UCB, 2013).

Phenytoin

Phenytoin is a hydantoin whose chemical structure is closely related to that of **barbiturates**. It is one of the drugs most commonly used to control epileptic seizures in the United States and around the world. **Phenytoin** is prescribed to treat various types of convulsions and seizures, including generalized tonic–clonic (grand mal), complex partial (psychomotor, temporal lobe) seizures, status epilepticus, non-epileptic seizures associated with Reye syndrome or after head trauma, and Bell's palsy.

Phenytoin inhibits the spread and frequency of seizure activity in the motor cortex by altering ion transport. More specifically, **phenytoin** acts on sodium channels on the neuronal cell membrane, limiting the spread of seizure activity and reducing seizure multiplication. By promoting sodium efflux from neurons, this drug tends to stabilize the threshold against hyper-excitability caused by excessive stimulation or environmental changes capable of reducing the membrane sodium gradient. This includes the reduction of post-tetanic potentiation at synapses. Loss of post-tetanic potentiation prevents cortical seizure foci from detonating adjacent cortical areas (Mantegazza, Curia, Biagini, Ragsdale, & Avoli, 2010).

Benzodiazepines

Benzodiazepines (**clonazepam**, **chlorazepate**, **diazepam**, **lorazepam**) are similar in pharmacologic action but have different potencies, and some benzodiazepines work better in the treatment of certain conditions than others. As a group, these medications are used as anticonvulsants, muscle relaxants, sedatives, and hypnotics, as well as for neurodegenerative disorders such as multiple sclerosis, ALS, and Parkinson's disease, which will be discussed in greater detail later in this chapter.

This class of agents works on the CNS, acting selectively on gamma-aminobutyric acid-A (GABAA) receptors in the brain (Rudolph et al., 1999). Benzodiazepines enhance the response to the inhibitory neurotransmitter GABA by opening GABA-activated chloride channels and allowing chloride ions to enter the neuron, making the neuron negatively charged and resistant to excitation.

Anticonvulsant Side Effects

Like all medications, anticonvulsants have potential side effects. Some effects are dose related and may become more likely as doses increase or during long-term therapy. The most common side effects seen with anticonvusants are drowsiness, irritability, nausea, rash, and unsteadiness. Some drugs may produce changes in behavior and emotions, and some patients may experience thoughts of suicide. At high doses or with toxicity, patients can demonstrate sedation, slurring of speech, sleep disturbances, double vision, and other symptoms (for more information, see, for example, the National Library of Medicine's MedlinePlus page describing specific drugs' characteristics).

Of all the anticonvulsants, the drug that should be monitored most carefully, or that should be considered "high priority" is phenytoin. At therapeutic doses, this drug can produce numerous side effects, but at higher drug levels, side effects of the drug become quite alarming. Phenytoin may accumulate in the cerebral cortex with chronic use and can cause atrophy of the cerebellum when administered at high doses. It inhibits the monoglutamate enzyme, thereby causing folate deficiency and predisposing patients

to megaloblastic anemia, agranulocytosis, and thrombocytopenia. Phenytoin is a known teratogen; it may produce craniofacial anomalies and a mild form of retardation in fetuses exposed to this drug. Due to the folate deficiency it produces, phenytoin has also been associated with drug-induced gingival enlargement, which may involve gingival bleeding and exudate, pronounced inflammatory response to plaque levels, and, in some instances, bone loss without tooth detachment. In addition, phenytoin has been known to cause hypertrichosis, rash, pruritus, exfoliative dermatitis, and autoimmune reactions such as drug-induced lupus, life-threatening skin reactions such as Stevens-Johnson syndrome, and toxic epidermal necrolysis. Like any antiepileptic drug, phenytoin carries an increased risk of suicide and other behavioral side effects. Despite all of these risks, the drug has a long history of safe use, making it one of the more popular anticonvulsants prescribed by primary providers and a common "first line of defense" in seizure cases.

Nursing Process

Assess

With any anticonvulsant medication, the dosage should be adjusted carefully, starting with low doses and increasing the amount given gradually until seizures are controlled, as long as there are no toxic effects. Monitoring plasma concentration levels assists in dosage adjustments. A few missed doses or a small change in absorption may result in a marked change in plasma concentration. Small dosage increases in some patients may produce large rises in plasma levels accompanied by acute toxic side effects.

Side effects such as acne and hirsutism, while mild, may be undesirable in adolescent patients. If ataxia, slurred speech, nystagmus, and blurred vision occur, notify the primary provider immediately, as these symptoms could be indications of toxicity or overdose. Avoid sudden withdrawal, as it can lead to serious side effects. Always taper anticonvulsant medications slowly.

Best Practices

Of all the anticonvulsants, **phenytoin** is the drug that needs the most careful monitoring, as its side effects become dangerous when the drug concentration reaches toxic levels.

Patients or their caregivers should be instructed regarding how to recognize signs of blood or skin disorders, and advised to seek immediate medical attention if symptoms of fever, sore throat, rash, mouth ulcers, bruising, or bleeding develop.

Instruct patients to take medications either after meals, or at least *with* food. Nurses should refer to the manufacturer's summary of product characteristics and to appropriate local guidelines. Encourage patients and their families to learn about the disorder being treated, the medication, and its potential side effects or drug interactions.

Neurodegenerative Diseases

Neurodegeneration is a blanket term for chronic, progressive diseases or disorders characterized by selective and often symmetrical loss, or death of, neurons in the motor, sensory, or cognitive systems. There are approximately 600 such disorders that afflict the nervous system. The area of the brain where neurons are affected is a way of determining the type of neurodegenerative disease. If the cerebral cortex is involved, typically diseases such as Alzheimer disease, Pick disease, and Lewy body dementias are seen. Cellular destruction or malformation in the basal ganglia is generally encountered in Parkinson's disease or Huntington disease. Degeneration occurring in the brain stem and cerebellum are characteristic of such disorders as Freidreich ataxia, multiple system atrophy, or spinocerebellar ataxia. When the motor areas are affected, diseases such as ALS and spinal muscular atrophy are seen.

Although many of the causes of neurodegenerative disorders are not known, research has found that many of these diseases are associated with genetic mutations, some of which are located in genes whose ultimate functions appear unrelated. In many of the different diseases, the mutated gene has one common origin: a repeat of the cytosine–adenosine–guanosine (CAG) nucleotide triplet. These triplets or "CAG repeats" encode for the addition of one glutamine residue to the polyglutamine tail in the huntingtin gene. When there are too many repeats, the tail becomes too long, creating problems for the resulting protein molecule and for the body as a whole.

When this pattern is repeated, polyglutamine tracts form. The extra glutamine residues can cause proteins to fold irregularly, disrupt neural pathways, alter subcellular localization, and cause abnormal interactions with other cellular proteins. Two examples of the nine reported neurodegenerative diseases that are affected by the CAG trinucleotide are Huntington disease and spinocerebellar ataxias.

Another protein, alpha-synuclein (α-synuclein), is an abundant synaptic protein in which four mutations have been found to cause an autosomal dominant form of Parkinson's disease (PD). It is also a major component of intraneuronal protein aggregates, designated as Lewy bodies (LB), a prominent pathological hallmark of PD (Wan & Chung, 2012).

How α-synuclein contributes to LB formation and PD is still not understood, but it has been proposed that aggregation of α-synuclein in cells contributes to the development of LBs that form insoluble fibrils in pathological conditions such as Parkinson's disease, dementia with Lewy bodies, and multiple system atrophy. An α-synuclein fragment, known as non-αβ component (NAC), also is found in the amyloid plaques commonly seen in Alzheimer disease. While treatments can sometimes slow the progression of these diseases or even alleviate certain symptoms, there are currently no cures for these devastating disorders.

This text cannot address all the neurodegenerative diseases and disorders in existence; therefore, the focus will be restricted to the most common medications used to slow progression and/or alleviate symptoms of three specific diseases. These diseases are Parkinson's disease, Alzheimer disease, and ALS. Other disorders may be mentioned in relation to the medications being addressed further in the chapter with regard to symptom relief.

Parkinson's Disease

Parkinson's disease (PD) is a disorder in which nerve cells in the areas of the brain that involve muscle movement (corpus striatum and substantia nigra) are affected. This disease is considered both chronic and progressive, meaning that once it develops, it does not go away, and symptoms generally get worse over time. In PD, brain cells are lost when an aggregation of α-*synuclein* binds to *ubiquitin* (a regulatory protein) in the damaged nerve cells. When these proteins bind, the complex that forms cannot be directed to the proteasome. This accumulation of proteins forms cellular inclusions called Lewy bodies. In Parkinson's disease, nerve cells that produce a neurochemical called **dopamine** die or become damaged.

Dopamine sends signals to the brain and normally acts to counter signals sent via **acetylcholine** (both then affect GABA), thereby coordinating movement. Symptoms that are characteristic of PD include tremors in the face, jaw, hands, arms, and legs. Stiffness of the extremities and trunk, slow movements, and altered coordination may also be seen. As symptoms worsen with progression of the disease, the patient may eventually lose the abilities to walk and speak; have difficulty chewing or swallowing; develop depression; and/or lose the ability to perform simple tasks. Sleep disturbances may be an early sign of PD, emerging even before motor symptoms have begun, and may include insomnia, excessive daytime sleepiness, restless leg syndrome, sleep apnea, and nocturia, among numerous other symptoms (**FIGURE 4-7**).

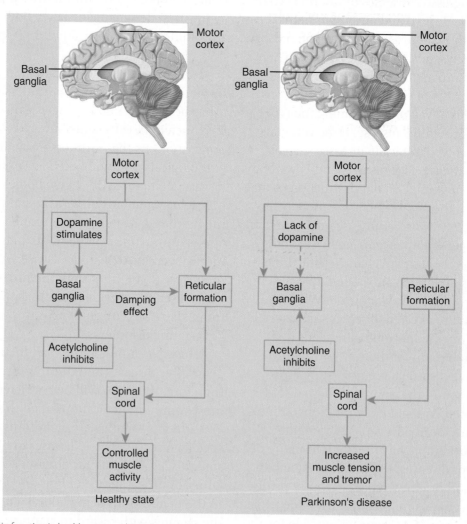

FIGURE 4-7 Brain function in healthy state and in Parkinson's disease.

Parkinson's disease usually begins around age 60 but may start earlier. It affects men more than women. Although there is no cure for PD, numerous medications are utilized to help control symptoms. The drugs and drug classes commonly used in treating PD are discussed next. The drug classes covered here are of two types: (1) those that increase dopamine in the nerves and (2) those that decrease acetylcholine in the nerves.

Carbidopa–Levodopa

The first and most effective drug for PD is carbidopa–levodopa, as levodopa, upon crossing the blood-brain barrier, is converted to dopamine, thus offering replacement therapy. Other dopamine agonists that may be prescribed for PD are pramipexole and ropinirole. Other drugs used are the monoamine oxidase B (MAO-B) inhibitor selegiline, the action of which enhances the effect of levodopa; the catechol-o-methyltransferase (COMT) inhibitor entacapone; and the anticholinergics benzatropine and amantadine, which decrease or block acetylcholine. Some of these drugs will be discussed in more detail here, chosen for their different actions.

Carbidopa-Levodopa

Carbidopa–levodopa is a catecholamine combination; it is considered the most effective medication for use in PD. Administration of dopamine itself is ineffective in the treatment of PD, as this agent does not cross the blood–brain barrier. However, levodopa, the metabolic precursor of dopamine, *does* cross the blood–brain barrier and is converted to dopamine in the brain. It therefore serves to supplement existing dopamine in affected neurons. Levodopa is rapidly decarboxylated to dopamine in extracerebral tissues so that only a small portion of a given dose is transported unchanged to the CNS. For this reason, large doses of levodopa are required for adequate therapeutic effect, but their administration may be accompanied by nausea and other adverse reactions, some of which are attributable to dopamine formed in extracerebral tissues. When levodopa is combined with carbidopa, however, decarboxylation of peripheral levodopa is prevented. The carbidopa does not cross the blood–brain barrier and does not affect the metabolism of levodopa within the CNS. Because its decarboxylase-inhibiting activity is limited to extracerebral tissues, administration of carbidopa with levodopa makes more levodopa available for transport to the brain (Merck & Co., 1999).

Carbidopa–levodopa combinations are used for PD or Parkinsonism-like syndrome caused by such factors as cerebral arteriosclerosis, carbon monoxide poisoning, and chronic manganese intoxication. These medications have also been used in restless leg syndrome. As with any drug, side effects are common, most of which are related to either dopaminergic or opposing cholinergic effects on motor movement, and have included dyskinesias, such as choreiform, dystonic, and other involuntary movements, and nausea. There is an increased risk of upper gastrointestinal bleeding in patients with a history of peptic ulcer disease who are being treated with carbidopa–levodopa formulations, just as when they are treated with levodopa alone. Dark brown, red, or black discoloration of urine, saliva, and sweat may also be seen; other side effects include anorexia, constipation, dry mouth, back and shoulder pain, dyspnea, fatigue, depression, psychosis, and bradykinetic episodes ("on-off" phenomenon), among others.

A more serious condition, neuroleptic malignant syndrome (NMS), is an uncommon but life-threatening condition characterized by fever or hypothermia. Neurologic findings include muscle rigidity, involuntary movements, altered consciousness, and mental status changes; other disturbances such as autonomic dysfunction, tachycardia, tachypnea, sweating, and hypertension or hypotension, along with laboratory findings such as creatine phosphokinase elevation, leukocytosis, myoglobinuria, and increased serum myoglobin, have been reported as well.

Early diagnosis of this condition is important for the appropriate management of affected patients, which may include intensive treatment and medical monitoring and treatment of any concomitant serious medical problems for which specific therapies are available. Dopamine agonists such as **bromocriptine** and muscle relaxants such as **dantrolene** are often used in the treatment of NMS; however, their effectiveness has not been demonstrated in controlled studies (Merck & Co., 1999).

Carbidopa–levodopa has been found to pass into breastmilk, so it is contraindicated for use during pregnancy or while breastfeeding. It is also contraindicated in patients with chronic wide-angle glaucoma, as it can affect intraocular pressure, which must be monitored during therapy. If there is any history of malignant melanoma or undiagnosed skin lesions resembling melanoma, the patient must be monitored carefully for development of melanomas. Epidemiological studies have shown that patients with PD have a higher risk (two to approximately six times higher) of developing melanoma compared to the general population (Huang, Yang, Chen, & Xiao, 2015).

Overdose with **carbidopa–levodopa** is rare, but treatment is the same as the management of acute overdosage with **levodopa**: General supportive measures are employed along with emergent gastric lavage. Intravenous fluids should be administered cautiously and a satisfactory airway maintained. Cardiac telemetry monitoring should be instituted and the patient carefully observed for arrhythmias. The healthcare provider should also investigate whether the patient may have taken other drugs in addition to **carbidopa–levodopa**.

Nursing Process for Carbidopa–Levodopa
Assess

Monitor the patient for any known PD symptoms such as tremors, "pill rolling" (a rhythmic, muscle contraction and relaxation involving to-and-fro movements of the fingers), drooling, akinesia, rigidity of extremities or trunk, or a shuffling gait. Obtain baseline vital signs and track the patient's blood pressure and respirations. Notify the primary provider if there are episodes of orthostatic hypotension, or changes in heart rate and rhythm. Be aware of any changes in the patient's affect, mood, and behavior; watch for onset of depression; and perform a complete suicide assessment. Muscle twitching or uncontrolled spasms of the eyelids may occur and indicate toxicity. Monitor renal, hepatic, and hematopoietic tests, as well as those for diabetes and acromegaly, in long-term use.

Administer

Carbidopa–levodopa is given orally as disintegrating tablets. When administering the medication to the patient, do not crush or let the patient chew the extended-release tablets, although they may be broken in half if necessary. The patient's dosage should be adjusted according to the response to the medication. The tablets are administered by gently placing them on the tongue and swallowing with saliva; after the tablet dissolves, liquids are not necessary.

Ask patients to take the medication with meals if GI symptoms occur; limit protein intake, as this can decrease the absorption of the drug. Do not initiate the drug until nonselective monoamine oxidase inhibitors have been discontinued for a minimum of 2 weeks. If the patient was previously on **levodopa**, discontinue it for at least 12 hours before changing to **carbidopa–levodopa**.

Pyridoxine (B_6) is required by the body for utilization of energy from the foods we eat, production of red blood cells, and proper functioning of nerves. It is a cofactor for the enzyme (among many) *DOPA decarboxylase*, which is responsible for converting 5-hydroxytryptophan (5-HTP) into serotonin (and then also melatonin), and for converting levodopa (L-DOPA) into dopamine (DA). DA, then, can be further converted to norepinephrine and epinephrine. Because pyridoxine is very ubiquitous in nature, deficiencies are not normally seen in humans, except in absorption deficiency diseases, such as alcoholism. A lack of pyroxidine in the body may lead to anemia, nerve damage, seizures, skin problems, and sores in the mouth when **carbidopa–levodopa** is administered. Pyridoxine is not effective in reversing the effects of **carbidopa-levodopa**, however.

Evaluate

Determine the therapeutic response of anti-Parkinson's medications based on the patient's decrease in "inner restlessness" or slowness of movement (akathisia/bradykinesis), tremors, rigidity, and improved mood.

Patient/Family Education

When educating the patient and family members, remind them that the patient should change positions or rise slowly to prevent orthostatic hypotension. If side effects are noted, report them to the primary provider immediately—especially such symptoms as twitching or blepharospasms, which may indicate overdose. Explain to the patient that his or her urine, sputum, or perspiration may darken, which could stain clothing. Instruct the patient to take the medication as prescribed, and advise the patient that discontinuing the medication abruptly could initiate Parkinson's crisis or NMS. If a patient needs to discontinue the medication, do so by tapering the medication gradually.

Encourage patients to continue physical activity or therapy to maintain mobility and function and to lessen muscle spasms. Remind them that improvement may not be seen for two to four months after initiation of **carbidopa–levodopa** therapy and that they may experience the "on-off phenomenon."

Ropinirole

Ropinirole is an anti-Parkinson's agent that acts as a dopamine receptor agonist in idiopathic PD; it is also used for the treatment of restless leg syndrome (RLS). It is a nonergot dopamine agonist with high relative *in vitro* specificity and full intrinsic activity at the D_2 subfamily of dopamine receptors, binding with *higher* affinity to D_3 than to the D_2

or D_4 subtypes; that is, this agent binds the dopamine receptors D_2 and D_3. Although the precise mechanism of **ropinirole's** action as a treatment for Parkinson's disease is unknown, it is believed to be related to the drug's ability to stimulate these receptors in the *striatum*. This conclusion is supported by electrophysiological studies in animals demonstrating that **ropinirole** influences striatal neuronal firing rates via activation of dopamine receptors in the striatum and the substantia nigra, the site of neurons that send projections to the striatum (Wishart et al., 2008).

Side effects of this medication are similar to those associated with other anti-Parkinson's drugs. **Ropinirole** should be avoided in pregnancy, and precautions should be taken with patients who experience dysrhythmias, cardiac disease, hepatic disease, renal disease, psychosis, or affective disorder.

Symptoms of overdose include confusion, agitation, chest pain, drowsiness, facial muscle movements, grogginess, increased jerkiness of movement, symptoms of low blood pressure (dizziness, lightheadedness) upon standing, nausea, and vomiting. It is anticipated that the symptoms of overdose with **ropinirole** will be related to its dopaminergic activity, so general supportive measures are recommended—for example, maintenance of vital signs or removal of any unabsorbed material (e.g., by gastric lavage).

Nursing Process for Ropinirole

Assess

Patient monitoring will be the same for **ropinirole** as for most anti-Parkinson's agents, such as monitoring for PD symptoms that either worsen or improve, obtaining a baseline of the patient's vital signs, and watching for possible changes during treatment, especially issues with hypertension or hypotension, and reporting them to the primary provider.

One symptom to be aware of with **ropinirole** is "*sleep attacks*" or *narcolepsy*. Sudden drowsiness or falling asleep without warning, especially during hazardous activities, should be reported immediately. Also monitor the patient's mental status for any changes in affect, mood, or behavior; watch for signs of depression; and perform a complete suicide assessment. Watch for worsening signs or symptoms in restless leg syndrome as well.

If the patient is on long-term therapy, provide testing for conditions such as diabetes mellitus and acromegaly, as these conditions may worsen with use of **ropinirole**. Monitor and report the therapeutic response for the patient, noting any improvement in movement and other symptoms of Parkinson's disease.

Administer

When administering **ropinirole**, provide it exactly as directed by the primary provider. Continue administering the medicine as ordered, unless or until the patient is NPO (nothing by mouth) prior to any surgery. Adjust the dosage according to the patient's response to medication and taper gradually when discontinuing. If the patient experiences GI symptoms, the medication should be taken with meals to reduce nausea. The extended-release tablets should not be chewed, crushed, or divided.

Patient/Family Education

When providing education to the patient, explain that when beginning a new medication, the therapeutic effects may take several weeks to a few months to be seen. If the patient will be changing positions or standing, he or she should do so slowly to prevent orthostatic hypotension. Explain to the patient that he or she must use the medication exactly as prescribed by the primary provider and

that abrupt discontinuation of the medication could lead to Parkinsonian crisis.

Recall that acetylcholine is released from a presynaptic neuron into the synaptic cleft (the space between the presynaptic neuron and postsynaptic neuron), where it then can bind the postsynaptic neuron at acetylcholine receptors. Effects on the sympathetic system are then ultimately through norepinephrine, via nicotinic receptorsfor acetylcholine, and on alpha and beta receptors for norepinephrine. Effects on the parasympathetic system are ultimately through muscarinic and nicotinic receptors. Acetylcholine receptors are subdivided into muscarinic- and nicotinic-types. Acetylcholine receptors—and therefore acetylcholine signal transmission—are found in the central and autonomic nervous systems (both muscarinic and nicotinic), and at neuromuscular junctions (muscarinic). Acetylcholine helps regulate various functions, including sleep, memory, muscle movement, and organ functions.

There are five known types of muscarinic receptors, and two types of nicotinic receptors. These are shown in TABLE 4-5. Acetylcholine is degraded by the enzyme acetylcholinesterase. Drugs may be introduced that either increase acetylcholine effects, or decrease acetylcholine effects. Some methods employ affecting acetylcholinesterase, usually inhibition, to slow the degradation of acetylcholine.

Benztropine

Benztropine is an anticholinergic agent that works by *blocking acetylcholine*. The action of acetylcholine is normally balanced by

TABLE 4-5	Acetylcholine Receptor Subtypes and Locations	
Acetylcholine Receptor	Subtype	Location
Muscarinic	M1	CNS
	M2	Heart
	M3	Smooth muscle
	M4	CNS
	M5	CNS
Nicotinic	N1	Neuromuscular junction
	N2	Autonomic ganglia; CNS; adrenal medulla

dopamine; in PD, however, because dopamine is depleted, decreasing the acetylcholine helps rebalance dopamine/acetylcholine actions on GABA neurons. This, in turn, helps in decreasing muscle rigidity, perspiring, and production of saliva, and works to improve ambulation in patients with Parkinson's disease. Benztropine is used to treat symptoms of PD as well as to diminish the involuntary movements arising from a variety of psychiatric drugs, such as the antipsychotics chlorpromazine and haloperidol. It is not helpful in treating problems with movement caused by tardive dyskinesia.

Potential side effects of benztropine are related to its anticholinergic activity and include drowsiness, dizziness, blurred vision, constipation, flushing, nausea, nervousness, and dry mouth. This medication is contraindicated in children younger than three years and in persons with tardive dyskinesia. Serious interactions have been reported with the medication pramlintide, a relatively new adjunct in the treatment of type 1 and 2 diabetes.

Symptoms of overdose may occur if too much benztropine is ingested. The specific effects of an overdose vary depending on how much of the medication was taken and whether it was ingested with other substances. As an anticholinergic medication, benztropine is prone to causing anticholinergic side effects, which may be more severe if too much is taken. These side effects include drowsiness, hallucinations, difficulty swallowing, muscle weakness, heart palpitations, blurred vision, and difficult or painful urination, among others.

Treatment for benztropine overdose may include gastric lavage if the overdose was recent, or administering certain medications to induce vomiting or absorb the medication from the digestive tract. An antidote, physostigmine, may be given to counteract the effects of the benztropine. Other measures include supportive care such as intravenous fluids, and cardiac monitoring and treatment of symptoms that result from the overdose.

Nursing Process for Benztropine

Assess

As with all medications, vital signs will be monitored while a patient is on benztropine, especially upon initiation of the drug. Blood work including monitoring of kidney and liver function is vital. Watch for a therapeutic response of documentable improvement of Parkinson's symptoms, while at the same time monitoring for any side effects or worsening symptoms.

Administer

Benztropine may be administered either with food or on an empty stomach. If the medication is ordered only once a day, it is recommended that it be taken at bedtime to avoid daytime drowsiness. Administer the medication at the same time each day to maintain constant blood levels. *Do not administer* injectable benztropine if the vial appears to be cloudy or have precipitate. Be sure to monitor the patient's blood work for renal or hepatic toxicity. Evaluate for a therapeutic response in the patient, including noticeable improvement of symptoms, and watch for any adverse effects of the medication.

Patient/Family Education

Teach the patient and family members that the medication should be taken exactly as directed; do not increase, decrease, or abruptly discontinue the drug without consulting a primary provider, as doing so could lead to serious side effects or worsening of symptoms. Benztropine should be taken at the same time each day to maintain constant blood levels; the medication may be taken with or without food. Do not use alcohol, prescription or over-the-counter sedatives, or CNS depressants without consulting a primary provider, as these substances could worsen side effects of the drug or affect the drug's efficacy.

The patient who is taking benztropine may experience drowsiness, dizziness, confusion, or blurred vision, so encourage patients not to drive, climb stairs, or operate machinery until their response to the drug is known. The medication should be used with caution in hot weather, as it can make the patient more susceptible to heat stroke due to the drug's side effect of decreasing perspiration; maintain adequate fluids and reduce exercise activity where possible. Report any unresolved nausea, vomiting, or gastric disturbances; rapid or pounding heartbeat, or chest pain; difficulty breathing; hallucinations; memory loss; anxiety; prolonged fever; pain; difficulty urinating; increased spasticity; or rigidity to the primary provider immediately.

Amantadine

Amantadine was serendipitously found to have anti-Parkinsonian effects in 1968, when it was seen to improve rest tremor, rigidity, and akinesia in a PD patient who had been prescribed the drug for influenza A prophylaxis. The female patient improved during the six-week duration of therapy and saw a return of symptoms when the drug was discontinued (Adler, 2002). Today, amantadine is used as prophylaxis or treatment of influenza type A, extrapyramidal symptoms, Parkinsonism, and Parkinson's disease.

Amantadine's mechanism of action in PD is not fully defined, but data from previous studies have suggested that amantadine hydrochloride *may* have *both direct* and *indirect* effects on *dopamine* neurons (Adler, 2002). Amantadine causes release of dopamine from the neurons, thereby rebalancing actions with acetylcholine. More recent studies have shown that it is a weak, noncompetitive **N-methyl-D-aspartate (NMDA)** receptor *antagonist* (Paquette et al., 2012). Although amantadine has not demonstrated direct anticholinergic activity, it does exhibit anticholinergic-like effects such as dry mouth, urinary retention, and constipation.

Nursing Process for Amantadine

Assess

As treatment is initiated and while it is ongoing, closely monitor the patient's intake and output ratios, reporting any frequency or hesitancy; also obtain baseline serum BUN and creatinine levels prior to beginning treatment. Be aware of patient allergies before initiation of treatment, and the potential reactions of amantadine with each medication that the patient is taking. Monitor hematologic status for signs of leukopenia or agranulocytosis. Be aware of the patient's bowel patterns before and during treatment. Watch the patient for signs of congestive heart failure (CHF), such as weight gain, dyspnea, crackles, and jugular vein distention. Monitor respiratory status, noting rate, quality, and presence of wheezing or tightness in the chest. After administering amantadine, watch for skin irritation and possible photosensitivity.

Question patients regarding symptoms and report to the primary provider if worsening gait, tremors, akinesia, or rigidity is noted. Monitor closely for signs of toxicity such as confusion, behavioral changes, hypotension, or seizures. Also be aware of a condition called livedo reticularis, characterized by mottling of the skin, usually red, with lower extremity edema and pruritus often present.

Administer

Administer the medication in divided doses to prevent CNS symptoms such as headache, dizziness, fatigue, and drowsiness. The patient should take amantadine after meals for better absorption and to decrease possible GI symptoms, and at least four hours before bedtime to prevent insomnia. Amantadine capsules should be stored in a tight, dry container.

Evaluate

Document the patient's response to the medication. The patient should be observed for the presence (or absence) of tremors and a shuffling gait as seen in Parkinson's disease.

Patient/Family Education

Teach patients that when repositioning themselves or beginning to rise from a lying or sitting position, they should do so slowly to prevent orthostatic hypotension. To avoid injury, they should also avoid any hazardous activities, including driving or climbing stairs, if dizziness or blurred vision occurs.

Explain to patients that they must take amantadine exactly as prescribed by the primary provider. They should not discontinue this medication abruptly, as Parkinsonian crisis may occur. If a dose is missed, the patient should be advised to take the medication if it is still within four hours after the missed dose. Otherwise, the patient should skip the missed dose and resume the regimen at the next regular dosing time. Capsules may be opened and mixed with food. If shortness of breath, sudden weight gain, dizziness, poor concentration, dysuria, or behavioral changes manifest, notify the primary provider immediately. Explain to patients that they should avoid alcohol while taking this medication, as adverse effects may occur.

Alzheimer Disease

Alzheimer disease (AD) is a neurogenerative disorder that is the most common form of *dementia*, a general term for loss of memory and other intellectual abilities serious enough to interfere with daily life. Alzheimer disease accounts for 50% to 80% of dementia cases (Alzheimer's Association, 2017).

Alzheimer disease is distinguished by the loss of nerve cells and synapses in the *cerebral cortex* and *subcortical* regions of the brain as well as the appearance of *plaques* and *tangles*, which make this disease unique (FIGURE 4-8). This loss results in profuse deterioration of the affected regions, including degeneration of the *temporal and parietal lobes*, and parts of the *frontal cortex* and *cingulate gyrus*. Aberrations in beta-amyloid, tau, and ApoE functionality have been associated intra- and extracellularly with AD. It is believed that these changes within and outside neurons lead to altered acetylcholine, glutamate, and other neurotransmitter concentrations and effectiveness.

Alzheimer disease is an irreversible, progressive brain disease that slowly destroys memory, reasoning, judgment, communication, and the ability to carry out simple tasks and activities of daily living. The disease worsens as it progresses and eventually leads to death. Most often, AD is diagnosed in people older than 65 years of age, although it is not just a disease of old age. As many as 5% of affected people have the less-prevalent early-onset AD, which can occur much earlier—when someone is in his or her 40s or 50s. Although some medications can slow the progression and help manage symptoms of the disease, there is currently no cure. AD affects women at approximately twice the rate as men. The reason for this is still not clear.

Although Alzheimer disease develops differently in every individual, there are many common symptoms. Early symptoms are often mistaken for "age-related" concerns, or manifestations of stress. In the disease's early stages, the most common symptom is difficulty in remembering recent events. When AD is suspected, the diagnosis is usually confirmed with tests that evaluate behavior and thinking abilities, and can be followed by a *positron emission tomography* (PET) scan if available (FIGURE 4-9). As the disease advances, symptoms may include confusion, irritability, aggression, mood swings, trouble with language, and long-term memory loss. As the patient declines, he or she often withdraws from family and society. Gradually, bodily functions are lost, ultimately leading to death (Waldemar, 2007).

The U.S. Food and Drug Administration (FDA) has approved *four* medications for the treatment of Alzheimer disease: donepezil, galantamine, memantine, and rivastigmine. *Three* of the FDA-approved medications are in the same drug class—namely, cholinesterase inhibitors. These drugs work to curb the breakdown of acetylcholine, a chemical in the brain that is important for memory and learning, by *inhibiting an enzyme*, acetylcholinesterase, that is responsible for the metabolism of acetylcholine; as a result, concentrations of

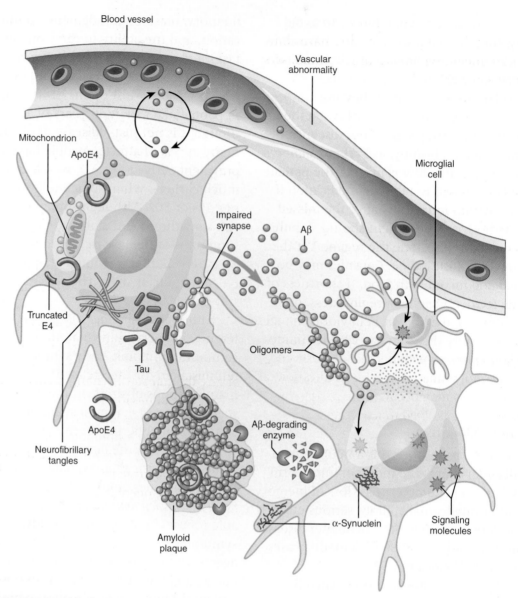

FIGURE 4-8 Some key players in the pathogenesis of AD.

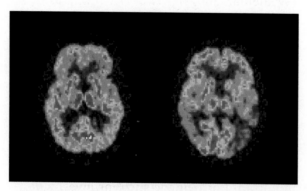

FIGURE 4-9 A brain scan comparison between a healthy brain and a brain afflicted with Alzheimer disease.

acetylcholine increase in the brain and symptomatic improvement is seen. While these drugs may reduce symptoms for approximately half the people taking them for a limited time, on average 6 to 12 months, the medications do not slow the progression of Alzheimer disease overall, and their effects are, for the most part, temporary.

Donepezil is the only cholinesterase inhibitor approved by the FDA for *all stages* (mild, moderate, and severe) of AD. The other listed cholinesterase inhibitors are used only in mild-to-moderate states of the disease. All cholinesterase inhibitors share common side effects, which are usually mild, such as nausea, vomiting, loss of appetite, and increased frequency of bowel movements due to cholinergic effects. Cholinesterase inhibitors also have *vagotonic effects* that may lead to bradycardia or complete heart block. Patients taking these drugs should be monitored for active gastrointestinal bleeding, weight loss, bladder outflow obstructions, and generalized convulsions. These drugs should be prescribed with care for patients with a history of asthma or chronic obstructive pulmonary disease (COPD).

The fourth FDA-approved drug, **memantine**, is used to treat moderate-to-severe AD, but its mechanism differs from that of the other approved drugs. **Memantine** is an (NMDA) receptor antagonist, acting by regulating the effects of glutamate, a chemical messenger involved in learning and memory. Glutamate is released in large amounts by cells damaged by AD and other neurologic disorders. Glutamate causes a magnesium ion in the NMDA receptor to dislocate. When the magnesium exits its NMDA receptor docking location, calcium influx is allowed, causing post-synaptic propagation. Slow leakage of glutamate from presynaptic neurons keeps NMDA receptors constantly activated. Over time, this leads to chronic overexposure to calcium, which can speed up neuronal damage and death, because the neurons are in a state of continuous stimulation. **Memantine** prevents this destructive chain of events by partially blocking the NMDA receptors (Alzheimer's Association, 2017), and is considered a **noncompetitive antagonist** (see Chapter 2).

The most common side effects seen with **memantine** are fatigue, dizziness, confusion, headache, hypertension, vomiting, constipation, back pain, hallucination, coughing, and shortness of breath. **Memantine** may cause a serious skin reaction called Stevens-Johnson syndrome. Co-occurring conditions in which

use of this drug should be avoided if possible include pregnancy, breastfeeding, renal disease, genitourinary conditions that affect or raise urine pH, history of seizures, and severe hepatic disease.

Nursing Process

Assess

When initiating medication for AD treatment, obtain the patient's baseline vital signs and then monitor them regularly, especially blood pressure for signs of hypertension. Continually assess GI status for signs of vomiting or constipation, and add bulk to the diet and increase fluids for issues with constipation. Monitor GU status for urinary frequency; monitor serum creatinine levels. Note whether the patient is having respiratory problems such as dyspnea. Be aware of any mental status changes such as affect, mood, and behavioral changes, and appearance of hallucinations or confusion. Assist the patient with ambulation during the onset of therapy, as dizziness may occur. Evaluate the therapeutic response of the patient, documenting decreased confusion and/or improved mood.

Administer

Instruct the patient to take the medication with a full glass of water and note that it may be taken without regard to meals. If the dose is greater than 5 mg, the total *daily* **memantine** should be divided into two doses. Adjust the dose according to the patient's response to medication, but no more than once a week. Patients should not crush, chew, or divide the extended-release capsules; instead, they should swallow the capsules whole or open them and sprinkle their contents on applesauce before swallowing. Remind patients that when using oral solutions of the drugs, they should use the dosing device provided with the medication and follow the instructions given. Oral solutions should not be ingested with any other liquids.

Patient/Family Education

Instruct patients to take their medication(s) regularly for best effect, and refill prescriptions before running out of the medication(s). If a dose is missed, the patient should take it as soon as remembered, unless it is almost time for the succeeding dose; in that case, the patient should skip the missed dose and take the medicine at the regularly scheduled time. The patient *should not* take extra medicine to make up for the missed dose. These are general guidelines regarding missed doses. Always refer to the literature regarding each drug's unique dosing requirements, *including* instructions for missed doses.

Remind patients to take the medication exactly as prescribed by the primary provider and explain that, while the drug will alleviate symptoms, it is not a cure for AD. Unless otherwise indicated by the drug's literature, medications should be taken with a full glass of water; they generally may be taken with or without food (again, refer to specific drug requirements). When taking oral suspensions, the included dispenser (where applicable) should be used, and other liquids should not be mixed with the medication. Capsules may be taken intact or opened and sprinkled over applesauce or pudding and then swallowed. **Memantine** must be stored at room temperature away from moisture and heat.

These medications may cause side effects that impair the patient's thinking or actions; consequently, patients should not participate in dangerous activities or driving until the effects of the medication are known. Instruct patients to report any side effects such as restlessness, psychosis, visual hallucinations, stupor, or changes in level of consciousness, as these symptoms may indicate overdose.

Amyotrophic Lateral Sclerosis

The final neurodegenerative disorder addressed in this chapter is amyotrophic lateral sclerosis (ALS). This disease, also known as Lou Gehrig disease or motor neuron disease (MND), is a progressive neurodegenerative disease with varied etiology characterized by rapidly progressive weakness, muscle atrophy and fasciculations, muscle spasticity, and difficulty speaking, swallowing, and breathing. ALS is the most common of the five motor neuron diseases.

The defining feature of ALS is the *death of both upper and lower motor neurons in the motor cortex* of the brain, the *brain stem*, and the *spinal cord*. Prior to their destruction, motor neurons develop proteinaceous inclusions in their cell bodies and axons; this may be partly due to defects in protein degradation. These inclusions often contain ubiquitin, and they generally incorporate one of the ALS-associated proteins: SOD1, TAR DNA binding protein (TDP-43, or TARDBP), or FUS. As motor neurons begin to deteriorate and die, the ability to initiate and send messages to the muscles in the body is lost. In turn, the muscles slowly lose their function, begin to atrophy, and demonstrate involuntary muscle contractions.

As with Alzheimer disease, studies of ALS have focused on the role of glutamate in motor neuron degeneration. It was mentioned previously that glutamate is one of the chemical messengers in the brain, but its importance in transmitting nerve impulses is not limited solely to the brain. Scientists have found that in comparison to healthy individuals, ALS patients have higher levels of glutamate in their serum and spinal fluid (Al-Chalabi & Leigh, 2000; Obál et al., 2016).

Commonly, the progression of ALS starts with the patient's speech being affected to the point that he or she is eventually unable to speak or vocalize. The disease then begins to affect the individual's ability to chew and swallow. This deteriorates to a point to where the patient may even be unable to swallow pureed foods or his or her own saliva, at which point the primary provider may recommend placement of a feeding tube so that the patient receives adequate nutrition. Finally, the individual begins to lose strength in the extremities, weakening with little activity or exertion, and losing the ability to perform tasks that require manual dexterity such as buttoning a shirt or unlocking the front door.

Although there is devastating loss of motor function, ALS does not affect a person's mind. The person's personality, intelligence, memory, and self-awareness, as well as the senses of smell, sight, touch, hearing, and taste, remain intact. While ALS initially may affect only one side of the body, or a single leg or arm, eventually the person is unable to walk, stand, or perform any activities without assistance, yet remains completely alert and aware of the changes taking place.

The majority of ALS cases diagnosed in the United States each year, approximately 90% to 95%, have no association with genetic inheritance. Worldwide epidemiological research has shown associations with ALS to occupations including heavy labor, exposure to heavy metals, or history of a traumatic head injury (Lacorte et al., 2016; Yu et al., 2014). With the exception of an unusually high frequency of cases in the western Pacific, particularly in Guam, there is no pattern of geographic clustering, nor is ALS associated with a particular race or educational level.

Currently, there is no cure for ALS. As with most incurable diseases, the main focus of treatment is symptom management or palliative care. As more research is carried out on brain diseases, scientists are learning more about what causes ALS and how best to treat it.

Riluzole, an *anti-glutamate agent*, is the first FDA-approved drug for the treatment of patients with ALS. Results in clinical trials have indicated that this drug shows some promise in prolonging lives. While its mechanism of action is relatively unknown, its pharmacologic properties include an inhibitory effect on glutamate release, inactivation of voltage-dependent sodium channels, and an ability to interfere with intracellular events that follow transmitter binding at excitatory amino acid receptors. **Riluzole** has also demonstrated neuroprotective properties in various *in vivo* experimental models of neuronal injury involving excitotoxic mechanisms. In *in vitro* tests, **riluzole** protected cultured rat motor neurons from the excitotoxic effects of glutamic acid and prevented the death of cortical neurons induced by anoxia. Due to its blockade of glutamatergic neurotransmission, **riluzole** also exhibits myorelaxant and sedative properties in animal models (Bellingham, 2011).

Numerous side effects can occur with **riluzole** therapy, the most common of which are asthenia, nausea, dizziness, decreased lung function, diarrhea, abdominal pain, pneumonia, vomiting, vertigo, circumoral paresthesia, anorexia, and sleepiness. There is no specific antidote or information on treatment of overdosage with **riluzole**, and experience with overdose in humans is limited. Neurologic and psychiatric symptoms including amnesic syndrome, acute toxic encephalopathy with stupor, coma, and methemoglobinemia have been observed in isolated cases (Cardoos, Inamori, Sanacora, Fava, & Mischoulon, 2013; Viallon, Page, & Bertrand, 2000). Treatment should be supportive and directed toward alleviating symptoms.

Nursing Process

Assess

Evaluate the patient for clinical improvement in neurologic function. Monitor hepatic studies such as AST, ALT, GGT, and bilirubin, along with liver function tests (LFTs), by obtaining baseline lab values and then performing follow-up lab work every month for three months, then every three months to adequately track liver function (**riluzole** is metabolized in the liver). Follow lab results for signs of neutropenia (i.e., neutrophils numbering less than 500 cells/mm^3).

Administer

Give the medication one hour before or two hours after meals; note that a high-fat meal will decrease **riluzole's** absorption. Evaluate the patient's response to the medication, watching for signs of neurologic improvement.

Patient/Family Education

Explain to patients the reason they are being given this medication and the expected results. Remind them that there is no current cure for ALS. Ask patients to report any febrile illness, signs of infection, or any cardiac or respiratory changes that may indicate neutropenia.

Other medications that may be used for ALS, or other neurodegenerative disorders, include *antidepressants* such as amitriptyline to reduce excess saliva production, *muscle relaxants* such as diazepam or baclofen, and *pain medications* for discomfort. As there is no known cure for ALS, these medications, along with proper nutrition, physical and occupational therapy, and use of braces, a wheelchair, or other orthopedic measures, are meant to maximize functioning, provide optimal general health to the patient, and prolong life.

Musculoskeletal Dysfunction

Neurologic musculoskeletal disorders stem from a variety of causes. Some are straightforward: An individual strains or overstretches a tendon or muscle during strenuous activity and experiences pain and, in the case of muscle injuries, spasm. Such injuries are usually acute and very common; indeed, low back and neck pain developing as a result of acute injury or, in many cases, from repetitive stress injury is among the top causes of work-related disability among adults (Theis, Roblin, Helmick, & Luo, 2017). Acute injuries can also evolve into chronic pain (pain lasting more than three months), which can be difficult to resolve. But the causes of other *CNS disorders* affecting the musculoskeletal system are harder to elucidate. Headache, an extremely common neurologic condition, may be transiently related to psychological or physiological stress (e.g., tension headache), but may also be more chronic in nature (e.g., migraine). Fibromyalgia, a condition characterized by widespread muscle and joint pain,

has multiple neurologic facets but its etiology is as yet unknown.

Because most musculoskeletal neurologic disorders are accompanied by pain and loss of function, the medications used to treat them seek to relieve symptoms and restore function. Thus, the most commonly administered medications for these indications are **muscle relaxants**, which seek to ease painful and involuntary contraction of injured or overstimulated muscle cells, and **anesthetics**, which obstruct nerve impulses to prevent the transmission of pain signals.

Muscle Relaxants

Muscle relaxants are drugs used to treat muscle spasm and spasticity. **Muscle spasm** is defined as a sudden involuntary contraction of one or more muscle groups and is usually an acute condition associated with muscle strain or sprain. By contrast, **spasticity** is a state of increased muscular tone with amplification of the tendon reflexes and is often associated with disease states, illness, or injury such as multiple sclerosis, stroke, and spinal cord injury. Spasticity can severely limit functioning due to weakness, spasms, and loss of dexterity. The goal of muscle relaxant therapy is to improve function as well as to alleviate pain and simplify activities of daily living.

The use of muscle relaxants in painful disorders is based on the *theory* that pain can induce spasms and spasms cause pain— although considerable evidence *contradicts* this theory (Beebe, Barkin, & Barkin, 2005). Generally, muscle relaxants are not approved by the FDA for long-term use, though rheumatologists often prescribe the drug cyclobenzaprine nightly to increase stage 4 sleep, which has been found to be beneficial for patients suffering with fibromyalgia.

Muscle relaxants may be used to alleviate symptoms such as muscle spasms, hyperreflexia, and pain, often in conjunction with NSAIDs. The term *muscle relaxant* is often used as a blanket term to refer to two major therapeutic groups: **neuromuscular blockers** and **spasmolytics**.

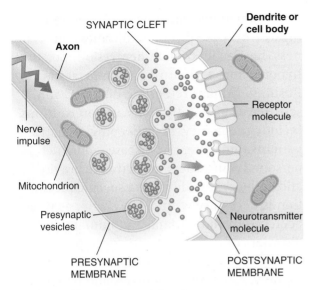

SYNAPTIC CLEFT

Dendrite or cell body

Axon

Receptor molecule

Nerve impulse

Mitochondrion

Presynaptic vesicles

Neurotransmitter molecule

PRESYNAPTIC MEMBRANE

POSTSYNAPTIC MEMBRANE

FIGURE 4-10 The path of transmission of neuromuscular impulses.

FIGURE 4-10 depicts neuromuscular transmission. Neuromuscular blockers act by preventing neuromuscular transmission at the neuromuscular junction, causing paralysis of the affected skeletal muscles. This occurs in two ways—either presynaptically or postsynaptically. In the presynaptic pathway, muscles are affected via the inhibition of *acetylcholine (Ach)* synthesis or release. Postsynaptically, these medications act at the *acetylcholine receptors* of the motor nerve endplate. Botulinum toxin and tetanus toxin are drugs that act presynaptically; the drugs of clinical importance that are used most often act postsynaptically. Neuromuscular blockers do *not* affect the CNS. They are most often administered during surgical procedures, intensive care, and emergency medicine to cause paralysis.

Spasmolytics or **antispasmodics** are referred to as "*centrally acting*" muscle relaxants. They are used to relieve musculoskeletal pain and spasms, and to diminish spasticity in a variety of neurologic disorders. While both types of agents are often grouped together as "muscle relaxants," the term commonly refers to spasmolytics only. Such drugs act by *blocking interneuronal pathways in the spinal cord* and in the *midbrain reticular activating system* by modifying the stretch reflex arc, or

by attenuation of excitation–contraction coupling process in the muscle itself.

Not every agent in this class has CNS activity, however; thus, even the label "centrally acting" is inaccurate. For example, **dantrolene**, which is a muscle relaxant, does not act on the CNS as the spasmolytics and antispasmodics do. This drug *belongs to its own distinct category*, directly acting agents.

Specific Drugs and Their Uses

Muscle relaxants such as **carisprodol**, **cyclobenzaprine**, **metaxalone**, and **methocarbamol** are often prescribed for tension headaches, myofascial pain syndrome, low back and neck pain, and fibromyalgia but are not considered first-line agents for pain. In *acute* pain, they are *no more* effective than NSAIDs, and even in conditions such as fibromyalgia, antidepressants are considered more beneficial. However, muscle relaxants are considered beneficial when used in *conjunction* with NSAIDs.

Carisprodol is a *centrally* acting skeletal muscle relaxant that depresses the CNS by interrupting neuronal communication within the descending reticular formation and spinal cord, resulting in sedation and alteration in pain perception. It is used as an adjunct in the symptomatic treatment of musculoskeletal conditions associated with painful muscle spasms.

Cyclobenzaprine is a *skeletal muscle relaxant and a CNS depressant*. It acts on the locus coeruleus, where it results in increased norepinephrine release, potentially through the gamma fibers that innervate and inhibit the alpha motor neurons in the ventral horn of the spinal cord. **Cyclobenzaprine** binds to the serotonin receptor and is considered a $5\text{-}HT_2$ receptor antagonist that reduces muscle tone by decreasing the activity of descending serotonergic neurons. It is commonly used as an adjunct with other medications for relief of pain and muscle spasms in several musculoskeletal conditions. **Cyclobenzaprine** has also been used for fibromyalgia.

Methocarbamol is a carbamate derivative that is a *centrally* acting skeletal muscle relaxant. It acts on the multisynaptic pathways by depressing them in the spinal cord, which in turn causes musculoskeletal relaxation. Methocarbamol is typically used as an adjunct with other medications to relieve spasms and pain in skeletal muscle conditions or in tetanus.

Baclofen is a *centrally* acting oral and injectable muscle relaxant and spasmolytic medication. It is a GABA chlorophenyl derivative. Baclofen, much like GABA, blocks the activity of nerves within the part of the brain that controls the contraction and relaxation of skeletal muscle. This agent is used for treating spasms of skeletal muscle clonus, rigidity, and pain caused by such conditions as ALS and multiple sclerosis.

Diazepam is a *centrally* acting, long-acting benzodiazepine that has antianxiety, anticonvulsant, and skeletal muscle relaxant properties. It heightens the actions of GABA, especially in the limbic system and reticular formation; it also inhibits reflexes, which are managed by control centers in the spinal cord. Diazepam is commonly used for anxiety, for acute alcohol withdrawal, and as an adjunct in seizure disorders. It has also been used preoperatively as a relaxant and for skeletal muscle relaxation, especially in conditions such as multiple sclerosis and ALS. Diazepam can be used rectally for acute repetitive seizures. Off-label uses have included agitation, insomnia, seizure prophylaxis, benzodiazepine withdrawal, and chloroquine overdose.

Dantrolene is a *direct-acting* skeletal muscle relaxant. Unlike the centrally acting drugs, it works by preventing intracellular release of calcium from the sarcoplasmic reticulum, which is necessary to initiate contraction. This drug also slows the breakdown of complex molecules in malignant hyperthermia. It is most commonly used for spasticity in multiple sclerosis, stroke, spinal cord injuries, cerebral palsy, and malignant hyperthermia.

Side Effects and Contraindications

Side effects produced by muscle relaxants as a group are similar. The most common effects a patient may experience when using any of these drugs are dizziness, drowsiness, headache, tremor, depression, postural hypotension, tachycardia, nausea, rash, flushing, urinary retention, diplopia, and seizures. Contraindications and precautions include pregnancy, breastfeeding, geriatric patients, renal/hepatic disease, addictive personality disorders, myasthenia gravis, and epilepsy. In addition, a specific precaution is necessary with dantrolene, as it has been observed that fatal and nonfatal liver disorders of an idiosyncratic or hypersensitivity type may occur with dantrolene therapy, especially in females and patients older than 35 years of age. Dantrolene should also be used with extreme caution with patients who have impaired pulmonary function or impaired cardiac function due to myocardial disease.

Nursing Process

Assess

While patients are on medications, monitor their vital signs such as blood pressure (both reclined and standing), pulse, and respiratory rate. Be aware that blood laboratory results can be affected by use of these products. Monitor CBC during long-term therapy for possible blood dyscrasias, though these conditions are rare. Due to the medications' effects on the liver, monitor hepatic laboratory results such as AST, ALT, bilirubin, creatinine, LDH, and alkaline phosphorus.

Assess the patient for relief of symptoms of pain and/or muscle spasms. If the patient has a history of seizures, monitor the type, duration, and intensity of seizures to dose these individuals appropriately. Regularly observe patients for degree of anxiety; attempt to ascertain factors that precipitate anxiety, and if the medication controls the symptoms. Observe patients' mental status for changes in mood, sensorium, affect, sleeping patterns, increased somnolence, vertigo, or suicidal tendencies.

If a patient has been prescribed a medication for alcohol withdrawal, observe and document changes in symptoms, which may include hallucinations (either visual or auditory), delirium, irritability, agitation, or fine to coarse tremors; these outcomes may indicate a need to adjust the dosage. In patients receiving intravenous medications, observe the IV site for any signs of thrombosis or phlebitis, which can occur during treatment.

Be observant for indicators that the patient may have become physically dependent on the medication. Likewise, monitor the patient for withdrawal symptoms, which may include headaches, nausea, vomiting, muscle pain, or weakness following long-term use.

Administer

Give oral medications with food or milk to prevent possible GI symptoms. Instruct the patient that medications may be crushed if the patient is unable to swallow the medication whole. If concentrated **diazepam** oral solutions are used, measure doses with calibrated droppers only. Liquid medications may be mixed with water, juice, pudding, or applesauce and should be ingested immediately. Remind patients that if they experience dry mouth, they should drink frequent sips of water or use sugarless gum or hard candy for relief.

Perform/Provide

At the beginning of therapy, assist patients with ambulation and standing as a safety measure and to prevent injury, in case they experience drowsiness or dizziness. Confirm that oral medication has been swallowed before leaving a patient.

Evaluate

Monitor the patient for an appropriate therapeutic response, which should include decreased anxiety, restlessness, and insomnia.

Patient/Family Education

Instruct patients that their medications may be taken with food or liquids. Patients should take the medication exactly as prescribed by the primary provider. Do not discontinue medication abruptly, but taper it gradually, as adverse reactions may occur otherwise.

Educate both patients and family members that these medications are not for "everyday stressors" and should not be used longer than four months unless directed by the primary provider. Instruct them to not take more than the prescribed amount and to recognize that such medications may be habit forming.

Explain to patients that drowsiness may occur or worsen at the beginning of treatment but should improve. Patients should be warned not to rise from a sitting position or lying position quickly, but rather to do so slowly, as dizziness or fainting may occur, especially with the elderly.

Remind patients to avoid concomitant use of over-the-counter medications unless first approved by their primary provider. Patients should not drive or perform any activities that require them to be alert, as these drugs may cause drowsiness. Nor should patients use alcohol or other psychotropic medications unless specifically allowed or ordered by the primary provider. Advise patients that smoking may decrease the effect of **diazepam** by increasing its rate of metabolism.

Local Anesthetics

Anesthetics are used for many different reasons. They can be used for pain that is not controlled using oral medications or other types of therapy, as well as for surgeries or other medical procedures. Types of anesthesia include general anesthesia, topical anesthesia, infiltration, plexus block, epidural block, and spinal anesthesia, among many others. Some of these are covered more in-depth in Chapter 15 ("Anesthetics").

Local anesthetics are drugs that cause reversible anesthesia in a specific location. They act mainly by *inhibiting the sodium influx* through sodium-specific ion channels in the neuronal cell membrane, in particular the voltage-gated sodium channels. When the influx of sodium is interrupted, an action potential cannot arise and the signal condition is inhibited. The drug receptor site is located at the cytoplasmic portion of the sodium channel.

Local anesthetic drugs produce an absence of pain sensation at a specific site, and though other local senses may be affected, this action occurs without changing the patient's awareness. When such agents are used on specific pathways (such as for nerve block), paralysis can be achieved as well. This is accomplished either by applying the anesthetic topically or by injecting a numbing medication into or on the area of interest, sometimes via several small injections; after a few minutes, the area should be numb. If the area is still sensitive, more anesthetic may be applied to achieve total numbness. Local anesthetics are most commonly associated with dental procedures, minor medical procedures such as receiving stitches, or for initiating IVs, but are used in many areas of the medical field for numerous other procedures as well.

Clinical local anesthetics belong to one of two classes: aminoamide and aminoester local anesthetics.

Synthetic local anesthetics are structurally related to cocaine. The difference is that the medications have no abuse potential and do not produce hypertension or local vasoconstriction, with the exception of ropivacaine and mepivacaine, which do produce mild vasoconstriction.

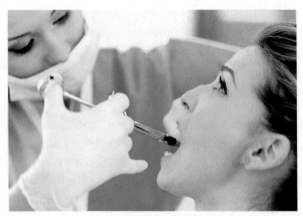

© Catalin Petolea/Shutterstock, Inc.

Specific Drugs and Uses

For the purpose of this chapter, only a few of the most commonly used local anesthetics will be discussed, as other forms of anesthesia are generally administered under fairly specific circumstances. The local anesthetics addressed here are procaine, lidocaine, and benzonatate.

Procaine is a local anesthetic drug of the *aminoester* group. It is primarily used to reduce the pain of intramuscular injection of penicillin but is also used in dentistry. Due to the ubiquity of the trade name Novocain, in many regions it is known generically as "novocain."

Procaine acts primarily by inhibiting sodium influx through *voltage-gated sodium channels* in the neuronal cell membranes of peripheral nerves. When the influx of sodium is interrupted, an action potential cannot arise; consequently, signal conduction is inhibited. The receptor site is thought to be located at the cytoplasmic portion of the sodium channel. Procaine has been shown to bind or antagonize the function of *NMDA receptors* as well as *nicotinic acetylcholine receptors* and the *serotonin receptor–ion channel complex* (Brau, Vogel, & Hempelmann, 1998), elaborated upon later in this text.

Side effects of procaine are minimal and mostly related to parenteral injection or spinal anesthesia uses. They may include adverse CNS and cardiovascular effects, under-ventilation, apnea, post-spinal headache, arachnoiditis, palsies, spinal nerve paralysis, hypotension, respiratory impairment, nausea, and vomiting.

Lidocaine is a local anesthetic and cardiac depressant that is used as an antiarrhythmic agent. It was the first *aminoamide*-type anesthetic synthesized. Lidocaine stabilizes the neuronal membrane by inhibiting the ionic fluxes required for the initiation and conduction of impulses, thereby effecting local anesthetic action. It alters signal conduction in neurons by blocking the fast voltage-gated sodium channels in the neuronal cell membrane that are responsible for signal propagation. With sufficient blockage, the membrane of the postsynaptic neuron will not transmit an action potential. This creates the anesthetic effect by not merely preventing pain signals from propagating to the brain, but rather by abolishing their origin (Muroi & Chanda, 2009).

Lidocaine is used topically to relieve itching, burning, and pain from skin inflammation; is injected as a dental anesthetic; and is used as a local anesthetic for minor surgery. Its side effects are generally mild and include flushing; redness of the skin; small red or purple spots on the skin; swelling at the site of application; unusually warm skin; bruising, burning, pain or bleeding at site of application; and itching of skin. Less common are symptoms of overdose, which would include change in consciousness, fainting, restlessness, coma, cardiac arrest, and rapid, bounding, or irregular heartbeat or pulse.

Benzonatate is a non-narcotic oral cough suppressant, or antitussive, with effects lasting six to eight hours. Because it is not an opioid, **benzonatate** is not prone to abuse like some other cough medications such as **codeine**. **Benzonatate** is a *butylamine*, so it is chemically related to other ester local anesthetics such as **procaine** and **tetracaine**. It acts as a *local* anesthetic, decreasing the sensitivity of *stretch receptors* in the lower airway and lung, thereby reducing the drive to cough after taking a deep breath.

Benzonatate acts *peripherally*, anesthetizing the stretch receptors of vagal afferent fibers in the alveoli of the lungs, bronchi, and pleura. Because these receptors are responsible for mediating the cough reflex, anesthetizing them results in inhibition of cough production. It also suppresses transmission of the cough reflex at the level of the *medulla*, where the afferent nerve impulse is normally transmitted to the motor nerves. When applied locally, **benzonatate** binds within the intracellular portion of voltage-gated sodium channels, decreasing the rate of membrane depolarization and increasing the threshold for electrical excitability (National Center for Biotechnology Information [NCBI], National Institutes of Health (NIH), & PubChem Compound, n.d.).

Numerous side effects are associated with **benzonatate**. The most common and milder adverse effects include burning sensation in eyes, constipation, dizziness, drowsiness, headache, itching, nausea, vomiting, and skin rash. More serious side effects and signs of overdose may include confusion, shortness of breath, hallucinations, tightness in the chest, wheezing, loss of consciousness, tremors in the extremities, and convulsions.

Nursing Process

Assess

During use of the medication, monitor the patient's blood pressure, pulse, and respirations. If the patient has a history of cardiac disease, obtain a baseline electrocardiogram and monitor it during parenteral or injectable therapies. Monitor the patient closely for possible allergic reactions, which may manifest as rash, urticaria, or itching.

Administer

Always use new solutions and discard any unused portions. Only use products that are *not cloudy* or have *no precipitate*. Protect the medication from *light*; keep it in a cool, dark place. Before administering medication, make sure that a crash cart and resuscitative equipment are nearby in case of emergency.

Evaluate

Ensure that an appropriate therapeutic response, providing sufficient anesthesia for the procedure, has been achieved.

Patient Education

Inform the patient about what to expect during the procedure, including what is being executed, expectations of the anesthetic, and possible transient or longer-lasting side effects. When the procedure is over, remind the patient not to arise too quickly to avoid possible dizziness due to orthostatic hypotension. Remind patients to call immediately if they experience side effects or notice areas of irritation or increased bleeding, warmth, or swelling at area of injection.

CHAPTER SUMMARY

This chapter has explored the CNS, touched briefly on the PNS, and discussed key conditions affecting the CNS as well as the drug classes most commonly used as treatments for specific CNS diseases and disorders. If there is one all-encompassing theme to this chapter, it is the principal necessity to support patients' ability to maintain physiological function and a sense of "normalcy" as they cope with the neurologic disorders for which they are being treated. Whether the problem is pain centered or focused on loss of memory (as in Alzheimer disease), physical capability (as in Parkinson's or ALS disease), or simply a matter of suppressing seizures, the therapeutic goal is the same: manage the condition with the goal of restoring normalcy to the extent possible. Where disease and/or symptom progression is inevitable, the goal becomes maintenance of high function and independence for as long as possible. In such cases (and, indeed, in any CNS disorder), medication is rarely used alone; it is most often supported with multiple adjunct therapies (or sometimes is better regarded as an adjunct to other modalities).

Key concepts include the importance of neurotransmitters such as *dopamine* and *acetylcholine* in brain-centered progressive disorders such as Alzheimer and Parkinson's disease, the function of glutamate and NDMA in memory and cognition, and the central role that prostaglandins play in inflammatory conditions. Management of pain is a challenging objective for the clinician because it is so often performed ineffectually. However, maintaining physiological function and supporting patients' ability to cope with various diseases and symptoms is as important as pain control.

Critical Thinking Questions

1. What are the advantages and disadvantages of NSAID analgesia versus opioid analgesia?

2. What distinguishes epilepsy from non-epileptic seizures? Why would therapy for each type of seizure disorder be different?

3. Name three common myths surrounding pain medications. How do these medications potentially affect therapy and clinical response to the patient?

4. In Alzheimer disease, the key diagnostic symptom is dementia; in Parkinson's disease, the most frequent identifying symptom is tremor and changes in gait. How do these differences alter the therapeutic approach to patients with these diseases?

5. What is the principal function of glutamate?

6. What are the roles of prostaglandins in inflammatory diseases? How do NSAIDs affect prostaglandin production?

7. Which of the following medications is most appropriate for a patient with a spinal cord injury who has a history of **benzodiazepine** addiction: **cyclobenzaprine**, **diazepam**, **aspirin**, or **dantrolene**?

8. ALS is a progressive neurodegenerative disease with varied etiology. What are typically the first symptoms seen in the progression of this disease?

9. What are the key symptoms or lab findings that would indicate toxicity in a patient on long-term **acetaminophen** therapy?

CASE STUDIES

Case Scenario 1

Ms. Smith, a 78-year-old woman with a history of gastric ulcers and stroke, comes into the clinic following an accident where her car was rear-ended. She is complaining of headache and pain in her neck and shoulders. The nurse takes the patient's vital signs: B/P, 123/68; P, 88; R, 18; T, 98.9. Ms. Smith states that she has allergies to **penicillin** and **codeine**, and has been taking Coumadin since her stroke three years ago. After a brief examination, the physician's assistant tells Ms. Smith that he believes she has whiplash and prescribes her **cyclobenzaprine** and **aspirin**.

Case Question

1. Is aspirin the best or most appropriate medication that should have been ordered?
   a. Yes, because it acts both as an anti-inflammatory and a pain medication.
   b. No, the patient would do better taking ibuprofen because it is less upsetting to the stomach.
   c. No, the patient should take acetaminophen because she has both a history of peptic ulcers and is currently taking warfarin.
   d. None of the above.

   Answer: The answer is c. Because Ms. Smith has a history of ulcers and is receiving anticoagulant therapy post stroke, aspirin should be avoided because it would both increase the anticoagulant effects of the warfarin and increase her risk of gastric ulcers.

CASE STUDIES

Case Scenario 2

Nathaniel, an EMT and girls' soccer coach in Connecticut, was flying home to Tulsa for a visit. When his father, Louis, picked him up at the airport, Nathaniel noticed that Louis seemed different. He didn't think much of it at the time, but as the week progressed, he noticed that his father was frequently confused, had difficulty organizing and planning, and was quite moody when normally he was always laughing and telling jokes. He had always loved making flies for his favorite hobby, fly-fishing, but Nathaniel's mother reported that he no longer made the flies or even went into his workshop anymore. She also stated that she noticed when they watched TV, Louis had difficulty following the plot of any of the shows they were watching.

Nathaniel felt that his father might have some mild dementia, which concerned him because his father was only 58. He made an appointment for his father with his doctor; following examination and testing, Louis was diagnosed with early-stage Alzheimer disease.

Case Questions

1. Because Louis is relatively young, and has been diagnosed with early-stage Alzheimer disease with what appear to be only mild symptoms, which medication would be *best* to start him on?

CASE STUDIES (CONTINUED)

    a. Namenda, because it has fewest side effects

    b. Vitamin E, as it is a supplement and much better than prescription medication

    c. Donepezil, as it is approved for all stages of Alzheimer disease

    d. Aspirin, because it acts as a "blood thinner" and should help improve blood flow to the brain

Answer: The answer is c.

2. Nathaniel's father has a history of vertigo and enlarged prostate. Which education should the nurse provide regarding donepezil?

    a. This medication has few side effects, so he doesn't need to worry about taking this medication in relation to his medical history.

    b. Donepezil can have side effects of dizziness and difficulty urinating, so he should rise slowly when getting up and avoid driving until he knows how he will react to this medication; he should also report any difficulty urinating to his primary provider immediately.

    c. If he has any side effects from the medication, he should stop taking it; he probably didn't need it anyway.

    d. None of the above.

Answer: The answer is b.

SUGGESTED READINGS

Avanzi, M., Uber, E., & Bonfa, F. (2004). Pathological gambling in two patients on dopamine replacement therapy for Parkinson's disease. *Neurologic Science, 25,* 98–101.

Copeland, R. L. (n.d.). Opioid agonists and antagonists. Retrieved from http://www.slideshare.net/jamal53 /opioid-agonists-and-antagonists

de Mey, C., Enterling, D., Meineke, I., & Yeulet, S. (1991). Interactions between domperidone and ropinirole, a novel dopamine D_2-receptor agonist. *British Journal of Clinical Pharmacology, 32*(4), 483–488.

Ernst, F. R., & Grizzle, A. J. (2001). Drug-related morbidity and mortality: Updating the cost-of-illness model. *Journal of the American Pharmacists Association, 41*(2), 192–199.

Gordon, D. B. (2003). Non-opioid and adjuvant in chronic pain management: Strategies for effective use. *Nursing Clinics of North America, 38,* 447–464.

Green, G. A. (2001). Understanding NSAIDs: From aspirin to –2. *Clinical Cornerstones, 3*(5), 50–60. doi: 10.1016/51098-3597(01)90069-9; PMID15208519

Grond, S., & Sablotzki, A. (2004). Clinical pharmacology of tramadol. *Clinical Pharmacokinetics, 43*(13), 879–923.

Gurkirpal, S. (1998). Recent considerations in nonsteroidal anti-inflammatory drug gastropathy. *American Journal of Medicine,* 31S.

Henry, T. R. (2003). The history of valproate in clinical neuroscience. *Psychopharmacology Bulletin, 37*(Suppl. 2), 5–16.

Hilal-Dandon, R., & Brunton, L. (2014). *Goodman and Gilman's manual of pharmacology and therapeutics* (2nd ed.). New York, NY: McGraw-Hill.

Kwan, P., & Brodie, M. J. (2004). Phenobarbital for the treatment of epilepsy in the 21st century: A critical review. *Epilepsia, 45*(9), 1141–1149.

McDonald, J., & Lambert, D. G. (2005). Opioid receptors. *Continuing Education in Anaesthesia, Critical Care, and Pain, 5*(1), 22–25.

Mehta, A. K., & Ticku, M. K. (1999). An update on GABAA receptors. *Brain Research: Brain Research Reviews, 29*(2–3), 196–217.

Meleger, A. (2006). Muscle relaxants and antispasticity agents. *Physical Medicine and Rehabilitation Clinics of North America, 17,* 401–413.

Millan, M. J. (2010). From the cell to the clinic: A comparative review of the partial D_2/D_3 receptor agonist and α_2-adrenoceptor antagonist, piribedil, in the treatment of Parkinson's disease. *Pharmacology and Therapeutics, 128*(2), 229–273.

National Library of Medicine (NLM), National Institutes of Health (NIH), & MedlinePlus. (n.d.). *Phenytoin.* Retrieved from http://www.nlm.nih.gov/medlineplus /druginfo/meds/a682022.html

Perucca, E. (2002). Pharmacological and therapeutic properties of valproate: A summary after 35 years of clinical experience. *CNS Drugs, 16*(10), 695–714.

Raghavendra, T. (2002). Neuromuscular blocking drugs: Discovery and development. *Journal of the Royal Society of Medicine, 95*(7), 363–367.

Raissy, H. H., & Harkins, M. (2017). Drug-induced pulmonary diseases. In J.T. Dipiro, R.L. Talbert, G.C. Yee, G.R. Matzke, B.G. Well, & L.M. Posey (Eds.), *Pharmacotherapy: A pathophysiological approach* (10th ed., pp. 431–433). Norwalk, CT: Appleton & Lange.

Rubinstein, D. C. (2006). The roles of intracellular protein-degradation pathways in neurodegeneration. *Nature, 443*(7113), 780–786.

Schwab, R. S., England, A. C., Poskanzer, D. C., & Young, R. R. (1969). Amantadine in the treatment of Parkinson's disease. *Journal of the American Medical Association, 208,* 1168–1170.

See, S., & Ginsburg, R. (2008). Skeletal muscle relaxants. *Pharmacotherapy, 28*(2), 207–213.

Skidmore-Roth, L. (2012). *Mosby's 2012 nursing drug reference* (25th ed.). St. Louis, MO: Elsevier Mosby.

Tortora, G. J., & Anagnostakos, N. P. (1990). *Principles of anatomy and physiology* (pp. 719–721). New York, NY: HarperCollins.

U.S. Department of Justice, Drug Enforcement Administration. (2011). *Drugs of abuse: A DEA resource guide* (Section V: Narcotics, pp. 34–41). Retrieved from https://www.dea.gov/pr/multimedia-library/publications/drug_of_abuse.pdf

Van Hecken, A., Schwartz, J. I., & Depré, M. (2000). Comparative inhibitory activity of rofecoxib, meloxicam, diclofenac, ibuprofen, and naproxen on COX-2 versus COX-1 in healthy volunteers. *Journal of Clinical Pharmacology, 40*(10), 1109–1120.

Webster, L.R., & Webster, R.M. (2005). Predicting aberrant behaviors in opioid-treated patients: Preliminary validation of the opioid risk tool. *Pain Medicine, 6*(6), 432–442.

West, J. B. (2011). *Respiratory physiology: The essentials* (9th ed.) (pp. 95–124). Philadelphia, PA: Lippincott Williams & Wilkins.

REFERENCES

Adler, C. H. (2002). Amantadine. In S. A. Factor & W. J. Weiner (Eds.), *Parkinson's disease: Diagnosis and clinical management.* New York, NY: Demos Medical Publishing.

Al-Chalabi, A., & Leigh, P. N. (2000). Recent advances in amyotrophic lateral sclerosis. *Current Opinion in Neurology, 13*(4), 397–405.

Alzheimer's Association. (2017). 2017 Alzheimer's Disease Facts and Figures. *Alzheimer's & Dementia, 13,* 325-373. Retrieved from https://www.alz.org/documents_custom/2017-facts-and-figures.pdf.

Beebe, F. A., Barkin, R. L, & Barkin, S. (2005). A clinical and pharmacologic review of skeletal muscle relaxants for musculoskeletal conditions. *American Journal of Therapeutics, 12*(2), 151–171.

Bellingham, M. C. (2011). A review of the neural mechanisms of action and clinical efficiency of riluzole in treating amyotrophic lateral sclerosis: What have we learned in the last decade? *CNS and Neuroscience Therapies, 17*(1), 4–31.

Bolden, J.L., Calixto, F., Beakley, B.D., Galan, V., Ripoll, J.G., Kaye, A.M., ... Manchikanti, L. (2017). Prescription opioid abuse in chronic pain: An updated review of opioid abuse predictors and strategies to curb opioid abuse: Part 1. *Pain Physician: Opioid Guidelines Special Issue, 20*(2S), S93–S109.

Brau, M.E., Vogel, W., & Hempelmann, G. (1998). Fundamental properties of local anesthetics: Half-maximal blocking concentrations for tonic block of Na^+ and K^+ channels in peripheral nerve. *Anesthesia and Analgesia, 87*(4), 885–889.

Cardoos, A., Inamori, A., Sanacora, G., Fava, M., & Mischoulon, D. (2013). Delayed amnesic syndrome after riluzole use in major depressive disorder: A case report. *Psychosomatics, 54*(5), 488–492. doi: 10.1016/j.psym.2013.02.002

Chan, F.K., Ching, J.Y., Tse, Y.K., Lam, K., Wong, G.L.H., Ng, S.C., ... Kyaw, M.H. (2017). Gastrointestinal safety of celecoxib versus naproxen in patients with cardiothrombotic diseases and arthritis after upper gastrointestinal bleeding (CONCERN): An industry-independent, double-blind, double-dummy, randomised trial. *The Lancet, 389*(10087), 2375–2382.

Chou, R., Deyo, R., Devine, B., Hansen, R., Sullivan, S., Jarvik, J.G., ... Turner, J. (2014). *The effectiveness and risks of long-term opioid treatment of chronic pain.* Rockville, MD: Agency for Healthcare Research and Quality. Retrieved from https://www.ncbi.nlm.nih.gov/books/NBK258809/

Epilepsy Foundation Michigan. (2011). Epilepsy & Seizure Facts. Retrieved from http://www.epilepsymichigan.org/page.php?id=358.

Gargallo, C.J., Sostres, C., & Lanas, A.I. (2014). Prevention and treatment of NSAID gastropathy. *Current Treatment Options in Gastroenterology, 12*(4), 398–413.

Hima, K., & Venkat, G. (2016). Study of gastrointestinal toxicity of selective COX-2 inhibitors in comparison with conventional NSAIDs. *International Journal of Research in Medical Sciences, 4*(12), 5180–5184. doi: 10.18203/2320-6012.ijrms20164010

Huang, P., Yang, X.-D., Chen, S.-D., & Xiao, Q. (2015). The association between Parkinson's disease and melanoma: A systematic review and meta-analysis. *Translational Neurodegeneration, 4,* 21. doi: 10.1186/s40035-015-0044-y

Lacorte, E., Ferrigno, L., Leoncini, E., Corbo, M., Boccia, S., & Vancore, N. (2016). Physical activity, and physical activity related to sports, leisure and occupational activity as risk factors for ALS: A systematic review. *Neuroscience & Biobehavioral Reviews, 66,* 61–79.

Mantegazza, M., Curia, G., Biagini, G., Ragsdale, D.S., & Avoli, M. (2010). Voltage-gated sodium channels as therapeutic targets in epilepsy and other neurological disorders. *Lancet Neurology, 9*(4), 413–424.

McNicol, E.D., Midbari, A., & Eisenberg, E. (2013, August 29). Opioids for neuropathic pain. *Cochrane Database Systematic Review, 8,* CD006146. doi: 10.1002/14651858.CD006146.pub2

Merck & Co, Inc. (1999). *Levodopa/carbidopa (Sinemat CR)* [Product package insert]. West Point, PA: Author.

Muroi, Y., & Chanda, B. (2009). Local anesthetics disrupt energetic coupling between voltage-sensors of the sodium channel. *Journal of General Physiology, 133*(1), 1–15.

National Center for Biotechnology Information (NCBI), National Institutes of Health (NIH), & PubChem Compound. (n.d.). *Benzonatate: Compound summary.* Retrieved from http://pubchem.ncbi.nlm.nih.gov/summary/summary.cgi?cid=7699

Obál, I., Klausz, G., Mándi, Y., Deli, M., Siklós, L., & Engelhardt, J. I. (2016). Intraperitoneally administered IgG from patients with amyotrophic lateral sclerosis or from an immune-mediated goat model increase the levels of TNF-α, IL-6, and IL-10 in the spinal cord and serum of mice. *Journal of Neuroinflammation, 13,* 121. doi: 10.1186/s12974-016-0586-7

Paquette, M.A., Martinez, A.A., Macheda, T., Meshul, C.K., Johnson, S.W., Berger, S.P., & Giuffrida, A. (2012). Anti-dyskinetic mechanisms of amantadine and dextromethorphan in the 6-OHDA rat model of Parkinson's disease: Role of NMDA vs. 5-HT1A receptors. *European Journal of Neuroscience, 36,* 3224–3234.

Rosenberg, G. (2007). The mechanisms of action of valproate in neuropsychiatric disorders: Can we see the forest for the trees? *Cellular and Molecular Life Sciences, 64*(16), 2090–2103.

Rosenquist, E.W.K. (n.d.). Overview of the treatment of chronic pain. UpToDate/Wolters Kluwer Health. Retrieved from http://www.uptodate.com/contents/overview-of-the-treatment-of-chronic-pain

Rudolph, U., Crestani, F., Benke, D., Brunig, I., Benson, J.A., Fritschy, J.M., … Mohler, H. (1999). Benzodiazepine actions mediated by specific big gamma-aminobutyric acid A receptor subtypes [Letter]. *Nature, 401,* 796–800.

Samad, T.A., Moore, K.A., Sapirstein, A., Billet, S., Allchorne, A., Poole, S., … Woolf, C.J. (2001). Interleukin-1β-mediated induction of COX-2 in the CNS contributes to inflammatory pain hypersensitivity. *Nature (Lond), 410,* 471–475.

Singh, G. (1998). Recent considerations in nonsteroidal anti-inflammatory drug gastropathy. *American Journal of Medicine, 105*(1B), 31S–38S.

Sostres, C., Gargallo, C.J., & Lanas, A. (2013). Nonsteroidal anti-inflammatory drugs and upper and lower gastrointestinal mucosal damage. *Arthritis Research & Therapy, 15*(Suppl. 3), 53.

Theis, K.A., Roblin, D., Helmick, C.G., & Luo, R. (2017). Prevalence and causes of work disability among working-age U.S. adults, 2011–2013, NHIS. *Disability and Health Journal, 11*(1), 108–115. doi: 10.1016/j.dhjo.2017.04.010

UCB. (2003). *KEPPRA XR* [Product package insert]. Smyrna, GA: Author.

Viallan, A., Page, Y., & Bertrand, J.C. (2000). Methemoglobinemia due to riluzole. *New England Journal of Medicine, 343,* 665–666.

Waldemar, G. (2007). Recommendations for the diagnosis and management of Alzheimer's disease and other disorders associated with dementia: EFNS guideline. *European Journal of Neurology, 14*(1), e1–e26.

Walker, E.P. (2012). Long-term opioid use questioned for chronic pain. *Medpage Today.* Retrieved from http://www.medpagetoday.com/painmanagement/painmanagement/33014

Wan, O.W., & Chung, K.K.K. (2012). The role of alphasynuclein oligomerization and aggregation in cellular and animal models of Parkinson's disease. *PLoS One, 7*(6), e38545.

Whittle, B.J. (2000). COX-1 and COX-2 products in the gut: Therapeutic impact of COX-2 inhibitors. *Gut, 47,* 320–325.

Wishart, D.S., Knox, C., Guo, A.C., Cheng, D., Shrivastava, S., Tzur, D., … Hassanali, M. (2008). DrugBank: A knowledgebase for drugs, drug actions and drug targets. *Nucleic Acids Research, 1*(36), D901–D906.

Yu, Y., Su, F.-C., Callaghan, B.C., Goutman, S.A., Batterman, S.A., & Feldman, E.L. (2014). Environmental risk factors and amyotrophic lateral sclerosis (ALS): A case-control study of ALS in Michigan. *PLoS ONE, 9*(6), e101186. doi: 10.1371/journal.pone.0101186

CHAPTER 5

Autonomic Nervous System Drugs

William Mark Enlow, Sue Greenfield, and Cliff Roberson

KEY TERMS

Acetylcholinesterase
Adrenal medulla
Adrenergic agonists
Adrenergic antagonists
Adrenergic nerves
Adrenergic receptors
Cardioselective
Catecholamine

Cholinergic agonists
Cholinergic antagonists
Cholinergic nerves
Craniosacral system
Direct-acting
Dual innervation
Effector organs
Enteric nervous system (ENS)

Epinephrine
Ganglia
Indirect-acting
Muscarinic acetylcholine
  receptors
Nicotinic acetylcholine
  receptors
Norepinephrine

Pheochromocytoma
Postganglionic neuron
Preganglionic neuron
Selectivity
Sympathomimetic
Synapse
Thoracolumbar system
Vasopressor

CHAPTER OBJECTIVES

At the end of the chapter, the student will be able to:

1. Identify the physiological functions the autonomic nervous system (ANS) controls.

2. Explain the mechanism of action for ANS drugs.

3. Compare the various classes of ANS drugs.

4. Describe common indications and contraindications of ANS drugs.

5. Discuss adverse effects of ANS drugs.

Introduction

The autonomic nervous system (ANS) controls a variety of involuntary regulatory responses that affect heart and respiration rates. It is responsible both for the "fight-or-flight" responses that represent the body's physiological response to crisis or stress and for the less crisis-driven functions of resting, repairing, digesting, and reproductive activities. Many of the drugs used to treat common conditions of the heart, circulation, and especially blood pressure do so by intentionally altering the functioning of the ANS.

The Three Systems of the ANS

An early view of the ANS described it as being separate from the central nervous system (CNS), which integrates sensory information in the brain and spinal cord. It is more accurate to say that the ANS carries out tasks that originate in the CNS (Blessing & Gibbins, 2008), but in some instances it acts more or less autonomously in doing so. It is important to recognize, though, that the ANS and the CNS are *not* separate systems; they simply have different key functional responsibilities. Whereas the CNS supervises all motor and cognitive functions, voluntary or otherwise, the ANS is primarily tasked with the involuntary functions of the body such as heartbeat, respiration, digestion, and so forth.

There are three key components to the ANS (**FIGURE 5-1**), two of which are of primary concern in this discussion: the sympathetic nervous system (SNS) and the parasympathetic nervous system (PNS). The third component, the **enteric nervous system (ENS)**, is intrinsic to the digestive system and carries out key functions that support systemic neurologic and immunologic well-being. The ENS is highly responsive to both physical and emotional stimuli. For purposes of this discussion, however, the focus will mainly be on the SNS and PNS.

Anatomy of the Autonomic Nervous System

The ANS is, in essence, an extension of the CNS that manages the involuntary functions

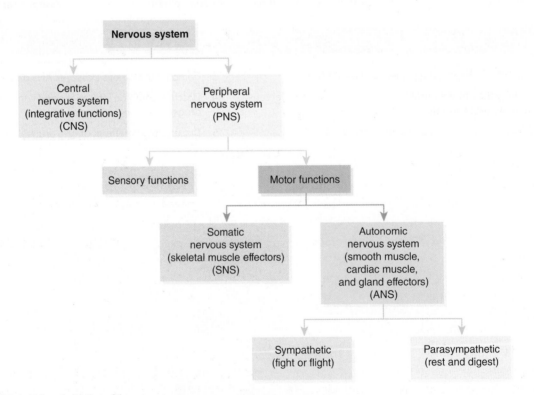

FIGURE 5-1 Major subdivisions of the nervous system.

of the body; thus, all signals that pass through ANS pathways originate in either the spinal cord (both SNS and PNS) or the medulla of the brain (PNS). These impulses pass through a **preganglionic neuron** to bundles of **synapses** called **ganglia**, most of which then synapse to **postganglionic neurons** that process the signal to the appropriate **effector organs**, muscles, and other structures that they innervate. In both the SNS and the PNS, acetylcholine is the key neurotransmitter facilitating the preganglionic synapse. In the SNS, **norepinephrine** stimulates postganglionic neurons while, conversely, postganglionic neurons in the PNS are activated once again by acetylcholine.

Although the SNS and PNS often innervate the same organs (**dual innervation**), the effects on that organ are often very different. For example, the heart is innervated by both sympathetic and parasympathetic nerves. Increased parasympathetic (PNS) stimulation of the heart will result in parasympathetic predominance and *decreased* heart rate, while decreased parasympathetic activation can result in unopposed sympathetic stimulation and *increased* heart rate. Conversely, increased sympathetic stimulation of the heart produces increases in heart rate and decreased sympathetic stimulation produces decreases in heart rate.

Integration of ANS Systems

The ANS can be thought of as being equivalent to a car racing team. The responsibility of one part of the team is driving the car, keeping the vehicle on the track, while dealing with the stresses and quick responses needed as circumstances change. The other part (the pit crew) is tasked with keeping fuel and repairs in place so that both the driver and the car can continue doing their jobs. In this metaphor, the SNS is the driver; it increases metabolism and stimulates the cardiovascular and pulmonary systems as the situation requires, whether that means maintaining a steady metabolic speed for normal activities or "revving the engine" in crisis situations. Meanwhile, the PNS functions are similar to the activities of the pit crew; the PNS produces more targeted responses that facilitate digestion, repair, and resting functions, enabling the body to maintain energy stores and recover from incidental damage. Finally, the ANS is more like the car itself; it responds to input from both the SNS and the PNS—it is nevertheless central to the operation of the whole team.

An important component of this metaphor is that the functions of the pit crew (PNS) and the driver (SNS) are rarely engaged at the same time. One operates under certain circumstances, while the other operates under different circumstances—yet together they can handle nearly all situations, whether it be routine maintenance, fueling, and upkeep or the critical stress of race time. The ANS, by comparison, is on the receiving end of signals from the PNS and SNS at any given moment; at the same time, it is always engaged and "running," even when at rest (just as the brain is).

Anyone who has seen cars race understands that the crew, the car, and the driver all need to work well and work *together* for the race to go well. Similarly, the ANS is a highly integrated system in which the major parts are mutually interdependent. Consequently, medications that alter how the ANS functions may be intended to act on one system, yet affect the others in unexpected ways. Understanding how the SNS and PNS interact will help the clinician to identify both how medical interventions may affect the ANS overall, and how those treatments may have more specific effects on the functions of certain components of the ANS.

Sympathetic Nervous System

SNS impulses are responses to a fairly specific set of stimuli requiring activation of the fight-or-flight response. When someone crosses a street and sees a car moving quickly toward him or her, or the car suddenly rounds a corner headed straight for the person—the rush of energy he or she experiences while jumping out of the way is exactly this type of impulse. It is, as may have been experienced by the reader, highly suited toward propelling the body into motion—it originates from the spine rather than the brain: the ganglia and nerves of the SNS connect the spinal cord to a specific set of organs. The sympathetic ganglia extend from the upper neck down to the coccyx and are found in paired chains close to and along each side of the thoracic and lumbar spine. Nerves carrying sympathetic fibers exit the spinal cord from T1 to L2. For this reason, the SNS is sometimes also referred to as the **thoracolumbar system**.

The nerves in the ANS release specific neurotransmitters that target a number of different receptors, listed in TABLE 5-1. Preganglionic sympathetic nerves release acetylcholine into synapses. Acetylcholine stimulates postganglionic **nicotinic acetylcholine receptors**, and impulses are propagated along postganglionic sympathetic nerves, which release adrenergic neurotransmitters—primarily norepinephrine—to produce systemic effects. Because these preganglionic sympathetic nerves release acetylcholine, they are classified as **cholinergic nerves** (FIGURE 5-2, and

also refer to **Figure 4-10**). Postganglionic sympathetic nerves release adrenergic neurotransmitters and, therefore, are classified as **adrenergic nerves**. Receptors responsive to adrenergic neurotransmitters—**adrenergic receptors**—include alpha (α), beta (β), and dopamine (D) receptors.

Parasympathetic Nervous System

The PNS, similar to the SNS, is composed of preganglionic and postganglionic nerves. However, preganglionic parasympathetic nerve fibers originate in cranial nerves—II, VII, XI, and X—and sacral spinal nerves (S2 through S4) (Johnson, 2013). For this reason, the PNS is sometimes referred to as the **craniosacral system** (see Figure 5-1).

The PNS is the "rest and repair" part of the ANS. Its essential job is to transition the body to those functions that support the body's ability to renew itself. Thus, it stimulates digestive secretions and gastrointestinal (GI) tract activity to promote processing of nutrients, and it slows the heart and constricts the pupils to promote resting. The principal route of PNS signaling is along the vagus nerve; in consequence, impulses tend to move more slowly through the PNS. This part of the nervous system is often conceived of as being "in opposition to" the SNS, but this is not entirely the case, although it is true that certain opposing functions are assigned

TABLE 5-1	Types of Autonomic Receptors		
Neurotransmitter	Receptor	Primary Locations	Responses
Acetylcholine (cholinergic)	Nicotinic	Postganglionic neurons	Stimulation of smooth muscle and gland secretions
	Muscarinic	Parasympathetic target: organs other than the heart	
		Heart	Decreased heart rate and force of contraction
Norepinephrine (adrenergic)	Alpha$_1$	All sympathetic target organs except the heart	Constriction of blood vessels, dilation of pupils
	Alpha$_2$	Presynaptic adrenergic nerve terminals	Inhibition of release of norepinephrine
	Beta$_1$	Heart and kidneys	Increased heart rate and force of contraction; release of renin
	Beta$_2$	All sympathetic target organs except the heart	Bronchoconstriction; blood vessel dilation

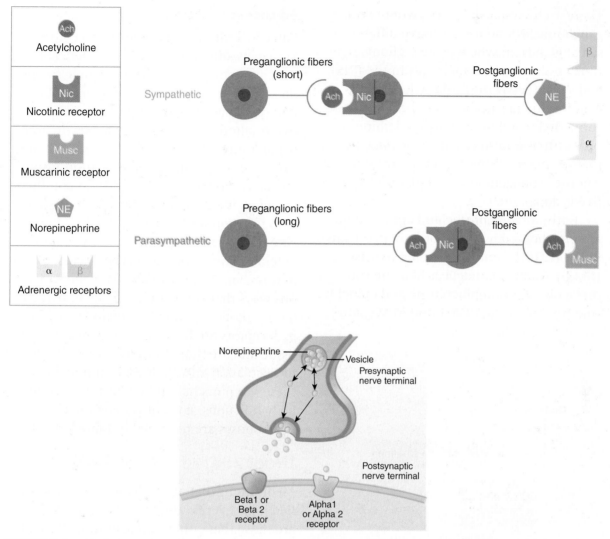

FIGURE 5-2 Acetylcholine interactions with sympathetic and parasympathetic innervation.

to each system. Increases (SNS) and decreases (PNS) in heart rate, for example, are two such "opposing" functions.

Neurotransmitters in the Autonomic Nervous System

Both the PNS and the SNS rely on two general types of neurotransmitters to pass nerve signals along. Preganglionic parasympathetic nerves in both systems are classified as cholinergic nerves and release acetylcholine. Acetylcholine attaches to nicotinic acetylcholine receptors on the postganglionic membrane, and impulses are propagated toward effector organs. Postganglionic parasympathetic nerves are also cholinergic nerves, and the acetylcholine they release attaches to **muscarinic acetylcholine receptors** at effector organs. Acetylcholine is rapidly metabolized to acetate and choline by the enzyme known as **acetylcholinesterase**, which is located on the postsynaptic membrane. Acetate diffuses away from the synapse and is metabolized in the liver, whereas choline is taken back up into the presynaptic membrane for synthesis of new neurotransmitters (**FIGURE 5-3**).

The postganglionic neurons of the SNS, unlike those in the PNS, primarily produce norepinephrine, a **direct-acting** neurotransmitter classified as a **catecholamine**.

There are two specific places where post-ganglionic SNS neurons behave differently: sweat glands, in which postganglionic neurons produce acetylcholine (as in the PNS), and the **adrenal medulla**, where norepinephrine (also called *noradrenaline*) is converted to a different catecholamine, **epinephrine** (also called *adrenaline*), by phenylethanolamine *N*-methyl transferase. Another endogenous catecholamine derivative is dopamine (**FIGURE 5-4**).

Both norepinephrine and epinephrine are metabolized by catechol-*o*-methyl transferase (COMT) and monoamine oxidase (MAO). Vanillylmandelic acid is the common metabolite for norepinephrine and epinephrine from both the COMT and MAO pathways (**FIGURE 5-4**).

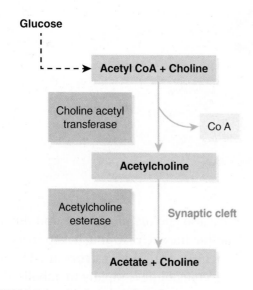

FIGURE 5-3 Acetylcholine metabolism.

Adrenergic Receptors

Catecholamines bind to specific receptors known as adrenergic receptors. There are two basic types of receptors: α-adrenergic receptors and β-adrenergic receptors. Each of these two types has various subtypes; there are two α-adrenergic receptor subtypes (α_1 and α_2) and three β-adrenergic receptor subtypes (β_1, β_2, and β_3). The action of neurotransmitters or **sympathomimetic** drugs upon these receptors is an important means of altering ANS function for therapy of different disease states—although this is not without its potential drawbacks, as will be discussed later in this chapter. **TABLE 5-2** identifies the various ways that stimulation acts upon particular receptors in particular organs. Note that β_3-receptors are found primarily in adipose tissue and are thought to play a role in thermoregulation and lipolysis; if stimulation of these receptors has an immediate effect on body functions, it is not yet identified. Thus, β_3 responses are not listed in Table 5-2.

Drugs That Affect the ANS

Medications that affect the ANS are classified into several categories. Adrenergic drugs are those that either mimic or interfere with the activity of neurotransmitters secreted by the adrenal medulla—for example, norepinephrine and epinephrine. Specifically, **adrenergic agonists** are drugs that stimulate the SNS, either by direct activation of receptors or by promoting the release of receptor-activating catecholamines, whereas **adrenergic antagonists** block the activity

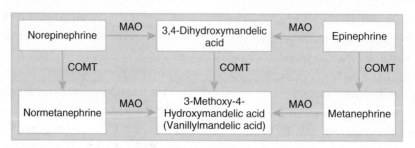

FIGURE 5-4 Catecholamine metabolism.

TABLE 5-2	Actions of Neurotransmitter Stimuli on Receptors in Various Organs	
Receptor	**Effector Organ**	**Response to Stimulation**
β_1	Heart	Increased heart rate
		Increased contractility
		Increased conduction velocity
	Fat cells	Lipolysis
β_2	Blood vessels (especially skeletal and coronary arteries)	Dilation
	Bronchioles	Dilation
	Uterus	Relaxation
	Kidneys	Renin secretion
	Liver	Glycogenesis
		Gluconeogenesis
	Pancreas	Insulin secretion
α_1	Blood vessels	Constriction
	Pancreas	Inhibition of insulin secretion
	Intestine and bladder	Relaxation
		Constriction of sphincters
α_2	Postganglionic (presynaptic sympathetic nerve ending)	Inhibition of norepinephrine release
	Central nervous system (postsynaptic)	Increase in potassium conductance (?)
	Platelets	Aggregation
D_1	Blood vessels	Dilation
D_2	Postganglionic (presynaptic) sympathetic nerve ending	Inhibition of norepinephrine release
Muscarinic	Heart	Decreased heart rate
		Decreased contractility
		Decreased conduction velocity
	Bronchioles	Constriction
	Salivary glands	Stimulation of secretions
	Intestine	Contraction
		Relaxation of sphincters
		Stimulation of secretions
	Bladder	Contraction
		Relaxation of sphincter
Nicotinic	Neuromuscular junction	Skeletal muscle contraction
	Autonomic ganglia	Sympathetic nervous system stimulation

of acetylcholine, norepinephrine, or other neurotransmitters.

Adrenergic Agonist Drugs

Adrenergic agonists can produce profound effects on the body's vital systems, typically requiring special care in their administration and monitoring of patient responses. Therapeutic activation of SNS receptors is useful for a range of clinical purposes, including cardiac stimulation, bronchodilation, and constriction of blood vessels. The clinical effects of adrenergic agonists, however, depend on the **selectivity** of the drug for the variety of receptor subtypes. For example, some agents may be used to treat hypotension, due to their preference for stimulation of α_1-adrenergic receptors (e.g., phenylephrine), whereas others may be used to treat hypertension, due to their selectivity for α_2-adrenergic receptors (e.g., clonidine).

Nonselective Agents

Nonselective adrenergic agonists act on particular adrenergic receptors anywhere in the body, producing a variety of systemic effects. Given their widespread action, they must be used with a fair amount of consideration for the possibility (or even probability) of unwanted or counterproductive effects, as well as careful review for the possibility of contraindications. TABLE 5-3 describes a selection of potential effects of adrenergic drugs, along with therapeutic goals associated with their use.

Best Practices

When administering a nonselective adrenergic agonist, keep in mind that the drug acts on receptors everywhere in the body, which may lead to unwanted adverse effects.

Epinephrine

Epinephrine is a direct-acting adrenergic agonist that stimulates all α-and β-adrenergic receptors (α_1, α_2, β_1, β_2, and β_3). As a pharmacologic agent, **epinephrine** is a potent cardiac stimulant that increases contractility and heart rate by β_1 receptor stimulation and characteristically leads to a dose-related increase in systolic blood pressure. **Epinephrine** also causes contraction of vascular smooth muscle and results in vasoconstriction due to activation of α_1-receptors. Conversely, stimulation of β_2-receptors by **epinephrine** leads to relaxation of respiratory and uterine smooth muscle, as well as skeletal smooth muscle vasculature. Because of these effects, **epinephrine** is used for circulatory support and treatment of airway swelling in severe acute anaphylactic reactions and shock, and for promotion of return of circulation in cardiac arrest during cardiopulmonary resuscitation. **Epinephrine** is also commonly added to local anesthetic solutions to diminish the rate of systemic absorption of the anesthetic by means of localized vasoconstriction, thereby prolonging the desired anesthetic effect while reducing the risk of systemic toxicity. **Epinephrine** may be administered by a range of routes—intravenous, intramuscular, subcutaneous, intraosseous, oral inhalation, endotracheal, and topical—depending on the indication and clinical situation; it is also given in a wide variety of doses.

Adverse effects include anxiety, headache, tremors, pallor, sweating, nausea, vomiting,

TABLE 5-3	Nursing Diagnoses Related to Use of Adrenergic Drugs and Associated Therapeutic Goals
Nursing Diagnoses	**Goals**
Impaired gas exchange related to bronchoconstriction	Patient will experience relief of symptoms. Goal: Bronchodilation
Altered tissue perfusion related to hypotension or vasoconstriction due to adrenergic drug therapy	Patient will attain adequate perfusion to the brain, heart, kidney, and peripheral tissue. Goal: vasodilation
Altered nutrition, less than body requirements, related to a loss of appetite	Patient will maintain his or her weight. Goal: increased appetite
Potential for injury related to cardiac stimulation: hypertension, dysrhythmias	Patient will not experience any adverse effects. Goal: prevent sympathomimetic adverse effects

hypertension, tachycardia, cardiac arrhythmias, cardiac ischemia, and intracranial hemorrhage. Administration of **epinephrine** can provoke chest pain in patients with underlying ischemic heart disease due to β-mediated cardiac effects and can cause urinary retention in males with enlarged prostates due to α-stimulation. Uterine relaxation caused by β_2-receptor activity can delay the second stage of labor.

Norepinephrine

Norepinephrine bitartrate is a potent **vasopressor** and cardiac stimulant that acts directly on α-and β-adrenergic receptors (α_1, α_2, and β_1). Like epinephrine, norepinephrine is a naturally occurring hormone in the body that mediates the stress response. It is also an important neurotransmitter within the SNS. Unlike **epinephrine**, however, **norepinephrine** bitartrate has little impact on β_2-receptors; its effects are primarily mediated by its interactions with alpha-receptors. As a result, **norepinephrine** has a profound effect on peripheral vascular resistance, increasing both systolic and diastolic blood pressures, and is utilized clinically most often as a vasopressor to restore blood pressure in acute hypotensive states. This medication is administered intravenously by means of an infusion pump, with careful titration and frequent systemic blood pressure measurements. Indications include hypotension and shock that are refractory to fluid volume replacement in septicemia, myocardial infarction, trauma, and burns.

Adverse effects of **norepinephrine** are similar to those of **epinephrine**. Given **norepinephrine's** potent vasoconstrictive properties, however, the risks of plasma volume depletion and organ damage to the bowel, kidneys, and liver are enhanced with this medication, especially in the context of hypovolemia or prolonged administration. Impaired circulation, tissue necrosis, and sloughing may occur at the infusion site even without demonstrable extravasation. Lower initial doses of **norepinephrine** are recommended for elderly patients because of their higher likelihood of concomitant organ dysfunction or coexisting disease.

Ephedrine

Ephedrine is a natural substance found in plants of the genus *Ephedra.* It has been widely used in traditional and modern medicine to treat symptoms of asthma and upper respiratory congestion. **Ephedrine** acts directly on α-and β-adrenergic receptors (α_1, α_2, β_1, and β_2), causing cardiac stimulation, bronchodilation, and vasoconstriction. **Ephedrine** also provokes an indirect effect by stimulating the release of **norepinephrine** from nerve terminals within the SNS. **Ephedrine** can cross the blood–brain barrier and enter the CNS, where it produces mild stimulatory effects; for this reason,this medication has been useful in the treatment of narcolepsy and depression. CNS effects have also resulted in the misuse and abuse of **ephedrine** as an athletic performance enhancer and as an appetite suppressant. A form of **ephedrine** used in nasal decongestants (**pseudoephedrine**) has been used in the illicit manufacture of methamphetamine, resulting in stricter controls of its over-the-counter sales. This agent is also used as a vasopressor in the treatment of hypotension during anesthesia.

Adverse effects of **ephedrine** include excessive CNS stimulation, which can manifest as anxiety, restlessness, headache, blurred vision, insomnia, and seizures. **Ephedrine** can cause palpitations, arrhythmias, pallor, tachycardia, chest pain, and severe hypertension. Nausea, vomiting, and anorexia can also occur with its use. Acute urinary retention can result from prolonged usage, especially in men with prostatism. **Ephedrine** can restrict renal blood flow with initial parenteral use and decrease urine formation. Caution must be exercised when prescribing this drug to patients with underlying hypertension, hyperthyroidism, ischemic heart disease, diabetes mellitus, and prostatic hypertrophy, because ephedrine can exacerbate these conditions. Severe hypertension from **ephedrine** can occur in patients who are taking MAO inhibitors. A reduced vasopressor response from **ephedrine** may be seen in patients taking **reserpine** and **methyldopa**, as well as those taking α-and β-adrenergic blocking agents. Due to the significant adverse effects experienced by patients, in 2004 the FDA removed ephedrine from the market, and banned the sale of all ephedrine-containing products, including the sale of dietary supplements containing ephedrine alkaloids.

Dopamine

Dopamine is a potent vasoactive agent that acts on a variety of adrenergic receptors in a dose-dependent manner. At low and moderate doses, **dopamine** causes dopaminergic and β_1-adrenergic effects, resulting in increased renal and splanchnic blood flow and increased cardiac contractility, respectively. At higher doses, this agent promotes vasoconstriction by directly stimulating α-adrenergic receptors and by causing the release of norepinephrine from sympathetic nerve terminals. **Dopamine** is an endogenous catecholamine and the immediate precursor of **norepinephrine**. Its therapeutic indications include the treatment of shock states, low cardiac output syndromes, and hypotension, and as an adjunct to increase cardiac output and blood pressure during cardiopulmonary resuscitation.

Adverse cardiac effects associated with **dopamine** include hypotension, hypertension, ectopic beats, tachycardia, palpitations, vasoconstriction, angina, dyspnea, and cardiac conduction abnormalities and widened QRS intervals. **Dopamine** can cause headaches, anxiety, nausea, and vomiting. Exaggerated effects can be seen in patients taking MAO inhibitors, tricyclic antidepressants (Chapter 14), and **methyldopa**. Administration of intravenous **phenytoin** to patients receiving **dopamine** may precipitate hypotension, bradycardia, and seizures. **Dopamine** extravasation can cause tissue

sloughing and necrosis. If this occurs, the tissue should be infiltrated immediately with 10–15 mL of normal saline with 5–10 mg of **phentolamine**.

Dopamine administration requires close monitoring of patient hemodynamics and careful titration of drug dosing using an infusion pump, based on the patient heart rate, blood pressure, peripheral perfusion, urinary output, and electrocardiogram (ECG) findings. **Dopamine** is contraindicated in hypovolemic states, pheochromocytoma, tachyarrhythmias, and ventricular fibrillation. It should be used with caution in patients with a history of occlusive vascular disease (atherosclerosis, arterial embolism, Raynaud disease, cold injury, diabetic endarteritis, or Buerger disease).

Selective Adrenergic Agents

Selective adrenergic agents act on adrenergic receptors in specific, targeted locations. Therefore, therapies including these agents are less likely than nonselective adrenergic drugs to produce undesired responses in the body.

Dobutamine

Dobutamine is a synthetic β_1-selective agonist that is used in the short-term management of patients with depressed cardiac contractility from organic heart disease, cardiac surgical interventions, and acute myocardial infarction. It is also used to treat low cardiac output states following cardiac arrest. **Dobutamine** acts on the β_1-adrenergic receptors in the heart, increasing the force of myocardial contraction. It causes a reduction in peripheral resistance and has a limited impact on heart rate. This agent is contraindicated in patients with hypovolemia, as well as those patients with idiopathic hypertrophic subaortic stenosis. Its use in the context of acute myocardial infarction is limited, but concerns about infarct extension have been articulated. **Dobutamine** increases atrioventricular conduction and may cause rapid ventricular responses in patients with atrial fibrillation, unless they have received digoxin prior to initiating **dobutamine** therapy.

Adverse effects of **dobutamine** include hypertension, increased heart rate, ectopic beats, and angina, as well as nausea, vomiting, headache, fever, and leg cramps. Increased effects may be seen with concomitant use of tricyclic antidepressants, **furazolidone**, and **methyldopa**. Patients require continuous monitoring of hemodynamics during **dobutamine** administration and careful titration of the medication based on their responses.

Phenylephrine

Phenylephrine is a potent synthetic vasopressor that acts predominately on α_1-receptors to produce vasoconstriction and dose-related elevations of both systolic and diastolic blood pressure. **Phenylephrine** is administered intravenously as an adjunct therapy to treat low vascular resistance states, hypotension, and shock, particularly the distributive shock seen in sepsis and spinal cord injury, after adequate fluid volume placement has been achieved. It is also commonly used to treat hypotension during spinal anesthesia, caused by a loss of vascular tone from the associated sympathectomy, and hypotension during general anesthesia, produced by the vasodilatory effects of anesthetic agents. Topical application of **phenylephrine** to the mucous membranes of the nasal passages is used to relieve nasal congestion from allergic conditions or the common cold. Oral administration of phenylephrine is used for its decongestant properties, and is taken either alone or in multidrug combinations with antipyretics and antihistamines in the treatment of upper respiratory symptoms. **Phenylephrine** is also an ingredient in many over-the-counter products for the treatment of hemorrhoids, as it can reduce the swelling of anorectal tissue through vasoconstriction.

Adverse effects of **phenylephrine** include anxiety, restlessness, tremor, pallor, headache, hypertension, and precordial pain. As a treatment for hypotension and

shock states, **phenylephrine** may cause severe peripheral and visceral vasoconstriction, and like **norepinephrine**, its use may result in plasma volume depletion and end-organ damage. **Phenylephrine** may cause severe bradycardia and reduced cardiac output, and should be used with caution in elderly persons and in patients with diminished cardiac reserve or history of myocardial infarction.

Self-medication with oral over-the-counter products containing **phenylephrine** should be avoided in patients with high blood pressure, thyroid disorders, cardiac disease, and urinary difficulties due to enlarged prostate. According to the U.S. Food and Drug Administration (FDA, 2016), children younger than age two years should not be given nonprescription oral cough and cold preparations due to the risk of overdose and death, and extreme caution should be used in children older than two years. Patients taking MAO inhibitors may experience life-threatening, exaggerated sympathetic responses to **phenylephrine** and other adrenergic agonists, resulting in severe headache, hypertension, hyperpyrexia, and precipitation of a hypertensive crisis.

Clonidine

Clonidine is a selective α_2-adrenergic agonist that is used as an antihypertensive and central analgesic. **Clonidine** stimulates α_2-adrenergic receptors in the CNS, mainly in the medulla oblongata, causing inhibition of the sympathetic vasomotor centers. This stimulation results in a reduction in peripheral SNS activity, peripheral vascular resistance, and systemic blood pressure. **Clonidine** produces a reduction in heart rate by inhibition of cardioaccelerator activity in the brain.

It also produces analgesia by activation of central pain suppression pathways in the brain and by inhibiting the transmission of pain signals to the brain through the spinal cord. Therapeutic indications for this medication include the treatment of hypertension and hypertensive urgencies, as well as in the multimodal management of chronic pain. **Clonidine** has also been used as a treatment for vascular headaches, dysmenorrhea, and vasomotor symptoms associated with menopause; in smoking cessation therapy; as treatment for opiate and alcohol dependency; and in attention-deficit/hyperactivity disorder (ADHD).

Adverse effects of **clonidine** include dizziness, drowsiness, sedation, dry mouth, fatigue, anxiety, nightmares, and depression. Cardiovascular effects can be pronounced, including palpations, tachycardia, bradycardia, orthostatic hypotension, and cardiac rhythm disturbances. **Clonidine** should not be discontinued abruptly because rebound phenomena can precipitate hypertension, tachycardia, and cardiac arrhythmias. Instead, therapy should be discontinued by gradual reduction of dosage tapered over several days. **Clonidine** should be used with caution in patients with severe coronary insufficiency, recent myocardial infarction, cerebrovascular disease, and chronic renal failure. Children are more likely to experience signs of CNS depression with **clonidine** than are adults.

Dexmedetomidine

Dexmedetomidine is a selective α_2-adrenergic agonist that has sedative, anxiolytic, and analgesic effects. **Dexmedetomidine** activates α_2-receptors in the locus ceruleus of the brain stem, suppressing firing of the noradrenergic neurons as well as activity in the ascending noradrenergic pathway. The inhibition by **dexmedetomidine** causes a decrease in the release of histamine, which then results in a hypnotic response, similar to that seen in normal sleep. Indications for the use of **dexmedetomidine** include sedation of mechanically ventilated patients in the intensive care unit (ICU), pediatric procedural sedation, and sedation for awake neurosurgical procedures. **Dexmedetomidine** has also been used as an anesthetic-sparing agent in a number of specialties, including bariatric and cardiac surgery, allowing for a reduction in the number of agents that cause postoperative respiratory depression while significantly attenuating postoperative pain.

Adverse effects of **dexmedetomidine** administration are primarily hypotension and bradycardia. Bradycardia can be profound when increased vagal stimuli are present, and in young individuals with high vagal tone, requiring modulation of vagal tone with intravenous anticholinergic agents (**atropine**, **glycopyrrolate**). Other adverse effects include hypertension, supraventricular and ventricular tachycardia, atrial fibrillation, anemia, pain, leukocytosis, and pulmonary edema. Caution should be exercised in patients who are volume depleted or who have high-degree heart block. The safety of this medication in lactating mothers has not been established.

Nursing Considerations for Adrenergic Drugs
Assessment

For patients with respiratory disease, the nurse should assess respiratory status, including respiratory rate, heart rate, blood pressure, color, use of accessory muscles, oxygen saturation, and breath sounds, when adrenergic drugs are prescribed. For patients who have diabetes mellitus, the baseline serum glucose level should be checked. For all patients, cardiovascular status should be assessed:

- Assess for potential contraindications to using adrenergic medications: angina, hypertension, and tachydysrhythmias.
- Before, during, and after treatment, monitor blood pressure, heart rate, respiratory rate, color, and temperature of skin.

There are also important life span considerations in using such drugs. Most adrenergic drugs should be used with caution, as they were previously classified as risk category C with regard to use during pregnancy, so healthcare providers should determine whether females of childbearing age are pregnant before giving such medications. Use adrenergic drugs with caution in infants and the elderly as well, as these patients are at higher risk for adverse effects.

Nursing Interventions

- For impaired gas exchange: Monitor oxygen saturation and/or arterial blood gases; check respiratory rate and breath sounds prior to administering adrenergic drugs and during treatment.
- For altered tissue perfusion: Monitor the level of consciousness, heart rate, blood pressure, ECG, chest pain, urine output, color and temperature of skin, and capillary refill.
- For altered appetite/nutrition concerns: Provide small frequent meals, feed when the medication effect is minimal, and serve foods the patient likes.
- For sleep pattern disturbances: Dim the lights, keep the area quiet, and offer a back rub.
- For the potential for injury: Monitor the ECG, blood pressure, heart rate, and any chest pain.

Patient Teaching

Patients should be taught to use adrenergic drugs as directed by their prescriber. Anxiety and insomnia are common feelings caused by the adrenergic drugs and should be reported to the prescribing clinician. Because of the potential for side effects or drug interactions, patients should be advised to check with their healthcare provider or pharmacist prior to taking any other medications, and to seek medical attention immediately if they experience chest pain. If the patient takes the medication as directed and has no relief of symptoms, he or she should let the prescriber know.

Patients who are prescribed epinephrine kits for emergency self-administration due to risk of anaphylaxis should be advised to read the instructions and practice using the pen on an orange or a stuffed animal prior to using it on themselves. (Self-injectable epinephrine kits are packaged with a practice syringe containing no needle or drug.) If the patient is a child younger than age 13, this instruction should be given to parents; if the patient is an adolescent or teen, and with the parent's consent, it may be helpful for the nurse to show the patient what to do and then monitor (and correct) as the patient mimics the procedure under the nurse's guidance. Patients should be advised to seek medical attention immediately after use of self-injectable epinephrine as epinephrine is short-acting and the source of the allergic response may still be present after the drug is metabolized if they have previous exposure to such medications.

Adrenergic Antagonists

Adrenergic antagonists are also known as adrenergic blocking agents or adrenergic blockers, and for good reason: When they interact with their respective receptors, the normal receptor response does not occur. They merely attach to receptors and block binding sites for their respective agonists by competitive inhibition or noncompetitive inhibition. Responses to adrenergic antagonists depend on the receptor classes and subclasses with which the antagonists interact. A review of adrenergic receptors and their *activation* or *stimulation* (see Table 5-2) is useful to facilitate understanding of the effects of blocking receptor activation using adrenergic antagonists.

Alpha-Adrenergic Antagonists

Drugs that attach to α-adrenergic receptors and block the effects of norepinephrine and epinephrine are categorized as α-adrenergic antagonists. Specific drug effects differ due to the degree of selectivity for α_1 or α_2 receptor subtypes. Moreover, patients' responses to these drugs may vary if they have had prior exposure to α-agonists or α-antagonists, or may reflect the concentration of endogenous catecholamines, receptor concentration on cell membranes (up- or down-regulation of receptors), or even simply a genetic variation in receptors. The following is an example: A typical response to endogenous catecholamines that stimulate α_1-receptors (e.g., norepinephrine) is vasoconstriction.

If an α_1-receptor antagonist is administered, vascular smooth muscle contraction and other α_1-receptor–mediated effects caused by **norepinephrine** are blocked, blood vessels dilate and blood pressure decreases.

Generally, α-adrenergic receptor antagonists are useful in the management of hypertension, benign prostatic hypertrophy, and heart failure. It has been observed, however, that repeated exposure to the same drugs *may* cause adaptive changes such that patients either no longer respond to the medication dose originally prescribed (tolerance) or perhaps become sensitized to it, meaning that the patient may develop an allergic reaction (sensitization). Studies of this phenomenon (Kojima et al., 2011) show that use of such drugs may lead to up-regulation of receptors over time, potentially changing the patient's response to the drug.

Selectivity

Alpha-adrenergic receptor antagonists may be nonselective or selective for α_1-receptors. With nonselective α-adrenergic antagonists, both α_1- and α_2-adrenegic receptors are blocked, resulting in reduced blood pressure as the major cardiovascular effect. While the inhibitory actions caused by α_2-receptor activation, such as decreased release of **norepinephrine**, are blocked by nonselective α antagonists, blockade of α_1-receptors produces profound hypotensive effects that mask the actions at α_2-receptors. The α_1-selective antagonists spare α_2-receptors of blockade and the predominant effect is, similarly, decreased blood pressure. Other favorable actions of α_1-specific antagonists include decreased urinary outflow obstruction caused by benign prostatic hypertrophy and beneficial effects on glucose and lipid metabolism.

Yohimbine, used primarily for the treatment of erectile dysfunction, is the only α_2-selective receptor antagonist available for clinical use. However, newer, more reliable medications that inhibit phosphodiesterase (e.g., **sildenafil**) have made this drug virtually obsolete.

Phenoxybenzamine

Phenoxybenzamine is a noncompetitive, nonselective α-adrenergic antagonist agent that is the prototype for α-antagonists. When the α-receptor–mediated effects of **norepinephrine** and **epinephrine** are blocked by **phenoxybenzamine**, peripheral vascular resistance decreases and blood pressure falls. Heart rate often increases due to a compensatory baroreceptor reflex–mediated effect (called reflex tachycardia) and perhaps to some extent due to increased circulating **norepinephrine** caused by α_2-receptor blockade. Additionally, **phenoxybenzamine** *irreversibly* binds to receptors and new receptors must be synthesized for termination of effects of the drug.

Phenoxybenzamine is primarily used in the preoperative management of episodic, dangerous hypertension in patients with **pheochromocytoma** prior to surgical excision. Beta-receptor antagonists are also useful in this setting but should be added *after* effective α blockade has been achieved to prevent unopposed alpha stimulation and possible pulmonary edema. Other indications include hypoplastic left heart syndrome and complex regional pain syndrome type 1.

Adverse effects of **phenoxybenzamine** include decreased blood pressure, which is an expected effect of the drug that can be detrimental if drug concentrations occur above the therapeutic range. Initiating **phenoxybenzamine** therapy at a low dose and increasing the dosage slowly over a period of several days may attenuate profound hypotension. As the peripheral vascular resistance decreases and the intravascular volume expands over several days, oral ingestion of fluids fills the expanded intravascular volume. Orthostatic hypotension may persist with associated increases in heart rate after slow initiation of therapy and appropriate volume repletion. Forced ejaculate is limited by α-receptor blockade, but orgasm and semen secretion are not impaired (Gerstenberg, Levin, & Wagner, 1990). Parasympathetic effects may become evident due to decreased α-adrenergic activity (e.g., nasal stuffiness, increased gastrointestinal motility, and increased glycogen synthesis).

Administration of exogenous catecholamines may be ineffective in treating hypotension due to **phenoxybenzamine**, as these drugs cannot compete with the irreversible phenoxybenzamine–receptor complex. **Phenylephrine** and **norepinephrine** may be completely ineffective. Because **epinephrine** is effective only at β-adrenergic receptors in individuals treated with nonselective α-receptor blockade, its administration will produce *hypotensive* responses due to unopposed vasodilation caused by β_2-receptor stimulation. This phenomenon, called "epinephrine reversal," may also be observed with other α_1-receptor *antagonists* due to stimulation of both β-adrenergic receptors and α_2-adrenergic receptors (Swan & Reynolds, 1971). Generous intravenous fluids administered to increase intravascular volume prior to and during **phenoxybenzamine** administration may prevent profound hypotension and reduce orthostatic hypotension and tachycardia. **Vasopressin** may correct hypotension due to **phenoxybenzamine** infusion proven to be refractory to **norepinephrine** administration (O'Blenes, Roy, Konstantinov, Bohn, & Van Arsdell, 2002).

Phentolamine

Phentolamine is a competitive, nonselective α-receptor antagonist. It differs from **phenoxybenzamine** in that its interaction with receptors is reversible and drug effects can be overcome by increasing the concentrations of an α-receptor agonist (e.g., **phenylephrine**, **norepinephrine**). **Phentolamine** also has affinity for serotonin (5-HT) receptors, blocks potassium channels, stimulates gastrointestinal motility, increases secretion of gastric acid, and causes mast cell degranulation. It is used systemically to treat hypertension and injected locally after extravasation of vasoconstrictor drugs (e.g., **dopamine**) to prevent soft-tissue necrosis (Bey, El-Chaar, Bierman, & Valderrama, 1998). **Phentolamine** should be used with

caution in patients with exaggerated histamine release or sensitivity to histamine effects (e.g., bronchoconstriction due to histamine, particularly in patients with asthma).

Prazosin

Prazosin is a competitive, selective α_1-receptor antagonist ($1000:1::\alpha_1:\alpha_2$). It also inhibits the phosphodiesterase enzyme, thereby decreasing smooth muscle contraction. This drug is used primarily in the treatment of hypertension. Antagonist effects at the α_1-receptor produce decreased peripheral vascular resistance and increased venous capacity, in turn leading to decreased preload and systemic blood pressure with little change in heart rate. Interestingly, **prazosin** increases the concentration of high-density lipoproteins and decreases the concentration of low-density lipoproteins via mechanisms that may be unrelated to α-receptor interactions. For this reason, it is sometimes prescribed for patients with both hypertension and hypercholesterolemia.

A number of **prazosin** analogs are also in use, including **terazosin**, **doxazosin**, and **tamsulosin**. **Terazosin** is a less potent, longer-acting analog of **prazosin** that is similarly selective for α_1-receptors. It is primarily used in the management of benign prostatic hyperplasia (BPH). **Doxazosin** is a selective α_1-receptor antagonist analog of **prazosin** that is used in the management of hypertension and BPH. Likewise, **tamsulosin** is a selective α_1-receptor antagonist analog of **prazosin**, but its effects are weaker in the vasculature and more selective for α-receptors in the prostate. This agent is used in the management of BPH.

Adverse effects for **prazosin** and its analogs include orthostatic hypotension and syncope, which may occur 30 to 90 minutes after the initial dose of any of these drugs, with the possible exception of **tamsulosin** (as noted earlier, **tamsulosin's** effects are weaker, so it is less likely to produce profound orthostatic hypotension than the other agents in this class). For this reason, the first dose is optimally taken just prior to bedtime. Postural hypotension may continue during long-term therapy with these drugs, so patients should be advised to rise from lying or sitting positions slowly to avoid dizziness and syncope. Headache and asthenia are common side effects.

Nursing Considerations for α-Receptor Antagonists

Because postural hypotension often persists with chronic therapy, it may be beneficial to assess and document the patient's standing, sitting, and recumbent blood pressures. Patients should be advised to take the first dose just prior to bedtime. Additionally, they should rise slowly from lying and sitting positions to avoid dizziness, syncope, and possible injury. Patients may be alarmed by some of the side effects (e.g., nasal stuffiness, increased gastrointestinal motility, abnormal ejaculate) and can be reassured with the understanding that these side effects are common.

Beta-Adrenergic Antagonists

Beta-receptor antagonists are drugs that attach to β-adrenergic receptors and block the effects of agonists (e.g., **epinephrine** and **norepinephrine**) at β-receptor sites. When β-receptors are stimulated, sympathetic responses occur. For example, β_1-receptor stimulation elicits increases in heart rate, while β_2-receptor stimulation elicits bronchodilation. Blockade of these receptors prevents cardiac and pulmonary excitation, respectively. The effectiveness of β-adrenergic antagonists, like the effectiveness of other adrenergic agents, may vary among individuals due to membrane receptor concentration (up- and down-regulation of receptors), catecholamine concentration, interactions with other agents, and receptor genetics.

Selectivity

Beta-antagonists are often classified as either nonselective or **cardioselective**. Nonselective β-antagonists block both β_1 and β_2-receptors. Cardioselective β antagonists

preferentially block β_1-receptors. The predominant cardiovascular effects for these antagonists at the β_1-receptor include decreased heart rate and myocardial contractility (see Table 5-3). The effects of β_2-receptor antagonists include *inhibition* of vascular dilation and inhibition of pulmonary bronchiole dilation, which may be problematic in patients with obstructive lung disease.

Beta-adrenergic antagonists are useful in the management of a number of illnesses, including hypertension, ischemic heart disease, arrhythmia, hypertrophic obstructive cardiomyopathy, chronic open-angle glaucoma, migraine, thyrotoxicosis, variceal bleeding due to portal hypertension, and "stage fright." More recently, β-antagonists have become important adjuncts in the management of chronic—*but not acute*—heart failure (Bristow, 2011; Javed & Deedwania, 2009).

Beta-antagonist drugs can produce a number of adverse effects. Common side effects include bradycardia, bronchospasm, fatigue, sleep disturbance, impotence in men, and attenuated responses to hypoglycemia. These drugs, particularly nonselective agents, are generally avoided in patients with asthma. More concerning effects include progressive heart block, bronchoconstriction, and heart failure. Additionally, abrupt discontinuation of long-term β-antagonist therapy may result in "rebound" increases in heart rate and blood pressure. These rebound effects can produce myocardial ischemia, infarction, or sudden death in susceptible individuals. Therefore, gradual tapering of the dose is recommended if β-adrenergic antagonist therapy must be terminated.

Symptomatic adverse effects of β-antagonist overdose may require intervention. Treatments for symptomatic bradycardia, hypotension, or heart block may include cessation of β-blocker therapy; administration of **atropine**, **glucagon**, or **isoproterenol**; or temporary cardiac pacing.

Administration of vasopressors such as **norepinephrine** and **epinephrine** in the context of β-antagonist pharmacotherapy or overdose may be harmful, as these agents' effects will be limited to α-receptor stimulation because β-receptors are blocked. The combination of α-receptor–mediated hypertension from vasopressor administration and decreased contractility from β blockade may produce iatrogenic heart failure and pulmonary congestion. When β-adrenergic–antagonist therapy is used during cocaine intoxication, it may result in unopposed α-receptor stimulation, leading to hypertension and pulmonary edema (Houston, 1991; Richards et al., 2016). Nonsteroidal anti-inflammatory agents (e.g., **ibuprofen, diclofenac sodium**) are not recommended in patients taking β-adrenergic antagonists for hypertension because they attenuate the antihypertensive effects of these agents.

Beta-adrenergic antagonist therapy is indicated in the presurgical management of pheochromocytoma only *after* α-adrenergic antagonist therapy has been initiated. These drugs are *not* indicated in the management of *acute* heart failure. Patients with diabetes may not experience the typical responses to hypoglycemia, putting them at higher risk for hypoglycemic crisis.

Propranolol

Propranolol is the prototype β-antagonist drug and has effects on both β_1 and β_2-receptors—it is a competitive, nonselective β-adrenergic antagonist. **Propranolol** has fallen out of favor since newer cardioselective β-antagonist agents have been developed. However, it remains useful in the management of intention tremor, thyroid storm, and pheochromocytoma.

Propranolol may interact with alcohol, α-antagonists, calcium-channel blockers, antiarrhythmic medications, α_2-agonists, digoxin, haloperidol, MAO inhibitors, nonsteroidal anti-inflammatory agents, thyroid medications, tricyclic antidepressants, and **warfarin**.

Other Commonly Used β-Adrenergic Antagonists

Metoprolol is a competitive, cardioselective β_1-receptor antagonist. It is effective in limiting heart rate increases during exercise in patients with ischemic heart disease. It is also useful in hypertension, angina, acute myocardial infarction, supraventricular tachycardia, chronic (but not acute) heart failure, hyperthyroidism, long QT syndrome, performance anxiety, vasovagal syndrome, and migraine headaches.

Esmolol is a competitive, cardioselective β_1-receptor antagonist with a unique structure that permits hydrolysis by erythrocyte esterases. This feature results in a drug with a short half-life, necessitating administration of this medication by intravenous infusion to achieve sustained effects.

Atenolol is a competitive, cardioselective β_1-receptor antagonist. It is eliminated unchanged in the urine and may accumulate in patients with impaired renal function, leading to overdose and toxicity.

Nadolol is a competitive, nonselective β-receptor antagonist with a long half-life, allowing for once-daily dosing. It is used in the management of angina, hypertension, migraine headaches, Parkinsonian tremors, and variceal bleeding.

Pindolol is a nonselective β-receptor antagonist. However, it is also thought to have some weak β-receptor–agonist effects, which limit the degree to which heart rate and blood pressure are reduced. This agent is sometimes used in patients who are sensitive to the bradycardic effects of other β-receptor antagonists.

Labetalol is unique among the β-adrenergic antagonists. It actually consists of several isomers that have α_1-antagonist and nonselective β-adrenergic–antagonist effects. **Labetalol** produces significant decreases in blood pressure without compensatory increases in heart rate and is most commonly used in the treatment of hypertension.

Carvedilol is a unique drug that acts as an antagonist at α_1-, β_1-, and β_2-adrenergic receptors. It also demonstrates antioxidant and antiproliferative properties. This agent is useful in the management of chronic heart failure and postmyocardial infarction. **Carvedilol** improves ventricular function and reduces morbidity and mortality in these populations.

Nursing Considerations for β-Adrenergic Antagonists

Assessment

A number of factors are contraindications to use of β-adrenergic antagonists. Women of childbearing age should be assessed for pregnancy or likelihood of pregnancy, as most β-adrenergic antagonists are considered to potentially carry some risk to the fetus. Elderly patients may be at higher risk for injury when such agents are prescribed, due to bradycardia, postural hypotension, and falls. The presence of conditions that might be worsened with these drugs—such as hypotension, bradycardia, unstable congestive heart failure, heart block, asthma, and COPD—should also be evaluated. Prior to, during, and after administration of β-adrenergic–antagonist medications, the nurse should monitor the patient's blood pressure and cardiovascular status.

In chronic treatment, the nurse should assess the patient for common effects such as fatigue, hypotension (especially orthostatic or postural), bradycardia, sleep disturbance, and depression. TABLE 5-4 lists nursing diagnoses associated with use of β-adrenergic antagonists and the goals associated with them.

Nursing interventions for β-adrenergic antagonists include the following:

- Monitor the blood pressure while the patient is supine, sitting, and standing for the possibility of postural hypotension.
- Teach the patient to minimize postural hypotension:

  - Dangle legs for a few minutes before standing.
  - Rise slowly and stand for a moment.
  - Move slowly and do not change positions readily.
- Tell the patient to check with his or her healthcare provider or pharmacist prior to taking any other prescription or over-the-counter medications.
- Tell the patient *not* to stop taking the medication abruptly, as this medication needs to be weaned.

Cholinergic Drugs   ↑PNS

Cholinergic drugs are divided into two classes: **cholinergic antagonists** and **cholinergic agonists**. Understanding the normal physiology of cholinergic nerves, acetylcholine, acetylcholinesterase, and cholinergic receptors is necessary to understand the actions of cholinergic drugs.

There are a number of conditions in which using cholinergic antagonists is not advised (TABLE 5-5). These contraindications arise because such medications may actually exacerbate a disease process in which stimulation of the receptors is already weak, or because the side effects of their use may exacerbate a condition related to the disease process.

Cholinergic Agents

Cholinergic agonists can be separated into two subclasses of drugs: direct-acting

TABLE 5-4	Nursing Diagnoses Related to β-Adrenergic Antagonist Use
Nursing Diagnoses	**Goals**
Activity intolerance related to fatigue, lethargy, or depression due to β-adrenergic antagonist administration	Patient will maintain his or her activity level.
Altered tissue perfusion related to hypotension or bradycardia related to β-adrenergic antagonist drug	Patient will maintain adequate tissue perfusion.
Risk for sleep pattern disturbance related to fatigue, lethargy, and depression	Patient will maintain his or her normal sleep and waking patterns.
Alteration in comfort: nausea related to β-adrenergic antagonist drug	Patient will maintain his or her weight.
Potential for injury related to potential postural hypotension	Patient will remain injury free and learn to change positions slowly.

TABLE 5-5	Contraindications to the Use of Cholinergic Antagonists
Contraindication	**Rationale**
Myasthenia gravis	Cholinergic antagonists will decrease the effects of the anticholinesterase medications, putting the patient at risk for a myasthenic crisis.
Tachydysrhythmias	Cholinergic antagonists block parasympathetic vagal stimulation, increasing the heart rate and increasing the myocardial oxygen demand.
Myocardial infarction	Cholinergic antagonists increase heart rate, increase myocardial oxygen demand, potentiate arrhythmias, and exacerbate a myocardial infarction.
Glaucoma	With narrow-angle glaucoma, cholinergic antagonists can increase the intraocular pressure and precipitate an occurrence of acute glaucoma.
Prostatic hypertrophy	Cholinergic antagonists affect the muscarinic receptors in the smooth muscle of the bladder and can cause urinary retention.
Hyperthyroidism	Cholinergic antagonists can aggravate the cardiac effects of tachycardia.
Pregnancy and lactation	Counsel patients according to the FDA Pregnancy and Lactation Labeling Rule (PLLR).

acetylcholine receptor agonists (e.g., bethanechol) and indirect-acting acetylcholinesterase enzyme inhibitors (e.g., neostigmine). The actions and adverse drug effects of this class of medications are listed in TABLE 5-6.

Directly Acting Acetylcholine Receptor Agonist

Bethanechol is the only commonly used cholinergic agonist. It stimulates muscarinic receptors on the bladder, causing contraction and urination. It also stimulates peristalsis of the urethra and relaxes the external sphincter. Spinal cord injury does not limit the use of bethanechol, as the drug is a direct-acting agonist. This agent is the drug of choice to treat postpartum and postoperative unobstructed urinary retention. In the gastrointestinal tract, bethanechol stimulates the muscarinic receptors to increase peristalsis and motility, causing defecation.

While drugs affecting the somatic (voluntary) nervous system are beyond the scope of this chapter, acetylcholine is also released at the neuromuscular junction and affects nicotinic acetylcholine receptors at or near postjunctional muscle membranes. When stimulated, nicotinic acetylcholine receptors cause skeletal muscle membrane depolarization and trigger a complex series of subsequent events resulting in muscle

contraction. Drugs with cholinergic activity in the ANS may have significant effects on neuromuscular transmission (cholinesterase inhibitors, e.g., neostigmine), and vice versa (neuromuscular blocking agents, e.g., pancuronium) (see also TABLE 5-6).

Acetylcholinesterase Inhibitors

Acetylcholinesterase inhibitors (or anticholinesterases) block the metabolic effects of the enzyme acetylcholinesterase in both the ANS and the neuromuscular junctions of voluntary skeletal muscle. Acetylcholinesterase breaks down (inactivates) acetylcholine (ACh); when ACh breakdown is blocked, the amount of acetylcholine increases. This inhibition allows acetylcholine to accumulate in synapses and subsequently increases acetylcholine receptor stimulation. It is important to note that acetylcholinesterase is not selective for cholinergic synapses. Therefore, cholinergic stimulation occurs in all autonomic ganglia, in parasympathetic end organs (muscarinic effects), and in neuromuscular junctions. Parasympathetic effects predominate due to increased acetylcholine activity at muscarinic sites.

Anticholinesterase agents are used in the management of Alzheimer disease, for the treatment of delirium,

↓ACh
↑acetylcholine

Best Practices

When acetylcholinesterase is blocked, the acetylcholine is not metabolized as quickly, allowing it to have a more prolonged effect at the cholinergic receptor sites.

TABLE 5-6	Cholinergic Agonist Actions and Adverse Effects	
	Cholinergic Agonist Action	Cholinergic Agonist Adverse Drug Effects (ADE)
Cardiovascular	↓ heart rate, vasodilation	Serious ADE: bradycardia, hypotension
Pulmonary	Bronchoconstriction, ↑ respiratory secretions, ↑ salivation	Serious ADE: bronchoconstriction, ↑ secretions → shortness of breath
Pupils	Constriction (miosis), ↓ intraocular pressure	
Gastrointestinal	↑ motility, ↑ secretions	Common ADE: ↑ gastric emptying, nausea, abdominal cramping, vomiting, diarrhea
Blood sugar	~	~
Sweating	↑ sweating	Diaphoresis, loss of fluids
Urinary	Voiding	Frequency of urination
CNS	~	~
Uses	Limited, but varied: Urinary retention or atony Paralytic ileus Diagnosis and therapy of myasthenia gravis Alzheimer disease Glaucoma "Wet" (salivation, lacrimation, urination, defecation)	Drying effects
Drugs	Bethanechol Neostigmine Pyridostigmine Edrophonium Donepezil	

and in the diagnosis and treatment of myasthenia gravis. They are also useful in the indirect reversal of certain paralytic agents by specially trained professionals.

Neostigmine

Neostigmine is the prototype of anticholinesterase drugs. It is used for the long-term treatment of myasthenia gravis. When used for this purpose, resistance may develop, necessitating administration of larger doses to achieve the same effect. Myasthenia gravis is an autoimmune disease in which antibodies destroy postsynaptic nicotinic acetylcholine receptors in the neuromuscular junction. The levels of acetylcholine are normal, but due to a lack of receptors, the acetylcholine cannot bind at a sufficient number of receptors

required to stimulate muscle contraction. This leads to muscle weakness, particularly of the voluntary muscles and often those muscles innervated by the cranial nerves. Symptoms usually include ptosis, diplopia, ataxia, dysarthria, difficulty swallowing, shortness of breath due to chest wall muscle weakness, and weakness in the arms, hands, and legs.

Neostigmine is indicated to treat urinary retention and paralytic ileus. It is also used as an antidote for nondepolarizing skeletal muscle relaxants (paralytic agents) used during surgery.

Physostigmine

Physostigmine is useful in the treatment of myasthenia gravis, glaucoma, and impaired gastric motility. Perhaps most importantly, it is useful in the treatment of central toxic effects of **atropine** and **scopolamine** because it is the only anticholinesterase drug that crosses the blood–brain barrier in an intact form. It also has been used in the management of delirium associated with anesthesia.

Edrophonium

Edrophonium is a short-acting cholinergic, making it ideal for the diagnosis of myasthenia gravis and to differentiate between myasthenic crisis and cholinergic crisis. When it is given in these situations, life support equipment such as **atropine** (the antidote), endotracheal tubes, oxygen, and ventilators must be available.

Pyridostigmine

Pyridostigmine is similar in actions, uses, and adverse drug effects to **neostigmine**. **Pyridostigmine** is the maintenance drug of choice for patients with myasthenia gravis, as it has a long duration of action. It is also available in a slow-release form that is taken at bedtime. Because this agent is effective for 8 to 12 hours, the patient with myasthenia gravis does not have to wake during the night to take their next dose of medication, and wakes strong enough to swallow a morning dose.

Donepezil

Donepezil is used to treat mild to moderate Alzheimer disease (see Chapter 4). Alzheimer disease is characterized by a loss of neurons that secrete acetylcholine in the brain. When acetylcholinesterase is blocked, the acetylcholine is not metabolized as quickly, allowing it to have a more prolonged effect at the cholinergic receptor sites. This can help improve memory, attention, reason, language, and the ability to perform simple tasks. **Donepezil** is given orally and can be taken without regard to meals.

Nursing Considerations for Cholinergic Agonists
Assessment

Assess the patient for possible contraindications such as uncontrolled asthma, active peptic ulcer disease, and cardiovascular disease. Female patients of childbearing age should be assessed for possible pregnancy or breastfeeding, as these drugs should be used only if no other alternatives are available in pregnant or lactating women. Elderly patients may be at greater risk for visual disturbances, so nurses should have a baseline knowledge of their visual capacity for comparison to the patients' experiences during treatment.

In patients with urinary retention, note the last time and amount of the previous urinary output. Note fluid intake and assess for bladder distention. In patients with paralytic ileus, assess for the presence or absence of bowel sounds, abdominal distention, pain, and regular bowel patterns. In patients with myasthenia gravis, assess for muscle weakness such as drooping of the eyelids (ptosis) and double vision (diplopia). In more severe stages of the illness, the patient should be assessed for any difficulty in chewing, swallowing, speaking, or breathing. Assess for respiratory rate, rhythm, and muscle use, as these patients can develop respiratory failure due to muscle weakness. In patients with Alzheimer disease, memory and cognitive functioning, as well as self-care abilities, should be assessed.

Nursing diagnoses and goals for patients taking cholinergic agonists and acetylcholinesterase inhibitors are found in TABLE 5-7.

Nursing Interventions

Nursing interventions for patients with urinary retention include the following:

- Ensure there is no obstruction of the urinary tract.
- Consider nonpharmacologic treatments such as providing privacy, bathing the perineum with warm water, and, if possible, allowing the patient to sit up to urinate or ambulate to the bathroom.

Nursing interventions for patients with paralytic ileus include the following:

- Ensure there is no obstruction in the gastrointestinal tract.

TABLE 5-7	Cholinergic Agonists and Anticholinesterases: Nursing Diagnoses and Goals
Nursing Diagnoses	**Nursing Goals**
Ineffective airway clearance related to increased respiratory secretions and bronchoconstriction	Patient will maintain effective oxygenation of tissues.
Ineffective elimination patterns	Patient will maintain or attain normal elimination patterns.
Knowledge deficit related to drug administration and effects	Patient will verbalize why this drug is being used and signs or symptoms to report to the healthcare provider.

- Implement preventive measures including early ambulation, adequate fluid intake, providing privacy, and, if possible, allowing the patient to sit up or ambulate to the bathroom.

Nursing interventions for patients with myasthenia gravis include the following:

- Schedule activities to allow for periods of rest.
- Encourage the patient to wear a medical alert bracelet.
- With the permission of the patient, involve family members in patient care.
- Suggest a family member be trained in cardiopulmonary resuscitation.

Nursing interventions for patients with Alzheimer disease include the following:

- Encourage self-care activities.
- Maintain a consistent routine.

Cholinergic Antagonists

Cholinergic antagonists are often referred to as anticholinergic drugs or antimuscarinic drugs. Their drug action is limited to muscarinic acetylcholine receptors, where they limit and block the actions of acetylcholine. Muscarinic receptors are located on most internal organs, such as those of the cardiovascular, pulmonary, gastrointestinal, and genitourinary systems. Stimulation of the muscarinic receptors causes an increase in secretions.

Muscarinic receptors are also found on smooth muscle. By blocking the action of acetylcholine at these receptors in the gastrointestinal and urinary tracts, anticholinergic drugs can relax the spasms of smooth muscles.

Clinical Indications for Use

Anticholinergic drugs have multiple actions, and their indications vary as well. For example, since anticholinergic drugs inhibit smooth muscle contraction and decrease gastrointestinal secretions, they are used to treat spastic and hyperactive conditions of the gastrointestinal and urinary tracts.

Anticholinergic agents are used preoperatively to decrease respiratory and gastrointestinal secretions and to prevent a drop in the heart rate caused by vagal stimulation during intubation. These drugs are also used in ophthalmology because they cause mydriasis (pupil dilation), which facilitates examination and ocular surgical procedures. Other uses of anticholinergic drugs include the treatment of Parkinson's disease, to decrease salivation, spasticity, and tremors; the treatment of asthma and COPD, as they produce bronchodilation and drying of the respiratory sections; and the treatment of symptomatic bradycardia.

The adverse effects of anticholinergic drugs are generally related to the dose administered. The major adverse anticholinergic drug effects include tachycardia, dried bronchial secretions, dry mouth, blurred vision, and decreased sweating. As noted in Table 5-5, there are specific conditions in which cholinergic antagonists are contraindicated because they may interact with pharmacotherapeutic interventions or worsen symptoms of the underlying pathology.

Individual Cholinergic Antagonists

Atropine

Atropine is the prototype anticholinergic drug. It is absorbed by the gastrointestinal tract and distributed throughout the body. **Atropine** crosses the blood–brain barrier. In the CNS, a therapeutic dose produces stimulant effects, whereas toxic doses produce depressant effects. When applied to mucous membranes, **atropine** is absorbed systemically. This agent has a short duration of action.

According to *Advanced Cardiac Life Support Guidelines*, **atropine** is the drug of choice in the treatment of symptomatic bradycardia. However, it is no longer recommended for the treatment of pulseless electrical activity or asystole (American Heart Association, 2010).

Atropine given preoperatively can avert the vagal stimulation that often accompanies endotracheal intubation, causing bradycardia and hypotension. This agent is also useful in drying respiratory secretions prior to head and neck surgery.

Atropine is used to treat the excessive cholinergic stimulation caused by anticholinesterase toxicity, mushroom poisoning, some nerve gases (Sarin) used for chemical warfare, and some organophosphate pesticide poisoning.

Glycopyrrolate

Glycopyrrolate does not cross the blood–brain barrier and, therefore, is devoid of central effects. This agent increases heart rate and blood pressure, but to a lesser extent than **atropine**.

Scopolamine

Scopolamine exerts minimal effects on heart rate and blood pressure. However, it has significant central effects and produces profound mydriasis. In high doses, it can cause central toxicity, which manifests as dry mouth, rubor, cycloplegia, and delirium. Central toxicity is an emergency and may be treated with the anticholinesterase drug **physostigmine**. Administration of **scopolamine** by cutaneous patch reduces nausea and vomiting due to anesthesia or motion (e.g., sea sickness, car sickness).

Ipratropium

Ipratropium can be used as an inhalation treatment for COPD to produce bronchodilation. It is also used as a nasal spray to relieve rhinorrhea. When **ipratropium** is administered by spray or inhalation, the bronchial secretions are decreased and there is less risk of mucous plugs forming.

Tiotropium Bromide

Tiotropium bromide is a long-acting antimuscarinic, anticholinergic agent that produces bronchodilation. It is administered as a dry-powder capsule with a HandiHaler device. This agent is indicated for use as a daily maintenance treatment in patients with COPD; it is not recommended for treating acute episodes.

Benztropine

Benztropine is a centrally acting anticholinergic drug. It is more selective for muscarinic receptors in the CNS, so it also produces fewer adverse drug effects. **Benztropine** can be used to decrease the symptoms of Parkinson's disease (see Chapter 4), such as tremors, spasticity, and salivation. This agent is usually prescribed in the early stages of the disease and in patients who have demonstrated a minimal response to **levodopa**, which is the treatment of choice for Parkinson's disease.

Oxybutynin

Oxybutynin increases bladder capacity and decreases voiding frequency by exerting a direct antispasmodic effect on smooth muscle and anticholinergic effects.

Nursing Process for Cholinergic Antagonists
Assessment

The assessment should identify whether the patient is on any other medications with anticholinergic effects, such as antihistamines, antipsychotic agents, or tricyclic antidepressants, as this combination could cause an adverse interaction. Similarly, the nurse should assess for any condition in which the anticholinergic drug would be contraindicated, such as glaucoma, myasthenia gravis, hyperthyroidism, prostatic hypertrophy, tachyarrhythmia, or myocardial infarction. Female patients of childbearing age should be

TABLE 5-8	Anticholinergic Drugs: Nursing Diagnoses and Goals
Nursing Diagnoses	**Nursing Goals**
Decreased cardiac output related to bradycardia	Patient will attain a heart rate of 60 to 100 beats per minute.
Ineffective airway clearance related to increased respiratory secretions and bronchoconstriction	Patient will maintain effective oxygenation of tissues.
Ineffective elimination patterns	Patient will maintain or attain normal elimination patterns.
Knowledge deficit related to drug administration and effects	Patient will verbalize why this drug is being used and signs or symptoms to report to the healthcare provider.
Risk for noncompliance related to adverse drug effects	Patient will verbalize the need to take the medication as prescribed.

assessed for pregnancy or breastfeeding, as these drugs should be used in such women only if no other alternatives are available. Elderly patients may be at greater risk for most adverse effects and heat stroke.

During the assessment, note the condition for which the patient was prescribed an anticholinergic drug, such as bradycardia, diarrhea, enuresis, Parkinson's disease, asthma, COPD, or other disorders. Note any indications of adverse drug effects such as tachycardia, dried bronchial secretions, dry mouth, blurred vision, and decreased sweating.

Nursing diagnoses and goals related to anticholinergic drugs are listed in TABLE 5-8.

Nursing Interventions

- Teach the patient why the drug is being prescribed and how to take it correctly.
- Teach the patient about the potential adverse drug effects.
- Have the patient protect his or her eyes from the sun with sunglasses.
- To alleviate a dry mouth and to prevent tooth decay, sip on cold water, suck on sugarless hard candies, chew sugarless gum, and use frequent oral hygiene.
- Increase fluid and fiber in the diet to prevent constipation.
- Avoid any over-the-counter or prescription drugs without first checking with the healthcare provider.

- Avoid overheating by staying in air conditioning, drinking fluids, and taking frequent showers or sponge baths.

CHAPTER SUMMARY

- The ANS is composed of three interconnected systems that manage involuntary functions: the SNS, the PNS, and the ENS.
- The SNS is responsible for fight-or-flight response, while the PNS is characterized as the rest-and-repair system; the two work in tandem, and the ENS (which innervates the digestive tract) interacts with both.
- The SNS is also called the thoracolumbar system, and the PNS is called the craniosacral system, reflecting the locations from which preganglionic nerves originate in each of the respective divisions.
- Preganglionic nerves may be sympathetic or parasympathetic, and in both cases they are cholinergic nerves that release acetylcholine.
- The receptors at ganglia for both the SNS and the PNS are nicotinic acetylcholine receptors.
- Postganglionic sympathetic nerves release norepinephrine, which stimulates adrenergic receptors at effector organs.
- Postganglionic parasympathetic nerves release acetylcholine, which stimulates muscarinic acetylcholine receptors at effector organs.
- Medications that affect the ANS often mimic or block the actions of acetylcholine or norepinephrine. These actions can provide therapeutic effects by either reducing stress on effector organs such as the heart, lungs, or kidneys, or increasing the output of these organs in cases where function is sub-par.
- Some medications that have generalized, rather than targeted, effects on receptors can also promote unwanted side effects. Understanding how each type of medication affects the receptors is therefore necessary for optimal disease management.

CASE STUDIES

Case Scenario 1

A 12-year-old boy is stung by a bee while playing in his backyard. In the past, he has had severe reactions to insect stings, which required emergency room visits and the dispensing of an epinephrine injector. On this occasion, by the time he reaches the door to tell his mother, he is covered in hives, is audibly wheezing, and passes out suddenly in the foyer. His mother immediately calls 9-1-1 and administers the prescribed intramuscular epinephrine dose into the boy's thigh. The child recovers consciousness rapidly; at the arrival of the ambulance, he is breathing easier and complaining of itching all over. Paramedics report normal blood pressure and tachycardia.

Case Questions

1. Given the patient's symptoms, what is the likely medical problem?
2. The administration of epinephrine caused a rapid improvement in the patient's symptoms. Which adrenergic receptors were likely stimulated by the medication, and what response did these invoke that improved his breathing?
3. Which adrenergic receptors were stimulated to restore the patient's normal blood pressure and return to consciousness, and what response did this invoke?
4. Which adrenergic receptors must be stimulated to relieve the patient's tachycardia, and what response would this invoke?

CASE STUDIES

Case Scenario 2

Mr. Walker enjoys cooking and prefers to eat locally grown food when it is available. While hiking on a trail through the woods, he finds a new crop of mushrooms growing by a log. Thinking about how good fresh sautéed mushrooms would be with his dinner that evening, Mr. Walker gathers the mushrooms.

When he arrives home, he cleans the mushrooms and eats a few of them as he works. Twenty minutes later, he is salivating and sweating, his vision is blurry, and he has difficulty breathing. He calls 9-1-1.

Case Questions

1. Which branch of the ANS has been stimulated?
2. What is causing the symptoms?
3. What is the antidote?
4. Why is the antidote effective in this case of mushroom poisoning?

CASE STUDIES (CONTINUED)

Discussion Questions

1. What are the components of the ANS? Which functions does the ANS control?
2. What does the SNS control? How does it differ from the PNS?
3. Where is acetylcholine released? Where is norepinephrine released? Which receptors do each of these neurotransmitters utilize?
4. Which types of drugs would have a positive effect on bronchoconstriction? Which drugs should be *avoided* in patients who suffer from bronchoconstriction?
5. Name the adrenergic receptors and identify a key function for each receptor.
6. Which conditions are contraindications for cholinergic antagonists?

SUGGESTED READINGS

Bellamo, R., Chapman, M., Finfer, S., Hickling, K., & Myburgh, J. (2000). Low-dose dopamine in patients with early renal dysfunction: A placebo-controlled randomised trial. *Lancet, 356,* 2139–2143.

Ichai, C., Passeron, C., Carles, M., Bouregba, M., & Grimaud, D. (2000). Prolonged low-dose dopamine infusion induces a transient improvement in renal function in hemodynamically stable, critically ill patients: A single-blind, prospective, controlled study. *Critical Care Medicine, 28,* 1329–1335.

REFERENCES

American Heart Association. (2010). 2010 American Heart Association guidelines for cardiopulmonary resuscitation and emergency cardiovascular care. *Circulation, 122*(18S), S640–S656.

Bey, D., El-Chaar, G.M., Bierman, F., & Valderrama, E. (1998). The use of phentolamine in the prevention of dopamine-induced tissue extravasation. *Journal of Critical Care, 13*(1), 13–20. doi: 10.1016/S0883-9441(98)90024-7

Blessing, B., & Gibbins, I. (2008). Autonomic nervous system. *Scholarpedia, 3*(7), 2787.

Bristow, M.R. (2011). Treatment of chronic heart failure with β-adrenergic receptor antagonists. *Circulation Research, 109,* 1176–1194.

Food and Drug Administration (FDA). (2016). *Use caution when giving cough and cold products to kids.* Retrieved from https://www.fda.gov/drugs/resourcesforyou/specialfeatures/ucm263948.htm

Gerstenberg, T.C., Levin, R.J., & Wagner, G. (1990). Erection and ejaculation in man: Assessment of the electromyographic activity of the bulbocavernosus and ischiocavernosus muscles. *British Journal of Urology, 65*(4), 395–402. doi: 10.1111/j.1464-410X.1990.tb14764.x

Houston, M.C. (1991). Nonsteroidal anti-inflammatory drugs and antihypertensives. *American Journal of Medicine, 90*(5 Suppl. 1), S42–S47. doi: 10.1016/0002-9343(91)90485-G

Javed, U., & Deedwania, P.C. (2009). Beta-adrenergic blockers for chronic heart failure. *Cardiology in Review, 17*(6), 287–292. doi: 10.1097/CRD.0b013e3181bdf63e

Johnson, J.O. (2013). Autonomic nervous system physiology. In H.C. Hemmings & T.D. Egan (Eds.), *Pharmacology and physiology for anesthesia: Foundations and clinical application* (pp. 208–218). Philadelphia, PA: Elsevier-Saunders.

Kojima, Y., Sasaki, S., Kubota, Y., Imura, M., Oda, N., Kiniwa, M., . . . Kohri, K. (2011). Up-regulation of alpha 1a- and alpha 1d-adrenoceptors in the prostate by administration of subtype-selective alpha 1-adrenoceptor antagonist tamsulosin for benign prostatic hyperplasia patients [Abstract #300]. International Continence Society Meeting, Glasgow, Scotland, August 29–September 2, 2011. Retrieved from http://www.ics.org/2011/programme/session/697

O'Blenes, S.B., Roy, N., Konstantinov, I., Bohn, D., & Van Arsdell, G.S. (2002). Vasopressin reversal of phenoxybenzamine-induced hypotension after the Norwood procedure. *Journal of Thoracic & Cardiovascular Surgery, 123*(5), 1012–1013.

Richards, J.R., Hollander, J.E., Ramosak, E.A., Fareed, F.N., Sand, S., Gomez, M.M., & Lange, R. A. (2016). β-Blockers, cocaine, and the unopposed α-stimulation phenomenon. *Journal of Cardiovascular Pharmacology and Therapeutics, 22*(3), 239–249.

Swan, K., & Reynolds, D. (1971). Adrenergic mechanisms in canine mesenteric circulation. *American Journal of Physiology—Legacy Content, 220*(6), 1779–1785.

CHAPTER 6

Cardiovascular Medications

Diane F. Pacitti and Blaine Templar Smith

KEY TERMS

ACE inhibitors
Angina pectoris
Angiotensin I
Angiotensin II
Angiotensin II receptor
  blockers (ARBs)
Angiotensin-converting
  enzyme (ACE)
Antidiuretic hormone (ADH)
Arrhythmias
Atherosclerosis
Beta-blockers
Beta-receptors
Blood pressure
Bradykinin
Calcium-channel
  blockers (CCBs)

Cardiac output (CO)
Cardiovascular system
Cholesterol
Congestive heart
  failure (CHF)
Coronary artery disease
Cytochrome P450 3A4
  (CYP3A4)
Deep vein thrombosis
  (DVT)
Diastolic
Direct renin inhibitors (DRIs)
Diuresis
Diuretic
First-dose effect
Fluid volume
Heart rate (HR)

High-density lipoprotein
  (HDL)
Hyperkalemia
Hyperlipidemia
Hypertension
Hypertensive emergency
Lipids
Low-density lipoprotein
  (LDL)
Myocardial infarction
Negative chronotrope
Peripheral dopamine-1
  agonists
Positive inotrope
Potassium-channel blockers
Prehypertension
Renin

Renin–angiotensin–
  aldosterone system (RAAS)
Selective α_1-blockers
Sodium-channel blockers
Statin
Systemic vascular
  resistance (SVR)
Systolic
Triglycerides
Vasodilators
Vasopressin antagonists
Very low-density
  lipoprotein (VLDL)

CHAPTER OBJECTIVES

At the end of the chapter, the student will be able to:

1. Define the key terms at the beginning of this chapter.

2. Describe the renin–angiotensin–aldosterone system and its impact on the cardiovascular system.

3. Discuss the most common cardiovascular conditions affecting patients.

4. Explain the rationales and approaches for treatments of common cardiovascular conditions.

5. Identify the mechanism of action for common drug classes used in treatment of cardiac conditions.

Introduction

Cardiovascular disease is the leading cause of death in the United States, for both men and women, according to the Division for Heart Disease and Stroke Prevention at the Centers for Disease Control (CDC). About 630,000 Americans die from heart disease each year—that is one in every four deaths. Each minute, more than one person in the United States dies from a heart disease–related event. Coronary artery disease (CAD) is the most common heart diseasein the United States: someone has a heart attack every 40 seconds. There are also 12 million yearly visits to physician's offices and close to 4 million hospital discharges for cardiovascular disease (Heron, 2014; Centers for Disease Control and Prevention, 2017). *Treatment* of cardiovascular disease and monitoring for therapeutic efficacy and side effects of the cardiovascular drugs used requires a comprehensive knowledge of the pharmacology of these medications. Nurses play a vital role in direct patient care; therefore, knowledge of cardiovascular medications, assessment of therapeutic and adverse effects, knowledge of drug effects on the body, and patient education are essential. It is the goal of this chapter to equip the nurse with not only a thorough understanding of the medication classes and mechanisms of action of the drugs used to treat these cardiac conditions, but more importantly, to provide the rationale for selecting appropriate drug regimens and ensure optimal therapeutic outcomes.

The Cardiovascular System

In broad terms, the **cardiovascular system** can be defined as a complex interrelated network composed of the heart and blood vessels (of the circulatory system). *Cardiovascular pharmacology* is the study of the *mechanism of action of drugs* used to treat pathologies of the heart, the circulatory system, and interrelated physiological systems which comprise the cardiovascular system.

It is *presupposed* the nurse has a working knowledge of the normal structure and function of the heart and vasculature (for review, the reader is referred to one of the many anatomy and physiology references and resources). Since *cardiovascular disease* is one of the leading causes of all deaths in the United States, it is important to distinguish that cardiovascular "disease" is actually a group of disorders that affect the heart, the blood vessels, or both (see FIGURE 6-1). For example, some disorders involve only the heart itself. Pathologies attributed to the *heart* include the following:

- Malfunctions of the heart's electrical impulses that result in rhythmic disturbances (**arrhythmias**)
- Poorly functioning valves, which result in blood "leakage" between chambers because of insufficient force to move blood forward
- Atrophy or hypertrophy of individual chambers, whether from congenital causes or disease processes, which can prevent adequate blood movement through the heart
- Acute infections, electrolyte imbalances, and fluid buildup around the heart, conditions that may create a cardiovascular crisis if not promptly treated

In contrast, conditions that affect *the circulatory* component of the cardiovascular system (including the blood vessels that feed the heart; see Figure 6-1B) include such cardiac disorders as **hypertension** (high blood pressure, which itself can have a variety of causative factors), **hyperlipidemia** (high cholesterol and/or triglyceride levels, which are generally lifestyle related but can also have genetic causes), and **congestive heart failure (CHF)**. Nearly all of these various conditions are treated with medication, although in some situations the medications are adjuncts to surgical and lifestyle interventions.

The number of medication classes used to treat cardiovascular disease is as varied as the

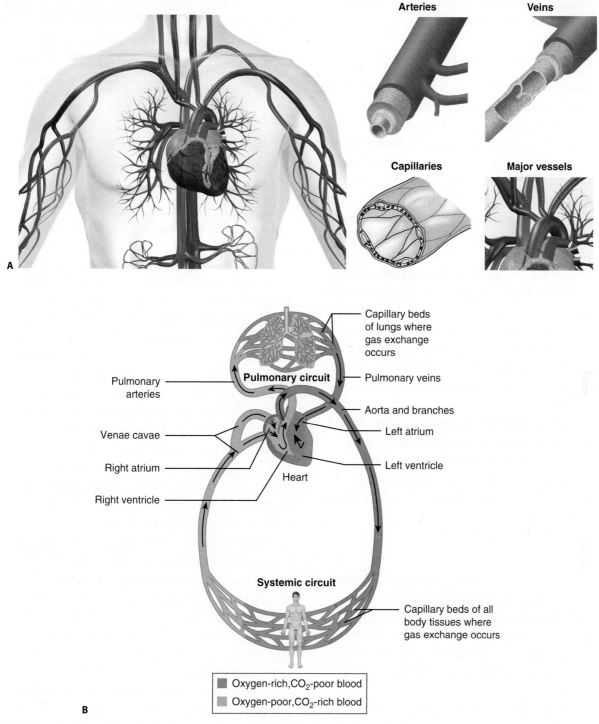

Arteries

Veins

Capillaries

Major vessels

A

Capillary beds of lungs where gas exchange occurs

Pulmonary circuit

Pulmonary arteries

Pulmonary veins

Aorta and branches

Venae cavae

Left atrium

Right atrium

Left ventricle

Heart

Right ventricle

Systemic circuit

Capillary beds of all body tissues where gas exchange occurs

■ Oxygen-rich, CO_2-poor blood
■ Oxygen-poor, CO_2-rich blood

B

FIGURE 6-1 Anatomy of the cardiovascular system. There are two physiological systems within this system: the circulatory system, which consists of the veins, arteries, and smaller vessels, and the heart. (A) The heart. (B) The circulatory system.

number of disorders themselves. The focus of this chapter, therefore, is restricted to the medication classes used in the treatment and long-term management of the cardiovascular conditions most commonly seen in the general population: *hypertension* (HTN), *angina*, *hyperlipidemia*, and *congestive heart failure*. The medications used to prevent *thrombosis* and stroke by reducing coagulation of blood are also discussed, as these agents are frequently used in conjunction with therapies to treat underlying diseases to prevent cardiovascular crises such as heart attacks (**myocardial infarction** [MI]) and *strokes*.

Treatment of High Blood Pressure

Blood pressure measures *the amount of force that blood exerts upon blood vessel walls as it flows* throughout the body. The two measurements of pressure are **systolic** blood pressure, which measures *the force of blood pressing against vessel walls while the heart is contracting* during a beat, and **diastolic** blood pressure, which is *the force exerted while the heart muscle is relaxed* between beats. The systolic measurement is typically anywhere from 40 to 50 mm Hg higher than the diastolic value.

When the force that pushes against blood vessels (pressure) remains consistently higher than the vessel walls can tolerate, the blood vessel becomes damaged. Left untreated, this could lead to serious cardiovascular pathologies such as heart attack, heart failure, and stroke.

Two significant factors that affect blood pressure are **cardiac output (CO)** and **systemic vascular resistance (SVR)**, as a function of **heart rate (HR)**. This relationship is often shortened to the following formula:

$$CO = HR \times SVR$$

Cardiac output is the amount of blood the heart is able to pump in one minute, and systemic vascular resistance is the resistance to blood flowing, present in the body from the vasculature, after the exit from the left ventricle (not including the pulmonary vasculature).

According to the preceding equation, *an increase in HR or SVR will cause blood pressure to increase; conversely, a decrease in the HR or SVR will cause a subsequent decrease in blood pressure.* It follows then, that a drug which decreases either the HR or the SVR would be a useful pharmacological agent to lower blood pressure.

According to the preceding equation, however, *all* physiological factors that

BP Formula

Blood pressure depends on cardiac output (CO) and systemic vascular resistance (SVR):

$$BP = CO \times SVR^*$$

Cardiac output depends on heart rate and stroke volume:

$$CO = HR \times SV^{**}$$

*SVR = total resistance of arterioles to flow of blood
**SV = the amount of blood pumped by the heart each cycle

contribute to CO and SVR must be considered. Key physiological factors that affect CO and SVR include fluid volume and vasoconstriction. **Fluid volume**, the volume of blood passing through the blood vessels, plays a significant role in the regulation of blood pressure. Specifically, the greater the amount (volume) of blood to be pumped, the greater the pressure will be on the vessel walls; the risk of damage to the vessel walls is increased. This can be likened to a garden hose (blood vessel) connected to a faucet (heart). If the faucet suddenly pumped three times *more* water than the hose could handle, the hose would be subjected to a significantly higher pressure than it was made to tolerate, which greatly increases the risk of damaging the hose. As a result of increased fluid in the body (blood volume), the heart must also work harder to compensate for the greater volume. *Excessive fluid, therefore, can be harmful to both the heart and the vessels.*

Vasoconstriction, similarly, affects blood pressure: less blood volume can pass through a constricted vessel than a dilated vessel; thus, there is an increased resistance to the passage of blood which can also damage blood vessels. Restriction of blood vessel walls, regardless of cause, impedes the flow of blood through that vessel, and causes the pressure inside the vessel walls to increase. *Persistent blood vessel constriction is associated with the development of hypertension.*

The autonomic nervous system (ANS), the kidneys, and the **renin–angiotensin–aldosterone system (RAAS)** are the key contributors in the control of blood pressure (TABLE 6-1). Hypertension may develop for any number of reasons, ranging from genetic factors to lifestyle factors (e.g., tobacco use, lack of exercise, high-sodium or low-potassium diet) to simple aging. Hypertension also accompanies a variety of chronic conditions, such as diabetes mellitus, renal disease, and sleep apnea (Story, 2012). In many instances, hypertension is a self-perpetuating condition in which high blood pressure damages renal blood vessels, leading to decreased blood flow to the kidney, which in turn triggers increased renin secretion (FIGURE 6-2). Because one of the responses to renin is vasoconstriction,

TABLE 6-1	Actions of the ANS, Kidneys, and RAAS for Regulation of Blood Pressure	
Autonomic Nervous System (ANS)	Kidneys	Renin-Angiotensin-Aldosterone System
• Responds to information received from baroreceptors located in the carotid sinus and aortic arch. • Sympathetic nervous system is stimulated when a decrease in blood pressure causes signals to be sent to the brain stem. • Epinephrine and norepinephrine are neurotransmitters released from the adrenal medulla (discussed in Chapter 5).	• Release renin (hormone) in response to need for increased blood pressure. • Regulate fluid and electrolyte balance in the body for long-term control of blood pressure.	• End products are angiotensin II and aldosterone, which elevate blood pressure through vasoconstriction of arterioles and volume expansion caused by increased sodium.

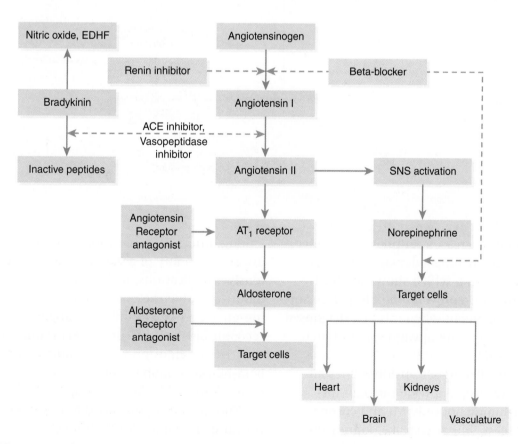

FIGURE 6-2 Actions of the ANS, kidneys, and RAAS for regulation of blood pressure.

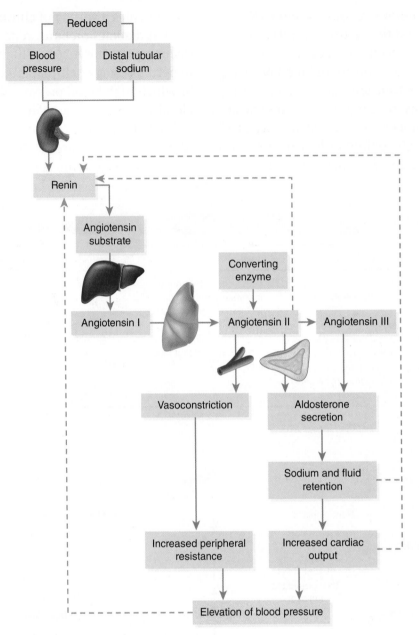

FIGURE 6-3 RAAS feedback loop: Renin is released from the kidney in response to a decrease in blood pressure.

this response increases peripheral resistance even further, creating a damaging feedback loop (see FIGURE 6-3, which shows the feedback loop). Thus, prevention of hypertension and early treatment when it is first diagnosed can help prevent the upward spiral of high blood pressure.

Uncontrolled hypertension carries an even greater risk of a wide range of diseases, including not only MI and coronary artery disease, but also stroke, kidney disease, aortic aneurysm, and heart failure,

among others. Hypertension is therefore addressed with any of a variety of antihypertensive medications, including drugs in the following categories: angiotensin-converting-enzyme (ACE) inhibitors, angiotensin II receptor blockers (ARBs), direct renin inhibitors (DRIs), aldosterone antagonists (AAs), beta-blockers, alpha-1-blockers, and calcium-channel blockers (CCBs).

The classes of drugs used to lower blood pressure are named for their mechanism of action. However, to understand *why*, for example, blocking beta-receptors or inhibiting the conversion of angiotensin will reduce blood pressure, one must understand the contributions these processes make toward cardiovascular function.

Given the relationship of CO, SVR, and HR in the equation given earlier, there are three ways to lower blood pressure: (1) lower CO (generally by reducing fluid volume); (2) reduce HR (generally by inhibiting signals that normally increase HR); or (3) decrease SVR (generally by expanding or dilating blood vessels). Most of the medications used in therapy for hypertension alter one or more of these factors.

Medication Naming Conventions

The generic names of the blood pressure medications can be helpful tools for recognizing the category to which "class" a medication belongs, and even its mechanism of action. For example, beta-blockers end in "lol" (propranolol, metoprolol, and atenolol); ACE inhibitors end in "pril" (benazepril, captopril, enalapril, or lisinopril); and ARBs end in "sartan" (candesartan, irbesartan, losartan). There are exceptions to every rule, and there are additional classes of medications that share similar suffixes as well.

What Is High Blood Pressure?
JNC 7: "Older" Guidelines for Treatment of Hypertension

The seventh report of the Joint National Committee (JNC 7) has served as the gold standard guideline for antihypertensive pharmacotherapy since it was published in 2003. Specifically, the JNC 7 defined and delineated "normal," "prehypertension," and "hypertension" blood pressure values and set treatment goals for initiating pharmacotherapy intervention accordingly. Their recommended guidelines for pharmacotherapeutic treatment goal was a resting systolic blood pressure *less than 120 mm Hg* and a resting diastolic blood pressure *less than 80 mm Hg*. **Prehypertension** was defined as a resting systolic value

in the range of 120–139 mm Hg and/or a diastolic value in the range of 80–89 mm Hg. *Hypertension* was defined as having *an average blood pressure of 140/90 mm Hg or higher most of the time.*

JNC 8: Updated Guidelines for Treatment of Hypertension

In 2014 panel members of the *Eighth* Joint National Committee published guidelines that do not recommend blood pressure guidelines numerically. In hypertensive persons younger than 60 years, there is not sufficient evidence to support a systolic goal; nor is there sufficient evidence to support a diastolic goal in those younger than 30 years. There panel therefore recommends a target blood pressure below 140/90 mm Hg for those groups (James et al., 2014).

The Renin-Angiotensin-Aldosterone System (RAAS)

The renin–angiotensin–aldosterone system is a *hormone system that regulates blood pressure and water (fluid) balance.* The second mechanism by which drugs act to lower blood pressure is to decrease angiotensin II levels, thereby suppressing its activity in the RAAS. As noted in FIGURE 6-4, hypertension is often a self-sustaining condition, as systemic vasoconstriction leads to increased renin production in the kidneys, which in turn raises the circulating level of angiotensin I. However, neither of these products is itself responsible for the vasoconstriction and increases in blood pressure. **Angiotensin II**, which is created by the conversion of **angiotensin I** by **angiotensin-converting enzyme (ACE)**, is the product that causes potent vasoconstriction and the release of aldosterone, which then increases the retention of sodium and consequently water. By *limiting the availability of angiotensin II*, vasoconstriction and aldosterone release are likewise limited, and volume expansion is curtailed. This reduces both the SVR and CO, thus lowering blood pressure.

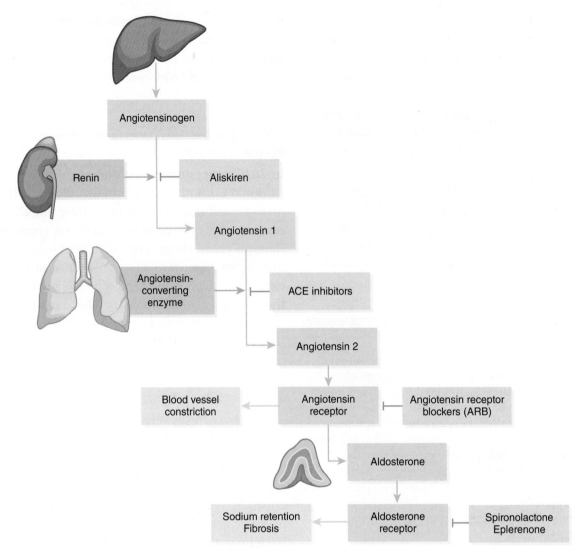

FIGURE 6-4 Drug targets: Renin–angiotensin–aldosterone system (RAAS).

The RAAS feedback regulation pathway presents multiple pharmacotherapy "targets," which can be exploited to lower blood pressure blood pressure. Each of these strategies is examined in turn.

There are several ways to go about reducing the activity of angiotensin II. One route is to limit its presence in the system, either by (1) reducing the availability of renin, thereby limiting the amount of angiotensin I available for conversion (drugs with this mechanism of action are called **direct renin inhibitors [DRIs]**), or (2) preventing ACE from acting on angiotensin I to produce angiotensin II (a class of medications called **ACE inhibitors** does exactly that). Another possibility is to focus instead on blocking the receptors where angiotensin II binds to cells, which is the mechanism of action of a class of drugs called **angiotensin II receptor blockers (ARBs)**. Note that using any of these methods does not mean there will be no angiotensin II available—angiotensinogen and angiotensin I are both converted to angiotensin II by means other than renin and ACE interactions. However, the goal of the therapy is not to *eliminate* the effects of angiotensin II (that would be harmful, rather than helpful) but rather to *reduce* them.

Direct Renin Inhibitors

As with many classes of medication, the name of this drug class is representative of the drug's mechanism of action. Direct renin inhibitors bind to the **renin** molecule and form a "renin-drug complex," which effectively *inhibits* renin activity. Recall that renin is responsible for the conversion of angiotensinogen to produce angiotensin I; decreasing renin levels and thereby reduces the amount of angiotensin I (see Figure 6-4). As the amount of angiotensin I in the RAAS decreases, the amount of the angiotensin II end product decreases as well. *As angiotensin II decreases, less vasoconstriction and volume expansion occur, causing blood pressure decrease as well.* Because the increase in renin secretion that accompanies hypertension tends to continually promote blood pressure increases (Farag, Maheshwari, Morgan, Sakr Esa, & Doyle, 2015), this drug class adds another option to the hypertension pharmacotherapy arsenal.

This class of antihypertensive medications is new, and there is currently only one FDA-approved DRI available; **aliskiren** was approved for use as an antihypertensive agent in 2007. DRI therapy for hypertension can be used as monotherapy, in conjunction with diuretics, or with other antihypertensive treatments, although combination therapy should be undertaken with caution. Initial research found **aliskiren** to be a safe and effective alternative to ACE inhibitors and ARBs for primary hypertension (Farag, Maheshwari, Morgan, Sakr Esa, & Doyle, 2015), and subsequent trials identified combined therapy with ACE inhibitors or ARBs plus **aliskiren** at low doses as having potential benefits for high-risk patients with type 2 diabetes (Riccioni, 2013).

Adverse Effects of Direct Renin Inhibitors

Patients taking DRIs are *much less likely to experience the side effect of dry cough and angioedema* than those receiving ACE inhibitors (Makani et al., 2012). Patients with renal insufficiency, diabetes, or who take a DRI in combination with an ACE inhibitor or an ARB have an increased risk of hyperkalemia. DRIs are contraindicated in pregnancy due to the increased risk of fetal complications and, therefore, are not used in pregnancy-induced hypertension.

Angiotensin-Converting-Enzyme Inhibitors (ACE Inhibitors)

As with the DRIs, the name of the angiotensin-converting-enzyme (ACE) inhibitor category of drugs is a helpful reminder of their mechanism of action. By limiting the production of the enzyme responsible for converting angiotensin I to angiotensin II, the amount of angiotensin II in the body decreases, which in turn lowers blood pressure. In addition to converting angiotensin I to angiotensin II, the angiotensin-converting-enzyme (ACE) breaks down **bradykinin**, an endogenous compound released in response to inflammation; bradykinin directly causes vasodilation. The *inhibition* of bradykinin breakdown decreases blood pressure by a different, yet significant, secondary mechanism of action. Increasing vasodilation reduces systemic vascular resistance (SVR), which leads to lower blood pressure (see BP Formula box). Patients most likely to benefit from ACE inhibitor drug therapy include those with hypertension, diabetic and nondiabetic nephropathy, coronary artery disease, and heart failure, as well as patients who have had a myocardial infarction (TABLE 6-2).

Adverse Effects of ACE inhibitors

Because this class of medications has "dual mechanisms of drug action" (inhibiting angiotensin-converting enzyme produces two distinct physiological effects), lowering angiotensin II *and* increasing bradykinin, it follows that use of this class of medications would produce multiple adverse effects. Indeed, adverse effects of ACE inhibitors can be grouped into two categories: (1) effects that are likely caused by the reduction in angiotensin II formation (hypotension, renal failure, and hyperkalemia) and (2) effects related to increased "kinins" (cough, angioedema, and anaphylaxis reactions); each is discussed in further detail.

TABLE 6-2	ACE Inhibitors Used in Hypertension*

Generic Name	Additional Uses and Notes
Benazepril	Also used for CHF and chronic renal failure. It is converted into its active molecule, benazeprilat, a non-sulfhydryl ACE inhibitor, by metabolism in the liver. Combinations of this drug with a thiazide diuretic and the calcium-channel blocker amlodipine are also available.
Captopril	Also used for CHF, post-MI left ventricular dysfunction, and diabetic nephropathy. Can be used with a thiazide diuretic or ARB. Patients with renal impairment may need dosing modifications. Like other medications in this class, captopril is a pro-drug, but its pharmacokinetic profile is distinguished by its poor bioavailability.
Enalapril	Also used for CHF and left ventricular dysfunction post MI. Enalapril is converted into its active molecule, enalaprilat, a non-sulfhydryl ACE inhibitor, by metabolism in the liver. Patients with renal impairment may need dosing modifications.
Fosinopril	Also used for heart failure. Because it is excreted via both renal and biliary pathways, fosinopril may be a safer choice for patients with renal impairment than other medications in this class that are excreted solely via the renal system. Like other medications in this class, fosinopril is a prodrug that is converted into its active form via metabolism in the body.
Lisinopril	Also used for CHF, post-MI left ventricular dysfunction, and diabetic nephropathy. This medication is one of the few in its class that is not a prodrug; it is excreted unchanged in the urine. Patients with renal impairment therefore may need dosing modifications.
Moexipril	Like most drugs in this class, moexipril is a prodrug. It has low oral bioavailability, but is lipophilic, which means it penetrates cell membranes better and has higher activity in blocking ACE in tissues as well as plasma.
Perindopril	Also used for stable coronary artery disease. Perindopril is a prodrug for the active metabolite perindoprilat.
Quinapril	Also used as an adjunct in treatment of heart failure. Quinapril is a prodrug for the active metabolite quinaprilat.
Ramipril	Also used in the treatment of post-MI heart failure and for prevention of MI, stroke, and cardiac death. Ramipril is a prodrug for the active metabolite ramiprilat.
Trandolapril	Also used in treatment of post-MI heart failure and left ventricular dysfunction. Trandolapril is a prodrug for the active metabolite trandolaprilat.

*All ACE inhibitors present a risk of fetal toxicity and, therefore, are contraindicated for the treatment of pregnancy-induced hypertension. Concomitant use in conjunction with aliskiren (a direct renin inhibitor) is contraindicated in many of these medications.

Adverse Effects Related to Decreased Angiotensin II Activity

Patients who begin an anti-hypertensive drug therapy regimen may experience adverse effects resulting from a significant *decrease* in their blood pressure. These symptoms are most commonly referred to the first-dose effect and include weakness, dizziness, and syncope, in addition to severe hypotension that may occur. Patients who have intravascular volume depletion (hypovolemia), as well as those who have high renin levels are at particular risk. For *these* patients, ACE inhibitor therapy initiation should be preceded with precautionary measures. If hypovolemia is a result of concurrent diuretic drug therapy (diuretics decrease blood volume; discussed later in this chapter), the diuretic therapy should be discontinued for a period of three to five days *before* starting ACE inhibitor therapy to ensure that the hypovolemia has been resolved. Additionally, caution must be used when treating patients with compromised renal activity. Patients taking an ACE inhibitor may experience a decrease in their glomerular filtration rate (GFR) severe enough to warrant discontinuation of therapy (Yusuf et al., 2008). Patients with known renal disease should be treated with an alternative antihypertensive drug class, if possible; if not, the patient's renal function should be closely monitored while taking an ACE inhibitor. ACE inhibitors block aldosterone release (the last step in the RAAS feedback loop); aldosterone increases urinary potassium excretion. As aldosterone levels decrease, the blood level of potassium increases. For patients with normal renal function, treatment with ACE inhibitors may not be a serious issue, as the amount of potassium in the body increases only minimally. However, ACE inhibitor therapy should be used with caution in patients with renal insufficiency, diabetes, receiving hemodialysis, and those taking other medications that can cause elevated potassium levels (such as a potassium-sparing diuretic) as **hyperkalemia** can occur.

Adverse Effects Due to Kinin Increase

A dry cough is the most frequent side effect associated with the use of ACE inhibitors. However, the literature is conflicting with respect to the number of patients that stop treatment of their ACE-inhibitor treatment due to cough. A study conducted by Sato and Fukuda in 2015 report that up to 20% of patients receiving an ACE inhibitor developed a dry, "hacking" cough. In this same study, the authors stated that although 5.1% of these patients discontinued treatment *due* to the cough, another 5% of patients reported that the cough either resolved naturally or completely disappeared as treatment with the ACE inhibitor continued. Once a patient develops a cough, if an additional ACE inhibitor is restarted at a later time, the patient will generally develop the cough again. Patients can be switched to an ARB medication (discussed in the next section), which has a much lower incidence of associated cough. Once a patient develops a cough, if an additional ACE inhibitor is restarted at a later time, the patient will generally develop the cough again.

Angiotensin II Receptor Blockers (ARBs)

As shown in Figure 6-3, *blockade of angiotensin II receptors* represents yet another pharmacological target along the RAAS feedback loop. Angiotensin II receptor antagonists (or ARBs; TABLE 6-3) compete with the endogenous ligand (angiotensin II) for binding sites on the angiotensin II receptor. While the antagonist (ARB) is bound to the receptor, angiotensin

TABLE 6-3	Angiotensin II Receptor Blockers (ARBs) Used in Hypertension*
Generic Name	
Azilsartan	
Candesartan	
Eprosartan	
Irbesartan	
Losartan	
Olmesartan	
Telmisartan	
Valsartan	

*All ARBs present a risk of fetal toxicity and, therefore, are contraindicated for the treatment of pregnancy-induced hypertension. Concomitant use in conjunction with aliskiren (a direct renin inhibitor) is contraindicated in many of these medications.

II cannot bind to its receptor, thus blocking the vasoconstriction and volume expansion caused by angiotensin II, leading to higher blood pressure. Patients who may benefit from ARB therapy include those with hypertension, diabetic and nondiabetic nephropathy, coronary artery disease, heart failure after developing MI, or scleroderma.

According to the JNC 8, when comparing ARBs to ACE inhibitors, the panel concluded that these two classes of drugs are comparable and thus interchangeable for the initial treatment of hypertension in patients who do not have heart failure (James et al., 2014). First, their side-effect profiles differ. Unlike ACE inhibitors, ARBs do not increase the levels of bradykinin; thus, patients taking ARBs are much less likely to experience the side effects of dry cough and angioedema than those taking ACE inhibitors. However, hypotension is *more* common with ARBs than with ACE inhibitors. ARBs are contraindicated in pregnancy due to the increased risk of fetal complications; they cannot be used in pregnancy-related hypertension (pre-eclampsia).

Aldosterone Antagonists (AAs)

The class of aldosterone-antagonist medications completes the pharmacological classes of medications that target the RAAS feedback loop. At present, two drugs are available: **eplerenone** and **spironolactone**, both of which are competitive antagonists at the aldosterone receptor (these drugs are also *potassium-sparing diuretics*; and are discussed later in this chapter). AAs work slightly differently in altering the RAAS than the three previously discussed classes. Angiotensin II causes both potent vasoconstriction *and* the release of aldosterone. Aldosterone signals to the kidneys *to conserve water and maintain fluid volume*. In normotensive individuals, this usually does not present a problem. For patients with hypertension, however, increasing fluid volume can indeed negatively impact blood pressure levels.

Recall CO and SVR were shown to be key factors in determining blood pressure. In patients with hypertension, both SVR and CO are increased due in part to increased blood volume related to heightened levels of aldosterone attributable to increased renin secretion. Reducing aldosterone activity can interrupt that sequence by decreasing water conservation and reducing fluid volume. Because AA are competitive antagonists at the aldosterone receptor, they prevent aldosterone from signaling the kidneys to conserve water, allowing any *excess fluid to be excreted as urine* (**diuresis**). Decreased levels of aldosterone also produce *increased potassium retention*, less sodium retention, less volume expansion, and lower blood pressure.

Adverse Effects of Aldosterone Antagonists

AAs block the aldosterone receptors, which decreases the sodium and water reabsorption and increases the potassium retention. Thus, hyperkalemia is a risk with these drugs.

Drug-Drug Interactions Within RAAS Feedback Loop

Of note: it should be clear that using more than one of these RAAS-focused medications simultaneously carries a risk of *overtreatment*—each drug class acts upon a different site along the RAAS feedback loop (Figure 6-3). Therefore, medications from different RAAS-drug classes should not be used together unless there is a proven medical benefit for doing so.

Drug-Drug Interactions Associated With AAs

Both AAs are also classified as potassium-sparing diuretics, so they should not be used in combination with other drugs in this class—namely, **amiloride** and **triamterene**—for fear of synergistic overtreatment leading to hyperkalemia. Similarly, use of supplemental **potassium**, whether taken over the counter (OTC) or by prescription, should be avoided with AAs, due to the likelihood of hyperkalemia. Less obvious, perhaps, is the potential interaction between vasopressin receptor antagonists ("vaptan" drugs), which should not be used with AAs for the simple reason that blocking the activity of vasopressin reduces the amount of circulating aldosterone; in conjunction with an AA, one would again expect synergism and overtreatment. **Cyclosporine** is contraindicated because it lowers serum aldosterone; similarly, **mifepristone** should not be taken within 14 days of AA usage due to its effects on mineralocorticoid receptors.

The Role of the Autonomic Nervous System in Blood Pressure Regulation

The autonomic nervous system (ANS) is the branch of the nervous system that regulates "involuntary" physiological processes, such as heart rate (**FIGURE 6-5**). The ANS is subdivided into the sympathetic nervous system (SNS) and parasympathetic system (PANS) (see Chapter 5). The ANS plays a significant role regulating cardiovascular function in addition to modulating the physiological control of blood pressure. In simplest terms, if the body suddenly requires more oxygen to support an activity or respond to danger, the ANS automatically signals the heart to beat faster and circulate blood more rapidly. Such signals are mediated by the neurotransmitters norepinephrine and epinephrine (formerly known as noradrenaline and adrenaline, respectively). Most readers have experienced an

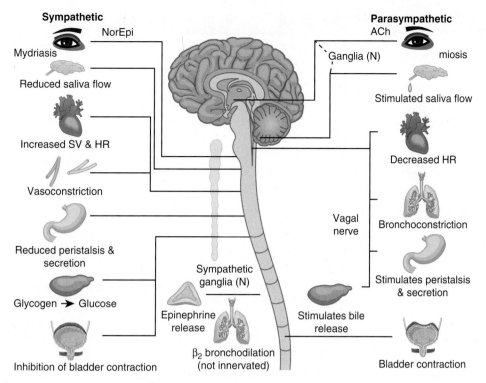

FIGURE 6-5 The autonomic nervous system (ANS).

"adrenaline rush" in response to danger, be it real or imagined—the heart rate increases (i.e., the heart "pounds"), breathing quickens, skin flushes, and muscles tense. This physiological response, known as the fight-or-flight response, is the result of the brain signaling (via the ANS) the adrenal glands to release norepinephrine (NE) and epinephrine (EPI), which bind to specific receptors located on the heart, called **beta-receptors** (β-receptors). When beta adrenoceptors (beta-receptors) are stimulated, automaticity in the sinoatrial (SA) node increases; the velocity of conduction through the atrioventricular (AV) node increases as well. These effects lead to a higher heart rate (HR) as well as increased myocontractility, producing more *forceful contractions* of the heart muscle. Norepinephrine and epinephrine are the natural ligands (agonists) for beta-receptors in the ANS (see Chapter 5). NE directly "activates" β-receptors on the heart, causing an increase in heart rate, which in turn increases blood pressure on the vasculature. Even when the body is *not* "stressed," norepinephrine circulates throughout the body. Because *activation*

of beta-receptors on the heart causes increased blood pressure levels, one would expect that an *antagonist* (or other chemical substance bound to the receptor site) would *prevent* receptor activation by blocking the endogenous ligand from binding to its receptor. Hence, one mechanism to reduce blood pressure is to restrict, or block, norepinephrine (and epinephrine) from binding to beta-receptors on the heart (which results in reduced heart muscle contractility and lower CO). This class of medications is known as **beta-blockers** (as their name implies) (TABLE 6-4).

Beta-receptors innervate organs *throughout* the periphery (see FIGURE 6-6), not just the heart (Chapter 5). Because this class of drugs blocks endogenous ligand-binding and receptor activation, it is critical to know precisely where *other β-receptors* in the body are located. Specific beta-receptors (β₁-receptors) are found not only in the heart, but also in the kidney. Blocking β₁-receptors in the kidney inhibits the release of renin (recall that this reduces the activity of the RAAS), which further decreases blood pressure. β₂-receptors have a less powerful effect on the heart

TABLE 6-4	Beta-blockers Used in Hypertension*		
Drug	Type of Beta-Blocker	Additional Uses and Notes	
Acebutolol	β_1 selective, cardioselective	Also used for treatment of angina and arrhythmias. May be used in patients with chronic obstructive pulmonary disease (COPD).	
Atenolol	β_1 selective, cardioselective	Also used for treatment of angina, tachycardias, and acute MI, as well as prevention of migraine and hereditary essential tremor. Use with caution in diabetes due to masking of hypoglycemia. May be used in patients with COPD.	
Betaxolol	β_1 selective, cardioselective	May be used in patients with COPD. Also frequently used as an ophthalmic solution to treat open-angle glaucoma.	
Bisoprolol	β_1 selective, cardioselective	Also used for treatment of angina and CHF. May be used in patients with COPD.	
Carvedilol	Nonselective β-blocker/ α_1-blocker	Primarily used in treatment of CHF, but may also be used to treat hypertension. Primarily used for "chronic" CHF. Not used in patients with "acute" CHF. Should not be used in patients with COPD, CHF, heart block, or bradycardia.	
Esmolol	β_1 selective, cardioselective	Short-acting, administered by injection; used more for treating arrhythmias than for hypertension. May be used in patients with COPD.	
Labetalol	Nonselective β-blocker/ α_1-blocker	Also used for angina, MI, and pregnancy-induced hypertension as well as acute forms associated with pheochromocytoma. Should not be used in patients with COPD, CHF, heart block, or bradycardia.	
Metoprolol	β_1 selective, cardioselective	Also used for treatment of angina, CHF, acute MI, and arrhythmias as well as prevention of migraine, treatment of tachycardia in hyperthyroidism, and hereditary essential tremor. Use with caution in diabetes due to masking of hypoglycemia. May be used in patients with COPD.	
Nadolol	Nonselective β-blocker	Also used for angina; often used off-label for long QT syndrome, migraine, attention-deficit/ hyperactivity disorder (ADHD; in adults), and essential tremor. Should not be used in patients with COPD.	
Nebivolol	β_1 selective, cardioselective	Has a nitric oxide–potentiating effect that promotes vasodilation. May be used in patients with COPD, but is contraindicated in patients with heart block, heart failure, or liver dysfunction.	
Penbutolol	Nonselective β-blocker	Should not be used in patients with COPD, and should be used with caution in diabetes due to its potential to mask hypoglycemia.	
Pindolol	Nonselective β-blocker	Also used for angina; is thought to have antiarrhythmic effects. Being investigated for depression and erectile dysfunction. Should not be used in patients with COPD.	
Propranolol	Nonselective β-blocker	Also used for treatment of angina and arrhythmias as well as prevention of migraine, treatment of tachycardia in hyperthyroidism, and hereditary essential tremor. Use with caution in diabetes due to masking of hypoglycemia. Should not be used in patients with COPD.	
Sotalol	Nonselective β-blocker	Used primarily for treatment of tachycardia due to its ability to inhibit potassium channels, but may be used for hypertension as well. Should not be used in patients with COPD.	
Timolol	Nonselective β-blocker	Also used for treatment of angina and arrhythmias as well as prevention of migraine; used off-label for mitral valve prolapse and hypertrophic cardiomyopathy. Should not be used in patients with COPD.	

*A variety of other beta-receptor antagonists are available that are used specifically for open-angle glaucoma, and not for hypertension. Some of the drugs listed here (e.g., carvedilol, esmolol, sotalol) are used more frequently for other indications than for treatment of hypertension.

when stimulated. Activation of β_2-receptors causes arterioles in the heart, lungs, and skeletal muscles to dilate; induces bronchial dilation, relaxation of the uterus in women, glycogenolysis in liver and skeletal muscle, and enhanced contraction of skeletal muscle; and promotes the movement of potassium into cells.

Therefore, following administration of either a β_1-receptor agonist *or* antagonist drugs produces a myriad of physiological effects, in addition to the desired therapeutic

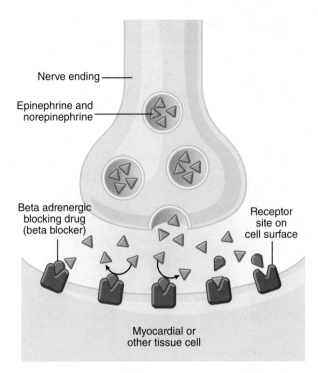

Nerve ending

Epinephrine and norepinephrine

Beta adrenergic blocking drug (beta blocker)

Receptor site on cell surface

Myocardial or other tissue cell

FIGURE 6-6 Beta-receptors innervate organs throughout the periphery.

effect for which the medication was given (in this discussion, to lower blood pressure). It is of utmost importance that the nurse be able to predict and/or anticipate these additional physiological responses following the administration of a β-blocker to a patient, due to antagonist blockade of beta-receptors at sites on different organs and tissues throughout the body.

Beta-blockers are further classified by their specific receptor-binding profile:

- *Nonselective beta-blockers* block *both* beta-one (β_1) *and* beta-two (β_2) receptors on tissues located throughout the body; not only those on the heart.
- *Selective beta-blockers* are selective about *which* beta-receptors they "block"; in other words, selective β-blockers bind to beta-receptors located on cardiac tissue (β1-blockers), but do *not* bind to beta-receptors located on all the other organs, throughout the body
- *First-generation beta-blockers* are nonselective and block both β1- and β2-receptors throughout the body.

- *Second-generation beta-blockers* are cardioselective drugs that block only β1-receptors at normal dosages
- *Third-generation beta-blockers* are typically mixed α1-/β-blockers and are therefore nonselective.

As evidenced by the most recent JNC 8 Guidelines, the use of beta-blockers for hypertension, despite their wide use, is *not* necessarily the best first-line treatment for this condition. These findings is corroborated by a 2017 Cochrane Database of Systematic Review conducted by the Cochrane Hypertension Group, which studied the overall efficacy of initiating treatment of hypertension with beta-blockers. The authors concluded that initiating treatment of hypertension with beta-blockers leads to modest CVD reductions, little or no effects on mortality, and are inferior to those of other antihypertensive drugs (such as diuretics, calcium-channel blockers, and rennin–angiotensin–system inhibitors) (Wiysonge, Bradley, Volmink, Mayosi, & Opie, 2017). It has been concluded that beta-blockers are not as effective preventing the number of deaths, strokes and heart attacks, as drugs in other classes of medications (used to treat hypertension).

While beta-blockers are not necessarily the best choice to treat hypertension, these medications are used to treat many other medical conditions. For example, long-term treatment of angina, coronary artery disease, heart failure, and dysrhythmias, and those who have recently experienced a myocardial infarction (MI). Medications of this class can also be used for the prevention of migraine headaches and anxiety attacks. In patients who have hypertension along with one or more of these other conditions, beta-blockers can offer a "two-for-one" option to potentially address both conditions simultaneously. However, clinicians should keep in mind (and inform patients) that abrupt beta-blocker discontinuation can cause a hyperadrenergic state that places the patient at increased risk for significant cardiovascular event or even death.

Gradual tapering of the beta-blocker will reduce this risk (Prescriber's Digital Reference [PDR], 2018).

Adverse Effects of Beta-Blockers

Blockade of β_2-receptors (on the lung) inhibits bronchodilation; for this reason, use of β-blockers has generally been avoided in patients with asthma over concerns regarding bronchoconstriction. Numerous studies report patients who have bronchospastic disease (e.g., asthma, chronic obstructive pulmonary disease [COPD]) should avoid nonselective beta-blockers, but can use cardioselective β_1-blockers with supervision (Morales et al., 2014).

Likewise, patients with significant peripheral artery disease (PAD) and Reynaud phenomenon should not be prescribed non-selective beta-blockers, for much the same reason: blockade of β_2-receptors will limit the arterioles' ability to dilate. Patients with mild to moderate PAD did not show an exacerbation of symptoms with beta-blockers (Radack & Deck, 1991), but even so, patients with these diseases should take beta-blockers with caution.

Beta-blockade prevents the normal response of tachycardia to low blood sugar and masks one of the classic signs and symptoms of hypoglycemia. Thus, medications based on this mechanism of action should be used with caution in patients with diabetes, particularly insulin-dependent type 2 or type 1 diabetes. Also, the body's responses to hypoglycemia are glycogenolysis and gluconeogenesis, which are slowed with beta-blocker medications, especially if the beta-blocker is noncardioselective.

Depression, fatigue, and sexual dysfunction were commonly reported as side effects of beta-blockers in early clinical trials. A review of 15 trials with more than 35,000 patients using such medications showed only a small increase in reports of fatigue or sexual dysfunction, however, and no difference in depressive symptoms (Ko et al., 2002). Beta-blockers have significant adverse effects when combined with certain common medications, as described in TABLE 6-5.

TABLE 6-5	Beta-Blocker-Drug Interactions
Drug	Possible Adverse Effects When Combined with Beta-Blockers
Aminophylline or isoproterenol	Inhibits both drugs
Amiodarone	May cause cardiac arrest
Digitalis	Potentiates bradycardia
Indomethacin	Inhibits the antihypertensive action of the beta-blocker
Lithium	Propanolol potentiates lidocaine levels
Phenytoin or quinidine	Potentiates the cardiac depressant effects
Rifampin or smoking	Increased metabolism of beta-blockers
Tricyclic antidepressants	Inhibits action of beta-blockers
Tubocurarine	Potentiates the action of the neuromuscular blocker

Blockade of α_1-Receptors

As mentioned earlier, some beta-blockers also block the α_1-receptors and thereby promote vasodilation, which helps to decrease SVR. However, certain medications block *only* the α_1-receptors without affecting β-receptors; these are, for obvious reasons, referred to as **selective α_1-blockers**. Drugs in this class include **terazosin**, **doxazosin**, and **prazosin**. Alpha-blockers act on the *postsynaptic* α_1-receptors. As antagonists, alpha-blockers bind to the ligand-binding site on alpha$_1$-receptors and thereby *block* receptor activation, preventing NE from binding to the smooth muscle receptors. When such agents are used to treat hypertension, the effect of blocking constriction of the arterioles and veins has the most significant impact on lowering blood pressure. Patients who may benefit from α_1-antagonist therapy include those with hypertension *and* benign prostatic hypertrophy (BPH). These agents are also often the drugs of choice for hypertensive crisis caused by pheochromocytoma (an adrenal gland tumor that causes hypersecretion of catecholamines).

Adverse Effects of Alpha-Blockers

Patients who take alpha-blockers may experience weakness, dizziness, and syncope caused by a significant decrease in their blood pressure and the loss of the reflex vasoconstriction upon standing, known as postural hypotension. The patient should be counseled not to sit or stand up from a lying position too quickly. In addition, there can be a **first-dose effect** characterized by severe hypotension. Patients who have intravascular volume depletion (hypovolemia) are at particular risk. *Reflex tachycardia* is seen most often with the use of nonselective alpha-antagonists, in response to the hypotension, as the body works to stabilize the blood pressure.

Nasal congestion due to the dilation of the nasal mucosal arterioles is caused by the α_1-blockers antagonizing those receptors. Alpha-blocking medications should be used with caution in the elderly and those with cataract surgery, as blockade of alpha-receptors in the eyes can lead to pupil dilation and blurred vision.

Drug–Drug Interactions

Some medications may increase the risk of hypotension and other adverse effects if used with α_1-antagonists. These agents include **alfuzosin**, **dutasteride/tamsulosin**, **silodosin**, **tadalafil**, and **tamsulosin**.

Calcium-Channel Blockers

The last major class of antihypertensive medications is not "antihypertensive." **Calcium-channel blockers (CCBs)** are, in truth, more of a broad-spectrum *vascular smooth muscle relaxant*, and this property can be exploited to provide a number of benefits to the heart and the cardiovascular system as a whole. This utility arises because calcium plays a major role in the mechanism of vascular smooth muscles contraction; calcium *channels*, which span the cell membrane channels, regulate the amount of calcium that enters the cell. *In the heart*, calcium levels affect the force and rate of contractions. *Calcium entry* causes *the heart to contract with more force*

(**positive inotrope**). It also increases the HR by affecting the rate in the SA node, and, the velocity of the conduction in the AV node. *Blocking calcium channels*, therefore, helps *lower CO by both reducing the force of contraction and decreasing the frequency of contractions.*

In the arteries, calcium-channel blockers impede the smooth muscle of arterial walls from contracting (i.e., constricting), resulting in smooth-muscle relaxation and the arterial dilation. Blood pressure levels decrease by decreasing SVR, while simultaneously increasing oxygen flow to the heart. In sum, CCBs act on all three of the factors related to blood pressure: CO, SVR, and HR.

The rationale that supports CCB use as antihypertensive agents make them (the CCBs) valuable agents for treatment of other cardiovascular pathologies (see TABLE 6-6). For example, they are used to treat chest pain and cardiac dysrhythmias. Three subclasses (based upon chemical structures) of CCBs—the dihydropyridines, phenylalkylamines, and benzothiazepines—are used to treat chest pain and hypertension. In addition, the phenylalkylamines and benzothiazepines may be given intravenously for atrial fibrillation, atrial flutter, and supraventricular tachycardia (SVT). The longer-acting CCBs are indicated for elderly patients with isolated systolic hypertension and one of the following coexisting conditions: angina pectoris, Raynaud phenomenon, asthma, or COPD; they may also be given to elderly patients who have not responded to other medications.

Adverse Effects of Calcium Channel Blockers

All CCBs carry a risk of hypotension, headache/weakness, and dizziness related to the vasodilatory effects necessary for lowering of the blood pressure. Edema of ankles and feet (peripheral edema) also may occur and is likely related to a redistribution of fluids from the intravascular space into the interstitial spaces. Unfortunately, diuretics may not be useful in resolving this type of edema.

Some specific effects are associated with particular classes of CCBs. Dihydropyridines

TABLE 6-6	Calcium-Channel Blockers Commonly Prescribed in the United States*	

Generic Name	Class	Additional Uses and Notes
Amlodipine	Dihydropyridine	Also used for coronary artery disease (e.g., chronic stable angina or variant angina). May be used in patients with heart failure, diabetes with or without renal failure, or hyperlipidemia.
Diltiazem[†]	Benzothiazepine	Also used in treatment of angina (chronic stable/variant), atrial fibrillation, superventricular tachycardia, atrial flutter.
Felodipine	Dihydropyridine	Generally used only for hypertension, as it has limited effects on cardiac muscle. Has significant interaction with components of grapefruit.
Isradipine	Dihydropyridine	Generally used only for hypertension. Use with certain medications, such as cimetidine, azole antifungals, macrolide antibiotics, rifamycin, and antiseizure medications such as carbamazepine and phenytoin can alter liver metabolism of this drug and lead to over/undertreatment.
Nicardipine[†]	Dihydropyridine	Also used for angina. Rifampin, phenobarbital, phenytoin, oxcarbazepine, and carbamazepine may reduce blood levels of nicardipine by increasing its metabolism in the liver.
Nifedipine	Dihydropyridine	Also used for treating angina, arrhythmias, and off-label for Raynaud phenomenon and migraine prevention. Patients using beta-blockers concomitantly with nifedipine may be at increased risk for CHF.
Nimodipine	Dihydropyridine	Infrequently used for hypertension because of its selectivity for cerebral vasculature, but for that reason, it is commonly used for treatment of subarachnoid hemorrhage. Contraindicated in patients with unstable angina or recent MI.
Nisoldipine	Dihydropyridine	Also used for angina.
Verapamil[†]	Phenylalkylamine	Also used for angina, arrhythmias, and migraine/cluster headaches.

*Many other drugs in this class are available outside the United States or on an experimental basis. The drugs in this table represent the most commonly used examples of this class.
[†]Also available in IV formulation for treatment of hypertensive crisis.

may cause reflex tachycardia due to arterial dilation, and large doses of short-acting nifedipine may increase the mortality of patients immediately following an MI (Furberg, Psaty, & Meyer, 1995). Phenylalkylamines and benzothiazepines reduce arterial pressure without as much reflex tachycardia as the dihydropyridines, but because of how these drugs act on the arterioles and the heart, a patient who has bradycardia or AV block is at risk. Constipation is also a concern with this group of medications, with verapamil being more likely to cause constipation than diltiazem.

CCBs are among the few medications with known interactions with nutrients—specifically, components of grapefruit juice (Sica, 2006). Certain flavonoid and nonflavonoid components of grapefruit juice interfere with presystemic clearance of these drugs, which means that less of the drug is metabolized before it enters the circulation; in turn, the overall bioavailability increases. The effects of this interaction are similar to what

might be seen if the patient took a higher dose of the medication than was prescribed; symptoms include hypotension, bradycardia, and peripheral edema. Patients should be warned not to drink grapefruit juice or eat grapefruit while taking these medications.

Diuretics

Recall earlier in this chapter it was said that another physiological mechanism which serves to lower blood pressure levels is to *decrease total body fluid*—or **fluid volume**. Diuretics, first discovered in 1957, are a class of medications used to reduce blood pressure by lowering the fluid volume in the circulatory system and are a mainstay in the treatment of hypertension. They have been shown, in placebo-controlled clinical studies, to significantly reduce cardiovascular morbidity and mortality (Salvetti & Ghiadoni, 2006). Commonly referred to as *water pills*, **diuretics** (TABLE 6-7) cause the kidneys to excrete sodium and water from the

TABLE 6-7	Diuretic Medications Used in Treating Hypertension and Other Cardiovascular Conditions	
Drug	**Class**	**Notes**
Amiloride	Potassium-sparing diuretic	Must not be used with another potassium-sparing diuretic or other medications that reduce potassium loss due to the potential for hyperkalemia. May be combined with thiazide diuretics or loop diuretics.
Bendroflumethiazide	Thiazide diuretic	
Bumetanide	Loop diuretic	
Chlorthalidone	Thiazide diuretic	
Eplerenone	Potassium-sparing diuretic/aldosterone antagonist	Must not be used with another potassium-sparing diuretic or other medications that reduce potassium loss due to the potential for hyperkalemia. May be combined with thiazide diuretics or loop diuretics.
Ethacrynic acid	Loop diuretic	
Furosemide	Loop diuretic	
Hydrochlorothiazide	Thiazide diuretic	
Hydroflumethiazide	Thiazide diuretic	
Methyclothiazide	Thiazide diuretic	
Metolazone	Thiazide diuretic	
Polythiazide	Thiazide diuretic	
Quinethazone	Thiazide diuretic	
Spironolactone	Potassium-sparing diuretic/aldosterone antagonist	Must not be used with another potassium-sparing diuretic or other medications that reduce potassium loss due to the potential for hyperkalemia. May be combined with thiazide diuretics or loop diuretics.
Torsemide	Loop diuretic	
Triamterene	Potassium-sparing diuretic	Must not be used with another potassium-sparing diuretic or other medications that reduce potassium loss due to the potential for hyperkalemia. May be combined with thiazide diuretics or loop diuretics.
Trichlormethiazide	Thiazide diuretic	

systemic circulation, which in turn lowers the fluid volume.

Diuretics have been used when initiating the stepped-care pharmacological treatment approach of antihypertensive drug therapy. FIGURE 6-7 illustrates the rationale for the use of diuretics to treat high blood pressure and both short-term and long-term effects using the thiazide class of medications. Several classes of diuretics are available to treat hypertension; diuretics are categorized into different drug classes based upon and the drugs' mechanism of action: thiazide diuretics, potassium-sparing diuretics, and loop diuretics.

Diuretics in the thiazide subclass also relax the walls of blood vessels, thereby reducing both CO and SVR.

As a class, diuretic drugs are attractive because they are well-tolerated and can be used in combination with other classes of antihypertensive medications. However, not all subtypes of diuretics behave in the same manner, so close attention should be paid to a drug's subclass and mechanism of action. (Another subclass of diuretics, carbonic anhydrase inhibitors, is not used for treating hypertension because these agents' effects are too weak; such drugs are used primarily to treat glaucoma.)

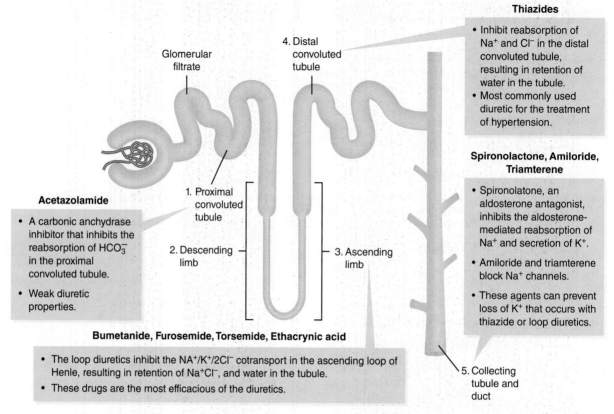

FIGURE 6-7 Treatment of hypertension: Mechanism of action of diuretics.

*Thiazide
1) safe
2) inexpensive
3) easy to use
+ minimal side effects*

Thiazide Diuretics

Thiazide diuretics (hydrochlorothiazide [HCTZ], chlorthalindone) are very commonly prescribed for several reasons. First, they have a long history of safe, successful use for hypertension. Second, they are relatively inexpensive. Third, they are easy to use and have fairly minimal side effects, which means patients are more likely to take them as prescribed. In addition, these agents' efficacy is quite good: thiazide diuretics are just as effective in reducing cardiovascular events in patients with hypertension as beta-blockers and ACE inhibitors, and they are actually better than either of the other classes in reducing stroke (Roush, Kaur, & Ernst, 2014). Of note, thiazide diuretics have been particularly successful in treating African American patients, in whom they tend to be the first-line therapy (see JNC 8 Guidelines; James et al., 2014). However, thiazide diuretics promote potassium loss and are thought to increase the risk of new-onset diabetes, especially when combined with beta-blockers; thus, use of these drugs in patients who are

at high risk for developing diabetes should be undertaken with caution. In such cases, the drugs should be prescribed at the lowest active dose and possibly in combination with ARBs, a pairing that has been shown to reduce the adverse impact on glucose tolerance. There is an association between glucose intolerance and hypokalemia, and some have suggested that treating hypokalemia might reverse insulin resistance or prevent diabetes (Sica, Carter, Cushman, & Hamm, 2011).

Loop Diuretics

Loop diuretics get their name from the loop of Henle in the kidney, which is where this class of drugs produces their effects. They bind to a carrier protein in the thick ascending limb of the loop of Henle that transports sodium, chloride, and potassium ions; by doing so, they prevent NaCl (salt) as well as water from being reabsorbed, lowering fluid volume (Wittner, Di Stefano, Wangemann, & Greger, 1991). The thick ascending limb of the loop of Henle is where a large proportion of the

bad effect = potassium loss

body's sodium transport occurs, so loop diuretics can reduce water reabsorption substantially more than thiazide diuretics (which work in the distal tubules of the kidney). The negative aspect of this capability is that it promotes potassium loss and, potentially, hypokalemia. **Furosemide** is perhaps the best-known drug in this class; it is much more often prescribed for congestive heart failure (CHF), an indication discussed later in this chapter.

Potassium-Sparing Diuretics

Potassium-sparing diuretics, unlike thiazide and loop diuretics, do not act on sodium transport mechanisms, so they avoid the problems associated with potassium loss. Two drugs in this class, **spironolactone** and **eplerenone**, are AAs (described earlier in the RAAS discussion) and produce a diuretic effect by that mechanism; the other two members of this class, **amiloride** and **triamterene**, act directly on sodium channels and likewise do not promote excretion of potassium. In patients for whom hyperkalemia is an issue, these medications will make the problem worse and should not be used. However, because potassium-sparing diuretics have relatively weak effects on overall sodium balance, they are often used in combination with other classes of diuretics as a way of maximizing fluid volume reduction while avoiding excessive potassium loss and hypokalemia. An important drug interaction occurs with concomitant use of trimethoprim-sulfamethoxazole antibiotic therapy, which acts similarly on the distal tubules as a potassium-sparing diuretic (Weir et al., 2010).

Hypertensive Emergencies

To this point, the discussion has been focused on the treatment of *chronic* hypertension stemming from a variety of causes. There is an additional form of hypertension that occurs in an *acute* form, known as a hypertensive emergency. **Hypertensive emergencies** are instances in which the patient has both severe hypertension and a risk of end-organ damage (e.g., myocardial infarction, unstable angina, acute left ventricular failure with pulmonary edema, acute aortic dissection, encephalopathy, stroke and life-threatening bleeding [intracerebral hemorrhage and subarachnoid hemorrhage]) (Chobanian et al., 2003; Perez & Musini, 2008). Careful management of the process of lowering the blood pressure is essential due to the risk of the antihypertensive treatment causing severe hypotension, which can lead to complications such as MI and stroke. Both oral and intravenous (IV) medications are available for these purposes, but the IV route is preferred for patients at risk of end-organ damage. IV medications for hypertensive emergencies include medications from the following categories: vasodilators, CCBs, peripheral dopamine-1 agonists, beta-blockers, and alpha-adrenergic blockers.

The primary goal of intervention in a hypertensive crisis is to safely reduce blood pressure. The appropriate therapeutic approach of each patient will depend on their clinical presentation. Patients with hypertensive emergencies are best treated in an intensive care unit with titratable, intravenous, hypotensive agents. Rapid-acting intravenous antihypertensive agents are available, including **labetalol**, **esmolol**, **fenoldopam**, **nicardipine**, and **sodium nitroprusside**. Newer agents, such as **clevidipine** and **fenoldopam**, may hold considerable advantages to other available agents in the management of hypertensive crises. **Sodium nitroprusside** is an extremely toxic drug and its use in the treatment of hypertensive emergencies should be avoided. Similarly, **nifedipine**, **nitroglycerin**, and **hydralazine** should not to be considered first-line therapies in the management of hypertensive crises because these agents are associated with significant toxicities and/or adverse effects.

Organs at Risk of Damage During a Hypertensive Crisis

- Eyes: Bleeding or swelling
- Brain: Complications from elevated intracranial pressure, stroke
- Kidneys: Renal failure
- Heart: MI, CHF

CCBs that are used for hypertensive emergencies are in the dihydropyridine category and include **clevidipine** and **nicardipine**. **Esmolol** is a predominantly cardioselective beta-blocker, and **labetalol** is a combined beta-receptor and alpha-adrenergic blocker. For emergency management, these drugs are given via the IV route. (See the previous sections for additional information on these drug categories.)

Vasodilators include **nitroprusside**, which dilates both arterioles and veins by releasing nitrous oxide (NO), which then activates smooth muscle guanylyl cyclase, to form cGMP. cGMP inhibits entry of calcium into cells, thereby causing smooth muscle relaxation, by virtue of the decreased calcium. **Nitroprusside** is a very effective drug for lowering blood pressure quickly. This effect occurs in less than 2 minutes and lasts for only 1 to 10 minutes, necessitating that the medication be administered as a continuous IV drip to maintain its effectiveness. In the body, **nitroprusside** is metabolized into cyanide; consequently, the patient must be monitored for signs of developing cyanide poisoning. The risk for cyanide poisoning correlates to both the length of therapy and the dosage level of medication administered. Patients should be monitored for signs of toxicity such as changes in mentation, miosis, tinnitus, gastrointestinal (GI) distress, methemoglobinemia, and metabolic acidosis. The patient should be on continual and accurate blood pressure monitoring to facilitate titration of the medication and to prevent severe hypotension. Pregnant women should not receive **nitroprusside**, as this drug may cross the placental barrier.

Another vasodilator is **hydralazine**, which works primarily on the vascular smooth muscles of the arteriolar vessels and has minimal impact on the venous vessels. This drug is considered safe and is widely used for the acute hypertensive treatment of pregnant women. However, its hypotensive episodes can be difficult to predict in comparison to other agents. **Hydralazine** can,

for instance, cause reflex tachycardia in response to the decrease in the arterial pressure. A beta-blocker may be considered to address this symptom. **Hydralazine** may also produce an increase in volume because the lowered blood pressure can cause an increase in sodium and, subsequently, water retention. A diuretic (see the earlier discussion) may be considered to address this increase in volume. Other adverse effects associated with **hydralazine** include chest pain, paradoxical hypertension, peripheral edema, anxiety, disorientation, further increase of intracranial pressure, GI disturbances, diaphoresis, lupuslike syndrome, and peripheral neuritis.

Peripheral dopamine-1 agonists are another class of medications that promote vasodilation and thereby relieve high blood pressure during an acute crisis. **Fenoldopam**, for example, activates the dopamine-1 receptors on the arterioles, which causes the vessels to vasodilate. It is as effective as **nitroprusside** and has even more benefits for the kidney because it acts on receptors in renal, coronary, mesenteric, and peripheral vessels. Acting as an antagonist, **fenoldopam** causes the renal arteries to dilate, which improves blood supply; it also promotes sodium and water loss. Like **nitroprusside**, this medication has a rapid onset (less than five minutes) and short duration (half-life of five minutes). Adverse effects include reflex tachycardia in response to the vasodilation and increased intraocular pressure; **fenoldopam** should not be administered, or should be given only with great caution, to patients with glaucoma.

Some high blood pressure medications, such as ACE inhibitors and the angiotensin II receptor blockers may harm a pregnant mother and developing fetus, so should not be used during pregnancy. **Reserpine**, an alkaloid that acts via monoamine depletion, should only be used when no alternatives exist, as it may also be harmful during pregnancy (Morelli, 2016). All pregnant patients should be counseled on medication use per the Pregnancy and Lactation Labeling Rules.

Cardiac Agents

Coronary Artery Disease

Coronary artery disease (CAD) is a condition that occurs when blood flow to the heart is restricted, or completely blocked, depriving cardiac muscle of oxygen. Coronary artery disease most commonly results from the buildup of cholesterol and other fatty materials (atherosclerotic plaques) in the wall of a coronary artery, in a process known as **atherosclerosis** (FIGURE 6-8). (Note: Fatty-plaque buildup occurs in arteries throughout the body; not just the coronary arteries of the heart.)

Chest Pain/Angina

Angina pectoris, known more commonly as *chest pain*, is characterized by the sudden onset of a "crushing" feeling of pressure, burning, squeezing, or suffocating pain in the chest. Chronic chest pain, or angina, generally occurs as a result of coronary artery disease (FIGURE 6-9). Pain from angina can also radiate to the arms, shoulders, neck, jaw, and throat, often leaving the patient uncertain of its origin. The "experience" of anginal pain varies among patients; symptoms also manifest differently depending upon *the type* of angina causing the chest pain. The three forms of angina discussed in this section are *exertional*, *variant*, and *unstable angina* (FIGURE 6-10).

Exertional Angina

Also called *chronic stable angina*, exertional angina usually has somewhat predictable triggers. Physical exertion, emotional stress, cold weather, or large meals are common examples of conditions that can trigger exertional angina in patients with underlying coronary artery disease. Each of these triggers places an increased workload on the heart, which in turn increases the heart's need for oxygen. The angina is the body's signal that the heart is not receiving adequate oxygen. The treatment goal is to balance the heart's oxygen needs with the available supply by decreasing the demand for oxygen.

Acute episodes of angina are usually treated with nitroglycerin, which, like nitroprusside, increases tissue cGMP, and is typically placed sublingually for rapid absorption but can also be administered orally or intravenously. Longer-term prevention and decrease of severity/number of angina attacks requires the use of any of several

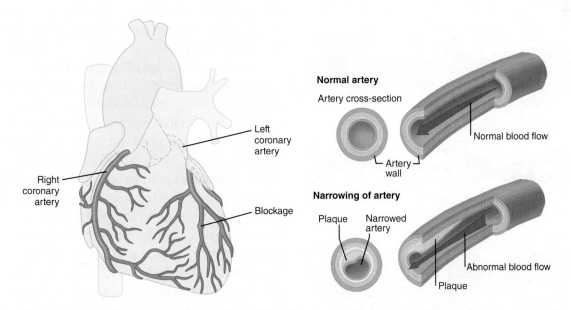

FIGURE 6-8 Development of coronary artery disease due to buildup of fatty deposits, called plaques, on the walls of coronary arteries, which restricts the flow of blood to the heart.

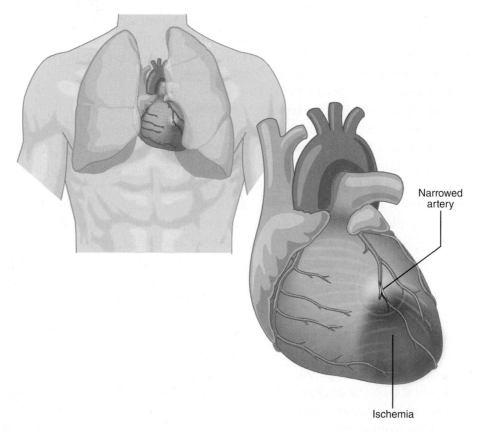

FIGURE 6-9 Oxygen deprivation in cardiac muscle results from restricted or blocked blood flow through the coronary arteries.

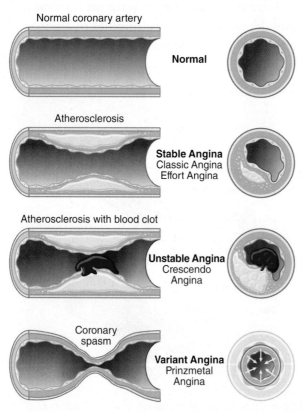

FIGURE 6-10 Three types of angina.

medications, primarily CCBs, beta-blockers, and **ranolazine**, a medication specific to angina pain.

Variant Angina

Also called *Prinzmetal angina,* variant angina is caused by vasospasm of the coronary arteries (which supply blood to the heart muscle). Exertion is *not* a trigger for variant angina. This is in direct contrast to stable angina (recall from the above discussion: chest pain occurs in a predictable pattern during exertion or exercise). Prinzmetal angina occurs *at rest,* often without a predictable pattern. The patient experiences pain as a result of coronary artery spasms, which decrease the amount of oxygen delivered to the heart. Therefore, the treatment goal for this type of angina is *to increase the blood flow and oxygen supply* to the heart. Medications used in the treatment of variant angina include nitrates and CCBs. Beta-blockers and ranolazine are not used to treat variant angina.

Unstable Angina

Unstable angina carries a much higher risk of mortality than chronic stable angina or vasospasm-related angina and is considered a medical emergency. The treatment recommendations are as follows:

1. Oxygen: Recommended for patients with an arterial saturation of less than 90%, patients in respiratory distress, or those at high risk for hypoxemia (Anderson et al., 2007).
2. Nitroglycerin: Either oral or IV nitroglycerine for patients who have continued hypertension or are in heart failure.
3. Morphine: IV morphine is recommended for pain relief and/or relief from anxiety. The morphine should be titrated while monitoring the patient.
4. Antiplatelet therapy: Unless there are serious contraindications, patients should receive antiplatelet therapy with aspirin and a P2Y12 receptor blocker (Anderson et al., 2007). Anticoagulants are discussed later in this chapter.
5. Anticoagulation: Anticoagulation therapy should be initiated to reduce the risk of MI or stroke.

Antianginal Agents

Most of the drugs used to treat angina are already familiar from the previous discussion of hypertension. Because the cause of angina is reduced oxygen to the heart, it stands to reason that drugs such as beta-blockers and CCBs, which cause vasodilation, can increase blood flow to the heart and thereby relieve the pain. Thus, there is no need to reiterate the activity of those drug classes here. However, two other drugs, **ranolazine** and (especially) **nitroglycerin**, have important roles in treating this condition, so they are discussed in more depth.

Ranolazine

The mechanism of action for **ranolazine** is not completely understood, but it can reduce the amount of sodium and calcium in the myocardial cells. As described in the earlier section on CCBs, the function of calcium in cardiac and vascular smooth muscle is to promote contraction and vasoconstriction; thus reducing the calcium level in these cells helps to relax both the vessels feeding the heart (increasing blood flow) and the heart muscle itself (reducing oxygen demand).

Adverse effects of this medication include alterations in heart function, specifically a dose-related increase in the QT interval that places the patient at an increased risk for serious dysrhythmias, including torsades de pointes. Patients with severe renal impairment may experience blood pressure elevation and should monitor their blood pressure closely. Other side effects include constipation, dizziness, nausea, and headache.

A few medications are known to have significant interactions with **renolazine**. Drugs that prolong the QT interval should not be combined with **renolazine** due to increased risk of developing torsades de pointes. CYP3A4 inhibitors can increase the serum levels of **renolazine**, because it is metabolized through that mechanism; patients taking this drug should be warned to avoid grapefruit and grapefruit juice.

Nitroglycerin

Nitroglycerin—or more correctly, glyceryl trinitrate—is a well-known therapy for chest pain. It works through a series of reactions that begin with the uptake of nitrates by the vascular smooth muscle to produce vasodilation, primarily in the veins but also in the arterioles. The obvious benefit of this response is an increased amount of blood remaining in the peripheral tissues, so that less blood returns to the heart. With this reduction in preload, the heart has a decreased demand for oxygen. Nitrates also lessen coronary artery spasm, thereby increasing the oxygen supply even more.

Nitroglycerin is typically (perhaps even stereotypically) administered sublingually as a spray or dissolving tablet; however, it may also be administered orally as a long-acting capsule, as a sustained-release patch, or, in unstable angina, intravenously. The development

> **Best Practices**
>
> Use of phosphodiesterase type 5 inhibitors (medications for erectile dysfunction) is absolutely contraindicated in patients taking nitroglycerin or other nitrate medications, as the interaction between the drugs may be life threatening.

of tolerance to the vasodilation effects of nitrates is one concern for patients receiving nitrate therapy. To minimize nitrate tolerance, the smallest effective dose should be utilized, and patients using sustained-release patches should allow for a consistent period of time each day that the patch is removed.

Nursing Considerations

Adverse effects associated with **nitroglycerin** include headache, which is caused by the direct vasodilation and can be treated with **acetaminophen**. Orthostatic hypotension may also result from the collecting or pooling of blood in the veins; patients should move from a lying or sitting position slowly to allow time for accommodation of their blood pressure. Reflex tachycardia may occur in response to the vasodilation as well, decreasing the patient's blood pressure.

Nitroglycerin's drug interactions include phosphodiesterase type 5 (PDE5) inhibitors, a group of medications used for erectile dysfunction; these medications are *absolutely contraindicated* with nitrates. Concomitant use of nitrates and PDE5 inhibitors can cause life-threatening hypotension. Care should be exercised with patients taking nitrates and other medications that lower blood pressure to decrease the risk of severe hypotension.

Hyperlipidemia

Lipids are a class of molecules that include a variety of substances: fatty acids, sterols (including **cholesterol**), certain fat-soluble vitamins (A, D, E, and K), and glycerides. The word *lipid* is often misconstrued as *cholesterol*, as *lipids* is the overall term most often blanketly associated with the "prevention of heart disease," along with **triglycerides**.

Cholesterol has also gained a bad reputation, yet the cholesterol molecule is *required* for key biochemical and physiological functions. For example, cholesterol is required for the synthesis of hormones (i.e., adrenal corticosteroids, estrogen, progesterone, and testosterone); it is essential for the synthesis of bile salts; and it literally makes up part of all cell membranes. In short, human beings could not live without cholesterol. The body obtains some of its necessary cholesterol from dietary sources, but the remaining amount is synthesized in the liver. However, too much of any molecular compound can become harmful.

Although most people know about two kinds of cholesterol (characterized in the media as "good" cholesterol and "bad" cholesterol), there are actually *six* major classes of lipoproteins. Only three of these six have been directly associated with the development of coronary artery sclerosis: **very low-density lipoprotein (VLDL)**, **low-density lipoprotein (LDL)**, and **high-density lipoprotein (HDL)**. An increase in LDL cholesterol—the type popularly identified as "bad" cholesterol—correlates with an increase in the risk of coronary heart disease (CHD). Conversely, an increase in HDL ("good") cholesterol correlates with a decrease in the risk of CHD. Remembering which is which is simply a matter of understanding that the names equate with the levels needed for health: LDL is the type of cholesterol which should be remain *low*, while HDL is the molecule that needs to stay *high*, to *avoid* dyslipidemia. VLDL is the principal transporter for other lipids, including triglycerides; a high triglyceride level generally equates to a high VLDL level and is a risk factor for heart disease. Because VLDL is not directly measured, it is not a target for medication in the same way that HDL and LDL are; however, the total amount of triglycerides *is* addressed with pharmacologic therapy due to its correlation with cardiovascular disease.

Cholesterol (and triglyceride) levels are best controlled via lifestyle alterations, in which high-fat foods are avoided and, in particular, cholesterol-bearing foods (meats, eggs, and dairy products) are limited. However, lifestyle modifications are not always successful. Some patients simply are not able to manage the dietary changes needed, while others, due to genetic factors, continue to have elevated cholesterol levels even with dietary modifications. For these situations, a variety of medical options are available. The goal of therapy is to reduce cholesterol and triglyceride levels so as to reduce risk of plaque buildup and the potential for thrombosis leading to MI or stroke. (Medical therapies specifically intended to prevent clot formation are discussed later in this chapter.)

Statin Drugs

Statin drugs (TABLE 6-8) are among the most widely prescribed medications for hyperlipidemia for one reason: this group of drugs is currently the most effective class available in terms of its ability to lower cholesterol levels, due to their mechanism of action (MOA). The MOA is exactly the same for each member of the statin class of medications. The cholesterol molecule is synthesized in the liver by an enzyme called HMG-CoA reductase; the statin drugs directly inhibit the action of this enzyme, HMG-CoA reductase, thus directly decreasing the synthesis of the cholesterol molecule. Lower cholesterol levels have been shown to slow the progression of CHD, and the complications of CHD. The enzyme, HMG-CoA reductase, is most active during the sleeping hours; thus, this class of medications is more effective when taken right before bedtime. These drugs are effective in decreasing the risk of CHD events in patients who have CHD as well as those who do not show evidence of CHD. Because the majority of cholesterol synthesis in the body occurs at night, it is recommended that the shorter half-life statins

be taken at bedtime so they can have the greatest effect in reducing cholesterol levels.

Adverse effects related to the use of statins vary. For some patients, muscle symptoms ranging from myalgia to myositis to rhabdomyolysis can begin to appear within weeks to months of starting statin therapy. Muscle injury is far less common when patients are taking statin therapy alone. There is also a risk of liver toxicity; elevation in the serum transaminase levels develops in 0.5% to 2% of patients who have been taking statins for a year or longer. While there is risk for liver injury, progression to liver failure is extremely rare. Liver function tests are recommended before the start of treatment and every 6 to 12 months. Some statin drugs may increase the risk of type 2 diabetes, particularly in women (Byrne & Wild, 2011), but recent studies suggest that this outcome occurs primarily in those patients who already have other risk factors for diabetes (Waters et al., 2013). Thus, a patient's baseline diabetes risk should be assessed carefully before using statin drugs and weighed against the risk of cardiovascular events (Nichols, 2013).

Statins are considered to be harmful to pregnant women and the developing fetus. They should not be taken by women who are pregnant or who plan to become pregnant.

Drug interactions of note include those with other lipid-reducing agents, which can increase the severity and incidence of statin-associated adverse events. Statins may also interact with drugs that inhibit CYP3A4 as statins are metabolized via this pathway; thus inhibition of CYP3A4 can elevate serum statin levels.

Best Practices

Because the majority of cholesterol synthesis in the body occurs at night, patients taking shorter half-life statins should be instructed to take their medication at bedtime.

TABLE 6-8	Statin Drugs
Generic Name
Atorvastatin
Fluvastatin
Lovastatin
Pitavastatin
Pravastatin
Rosuvastatin
Simvastatin

Fibrates

Fibrate drugs (TABLE 6-9) are derived from fibric acid, which lowers lipid levels, at least in part, by activating peroxisome proliferator-activated receptors (PPARS) (Staels et al., 1998). Activating these receptors promotes the

TABLE 6-9	Fibrate Drugs
Generic Name	Notes
Bezafibrate	Not marketed in the United States.
Ciprofibrate	Not marketed in the United States.
Clofibrate	No longer commonly used due to its side-effect profile, which includes the production of gallstones. Dosing adjustment is needed in patients with renal dysfunction.
Fenofibrate	Contraindicated in patients with liver or severe renal dysfunction, unexplained persistent liver function abnormalities, or preexisting gallbladder disease.
Gemfibrozil	Patients with Type IV hyperlipoproteinemia may see their serum LDL increase rather than decrease. May potentiate action of warfarin.

breakdown of fatty acids. Fibrates can lower serum triglycerides by 35% to 50% and raise serum HDL by 5% to 20%—a substantial improvement in patients with significantly elevated triglycerides.

Adverse effects of fibrate drugs include muscle toxicity, especially when taken concomitantly with a statin. Patients taking fibrates have also been identified as experiencing elevations in their serum creatinine levels. Dyspepsia and formation of gallstones have been identified as common side effects of this drug class, with clofibrate in particular marked as causing the latter problem.

Known drug interactions include exacerbation of muscle toxicity when fibrates are taken with statins, especially those that are metabolized by the CYP3A4 pathway; caution should be used when taking fibrates alongside any CYP3A4-inhibiting drug, or any other agent that likewise relies on this metabolic mechanism. Fibrates interfere with **warfarin** metabolism and increase this medication's circulating levels (Dixon & Williams, 2009), so patients on **warfarin** should have their International Normalized Ratio (INR) monitored while taking fibrate drugs. **Fenofibrate** increases the clearance of **cyclosporine**, and patients can experience a significant reduction in their serum cyclosporine levels.

Niacin

Niacin, also known as vitamin B_3 or nicotinic acid, is an essential nutrient that offers benefits for patients with dyslipidemia. In the liver, niacin inhibits the production of VLDL, which helps to lower LDL levels. It also raises HDL levels by decreasing the lipid transfer of cholesterol from HDL to VLDL and slows down HDL clearance. In this way, niacin both lowers LDL levels and causes a reduction in plasma fibrinogen levels. It is effective in patients with elevated cholesterol levels and those who have elevated lipids and low HDL levels. Some studies have suggested that niacin may be useful in decreasing mortality when used with patients for secondary prevention of CHD.

Niacin (vitamin B_3) is available as an OTC product in the same strength as the prescription medication, but it comes in several different forms: nicotinic acid, inositol hexanicotinate, and nicotinamide. Neither nicotinamide nor inositol hexanicotinate has been shown to lower lipid levels; thus, if patients are told to take **niacin** and wish to purchase it on an OTC basis rather than obtaining it by prescription, it is imperative that they be instructed to read the label and purchase nicotinic acid—otherwise, they will not get the benefit of the medication. A helpful pointer to patients is to avoid brands that advertise themselves as "no-flush niacin," because these are almost universally made with inositol hexanicotinate. Such products are able to make "no flush" claims precisely because they *lack* nicotinic acid, the very substance needed to lower cholesterol!

Flushing is the most common adverse effect of **niacin**, and it can last from a few minutes to several hours. Flushing is more prevalent with the crystalline preparation versus the controlled-release formulation. This side effect is a minor consideration, however; of greater concern is the fact that niacin can elevate serum glucose levels, which can be particularly problematic for those patients with diabetes. Nicotinic acid can also cause hyperuricemia, so patients with a history of gout should not take nicotinic acid. Pruritus, paresthesias, and nausea are other potential adverse effects. Also, in patients who are on vasodilators for unstable angina pectoris, nicotinic acid can cause further hypotension, which can exacerbate chest pain.

Bile Acid Sequestrants

Bile acids are by-products of cholesterol and are excreted in the feces, but often a substantial amount of these acids are reabsorbed in the intestines. By binding bile acids in the intestines, bile acid sequestrants inhibit the reabsorption of bile acids. This lowers the cholesterol in the liver, which in turn encourages LDL receptors to be created; their proliferation then leads to additional reduction in serum cholesterol. Examples of this drug class include cholestyramine, colestipol, and colesevelam.

Patients with mild to moderately elevated LDL cholesterol levels are best served with this group of cholesterol-lowering agents. For patients with significantly higher serum LDL

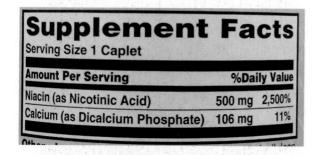

Supplement Facts

Serving Size 1 Caplet

Amount Per Serving		%Daily Value
Niacin (as Nicotinic Acid)	500 mg	2,500%
Calcium (as Dicalcium Phosphate)	106 mg	11%

levels, bile acid sequestrants are more effective when taken concomitantly with statins or nicotinic acid.

GI disturbances are the most common adverse effects with these drugs, including nausea, bloating, and cramping. Of note in regard to drug interactions are those with **digoxin** and **warfarin**. Both of these agents may bind to bile acid sequestrants in the gut, which can impair the absorption of these two drugs and result is less-than-therapeutic serum levels.

Congestive Heart Failure

CHF is a progressive disease in which the heart is unable to pump with sufficient force to push blood through the blood vessels. When this happens, fluid backs up in the vessels and leaks into the tissues and organs, particularly the lungs, leading to the shortness of breath and "congestion" that characterize CHF. Heart failure usually develops in the ventricles and can occur on one side of the heart or the other, or both sides simultaneously.

CHF has been described in terms of four stages of increasing severity (TABLE 6-10). Symptoms of heart failure include reduced CO, shortness of breath with or without exertion, pulmonary edema, peripheral edema, angina, and jugular vein distention caused by the heart's decreased inotropic strength.

Best Practices

Make sure patients understand that if they are buying niacin on an OTC basis, they must look for "nicotinic acid" on the label.

TABLE 6-10	Four Stages of Congestive Heart Failure
Stage	**Characteristics**
AHA Stage A/NYHA Stage I*	No symptoms or minimal/absent structural/functional cardiac abnormalities. Patient experiences no limitation of physical activity or symptoms such as dyspnea, fatigue, or palpitations.
AHA Stage B/NYHA Stage II	Structural heart disease associated with the development of heart failure is present. Patient experiences no symptoms at rest, but mild symptoms and slight limitation that increase with activity. Strenuous activity may produce anginal pain.
AHA Stage C/NYHA Stage III	Structural heart disease is moderate to severe. Patient experiences marked limitation and symptoms such as dyspnea, fatigue, arrhythmia, or angina even with mild activity, but is comfortable at rest.
AHA Stage D/NYHA Stage IV	Severe structural heart disease. Patient experiences discomfort even at rest; limitations on physical activity are considerable, as any activity exacerbates symptoms.

*There are two standard classification systems used to identify CHF stages. The American Heart Association's A–D classification is based on objective, clinical criteria. The NYHA I–IV classification is based on patient symptoms. Both are equally valid measures and are often used side-by-side.

Appropriate pharmacologic treatment is selected based on the patient's stage of CHF and response to the medication. Controlling volume overload can help alleviate left ventricular dysfunction. To reduce ventricular wall stress, drugs that affect the RAAS, and those that target the sympathetic nervous system effects on the heart can be employed. Three main groups of drugs are considered first-line therapy for CHF: diuretics, ACE inhibitors or ARBs, and beta-blockers (all of which were discussed in detail in the earlier section on hypertension). The reason for using these medications should be clear: They reduce the workload of the heart and lower overall fluid volume, both of which are important considerations in patients with CHF.

Additionally, angiotensin receptor antagonists (AAs), inotropic agents (which include cardiac glycosides [**digoxin**]), and vasodilators can be considered if treatment with the three main categories of drugs is not adequate. AAs and vasodilators were discussed previously; thus inotropic agents will be considered here.

Inotropic Agents

Inotropic agents affect contractions of the heart muscle. Inotropes can be either *positive* or *negative*. Positive inotropes cause increased cardiac contraction force, increasing cardiac workload, but improve cardiac function. Negative inotropes decrease cardiac contraction force, which decreases cardiac workload. Positive inotropes, primarily cardiac glycosides, have found utility for the treatment of CHF.

Cardiac Glycosides

The class of drugs known as cardiac glycosides is represented by the commonly prescribed medication **digoxin** (derived from the foxglove plant *Digitalis*), acts on the heart both as a positive inotrope (leading to increased force of contraction) and a **negative chronotrope** (leading to altered impulse conduction) in the heart.

Each time the heart contracts, sodium and calcium ions move into myocyte intracellular space. The calcium ions cause release of stored calcium ions within the cell to interact with the myocyte contractile proteins, leading to contraction. This intracellular calcium is re-stored during repolarization and relaxation. Cardiac glycosides bind the ATPase responsible for sodium and potassium movement, resulting in a decrease in the amount of sodium that moves out of the cell, resulting in less calcium recycled out of the myocyte, and increasing the amount of usable calcium inside the myocyte. By increasing usable calcium, myocardial contractility is improved. The increased force raises the CO and arterial pressure. When arterial pressure increases, the baroreceptor reflex decreases the sympathetic stimulation of the heart and blood vessels, allowing the heart to pump more efficiently and in a more organized manner. This reduces the symptoms of CHF and can treat some cardiac dysrhythmias. Increases in extracellular potassium ion concentration interfere with cardiac glycoside binding of the ATPase, inhibiting the effectiveness of cardiac glycosides (such as **digoxin**).

Digoxin has a narrow therapeutic index, which facilitates the potential for undertreatment or toxicity. Because of the significant potential for under- or overtreatment with this agent, **digoxin** is now considered a secondary treatment for CHF, to be used only if primary treatment is not adequate. Because of its *negative* chronotropic action, **digoxin** can also be useful in the treatment of atrial fibrillation, atrial tachycardia, and supraventricular tachycardia. However, in patients who are being treated with this drug for CHF, digoxin's negative chronotropic effects can severely decrease HR and impact cardiac rhythm.

Nursing Considerations

The patient's pulse should be checked before the administration of each dose, if not more often. A low potassium level places the patient at increased risk for **digoxin** toxicity, so caution should be used in patients who have chronic hypokalemia; extreme caution should be used in patients with partial AV block or renal failure. Conversely, hyperkalemia reduces the drug's effectiveness in such a way that if used in conjunction with medications that promote potassium retention, digoxin may prove less effective or completely ineffective.

A number of key drug interactions with digoxin have been identified. Diuretics that can cause hypokalemia put the patient at increased risk for digoxin toxicity. ACE inhibitors and ARBs, in contrast, can increase potassium levels and decrease the response to digoxin. **Quinidine**, an antidysrhythmic drug, can elevate **digoxin** levels and increase the risk of toxicity. Patients on **quinidine** may need **digoxin** dosage adjustments. Also, the CCB **verapamil** can elevate digoxin levels and increase the risk of digoxin toxicity.

Vasodilators are discussed in other parts of this chapter, and so are not discussed here, other than to point out that arterial and venous dilatation improves the hemodynamic status of patients, decreasing resistance to blood flow, and cardiac workload.

Vasopressin, also called **antidiuretic hormone (ADH)**, is released by the pituitary gland, and induces increased water resorption by the kidneys. Elevated vasopressin concentrations may increase peripheral vascular resistance and pulmonary capillary wedge pressure via free water resorption in the kidneys, leading to worsening of congestive heart failure. There are three known vasopressin receptors: V_{1a}, V_{1b}, and V_2. V_{1b} receptors are located in the central nervous system, V_{1a} receptors are found both centrally and peripherally, and V_2 receptors peripherally. V_{1a} are involved in blood pressure regulation, while V_2 receptors affect renal function.

One goal for treatment of CHF is to increase fluid elimination, while minimizing electrolyte loss, particularly of sodium (leading to hyponatremia). Vasopressin antagonism, especially of V_2 receptors, increases urine output without associated sodium loss. Thus, **vasopressin antagonists** are sometimes employed as part of the strategy to combat CHF. Two approved vasopressin antagonists are **tolvaptan** and **conivaptan**.

The resulting sodium retention can lead to an anticipated adverse effect of increased thirst. Hyperkalemia (potassium) may also be seen in patients taking these medications. Though these drugs do decrease patient body weight, and improve sodium concentrations, their benefits for patients with CHF appear to be marginal (Nistor et al., 2015).

Prevention of Thrombosis and Stroke: Anticoagulant Therapy

Earlier, we discussed therapy to reduce cholesterol levels. The reason these therapies are so widely used is that the long-term consequences of uncontrolled hyperlipidemia include two of the most dreaded acute cardiac dysfunctions—stroke and MI. Plaque buildup in the arteries promotes the formation of blood clots, which can block blood vessels and lead to tissue death locally. Often, this condition occurs in the deep veins of the legs (**deep vein thrombosis [DVT]**), which can provide a warning to patients of the need to address a propensity toward clotting before such an event takes place in the brain, the lungs, or the heart, which may prove fatal.

Prevention of strokes/MI, DVT, or pulmonary thrombosis relies on several classes of medications. Among the best known are the anticoagulants; some of these agents, such as heparin, are given intravenously, while others are taken orally (e.g., **warfarin**).

Anticoagulants
Heparin

Heparin, also known as unfractionated heparin, binds to antithrombin III (AT-III, part of the body's anticoagulant system). When this occurs, a sequence of associated responses increases the efficacy of the body's anticoagulant system and decreases the blood's ability to clot. **Heparin** is therefore used to treat individuals with the potential for or past history of experiencing harmful clots. Indications that increase the risk of clotting include acute coronary syndromes, percutaneous coronary interventions, venous thromboembolism, and maintenance of IV catheter patency. Unfractionated heparin therapy is reserved for the inpatient setting.

Special Note

The concentrations of heparin that are available range from 1 unit/mL to 20,000 units/mL. Effective May 1, 2013, manufacturers of Heparin Lock Flush Solution, USP and Heparin Sodium Injection, USP were required to clearly state the strength of the entire container of heparin followed, in parentheses, by the amount of the medication contained in 1 mL (Lexicomp, 2012).

Heparin is not absorbed well from the gut. Therefore, administration of this drug is limited to IV and subcutaneous injection; it is not given intramuscularly, to decrease the possibility of bruising. The subcutaneous injections should be given in the abdomen, rotating between the left and right sides above the iliac crest. It is also important to make sure *not* to aspirate before depressing the plunger on the syringe. In addition, the site should *not* be rubbed after removing the needle from the abdomen.

As with all anticoagulants, excessive bleeding is a primary concern. Frequent complete blood counts (CBC) and activated partial thromboplastin times (aPTT or APTT) tests are required to monitor the impact of the heparin therapy. The complete blood count will provide hemoglobin, hematocrit, and platelet levels. The aPTT measures the efficacy of the contact activation pathway and the common coagulation pathways.

Heparin can cause two types of thrombocytopenia. The first type, simply referred to as heparin-induced thrombocytopenia (HIT), is benign and is the most common. Three factors that increase a patient's risk of developing HIT are unfractionated heparin therapy versus use of low-molecular-weight heparin (LMWH), surgical versus medical patient, and female versus male

patient (Coutre, 2012). The second type of thrombocytopenia associated with heparin use, immunological HIT, is less common but far more serious. This form of HIT is an immunological reaction to heparin therapy in which the body's platelets are attacked. The condition is usually reversible if the heparin is discontinued. However, serious side effects such as skin necrosis, pulmonary embolism, gangrene of the extremities, stroke, or MI can occur (Lexicomp, 2012). Two additional side effects associated with heparin use include elevation of aminotransferase levels and hyperkalemia due to heparin-induced aldosterone suppression.

The antidote for an overdose of heparin is protamine sulfate. After administration, the protamine sulfate combines with heparin to form a stable complex (salt), which neutralizes the anticoagulant activity of the drugs.

Heparin may be given simultaneously with other anticoagulant agents when transitioning a patient to an outpatient regimen. In such a case, it is important to keep in mind that the heparin is likely to enhance the anticoagulation effect on the body when given in combination with these other drugs. Examples of some of the drugs that interact with heparin include other anticoagulants, antiplatelets, aspirin, NSAIDs, certain herbs, nitroglycerin, thrombolytic agents, and vitamin E.

Low-Molecular-Weight Heparin

LMWHs are not interchangeable with unfractionated heparins, and the two groups of drugs have different pharmacologic properties. Two examples of LMWH are enoxaparin (1 mg = 100 units of anti-Xa activity; World Health Organization First International Low Molecular Weight Heparin Reference Standard) and dalteparin (1 mg = 70–120 units of anti-Xa activity; World Health Organization First International Low Molecular Weight Heparin Reference Standard). As their name suggests, LMWHs have smaller heparin molecules than the unfractionated heparins. The mechanism of action for LMWH is to have a small effect on the aPTT and a strong anti-factor Xa ability.

LMWH drugs are becoming widely prescribed because they are much more predictable than the unfractionated heparins, have longer half-lives, are just as effective, and do not require the blood test monitoring necessary when unfractionated heparin is administered. Also important is that these medications, with the appropriate patient education, can be successfully managed in an outpatient setting.

Some examples of the uses of LMWH enoxaparin include DVT prophylaxis and treatment, percutaneous coronary intervention, and treatment of pulmonary embolism, ST elevation MI (ST-segment elevation myocardial infarction [STEMI]), and unstable angina or non-ST elevation MI (non-ST-segment elevation myocardial infarction [NSTEMI]). **Enoxaparin** should not be administered intramuscularly. Administration should be subcutaneous only to the left or right anterolateral or posterolateral abdominal wall. It is important *not* to expel the air bubble in the syringe before administration, to prevent inaccurate dosing. As with unfractionated heparin, the site should *not* be rubbed after injection. The patient may experience a burning sensation upon subcutaneous injection at the entry site. A single IV dose may be given to patients experiencing STEMI.

Enoxaparin has not been approved for use with dialysis patients by the Food and Drug Administration (FDA). If the patient has chronic kidney disease, the dosage should be decreased and the anti-Xa levels checked frequently. Elderly patients may have increased sensitivity to LMWH, and these drugs are not recommended in patients with renal impairment and age older than 70 years.

Patients receiving **enoxaprin** are at risk for excessive bleeding (may be increased in women weighing less than 45 kg and men weighing less than 57 kg), HIT, thrombocytopenia, and hyperkalemia. Morbidly obese patients (body mass index greater than 40 kg/m^2) will likely need adjusting/correcting of the weight-based dosage, but there is no consensus on specific recommendations.

Examples of some of the drugs that interact with LMWH heparin include anticoagulant drugs, antiplatelet agents, aspirin, NSAIDs, certain herbs, thrombolytic agents, and vitamin E.

Oral Anticoagulants

While injectable anticoagulants are used in critical situations, for patients in whom thrombosis is merely a risk, preventive use of oral anticoagulant drugs is commonly undertaken. The drugs most often used for this purpose are the vitamin K antagonist **warfarin** as well as a class of drugs called direct thrombin inhibitors (DTIs).

Warfarin

Warfarin blocks the availability of vitamin K in the body. With less vitamin K available, the liver's production of clotting factors declines. The decreased amount of clotting factors increases the amount of time it takes for the blood to form a clot, which can be beneficial in people at risk of thrombosis.

The most harmful adverse effect of **warfarin** therapy is excessive bleeding, which is also the reason that lab work is necessary for patients on therapy. Patients receiving **warfarin** require close monitoring of their prothrombin times (PTs) and INR. The PT is particularly dependent on the clotting factors affected by **warfarin**, while the INR is a standardized value that is calculated from the PT results. The exact target range will be determined by the healthcare provider. The dosage of the medication should be adjusted to meet this goal. A PT that is below the target will require an increase in the dosage; a PT or INR that is above the target will require a decrease in the dosage and monitoring for bleeding. In addition, patients should seek medical evaluation following any serious fall or head injury.

Patients should also take precautions to minimize the risk of harm from bleeding such as using a soft-bristle toothbrush, proactively reducing their risk of falling in the environment, using an electric razor instead of a blade, and <u>avoiding activities that involve or have the risk of intense traumatic physical contact</u>.

Alcohol should be limited to no more than one to two servings occasionally. Chronic alcohol abuse affects the body's ability to handle **warfarin** and also increases the risk of falls (Hull, Garcia, & Vazquez, 2018).

Signs of Bleeding

- Nosebleeds
- Bleeding gums
- Coffee-ground emesis
- Persistent nausea or stomach pain
- Blood in stool or tarry stools
- Blood in urine or dark brown urine

Drug-Drug Interactions

Many drugs interact with **warfarin**, both prescription and OTC (TABLE 6-11). Because of this, patients who are receiving **warfarin** therapy should contact their healthcare provider before taking any new OTC medications, prescription medications, or vitamin supplements. It is especially important that vitamin K supplements be avoided in patients taking **warfarin**, as vitamin K promotes clotting and counteracts the effects of the drug.

Dietary Guidelines

Significant dietary guidelines must be followed while a patient is taking a vitamin K antagonist. A consistent vitamin K dietary intake is essential for maintaining a therapeutic **warfarin** level. Patients need significant dietary and safety education on ways to maintain a consistent vitamin K dietary intake and to prevent falls and traumatic injuries. Most patients, unless they are very conscientious about consuming a healthy diet, will not know which foods contain vitamin K, or they may understand the "dietary guidelines" portion of the therapeutic intervention to

TABLE 6-11	Drugs That Affect Warfarin Therapy
Drug Name	**Effect on Warfarin**
Acetaminophen	Increases effects; potential for bleeding
Amiodarone	Increases effects; potential for bleeding
Antithyroid drugs	Decreases effects; potential for clotting
Carbamazepine	Decreases effects; potential for clotting
Cephalosporins	Increases effects; potential for bleeding
Ciprofloxacin	Increases effects; potential for bleeding
Haloperidol	Decreases effects; potential for clotting
Levothyroxine	Increases effects; potential for bleeding
Macrolide antibiotics (e.g., clarithromycin)	Increases effects; potential for bleeding
Metronidazole	Increases effects; potential for bleeding
NSAIDs (e.g., ibuprofen, naproxen)	Increases effects; potential for bleeding
Oral contraceptives	Decreases effects; potential for clotting
Phenobarbital	Decreases effects; potential for clotting
Rifampin	Decreases effects; potential for clotting
Vitamin E	Increases effects; potential for bleeding
Vitamin K	Decreases effects; potential for clotting

mean that they must *avoid* foods rich in this vitamin. That is not actually the case: What is needed is maintenance of *consistency* in eating leafy green vegetables and other common food sources. This may be challenging in areas where access to such vegetables is limited due to climate; if the patient's intake falls (or increases) due to seasonal availability of certain foods, it may adversely affect the therapeutic efficacy of the **warfarin** regimen. Regular PT and INR lab work should be performed and evaluated by a healthcare provider to ensure safe and therapeutic levels if the patient has difficulty maintaining dietary consistency.

Direct Thrombin Inhibitors

An alternative to warfarin is the DTI dabigatran etexilate. Although there are other drugs in this class, dabigatran etexilate is the first DTI that can be given orally. The body converts this prodrug into dabigatran, which binds directly to thrombin. The benefit of this drug over other, similar medications is that dabigatran can actually bind to clot-bound thrombin, which is an effect not even IV heparin can achieve. Blocking the effect of thrombin decreases the probability of a dangerous clot developing. Another benefit is that there is no need for lab work monitoring with dabigatran etexilate, unlike that required with heparin and warfarin therapy.

Dabigatran etexilate has been used for the prevention and treatment of venous and arterial thromboembolic disorders. It has been used primarily to treat venous thromboembolism (VTE) after orthopedic surgery. In 2010 the FDA approved the drug for the prevention of stroke and blood clots for patients who experience chronic atrial fibrillation.

The most significant adverse effect associated with this DTI is excessive bleeding. However, preapproval studies of the medication showed comparable rates of serious bleeding in patients taking dabigatran etexilate and patients receiving warfarin. Patients with liver or renal impairment should either avoid this medication or use it with extreme caution and medical oversight due to their increased risk of developing excessive bleeding. Other side effects include GI disturbances. In December 2012 the FDA issued a warning against the use of dabigatran etexilate in patients with mechanical prosthetic heart valves, as a RE-ALIGN study indicated that these individuals may be at increased risk of experiencing stroke, MI, and mechanical valve thrombosis compared to patients taking warfarin ("Pradaxa," 2012).

Drug-Drug Interactions

Drugs that cause P-glycoprotein to increase or decrease its pumping rate impact the amount of dabigatran etexilate that is available in the bloodstream. Such medications include antacids, drugs that decrease gastric acid secretion, and rifampin. Medications that reduce the drug's metabolism and, therefore, increase its presence in the bloodstream include verapamil, amiodarone, dronedarone, ketaconazole, quinidine, clarithromycin, and clopidogrel (Bussey & Edith, 2012).

Other drugs that affect platelets, such as NSAIDs and other antiplatelet agents, should be avoided when taking dabigatran etexilate. Concomitant use of dabigatran etexilate with anticoagulants also increases the risk of excessive bleeding.

Direct Factor Xa Inhibitors

Factor Xa activates conversion of prothrombin to thrombin in the coagulation pathway. The end result of this pathway is the development of a clot. The inhibition of factor Xa decreases the probability of developing life-threatening clots or from current ones becoming larger. Two drugs, rivaroxaban and apixaban, are specific inhibitors of activated factor X; both have excellent oral bioavailability.

Factor Xa inhibitors have a fast onset of action and consistent pharmacokinetic and pharmacodynamic actions (Kubitza, Becka, & Voith, 2005). Rivaroxaban reaches peak plasma concentrations within 2.5 to 4 hours after taking the medication orally (Lawrence, 2014). Rivaroxaban was found to be equivalent to enoxaparin followed by vitamin K antagonist treatment in patients with DVT (Lawrence, 2014).

There is no coagulation monitoring lab work required, and no known dietary restrictions with either rivaroxaban or apixaban. Both drugs have been approved for the treatment and/or prevention of clots in patients with atrial fibrillation, after knee or hip replacement, in DVT, and with pulmonary embolism (PE). **Rivaroxaban** is approved in the United States for treatment and prevention of acute pulmonary embolism and DVT. **Apixaban**, meanwhile, is indicated for prevention of stroke and thromboembolism in patients with atrial fibrillation.

As with all anticoagulants, adverse effects with **rivaroxaban** and **apixaban** include an increased risk of excessive bleeding. Because there is no known antidote to these drugs, and given that dialysis is not likely to reduce their presence in serum, patients should be given careful dosing instructions to help avoid overdose. Similar to patients taking the other anticoagulant medications, patients on **rivaroxaban** should avoid other antithrombic agents, aspirin, NSAIDs, combined P-gp and CYP3A4 inhibitors, P2Y12 platelet inhibitors, and fibrinolytic therapy, all of which could further increase the risk of excessive bleeding.

Antiplatelet Agents

A variety of oral medications inhibit platelet function directly. These drugs include **aspirin**, which inhibits the enzyme cyclooxygenase, reducing the production of thromboxane A_2 (stimulator of platelet aggregation). Use of low-dose **aspirin** as a "blood thinner" to prevent clotting is widespread as a result. However, there are alternatives. Thienopyridines (**clopidigrel**, **pasugrel**) inhibit ADP-dependent platelet aggregation; the PDE5 inhibitor **dipyridamole** impairs platelet function by inhibiting the activity of adenosine deaminase and phosphodiesterase (it may also cause some vasodilation).

Aspirin is the most commonly used antiplatelet medication and is used to prevent ischemic stroke and cardiovascular events, despite evidence that it is not always the best medication for the job. For example, the CAPRIE study showed that a composite outcome of stroke, MI, or vascular death was significantly reduced with **clopidogrel** treatment versus **aspirin** use (Cucchiara &

Messe, 2018). However most of the benefit was observed in patients with PAD (Cucchiara & Messe, 2018). The combination of **aspirin** and **dipyridamole** for secondary stroke prevention appears to be additive, and **aspirin-extended-release** with **dipyridamole** is significantly more effective than **aspirin** alone for stroke prevention (Cucchiara & Messe, 2018).

All antiplatelet medications carry a risk of excessive bleeding. **Aspirin** is known to increase the risk of GI distress and bleeding. These risks can be decreased with lower dosages or enteric coatings. Also, patients may experience **aspirin toxicity**, which, in addition to increased bleeding risk, may present as tinnitus or ringing of the ears. Patients who experience **aspirin** allergies should also avoid a cross-allergy to NSAIDs.

Clopidogrel is associated with a slightly lower occurrence of GI upset or bleeding than **aspirin** (Cucchiara & Messe, 2018). With **dipyridamole**, headache is the most frequently reported adverse effect.

Similar to patients taking the other anticoagulant medications, patients on antiplatelet medications should avoid the use of other antiplatelet medications, antithrombic agents, NSAIDs, and fibrinolytic therapy, all of which could further increase the risk of excessive bleeding. Patients on long-term anticoagulation therapy may also be receiving antiplatelet therapy, but only under the close supervision and monitoring of a healthcare provider.

Antiarrhythmic Agents

Cardiac cells depolarize and repolarize about once per second. Multiple proteins, affected by ion concentration fluctuations, are responsible for maintenance of cardiac rhythms. Outside of the proximal electrophysiology, the heart is affected by input from the sympathetic and parasympathetic systems. When improper rhythms (arrhythmias) occur, pharmacologic intervention is sometimes indicated.

Ions move through specific channels or transporters in response to changes in electrical stimulation and ion concentration gradients. Important ions for cardiac conduction include sodium, potassium, and calcium. At rest, potassium is allowed in myocytes, while sodium is excluded. Depolarization of myocyte membranes briefly allows sodium ions in and potassium ions out, propagating the conduction signal, then sodium is once again excluded from cells, while potassium returns. Also involved in ion exchange is calcium. Improper ion transport can result in improper cardiac rhythm. For a more complex review of cardiac conduction, signal transmission and muscle contraction, the reader is referred to physiology textbooks.

An arrhythmia occurs when the normal sequence of impulse initiation and propagation is disturbed. Arrhythmias include rapid heart rhythms (tachycardia), premature depolarizations, flutters, fibrillations, and signal re-entry, and can involve the atria (atrial) or ventricles (ventricular).

Antiarrhythmic drugs are sometimes unpredictable in their effects on patients, in part because arrhythmias often involve multiple mechanisms, and in part because drugs can affect multiple targets. These drugs usually act by one of three mechanisms: by altering conduction velocity; by changing cardiac cell excitability via altering the length of impulse refractory time; by suppressing abnormal automaticity. Drugs are utilized to alter ion (sodium, potassium, calcium) channels and conduction velocity, or affect sympathetic or parasympathetic actions on the heart. Antiarrhythmics are usually classified as members of four or five groups, though members of groups sometimes can be classified in more than one group. The four main groups include **sodium-channel blockers**, beta-blockers, **potassium-channel blockers**, and **calcium-channel blockers**. A fifth grouping includes drugs that act by a variety of mechanisms.

Group I Antiarrhythmics: Sodium-Channel Blockers

Blockade of fast sodium channels slows electrical conduction in the heart. Group I antiarrhythmics bind to fast sodium channels (which are involved in the rapid depolarization [phase 0] of fast-response cardiac action potentials). The result is a reduction of inward-moving sodium, but utilizing drug concentrations that do not affect resting membrane potential (FIGURE 6-11).

This reduces the action potential transmission velocity, which can counter tachycardias caused by mechanisms including signal re-entry. Sodium-channel blockers also can affect refractory period. Therefore, there are

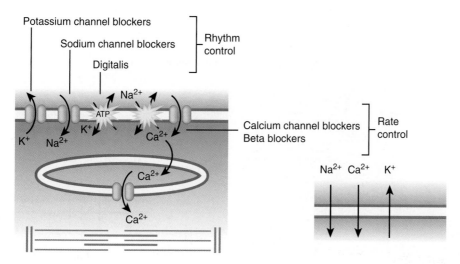

FIGURE 6-11 Group I antiarrhythmics: Sodium-channel blockers.

three subclasses of sodium-channel blockers, categorized as groups IA (increase refractory period), IB (decrease refractory period), or IC (no effect on refractory period).

Examples of group IA drugs include quinidine, procainamide, and disopryamide, and can be useful for treating atrial fibrillation and flutter, and supraventricular and ventricular tachyarrhythmias. Examples of group IB drugs include lidocaine, tocainide, and mexilitine. Group IB drugs tend to be useful for the treatment of ventricular tachycardias. Examples of Group IC drugs include flecainide, propafenone, and moricizine, and can be useful for treating supraventricular and ventricular tachyarrhythmias.

Group II Antiarrhythmics: Beta-Blockers

Beta-1 antagonists (beta-blockers) affect beta-1-receptors located in the heart, eyes, and kidneys. When utilized as antiarrhythmics, they act by inhibiting sympathetic stimulation, especially by epinephrine and norepinephrine, of cardiac impulses. Normally, sympathetic nerves increase pacemaker currents, causing increased heart rate. Sympathetic stimulation of the heart can also be a cause of aberrant pacemaker activity from increasing conduction velocity. β_1-blockers can reduce these effects by decreasing reactivity of pacemaker cells to adrenergic sympathetic

stimulation (FIGURE 6-12). Examples of beta-blockers (though not necessarily β_1-selective) that can be useful antiarrhythmics include acebutolol, propranolol, and esmolol.

Group III Antiarrhythmics: Potassium-Channel Blockers

Most drugs in Group III have potassium-channel blocking activity, but may also affect other ion channels, and so are not necessarily *purely* targeting potassium transport. Blocking potassium channels causes delayed repolarization of myocardial cells, increasing the refractory between beats (FIGURE 6-13). They can

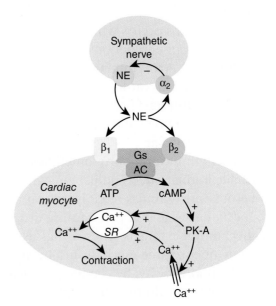

FIGURE 6-12 Group II antiarrhythmics: Beta-blockers.

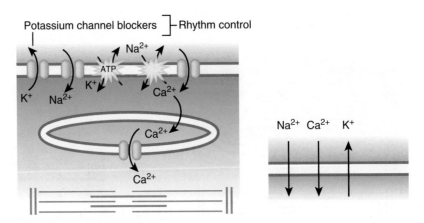

FIGURE 6-13 Group III antiarrhythmics: Potassium-channel blockers.

be useful for treatment of tachyarrhythmias caused by reentry signals. Examples of Group III drugs include amiodarone, dofetilide, dronedarone, bretylium, sotalol, ibutilide, and dofetilide.

Group IV Antiarrhythmics: Calcium-Channel Blockers

Group IV antiarrhythmics are calcium-channel blockers (CCBs), and, by inhibiting calcium from crossing cell membranes, decrease firing rate of aberrant sites in the heart, decrease conduction velocity at the AV node, and reduce heart rate. Action at the AV node is useful for treating supraventricular tachycardias caused by reentry impulses (FIGURE 6-14).

Calcium channel blockers are subdivided into two categories, dihydropyridines and non-dihydropyridines, the latter being useful for arrhythmias. Dihydropyridines are more vascular-selective, and so more useful for treating hypertension via calcium channel blockade. The non-dihydropyridine class includes the drugs diltiazem and verapamil.

Group V Antiarrhythmics: Miscellaneous

Group V antiarrhythmics include drugs that act via a variety of mechanisms other than those recognized as Groups I–IV. Included in this class are adenosine and digoxin. Adenosine binds adenosine type-1 receptors on the heart, which opens potassium channels, and blocks calcium channels. The result is hyperpolarization of cells, and decreased conduction velocity. Adenosine, which is very short-lived in the body, can be used for rapid treatment of SVTs. Digoxin, which was previously discussed, is useful for arrhythmias because it reduces heart rate, and can be useful for treating atrial fibrillation and flutter.

CHAPTER SUMMARY

This chapter has touched upon the most common subsets of cardiovascular disorders seen by healthcare providers. It is nowhere near a comprehensive overview of cardiovascular disease—a topic that could fill numerous volumes—but rather highlights the classes of medications used most frequently in addressing the commonly seen problems. Of key importance is an understanding of which drugs may be used in conjunction with one another to support cardiovascular function, and which may not; understanding how drug classes act upon particular receptors, and how they are metabolized in the body, is an important topic for identifying potentially dangerous drug interactions.

Critical Thinking Questions

1. Describe the three factors that affect blood pressure, and name specific classes of drugs that can alter each factor to reduce hypertension.

2. How does the RAAS impact the cardiovascular system? Which classes of drugs are used to alter it, and how does each drug class do so to lower blood pressure?

3. Which factors affect CO? How does the clinician seek to change CO in (1) hypertension and (2) CHF?

4. How do medications that inhibit cytochrome P450 3A4 affect the metabolism and serum levels of eplerenone? Why does this effect not occur with spironolactone?

5. Why should patients who are taking statins avoid grapefruit?

6. Which medications are the best first-line therapy for chronic hypertension? Which are best used in hypertensive crisis? Why is there a difference?

7. Which major classes of medications should not be used with anticoagulants?

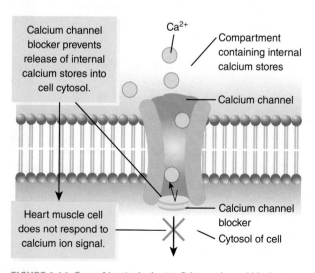

Calcium channel blocker prevents release of internal calcium stores into cell cytosol.

Ca²⁺

Compartment containing internal calcium stores

Calcium channel

Heart muscle cell does not respond to calcium ion signal.

Calcium channel blocker

Cytosol of cell

FIGURE 6-14 Group IV antiarrhythmics: Calcium-channel blockers.

CASE STUDY 1

Hypertension Management

A 62-year-old Caucasian male, CW, is an established patient at a free primary care clinic where you are volunteering. The clinic serves only persons without health insurance. CW works as a general handyman in a rural farming community and is quite physically active most days of the week doing his jobs. He did not complete high school and reads at approximately a sixth-grade level. He is single, does not use tobacco products or recreational/illicit drugs, and rarely drinks alcohol. His medical history is significant for primary or essential hypertension, prediabetes, and osteoarthritis; he is extremely hard of hearing. He was last seen six months ago for a routine check-up; his BP at that time was 140/84. Today CW is worried about his blood pressure after discovering it was 200/110 when he checked it last night at the local grocery store. He denies headache, dizziness, palpitations, chest pain, or shortness of breath. On further questioning, he tells you that he has not taken his blood pressure medicine for "several months" because "I ran out and couldn't afford to buy more." He admits that he has "not been eating right" for the last few months. He drinks only coffee for breakfast, then typically stops at a convenience shop for lunch choosing a packaged snack food, Coke, and a fried meat product. For supper, he eats scrambled eggs with sausage or frozen burritos most nights. He drinks four to five caffeinated beverages daily.

Medication list:
Lisinopril 20 mg one tab daily in AM, initiated 2 years ago
Ibuprofen 200 mg (OTC) 1–2 tabs every 6 hours prn joint pain
Allergies: NKDA
Vital signs: BP: left arm: 200/110, right arm: 190/110; P: 86/minute, regular; Respirations: 12/min, regular; Oral temperature 98.4°F; Weight: 185#; Ht: 69″; BMI 27.3.

Upon assessment, you notice that CW is sitting comfortably and is in no acute distress. The healthcare provider reports no unusual findings upon funduscopic exam and evaluation of heart sounds, peripheral pulses, lungs, abdomen, and extremities.

Lab values from today's visit: CMP all within normal range; hemoglobin A1c 5.7% (consistent with prediabetes); Lipid panel all values within normal range (normal values in parentheses). Total cholesterol: 152 (125–200 mg/dL); LDL-c: 75 (<130 mg/dL); HDL: 54 (≥40 mg/dL); Triglycerides: 114 (<150 mg/dL)

The healthcare provider decides to prescribe two antihypertensive agents: Lisinopril 40 mg and hydrochlorothiazide 12.5 mg daily. CW is to return in two weeks for a nurse visit to recheck his blood pressure and assess for adherence. He asks you to instruct the patient regarding the importance of adherence to this regimen, expected side effects, and any other relevant teaching points. He also asks you to teach CW about the DASH diet.

Case Questions

1. What are two nursing diagnoses (NANDA format) you would make concerning CW's hypertension management and eating patterns?

2. According to current hypertension management guidelines, what is the target blood pressure for this patient?

3. What will you tell CW about why the provider has prescribed two medications instead of one for his blood pressure?

4. Explain the difference between the two medication classes in clear language appropriate for someone with a sixth-grade reading level.

5. Knowing that CW is uninsured, what formulation of these medications would be most appropriate to decrease cost and thus promote adherence?

6. What is one open-ended question you can ask CW to initiate a conversation about medication adherence?

7. What precautionary information should you provide for CW regarding this medication? What would be the expected results?

CASE STUDY 1 (CONTINUED)

8. What are the basic principles of the DASH diet that you would communicate to CW?

9. Write one long-term and one short-term goal for one of the two nursing diagnoses that you made.

10. What action step can you take at today's visit as an intervention to meet the short-term goal?

11. When CW returns for his follow-up appointment in two weeks, how will you evaluate the effectiveness of your intervention?

CASE STUDY 2

Dyslipidemia Management

CW is a 62-year-old Caucasian male and an established patient at a free primary care clinic where you are volunteering. The clinic serves only persons without health insurance. He presents today for a two-week follow-up nurse visit to evaluate the effectiveness of and adherence to his new blood pressure medication regimen. CW works as a general handyman in a rural farming community and is quite physically active most days of the week doing his jobs. He did not complete high school and reads at approximately a sixth-grade level. He is single, does not use tobacco products or recreational/illicit drugs, and rarely drinks alcohol. His medical history is significant for primary hypertension, prediabetes, and osteoarthritis; he is extremely hard of hearing. He tells you that he has taken his prescribed medications daily since his last visit. He went to the health department once last week to have his BP checked, and "they said it was ok." He denies headache, dizziness, palpitations, chest pain, or shortness of breath. He thanks you for the time you spent at the last visit explaining about the DASH diet; then he says, "I don't hear so good, so I missed some things you said." He still drinks coffee, but he has cut down to one cup daily. He continues to eat packaged snack foods such as chips, cinnamon rolls, and cookies because of convenience.

Medication list:
Lisinopril 20 mg one tab daily in AM, hydrocholorthiazide 12.5 mg daily in AM started 2 weeks ago
Ibuprofen 200 mg (OTC) 1–2 tabs every 6 hours prn joint pain
Allergies: NKDA
Vital signs: BP: left arm: 140/86, right arm: 142/88; P: 76/minute, regular; Respirations: 12/min, regular; oral temperature 98.4°F; Weight: 183#; Ht: 69"; BMI 27.02.
His lipid panel values from his visit 2 weeks ago are in normal range as follows (normal values in parentheses): Total cholesterol: 152 (125–200 mg/dL); LDL-c: 75 (<130 mg/dL); HDL: 54 (≥40 mg/dL); Triglycerides: 114 (<150 mg/dL).

CW is sitting comfortably and is in no acute distress. He turns his left ear toward you when you speak.

You have learned how to use the online ACC/AHA ASCVD Risk Calculator, so you invite him to watch as you enter his lipid and blood pressure values. The risk calculator shows that CW has a 9.9% 10-year risk of heart disease or stroke. CW sits up straight, looks directly at you, and says, "Does that mean I could have a heart attack or stroke? What can I do to prevent this?"

Case Questions

1. Is CW's blood pressure at JNC-8 goal for his age and medical history? He has no chronic kidney disease, and he does not have diabetes.

2. Even though CW's lipid panel is in normal range, he has a fairly high risk for an atherosclerotic cardiovascular disease (ASCVD) event, such as heart attack or stroke, within the next 10 years. How will you answer his two questions?

(continues)

CASE STUDY 2 (CONTINUED)

3. CW is experiencing the proverbial "teachable moment" as he learns about his risk for ASCVD. According to guidelines, might he benefit from taking a statin drug for lowering cholesterol?

4. What will you tell CW about the class of statin drugs when he asks how they work?

5. What is one open-ended question you can ask CW to initiate a conversation about making lifestyle modifications?

6. Write one nursing diagnosis (NANDA format) related to patient education that addresses CW's known hearing deficit.

7. Write one short-term goal to reflect CW's patient education needs.

8. What action will you take today to meet the short-term goal?

9. You work together with CW to arrive at one change in his diet patterns he could make in the next three months. Write one long-term goal for this using the SMART (Specific, Measurable, Attainable, Relevant, Time-Based) goal format.

10. When CW returns for his follow-up appointment in three months, how will you evaluate the effectiveness of your intervention?

REFERENCES

Anderson, J., Adams, C., Antman, E., Bridges, C.R., Califf, R.M., Casey, D.E. Jr., . . . Smith, S.C. Jr. (2007). ACC/AHA 2007 guidelines for the management of patients with unstable angina/non-ST-elevation myocardial infarction: A report of the American College of Cardiology/American Heart Association Task Force on Practice Guidelines. *Journal of the American College of Cardiology, 50*, e1.

Bussey, H.I., & Edith, N.A. (2012). Dabigatran demystified: What warfarin patients should know about this new anticoagulant. Retrieved from http://www.clotcare.com/dabigatran_demystified.aspx

Byrne, C.D., & Wild, S.H. (2011). Increased risk of glucose intolerance and type 2 diabetes with statins. *British Journal of Medicine, 343*, d5004.

Centers for Disease Control and Prevention (CDC). (2017). Multiple cause of death 1999-2016. *CDC WONDER Online Database.* Accessed at https://wonder.cdc.gov/mcd.html.

Chobanian, A., Bakris, G., Black, H., Cushman, W.C., Green, L.A., Izzo, J.L. Jr., . . . Roccella, E.J. (2003). The Seventh Report of the Joint National Committee on Prevention, Detection, Evaluation, and Treatment of High Blood Pressure: The JNC 7 report. *Journal of the American Medical Association, 289*, 2560. Retrieved from https://www.nhlbi.nih.gov/files/docs/guidelines/jnc7full.pdf

Coutre, S. (2012). Heparin-induced thrombocytopenia. *UpToDate.* Retrieved from https://www.uptodate.com/contents/clinical-presentation-and-diagnosis-of-heparin-induced-thrombocytopenia

Cucchiara, B.L., & Messe, S.R. (2018). Antiplatelet therapy for secondary prevention of stroke. *UpToDate.* Retrieved from https://www.uptodate.com/contents/antiplatelet-therapy-for-secondary-prevention-of-stroke

Dixon, D.L., & Williams, V.G. (2009). Interaction between gemfibrozil and warfarin: Case report and review of the literature. *Pharmacotherapy, 29*(6), 744–748.

Farag, E., Maheshwari, K., Morgan, J., Sakr Esa, W.A., & Doyle, D. (2015). An update of the role of renin angiotensin in cardiovascular homeostasis. *Anesthesia & Analgesia, 120*(2), 275–292.

Furberg, C., Psaty, B., & Meyer, J. (1995). Dose-related increase in mortality in patients with coronary heart disease. *Circulation, 92*(5), 1326–1331.

Heron M. (2014). Deaths: Leading causes for 2014. [PDF-4.4M] *National vital statistics reports.* 2016; 65(5).

Hull, R.D., Garcia, D.A., & Vazquez, S.R. (2018). Patient education: warfarin (Coumadin) (beyond the basics). *UpToDate.* Accessed at https://www.uptodate.com/contents/warfarin-coumadin-beyond-the-basics?search=Patient%20information:%20Warfarin%20(Coumadin)%20(beyond%20the%20basics)&source=search_result&selectedTitle=1~150&usage_type=default&display_rank=1.

James, P.A., Oparil, S., Carter, B.L., Cushman, W.C., Dennison-Himmelfarb, C., Handler, J., . . . Ortiz, E. (2014). 2014 evidence-based guidelines for the management of high blood pressure in adults: Report from the panel members appointed to the Eighth Joint National Committee (JNC 8). *JAMA, 311*(5), 507–520.

Ko, D., Hebert, P., Coffey, C., Sedrakyan, A., Curtis, J.P., & Krumholz, H.M. (2002). Beta-receptors blocker therapy and symptoms of depression, fatigue, and sexual dysfunction. *Journal of the American Medical Association, 288*(3), 351–357.

Kubitza, D., Becka, M., & Voith, B. (2005). Safety, pharmacodynamics, and pharmacokinetics of single doses of BAY 59-7939, an oral, direct factor Xa inhibitor. *Clinical Pharmacological Therapy, 78*, 412–421.

Lawrence, L.L. (2014, August 14). Anticoagulants other than heparin and warfarin. PharmaGuide. Accessed at http://pharmaguide.co/anticoagulants-heparin-warfarin/

Lexicomp. (2012, December). Heparin: Drug information. Retrieved from http://ultra-medica.net/Uptodate21.6/contents/UTD.htm?39/34/40489?source=see_link

Makani, H., Messerli, F., Romero, J., Wever-Pinzon, O., Korniyenko, A., Berrios, R., & Bangalore, S. (2012, August 1). Meta-analysis of randomized trials of angioedema as an adverse event of renin–angiotensin system inhibitors. *American Journal of Cardiology, 110*(3), 383–391. DOI: https://doi.org/10.1016/j.amjcard.2012.03.034

Morales, D.R., Lipworth, B.J., Guthrie, B., Jackson, C., Donnan, P.T., & Santiago, V.H. (2014). Safety risks for patients with aspirin-exacerbated respiratory disease after acute exposure to selective nonsteroidal anti-inflammatory drugs and COX-2 inhibitors: Meta-analysis of controlled clinical trials. *Journal of Allergy and Clinical Immunology, 134*, 40. http://dx.doi.org/10.1016/j.jaci.2013.10.057

Morelli, J. (2016). High blood pressure (hypertension) medications. *RxList*. Retrieved from http://www.rxlist.com/high_blood_pressure_hypertension_medications-page9/drugs-condition.htm#is_it_safe_to_take_high_blood_pressure_medication_during_pregnancy

Nichols, G.A. (2013, April 8). Are statins worth the diabetes risk? *Medscape*. Retrieved from https://www.medscape.com/viewarticle/781684

Nistor, I., Bararu, I., Apavaloaie, M.C., Voroneanu, L., Donciu, M.D., Kanbay, M., . . . Covic, A. (2015). Vasopressin receptor antagonists for the treatment of heart failure: A systematic review and meta-analysis of randomized controlled trials. *International Urology and Nephrology, 47*(2), 335–344. doi: 10.1007/s11255-014-0855-2

Perez, M.I., & Musini, V.M. (2008). Pharmacological interventions for hypertensive emergencies: A Cochrane systematic review. *Journal of Human Hypertension, 22*, 596–607. doi:10.1038/jhh.2008.25

Pradaxa (dabigatran etexilate mesylate) should not be used in patients with mechanical prosthetic heart valves. (2012). *FDA Drug Safety Podcast*. http://wayback.archive-it.org/7993/20161022043202/http://www.fda.gov/downloads/Drugs/DrugSafety/DrugSafetyPodcasts/UCM333208.mp3

Prescriber's Digital Reference (PDR). (2018). Atenolol—Drug summary. Retrieved from http://www.pdr.net/drug-summary/tenormin?druglabelid=1128

Radack, K., & Deck, C. (1991). Beta-receptors adrenergic blocker therapy does not worsen intermittent claudication in subjects with peripheral arterial disease: A meta-analysis of randomized controlled trials. *Archives of Internal Medicine, 151*, 1769–1776.

Regulski, M. Regulska, K., Stanisz, B., Murias, M., Gieremek, P., Wzgarda, A., & Niznik, B. (2015). Chemistry and pharmacology of angiotensin-converting enzyme inhibitors. *Current Pharmaceutical Design, 21*(3):1764-1775.

Riccioni, G. (2013). The role of direct renin inhibitors in the treatment of the hypertensive diabetic patient. *Therapeutic Advances in Endocrinology and Metabolism, 4*(5), 139–145.

Roush, G. C., Kaur, R., & Ernst, M.E. (2014). Diuretics: A review and update. *Journal of Cardiovascular and Pharmacologic Therapy, 19*(1), 5–13.

Salvetti, A., & Ghiadoni, L. (2006). Thiazide diuretics in the treatment of hypertension: An update. *Journal of the American Society of Nephrology, 17*(4 Suppl.2), S25–S29.

Sato, A., & Fukuda, S. (2015). A prospective study of frequency and characteristics of cough during ACE inhibitor treatment. *Clinical and Experimental Hypertension, 37*(7), 563–568.

Sica, D. A. (2006). Interaction of grapefruit juice and calcium channel blockers. *American Journal of Hypertension, 19*(7), 768–773.

Sica, D.A., Carter, B., Cushman, W., & Hamm, L. (2011). Thiazide and loop diuretics. *Journal of Clinical Hypertension (Greenwich), 13*(9), 639–643.

Staels, B., Dallongeville, J., Auwerx, J., Schoonjans, K., Leitersdorf, E., & Fruchart, J.C. (1998). Mechanism of action of fibrates on lipid and lipoprotein metabolism. *Circulation, 98*, 2088–2093.

Story, L. (2012). *Pathophysiology: A practical approach*. Burlington, MA: Jones & Bartlett.

Waters, D.D., Ho, J.E., Boekholdt, S.M., DeMicco, D.A., Kastelein, J.J., Messig, M.,... Pederson, T.R. (2013). Cardiovascular event reduction versus new-onset diabetes during atorvastatin therapy: Effect of baseline risk factors for diabetes. *Journal of the American College of Cardiology, 61*, 148–152.

Weir, M.A., Juurlink, D.N., Gomes, T., Mamdani, M., Hackam, D.G., Jain, A.K., & Garg, A.X. (2010). Beta-receptors blockers, trimethoprim-sulfamethoxazole, and the risk of hyperkalemia requiring hospitalization in the elderly: A nested case-control study. *Clinical Journal of the American Society of Nephrology, 5*, 1544–1551.

Wittner, M., Di Stefano, A., Wangemann, P., & Greger, R. (1991). How do loop diuretics act? *Drugs, 41*(Suppl. 3), 1–13.

Wiysonge, C.S., Bradley, H.A., Volmink, J., Mayosi, B.M., & Opie, L.H. (2017). Beta-blockers for hypertension. *Cochrane Database of Systematic Reviews, 1*, CD002003. doi: 10.1002/14651858.CD002003.pub5

Yusuf, S., Teo, K., Pogue, J., Dyal, L., Copland, I., Schumacher, H., . . . Anderson, C. (2008). ONTARGET: Telmisartan, ramipril, or both in patients at high risk for vascular events. *New England Journal of Medicine, 358*(15), 1547–1559.

CHAPTER 7

Respiratory Medications

Amy Rex Smith and Blaine Templar Smith

KEY TERMS

Allergen
Alveoli
Anticholinergics
Asthma
Atopy
β_2-receptor agonists
Bronchioles
Bronchoconstriction
Chronic bronchitis
Chronic obstructive pulmonary disease (COPD)
Corticosteroids

Cyclic adenosine monophosphate (cAMP)
Cysteinyl leukotriene type-1 (CysLT-1) receptors
Dry-powder inhaler (DPI)
Dyspnea
Early response
Emphysema
FEV_1:FVC ratio
Immunoglobulin E (IgE)
Late response
Leukotrienes (LT)

Leukotriene synthesis and receptor blockers
Metered-dose inhaler (MDI)
Mixed obstructive/restrictive airway disease
Monoclonal anti-IgE antibody
Obstructive airway disease
Peak expiratory flow rate (PEFR)
Peak flow (PF)
Peak flow meter
Preventive medications

Primary mediators
Rescue medications
Restrictive airway disease
Secondary mediators
Slow-reacting substance of anaphylaxis (SRSA)
Spirometer
Thromboxanes (TXAs)
Type I hypersensitivity

CHAPTER OBJECTIVES

At the end of the chapter, the reader will be able to:

1. Differentiate among the major classes of respiratory drugs.

2. Relate the mechanisms of action of each class of respiratory drugs to the pathophysiological changes in the immune system and inflammatory response that each one treats.

3. Analyze patient characteristics that indicate appropriate responses to respiratory medications, focusing on symptoms, patterns of airflow, and changes in physical examination.

4. Identify the role of the nurse in the administration of respiratory medications.

5. Recognize typical profiles of a home-medication regimen for patients with asthma and chronic obstructive pulmonary disease (COPD).

6. List essential features of patient education about respiratory medication regimens that will improve patient adherence.

Introduction

Great progress has been made in the scientific understanding of the immune system and the inflammatory responses specific to common conditions of the respiratory system. Identification of the molecular mechanisms of these conditions has led to the development of new medication categories based on what is now known to be occurring. In addition, respiratory medications are now often delivered directly to the airways using a variety of novel medication administration devices. These new approaches to the treatment of respiratory conditions require many patients to use medications on a daily basis.

Most patients are willing to take medications to treat troubling symptoms but are reluctant to use medications to treat an unseen condition. However, prevention of the symptoms of respiratory diseases is important for attaining and maintaining the best control over the disease processes. Because many of the pulmonary medications are self-administered, much of the nursing role regarding medications for the respiratory system focuses on patient education—that is, teaching correct methods of medication administration for adults and children (especially the proper use of inhalation devices), and the reasons for scheduled dosing. These two nursing interventions can profoundly improve outcomes for patients. It is essential that nurses understand the mechanisms of the immune dysfunction (where applicable), or other pulmonary disease processes, and recognize how each medication contributes to treatment of the underlying disease.

Most pharmacology of the pulmonary system can be illustrated using two common diseases: **asthma** and **chronic obstructive pulmonary disease (COPD)**. Many of the medications used for one of these conditions are used for the other as well, and for many other pulmonary conditions. Asthma and COPD differ in that asthma is a purely **obstructive airway disease**, while COPD is a more complex condition, being a **mixed obstructive/restrictive airway disease**. Obstructive airway disease is relatively common, including asthma (which is widespread), bronchiectasis, and cystic fibrosis; COPD is generally included among obstructive airway disorders despite also having elements of restrictive lung disease. Purely **restrictive airway disease** is uncommon and usually relates to damage of the airways from other initiating causes; it includes conditions such as pneumonia and myasthenia gravis, or can result from the use of certain medications such as methotrexate. It is far more likely that nurses will encounter restrictive airway disorders in the context of COPD; however, the key therapy in restrictive lung disease is supplemental oxygen to offset the inability of the lung tissue to adequately oxygenate on room air. Medical therapy is generally useful only in obstructive or mixed obstructive/restrictive disorders. Thus, focusing on how asthma and COPD are treated allows for an in-depth understanding

What About Lung Cancer?

It might seem strange to have a chapter on respiratory disease that does not address lung cancer. In fact, lung cancer is not, strictly speaking, a disease of respiration because it does not represent a functional issue with the mechanics of breathing. Instead, it is a neoplastic disorder that happens to occur in lung tissue. This disease can create problems with respiratory function if cancer obstructs the airways or reduces the ability of the lung to oxygenate blood. Even then, treatment generally does not focus on improving function of the airways themselves but rather comprises combined medical, surgical, and radiotherapy interventions to remove the cancerous tissue. Such interventions are generally undertaken in the care of a specialist in pulmonary oncology and are not applicable to the general population of patients who develop chronic respiratory disorders.

of respiratory pharmacology that can then be applied in many clinical situations.

Assessment of Lung Function

Before discussing pharmacotherapy, it is helpful to understand how lung diseases are diagnosed and assessed. A **spirometer** can be helpful for diagnosing and staging both restrictive and obstructive lung disorders (FIGURE 7-1). Spirometry measures both volumes and airflow. Volume measures include the complete volume, called the total lung capacity (TLC); the amount of air exchanged with each breath, called the tidal volume (V_T); and the amount of air left in the lungs after a maximal exhalation, called the residual volume (RV).

Simply measuring the amount of air exchanged does not necessarily diagnose a disease. However, spirometry helps assess a person's ability to breathe not only by measuring how much air he or she is able to exhale, but also by the rate—how fast it comes out. Three specific measurements are made:

- FEV_1 = Forced expiratory volume in 1 second. This measures how much air a patient can blow into the tubing in 1 second.
- PEFR = **Peak expiratory flow rate**. This measures how fast a patient can exhale a volume of air (measured in liters/minute).

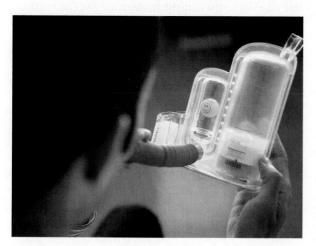

FIGURE 7-1 Spirometry for the diagnosis of respiratory disorders.
© age fotostock/Alamy

- FVC = Forced vital capacity. This measures the total volume of air expired after a full inspiration.

With obstructive airway disease, normal volumes of air pass through the airways, but the ability of the lungs to push out air quickly is reduced. Thus, one would expect to see low FEV_1 and PEFR, but a normal FVC, in a person with an obstructive disease such as asthma. Restrictive airway disease prevents the lungs from filling to their full capacity, so one would expect a smaller volume of air to pass through the airways, with normal values for the speed at which it can be exhaled. Thus, in restrictive lung disease, FEV_1 may be normal, FVC would be reduced, and PEFR may be normal, but the total volume of air expired would be smaller. Some patients have characteristics of both restrictive and obstructive disease, but diagnosis can be confirmed by comparing FEV_1 to FVC—in essence, determining how much of the total amount of air the person has to exhale *is* exhaled within the first second. In obstructive disease, FEV_1 is low in relation to FVC, so the ratio tends to be smaller than normal values. "Normal," however, can vary by age; a reading of less than 75%, for instance, would be diagnostic of asthma in anyone younger than 60 years, but not necessarily in an older adult. In restrictive disease, the amount of air available is small and there is generally little obstruction to exhalation, so normal or near-normal results (75–80%) would be seen.

COPD paints a more complex picture, because of the chronic hyperinflation of the lungs. In addition to the expected obstructive airflow pattern results, abnormal volumes are seen—most significantly an increase in the residual volume, which results in a decreased **FEV1:FVC ratio**. Effective tidal volumes are reduced, which may contribute to the sensation of **dyspnea** (shortness of breath) so often reported by these patients. This is why, as mentioned earlier, COPD is considered a mixed obstructive/restrictive airway disease.

At the bedside, a **peak flow meter** is used (**FIGURE 7-2**). This device registers, in cubic centimeters (cc), the volume of airflow. The resulting value is referred to as the patient's **peak flow (PF)**; it is usually measured each shift in an acute care setting, and daily at home and in long-term care settings. The PF value provides real-time objective data as to how effective the medications are at reversing the resistance to airflow. It is important to know the patient's baseline PF so that individualized realistic treatment goals can be achieved.

Cystic Fibrosis

One chronic obstructive airway disease that is distinct from either asthma or COPD is *cystic fibrosis*. This disease is caused by a genetic defect in a particular protein that leads to the buildup of sticky mucus in the lungs. It generally manifests in infancy, but genetic testing allows for prenatal identification and early intervention, which has increased the life span and improved the prognosis for individuals with this disorder. Cystic fibrosis is treated primarily with **ivacaftor** and **dornase alfa**, medications specific to the biochemistry of the disease. A variety of mechanical methods are also used to loosen and break up the mucus. Because this disease is so specialized, most of what is discussed in the context of asthma/COPD is not directly relevant to cystic fibrosis, and the nursing student is encouraged to find further reading if interested in this disorder.

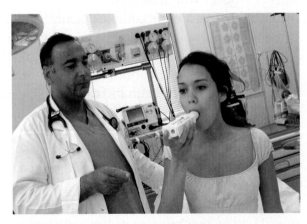

FIGURE 7-2 Use of handheld (bedside) peak flow meter.
© BSIP SA/Alamy Stock Photo

Asthma

Asthma is not, strictly speaking, a respiratory disorder—it is actually an immune system dysfunction that manifests in the respiratory system. The patient with asthma does not have an anatomical abnormality of his or her airways; instead, he or she has an inappropriate and exaggerated immune response that is dysfunctional, and that produces symptoms in the airways. The term "reactive airway disease" (RAD) is often used interchangeably with "asthma," and sometimes "asthma" is thought of as a part of RAD. In fact, RAD is ill-defined, and only "asthma" will be considered a true disease condition in this text.

As an immune disorder, asthma is classified as a **type I hypersensitivity**—an excessive response of the immune system to an encounter with a nonpathogenic substance to which it has been sensitized. Type I hypersensitivities (also known as **atopy**) are mediated by **immunoglobulin E (IgE)**. Upon exposure to a specific **allergen**, bound IgE on mast cells and basophils is cross-linked by the allergen. This leads to signals to the respective cells that allow calcium ion influx, which is thought to lead to decreased concentration of **cyclic adenosine monophosphate (cAMP)** in the cell. Decreased cAMP permits degranulation of the membrane, releasing **primary mediators** and **secondary mediators**, including histamine, serotonin, leukotrienes, prostaglandins, and cytokines, among others.

These primary and secondary mediators are the cause of overt respiratory symptoms, including bronchoconstriction (resulting from smooth muscle contraction), vasodilation, and increased mucus secretion. Together, these responses cause trapping of air in the lower (distal) respiratory tract. Thus, during an asthmatic episode, the lungs will be near their maximum inflated volume, but there will be resistance to *exhaled* air.

Until this point, the reaction (type-I hypersensitivity) is considered an **early-response** reaction, meaning one that occurs within minutes to hours after exposure to the allergen. In contrast, **late-response** asthmatic reactions can occur hours after the early phase, and are much more pharmacologically complex than are the early-response reactions. If the reader is unfamiliar with hypersensitivity reactions and the pathophysiology of asthma, he or she is referred to immunology and pathophysiology textbooks for in-depth reading. Late-response reactions require specialized (emergency department) care. Outpatient asthma management is aimed at prevention and treatment of early-response reactions. If managed properly, the occurrence of late-response reactions can be largely avoided in most patients.

While most asthmatic attacks can be traced to antigen exposure, it is well known that acute symptom onset can be induced in some patients by exercise, cold air, and even emotional distress. These non-allergen-induced attacks are believed to occur when membrane cAMP levels are close to the "threshold" concentration required for degranulation that exists in some patients' mast cell and basophil cell membranes. In this scenario, anything that might disturb the cell membranes may be sufficient to lower cAMP to "sub-threshold" concentrations, thereby allowing the pharmacology of asthma to proceed—without direct allergen exposure.

Approach to the Treatment of Asthma

It is a general principle that prevention of a disease is often better than treating disease after it develops. This principle explains why the emphasis for asthma therapy is on daily treatment of the underlying inflammation. If a medication can intervene in the body to prevent symptoms, then this is the optimal outcome. Thus, the treatment protocol for asthma is to practice allergen avoidance to the greatest extent possible, to use agents that suppress the immune response appropriately, and to carry fast-acting agents to reverse symptoms if and when they occur.

Based on this understanding, medications can be grouped into two conceptual categories: (1) those that prevent the immune response and/or restrict the actions of initial (primary and some secondary) mediators and (2) those used after the release of histamine and other early-phase mediators to treat the resulting symptoms.

In the past, asthma was considered a disease of "attacks": acute exacerbations were recognized only as a person started to audibly wheeze, an obvious sign of airway obstruction. In recent years, however, a new understanding of asthma has emerged, so that asthma is now best understood as a chronic disease with the main feature being an ongoing, underlying inflammatory process. In turn, the approach to treating asthma has changed; instead of focusing solely on treating the acute symptoms by reversal of airway obstruction, treatment protocols now recognize the need to address the underlying inflammation on a daily basis.

An important method of prevention is removing the allergen from the vicinity of the patient, or removing the patient from the vicinity of the allergen, as much as is practical. Smoking is a common and serious source of allergens that is best totally avoided, by discontinuation of smoking by the patient and/or minimizing or eliminating smoke in the environment in which the patient lives and works. However, not all allergens can be avoided; a patient who is allergic to cat dander, for example, can avoid keeping or touching cats, but that will not keep the person entirely away from cats throughout his or her life span—sooner or later, the allergen will be encountered. It is important to be able to respond to such encounters (when they arise) with medication to reduce the response of the immune system.

As described earlier, from a pharmacologic point of view, reactions can be categorized as early and late responses. The pharmacologic categories of early-response asthma prevention and treatment include β₂-**receptor agonists** (both long- and short-acting), **corticosteroids**, **leukotriene synthesis and receptor blockers**, and a **monoclonal anti-IgE antibody** designed to bind circulating IgE, preventing it from proceeding to bind to surface receptors. Management may also include inhaled muscarinic cholinergic receptor blockers, (**anticholinergics**), and agents aimed at stabilizing mast cell and basophil cell membranes (mast cell stabilizers).

Drugs that stimulate β₂-receptors (β₂-receptor agonists) have structures similar to those of the naturally occurring catecholamines, epinephrine and norepinephrine. **Epinephrine** and **norepinephrine** have short durations of action before being metabolized. Differences made in the structures of the drugs used for β₂ stimulation allow them to avoid quick degradation (by COMT), and to improve their utility for respiratory use. Stimulation of β₂-receptors activates their cells' Gₛ-adenyl cyclase-cAMP-PKA pathway, which ultimately leads to bronchial smooth muscle relaxation, regardless of the original cause of constriction. There are β₂-receptors in the peripheral circulation. Stimulation of these receptors causes vasodilation, which is the genesis of some of the side effects of these drugs.

The anti-inflammatory mechanisms of corticosteroids are complex. After entering target cells, corticosteroids bind intracellular glucocorticoid receptors; drug-bound receptors then move to the nucleus, bind to DNA and alter gene transcription, which may also directly affect protein functions. The result is decreased, or inhibited, transcription factors responsible for activation of inflammatory processes, including inhibition of several cytokines and immune inflammatory cells.

Ideally, asthmatic patients can be managed with minimal, basic drug intervention. This approach depends on the severity of daily symptoms, of course, as well as the propensity of the patient to have more exacerbated symptoms when attacks do occur. Many patients are able to restrict the disease with **preventive medications**. These drugs include antagonists of primary mediators or primary mediator effects (such as β₂-adrenergic bronchoconstriction). Preventive agents include medications that are orally administered, inhaled, or injected.

For times when symptoms progress, or for patients whose symptoms are not well controlled, **rescue medications** are available. Rescue medications, by their nature or by design, act more rapidly than preventive medications. These agents include inhaled and injected medications.

Patients should understand that preventive medications are of little value in treating acute asthmatic episodes. Patients and practitioners should be fully knowledgeable of the applications and limitations of both categories of medications. In practice, attaining optimal outcomes for patients can be a "trial and error" process, in which practitioners experiment with various single- or multiple-drug regimens, aiming to achieve the best control over the disease.

Oral Preventive Medications

A variety of daily oral medications is available to address the underlying immune response that leads to asthma. These drugs need to be taken daily by the patient according to instructions. In turn, patient education must emphasize the need to use the medication, even in the absence of overt symptoms.

Several of these medications focus on suppressing the action of **leukotrienes (LT)** (Berger, 1999). These inflammatory molecules are products of phospholipid breakdown via arachidonic acid metabolism, usually from host cells, including mast cells and eosinophils. Two "families" of leukotrienes exist, but the one that is important in asthma comprises the cysteinyl-leukotrienes, which bind to **cysteinyl leukotriene type-1 (CysLT-1) receptors** found in smooth muscle cells, airway macrophages, and eosinophils. Beyond their more "asthma-specific" origins and effects mentioned previously, leukotrienes can be secreted by activated macrophages, exhibit cytotoxicity, participate in febrile responses via the hypothalamus, and have hematopoietic effects. Those particularly important in inducing asthmatic symptoms include LTC$_4$, LTD$_4$, and LTE$_4$. These leukotrienes traditionally have been recognized as components of the **slow-reacting substance of anaphylaxis (SRSA)**. The negative asthma-related effects for which leukotrienes are responsible include **bronchoconstriction** (they may exhibit up to 1,000 times the potency of histamine), increased vascular permeability, and increased mucus production.

Leukotriene-Receptor Antagonists

A preventive approach to dealing with leukotriene actions is to block (antagonize) leukotriene receptors, with the goals of decreasing airway edema, smooth muscle constriction, and the general inflammatory process associated with asthma (Scow, Luttermoser, & Dickerson, 2007). Currently available leukotriene receptor agonists (LTRAs) are zafirlukast and montelukast tablets for oral administration (TABLE 7-1). **Zafirlukast** antagonizes LTC$_4$, LTD$_4$, and LTE$_4$ receptors and can be effective in both early and late responses, although it has found application mainly as a preventive medication. **Montelukast** binds CysLT1 receptors, and blocks the binding of LTD$_4$ to CysLT1 receptors, without itself stimulating the receptors.

Nursing Notes for LTRAs

Even when patients are not symptomatic, they should continue to take LTRAs, as these agents are preventive medications. Conversely, patients should not use LTRAs for acute asthmatic attacks, as they do not work quickly enough; be sure to emphasize that these are not rescue medications.

Thromboxane Antagonists

Thromboxanes (TXAs) are eicosanoids (lipids) derived from arachidonic acid, but from the prostaglandin-producing side of the cascade. TXA$_2$ is of particular importance in asthma, as it is a vasoconstrictor, a potent hypertensive agent, and facilitates platelet aggregation (which can be of concern especially in late-response reactions). Inhibition of TXA$_2$ is aimed mainly at stopping airway bronchoconstrictive and vasoconstrictive actions. Inhibition of leukotriene formation also decreases neutrophil and eosinophil migration, along with the aggregation of neutrophils and monocytes. In addition, it decreases leukocyte adhesion, cell–cell permeability, and smooth muscle contraction.

One example of a thromboxane receptor antagonist (TxRA) is zileuton. Zileuton inhibits 5-lipooxygenase, the enzyme that catalyzes the conversion of arachidonic acid to leukotrienes. Thromboxane inhibitors act by blocking the formation of leukotrienes, which in turn decreases inflammatory cell migration and the inflammatory process. Symptomatically, these actions lead to decreased edema, reduced mucus secretion, and less (smooth muscle) bronchoconstriction in the airways of asthmatic patients.

Nursing Notes for TxRAs

Because they are preventive medications, TxRAs should be taken regularly, even during asymptomatic periods. For optimal action, zileuton should be taken within an hour of a meal, and should not be crushed, cut, or chewed. In some patients, zileuton metabolism elevates some liver enzymes (AST or ALT). Therefore, periodic liver enzyme laboratory values should be obtained.

Oral Corticosteroids

Oral corticosteroids have well-known anti-inflammatory properties. Some patients may need low-dose corticosteroids (TABLE 7-2)

TABLE 7-1	Examples of Leukotriene-Receptor Antagonists
Generic Name	**Mechanism**
Montelukast	Binds CysLT1 receptors, and blocks the binding of LTD$_4$ to CysLT1 receptors
Zafirlukast	Antagonizes cysteinyl-leukotrienes receptors, especially LTC$_4$, LTD$_4$, and LTE$_4$

TABLE 7-2	Examples of Oral Corticosteroids
Generic Name	
Prednisolone	
Prednisone	
Dexamethasone	
Methylprednisolone	

to remain free of attacks, or to reduce the frequency and severity of those attacks that do occur. The general mechanisms by which corticosteroids act are discussed later in this chapter. Clinicians may prescribe a continuous low-dose corticosteroid, or a "burst and taper" dosing regimen, in which a higher dose is used to quickly resolve inflammation and then the dose is gradually reduced, as, once inhaled, the anti-inflammatory effects of glucocorticoids persist past the duration of dosing. The taper approach is most often used to treat intermittent flare-ups of asthmatic symptoms, while the continuous dosing approach is most often used as maintenance medication.

Nursing Notes for Oral Systemic Steroids

Long-term use of systemic steroids can lead to many serious adverse effects, including increased vulnerability to infection, development of insulin resistance or frank diabetes, complications in patients who already have diabetes, osteoporosis, adrenal insufficiency, and hyperlipidemia, among others. That is why "burst and taper" dosing is used if at all possible. If continuous steroid administration is required, the lowest dose of steroids possible is used, but patients should still be closely monitored for signs of adverse effects. Patients who have diabetes, particularly insulin-dependent diabetes (type 1), should use oral corticosteroids with caution, as even short-term therapy can produce excessively high blood glucose values (Caughey, Preiss, Vitry, Gilbert, & Roughead, 2013).

Inhaled Preventive Medications

Inhalation of drugs provides delivery of medication directly and quickly to the affected tissues. Inhaled drugs are used to prevent asthma attacks, thin mucus secretions, provide bronchodilation, act as anti-inflammatories, and stimulate respiration. Like other preventative medications, the preventive inhaled products provide optimal results when used on a consistent basis, but are not useful for acute attacks.

The use of drugs directly delivered to the desired site of action is attractive, and often very effective. However, the **metered-dose inhaler (MDI)** devices used to deliver the drugs require proper timing between inspiration and actuation of the device to be effective, and **dry-powder inhaler (DPI)** devices must be correctly loaded and primed. Thus, the patient's ability to use the device correctly to self-medicate plays a large role in the success or failure of the treatment (Aydemir, 2015; The Inhaler Steering Committee, et al., 2013; Yawn, Colice, & Hodder, 2012). Patients need teaching regarding proper technique for self-administration of inhaled medications (FIGURE 7-3). Taking time to educate patients about the proper technique can have a great impact on the successful use of inhalers. In most cases, a spacer can compensate for patients who are unable to use the proper technique due to a lack of physical coordination; such patients may include children, older adults, or individuals who suffer from neuromuscular disorders that limit their capacity for fine manual maneuvers. Use of nebulizers and facemasks is important in small children,

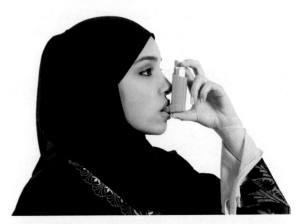

FIGURE 7-3 Delivery of medications via self-administered inhaler.
© Antonio Guillem/Shutterstock

TABLE 7-3	Common Devices Used to Deliver Respiratory Medications		
Name of Device	Advantages	Disadvantages	Types of Drugs Delivered by This Device
Nasal sprays	Direct delivery to nasal passages; easy to use correctly; small, convenient to carry	Delivery of medication to airways may be inadequate in patients with congestion	Corticosteroids
Dry-powder inhalers	Direct delivery of the appropriate dose of medication to the lungs via inhalation; small, convenient to carry	If patient cannot inhale strongly or quickly enough due to congestion or COPD, patient may not get full dose or adequate relief; accidental exhalation can blow medication away	Often used for delivery of combination medications (e.g., fluticasone/salmeterol)
Metered-dose inhalers	Direct delivery of the appropriate dose of medication to the lungs via chemical propellant; small, convenient to carry	If timing of inhalation is incorrect, patient may not get full dose or adequate relief	Bronchodilators Corticosteroids
Metered-dose inhalers + spacers	Support correct inhaler technique, particularly in children	Not convenient to carry; may harbor bacteria if not properly cleaned	Bronchodilators Corticosteroids
Handheld nebulizers	Turn medication into a mist that may be easier to inhale, particularly for young children or very ill people; work with low inspiratory capacity	Equipment may be expensive or cumbersome, and treatment time may be longer; external power source is needed	Any medication that can be obtained as or compounded into a solution that can be aerosolized

and all children may benefit from the use a spacer so that they receive full dose of the medication.

Inhaled medications come in a variety of forms (TABLE 7-3). The type of delivery device used depends partly on the medication's availability in a particular form, and partly on the capacity of the patient to use it correctly.

Inhaled Corticosteroids

Corticosteroids have multiple and complex actions. Their usefulness for prevention of asthma symptoms is mostly by virtue of their glucocorticoid-receptor agonist action, resulting in several anti-inflammatory effects. Importantly, inhaled corticosteroids inhibit multiple inflammatory cell types, including mast cells and basophils, among others. Inhaled corticosteroids also inhibit asthma-related mediator production or secretion. Some of these effects include decreased histamine production by target cells; increased cAMP production, which helps stabilize membranes of granule-containing cells; and decreased production of cytokines. This action then results in reduced

TABLE 7-4	Examples of Inhaled Corticosteroids
Generic Name	
Fluticasone	
Budesonide	
Mometasone	
Flunisolide	
Beclomethasone	

eosinophil infiltration, inhibition of macrophage and eosinophil function, reduction of vascular permeability, and production of leukotrienes.

Inhaled corticosteroids (like the ones listed in TABLE 7-4) are not for immediate ("rescue") use because their effects may not appear until up to two weeks after initiation of therapy. Patients benefit most from consistent daily use of these drugs rather than sporadic dosing. As with systemic corticosteroids, there is an increased risk of developing diabetes using inhaled corticosteroids, but it is much smaller than with oral delivery.

Nursing Notes for Inhaled Corticosteroids

Inhaled corticosteroids are used for prevention of symptoms, not for treatment of acute asthma exacerbations. Daily use, even during asymptomatic periods, is important. Careful instruction in the proper use of MDI or DPI inhalers is essential; patients should be able to demonstrate correct use to the nurse. If the patient cannot demonstrate correct use, additional teaching and/or a spacer should be provided.

Because some of the inhaled product may remain in the mouth after administration, patients should rinse after each administration to decrease the likelihood that corticosteroid-induced fungal infections may occur in the mouth. If a fungal infection (such as oropharyngeal candidiasis) occurs, the inhaled corticosteroid should be discontinued for the duration of antifungal treatment. Patients may also be more susceptible to onset or worsening of existing tuberculosis, fungal, bacterial, viral, or parasitic infections. If using a spacer or nebulizer, patients or caregivers should be given written instructions regarding care and cleaning of the device, and a schedule of frequency of maintenance if applicable.

Inhaled Long-Acting Beta Agonists

Receptors in the respiratory tract include β_2-receptors, as discussed in the preceding sections and Chapter 5. Stimulation (agonism) of these receptors causes smooth muscle relaxation, and results in bronchodilation (reverse of bronchoconstriction). Inhaled β_2 agonists are important drugs used for asthma because they are very effective bronchodilators. When used correctly, side effects can be minimized. Depending on modifications made to the chemical structure, β_2 agonists can be synthesized that are short or long acting. Short-acting β_2 agonists (SABAs) typically act for up to six hours, whereas long-acting β_2 agonists (LABAs) act for more than twelve (12) hours. Short-acting β_2 agonists are more useful for rescue ("attacks," discussed later in this chapter), whereas long-acting β_2 agonists

are more effective for prevention of attacks. Both the short- and long-acting β_2 agonists utilize the same mechanism: They occupy and stimulate β_2 receptors in much the same fashion as **epinephrine** and **norepinephrine**. Like the natural catecholamines, β_2 agonists activate the Gs-adenyl cyclase-cAMP-PKA pathway, leading to bronchial smooth muscle relaxation. Adenyl cyclase catalyzes the conversion of adenosine triphosphate to cAMP, and it is the increased concentration of cAMP that induces smooth muscle relaxation. In addition, increasing cAMP inhibits primary mediator release, especially from mast cells. Examples of long-acting β_2 agonists include **salmeterol** and **formoterol**.

Nursing Notes for LABAs

Adrenergic stimulation, even by long-acting β_2 agonists, may cause the patient to experience nervousness, tachycardia, palpitations, and difficulty sleeping, much of these due to vagal responses, and some β_2 cardiac stimulation (see the following discussion). Adjustment of the timing of administration may alleviate some of these effects. If they are intolerable, alternative medications may be necessary.

Inhaled LABAs are to be used for prevention of symptoms, not the treatment of acute attacks. Even though LABAs act via the same pharmacology as short-acting β_2 agonists, they are designed to act over long periods of time and, therefore, do not work for "rescue" applications.

Careful instruction in the proper use of MDI or DPI devices for delivery of LABAs is warranted; patients should be able to demonstrate their correct use to the nurse. If the patient cannot demonstrate correct use, additional teaching and/or a spacer should be provided.

Combination Inhalers (Corticosteroid + LABA)

As the category name implies, combination inhalers provide medications from more than one pharmacologic category. Combination inhalers for asthma provide a long-acting β_2

agonist with a corticosteroid, enabling the patient to benefit from both drugs with a single administration. As with other preventive medications, the combination inhalers are intended to be used daily, rather than as "rescue" medications.

Examples of combination inhalers for asthma include the combination of **fluticasone** and **salmeterol**, and the combination of **budesonide** and **formoterol**. For each, the corticosteroid is named first, followed by the LABA.

Nursing Notes for Combination Inhalers

The advantage of the combination inhaler is increased compliance: The patient has to administer the medication from only one device instead of two. As with other preventive medications, combination inhalers are not intended to be used for "rescue" of acute exacerbations of asthmatic symptoms. Side effects to anticipate for the combination inhalers are the same as those for both the inhaled corticosteroids and the inhaled LABAs.

Again, careful instruction in the proper use of MDI or DPI devices is essential; patients should be able to demonstrate their correct use to the nurse. If the patient cannot demonstrate correct use, additional teaching and/or a spacer should be provided.

Injected Preventive Therapies
Monoclonal Antibodies

An injected antibody is available for prevention of asthma and other type I hypersensitivity reactions. **Omalizumab** is a recombinant humanized IgGκ monoclonal antibody that binds circulating IgE antibodies, reducing the amount of IgE available to bind to high-affinity IgE receptors (FcåRI) on the surface of mast cells and basophils. This medication is injected subcutaneously every two to four weeks, with the dose based on the patient's serum IgE concentration each time. As this therapeutic approach relies on passive immunization, injections must be repeated every two to four weeks to maintain an effective serum concentration.

Other, recently approved monoclonal antibodies for asthma treatment include **reslizumab** and **mepolizumab**. These antibodies are directed at IL-5, which normally promotes eosinophil growth and inflammatory actions. **Reslizumab** and **mepolizumab** bind IL-5, thereby reducing its ability to bind IL-5 receptors on eosinophils.

Nursing Notes for Omalizumab

Omalizumab should be kept in a refrigerator and not used after the expiration date stamped on the product carton. Also, once reconstituted, the drug should be administered within eight hours following reconstitution if kept in the refrigerator, or within four hours if kept at room temperature, and vials need to be protected from direct sunlight. As with any product containing foreign protein, there is a risk of life-threatening anaphylaxis with **omalizumab**, even up to four days after its administration. Therefore, patients should be observed for signs and symptoms of anaphylaxis after injections. Also, as **omalizumab** is a preventive medication, patients should be told that improvement in asthma symptoms from this drug may be delayed.

Methylxanthines

Methylxanthines are structurally related to other xanthines, such as **caffeine** and **theobromine**, found in coffee and chocolate. Although the exact mechanisms of action of the methylxanthines used as drugs, **theophylline** and **aminophylline**, are not completely understood, some important effects of these drugs for asthma treatment include an elevation of cell membrane cAMP concentration and antagonism of adenosine receptors (adenosine induces bronchoconstriction). It is thought that the elevation of cAMP results from blocking of cAMP breakdown. The cAMP effect, then, would hinder degranulation of cells responsible for asthma mediator release, and would induce relaxation of the smooth muscles around the airways.

Theophylline (and its derivative, aminophylline)*, can easily cause toxicity in patients, so monitoring of drug concentrations in patients' blood is required. For this reason, the methylxanthines are not as commonly used as they were in the past, being replaced largely by inhaled β_2-agonists. Nevertheless, they remain a viable alternative drug choice for patients whose asthmatic (or COPD) symptoms are resistant to other drug regimens. Theophylline can be delivered either intravenously or orally, but absorption and metabolism of the drugs is inconsistent via the oral route, which is why it is not a favored regimen.* [Aminophylline is generally no longer available in the United States.]

Theophylline induces both smooth muscle relaxation, leading to bronchodilation, and suppression of airway responses to triggering stimuli. As a result, it has both immediate and prophylactic actions. The bronchodilation is suspected to be caused by theophylline's ability to inhibit two isozymes of phosphodiesterase (PDE), PDE III, and PDE IV. PDE III and PDE IV are enzymes that metabolize (hydrolyze) cAMP, so inhibition of PDE III and/or PDE IV by theophylline increases the availability of cAMP. Theophylline is also known to antagonize adenosine receptors. This medication's prophylactic actions are less clearly understood.

Nursing Notes for Methylxanthines

Adverse effects of theophylline include hypotension, tachycardia, headache, emesis, and possibly cardiac arrhythmias and convulsions. These may be related to theophylline's PDE III actions. Because methylxanthines (i.e., theophylline) have a narrow therapeutic index (Chapter Two), serum theophylline concentrations must be closely monitored to avoid toxicity. Dosing is adjusted based on this drug's serum concentration, as well as therapeutic responsiveness.

Fast-Acting "Rescue" Medications

Specific medications have been designed to be of help during an asthmatic attack and are used for "rescue," rather than for preventive reasons. These drugs, which have a rapid onset of action, are intended for short-term use. Rescue medications are used to counter an acute attack or to prevent exercise- or stress-induced attacks. Because rapid onset is a primary goal for these medications, none is administered orally, as the requirement for an absorption step would delay the desired drug effects. All of these medications are administered either by some type of inhaler or by injection to ensure rapid effect.

Short-Acting Inhaled Beta Agonists

Short-acting β_2 agonists act by the same mechanism as the long-acting β_2 agonists, except that the SABAs are designed to have immediate or rapid onset of action and a short duration of action. Although they are considered "rescue" medications, it is common practice to prescribe SABAs as "prn" (*pro re nata*, meaning "as circumstances arise") preventive medications, especially for patients who may be predictably susceptible to specific, irregular stimuli such as cold air, exercise, and animal dander, or those who do not have severe asthma and can be maintained on nominal β_2 agonism. For these patients, many practitioners consider SABAs the first medication to prescribe patients, and all are supplied via inhaler, usually MDI. Some examples of SABA inhaled medications are shown in TABLE 7-5.

Nursing Notes for SABAs

The SABAs have a shorter duration of action than do the LABAs. Therefore, it is important to understand why the patient is

TABLE 7-5	Inhaled Short-Acting β_2 Agonists
Generic Name	
Albuterol	
Levalbuterol	
Pirbuterol	

prescribed a SABA. Often, SABAs find use among patients such as athletes, who may have exercise-induced bronchoconstriction, or persons with mild asthma who experience periodic or seasonal difficulties, rather than continuous problems. Because they are short acting, for SABAs to be useful throughout the day, they may need to be used as often as four times daily, (but not more than every three to four hours). Therefore, some clinicians may opt for a LABA, whereas others may prefer the acute dosing control of SABAs. One advantage of SABA use in some patients may be the ability to avoid evening doses, thereby lowering the potential for sleep disturbance.

It is especially important that patients who are prescribed these medications receive training in correct use of inhaler devices; patients should be able to demonstrate their correct use to the nurse. If the patient cannot demonstrate correct use, additional teaching and/or a spacer should be provided.

Anticholinergic Agents

Acetylcholine has direct constrictor effects on bronchial smooth muscle via muscarinic cholinergic receptors. By blocking muscarinic cholinergic receptors, anticholinergic agents cause bronchodilation, albeit not as effectively as β_2-agonists; consequently, these drugs are typically used as adjunct agents for asthma. Drugs that exhibit muscarinic cholinergic antagonism can be useful for reversing the bronchoconstriction associated with asthma. Two drugs that act in this fashion are ipratropium and tiotropium, both of which are supplied as inhaled medications; ipratropium is delivered via an aerosol inhaler, while tiotropium is delivered via DPI. These drugs antagonize acetylcholine's binding to muscarinic cholinergic receptors, specifically the M_3-receptors on smooth muscles in airways, inhibiting intracellular calcium ion increases caused by acetylcholine. Additionally, anticholinergic agents possess the benefit of countering histamine effects, due to muscarinic receptor antagonism actions on vagal reflex bronchoconstriction.

Nursing Notes for Anticholinergics

As these drugs are anticholinergic in nature, they can induce anticholinergic side effects, even systemically. These side effects include dry mouth and decreased saliva production, blurred vision, drowsiness, constipation, difficulty urinating, decreased sweating, and memory impairment, among others. Care should be taken to avoid spraying or rubbing the medications in the eyes for this reason as well. Training in correct use of the type of inhaler supplied (DPI versus MDI) must be provided.

Intravenous Corticosteroids

In some circumstances, injectable corticosteroids can enhance asthma treatment, but they are usually reserved for emergency situations. The actions of corticosteroids have been discussed previously. Examples of injectable corticosteroids include methylprednisolone and triamcinolone.

Epinephrine

One of the staples in emergency treatment of asthma attacks is epinephrine (adrenaline.) It acts on both alpha and beta receptors (see Chapter 5). Injectable epinephrine is usually reserved for emergency situations, where direct physician oversight can occur. One patient-administered product is the epinephrine self-injection pen, whose use is reserved for acute, severe attacks. Epinephrine is an agonist at both alpha and beta receptors. Agonism of α_1 and α_2 receptors reverses asthma-induced vasodilation and vascular permeability. Agonism of β_2 receptors reverses bronchial smooth muscle constriction. Epinephrine also increases cAMP concentrations in several cell types, including mast cells, which prevents further degranulation. When administered via injection (subcutaneously or intramuscularly), this drug has a rapid onset and short duration of action.

Nursing Notes for Epinephrine

Patients should be advised that, if they use their **epinephrine** self-injection pen, they should proceed to an emergency provider, as the asthmatic reaction may not be permanently controlled by the self-injection treatment. Also, with any injection of **epinephrine**, patients should be aware the drug will induce multiple adrenergic-related effects, which may be unpleasant, including "shakiness" (muscle tremor, due to presence of β_2-receptors on skeletal muscle), tachycardia (both from the direct effect of β_1-receptor presence in the cardiac atrium, and from peripheral vasodilation resulting from β_2 stimulation on blood vessels), palpitations, sweating, nausea and vomiting, dizziness, and feelings of panic. Cardiac arrhythmias are also possible after **epinephrine** administration. The **epinephrine** self-injection kit is supplied with a "practice" syringe, which does not have a needle or contain medication. The purpose of the device is to allow patients to practice self-administration. Patients should demonstrate the ability to self-administer the self-injection pen practice device to the nurse.

Late-Phase Asthma Treatment: Emergency Room Only

Acute (rescue) events are troubling. It is frightening to patients to be unable to breathe. Not surprisingly, then, anxiety and even panic commonly accompany an acute asthma exacerbation. This makes the psychosocial care of patients a focus while they are receiving emergency treatment of rescue medications. Emergent care may not be enough to resolve the attack; often, hospitalization may be needed. A patient hospitalized for an acute exacerbation of asthma requires close surveillance by nurses. This is a serious condition; the most severe events require intensive care unit care, and death can result from asthma attacks. The hospitalization event is a critical time for nurses to provide essential teaching about medication use to prevent another exacerbation and subsequent hospitalization.

Chronic Obstructive Pulmonary Disease

Like asthma, COPD is a disease in which patients struggle to breathe. However, the mechanisms are slightly different. COPD does appear to have an immunological component, in that there is an exaggerated immune response to the presence of foreign bodies such as particles and pollutants, usually from smoke (Hassett, Borchers, & Panos, 2014; Zuo et al., 2014). A second key factor is the progressive breakdown of the mechanical processes of breathing due to damage to the **bronchioles** and **alveoli** (air sacs) in the lungs. COPD is almost always a result of smoking, although exposure to heavily polluted air and secondhand smoke can also contribute to its development. Another area of difference lies in the fact that, whereas in asthma there is no difficulty inhaling, only obstruction on exhaling, COPD is characterized by a restrictive element as well as an obstructive element—that is, patients are unable to take in adequate air, and they are unable to exhale what they take in.

There are two major forms of COPD: **emphysema** and **chronic bronchitis**. In emphysema, the alveolar walls are damaged in such a way that the alveoli lose their shape and elasticity, which provides less surface area for gas exchange and makes it both more difficult for the sacs to fill with air and more difficult for gas exchange to occur over the damaged areas. As a consequence, patients with emphysema receive less oxygen and suffer all of the effects of poor oxygenation—weakness, fatigue, and general debility. In chronic bronchitis, inflammation of the bronchi and mucus-producing glands leads to excessive mucus secretion, which in later stages can contribute to obstruction.

Like their counterparts with asthma, COPD patients may experience critical exacerbations of their condition. With bacterial infections, antibiotic therapy may be required; viral infections are best treated via preventive measures (vaccination, hand washing, crowd avoidance) and supportive measures should the patient become ill.

Patients with COPD are chronically ill, are vulnerable, and experience chronic dyspnea. They are often oxygen dependent at home and live with chronic hypoxemia and hypercapnea. Often, they are admitted for acute exacerbations of COPD, for which they receive many of the same medications used in asthma treatment. These medications work in COPD for the same reasons they work in asthma. However, because of the restrictive factor involved in COPD, inhaled delivery may be less effective; in turn, systemic, injected medications—particularly corticosteroids—are used more often in COPD than in asthma. Unfortunately, an optimal regimen for corticosteroid continues to be debated, and further data are needed to determine the most effective approach and optimal doses (Kiser et. al., 2017; Woods, Wheeler, Finch, & Pinner, 2014), although results of the REDUCE clinical trial support a five-day course of glucocorticoid treatment for acute exacerbations of COPD (Leuppi et al., 2013).

Most often the medications used include SABAs and anticholinergic agents for bronchodilation. In acute exacerbations, the bronchodilators are generally administered using handheld nebulizer devices instead of MDIs. Patients may require systemic steroids as well, often given intravenously with a burst during hospital stay and a tapering dose to be followed after discharge. Patients with COPD often develop lung infections, resulting in pneumonia or bronchitis that require antibiotics (discussed later in this section). They also will usually be prescribed LABAs and inhaled steroids upon discharge.

COPD Adjunct Therapies

A number of medical therapies are used in COPD as need arises. These treatments include antibiotics, smoking cessation, and mucoactive medications.

Antibiotics

Most COPD exacerbations are associated with a microbial infection. Nearly half of these (40–50%) are bacterial, and most of the remainder are assumed viral (Siddiqi & Sethi, 2008), although the cause of up to one-third of severe COPD exacerbations remains unknown (Ouanes, Ouanes-Besbes, Abdallah, Dachraoui, & Abroug, 2015). Vaccinations, such as "flu shots," and preventive hygiene (hand washing, crowd avoidance) are prophylactic measures that can protect against many of the most common viruses, which include rhinovirus (40–50%), influenza (10–20%), respiratory syncytial virus (RSV; 10–20%), coronavirus (10–20%), and adenovirus (5–10%) (Siddiqi & Sethi, 2008). For bacterial infections, however, antibiotic therapy is generally required.

A wide range of antibiotics is used to combat bacterial respiratory infections in COPD patients, with **cefuroxime** and **ciprofloxacin** being the two most commonly selected drugs (TABLE 7-6). Antibiotic therapy has been associated with improved outcomes in a number of studies, although not

TABLE 7-6	Antibiotic Treatment for Bacterial Respiratory Infections in COPD

Amoxicillin-clavulanate
Azithromycin
Aztreonam
Cefepime
Ceftriaxone
Cefuroxime
Ciprofloxacin
Doxycycline
Levofloxacin
Piperacillin-tazobactam

Data from Anderson, J. (2017). Antibiotic Guidance for Treatment of Acute Exacerbations of COPD (AECOPD) in Adults. University of Nebraska Medical Center. Accessed at https://www.nebraskamed.com/sites/default/files/documents/for-providers/asp/COPD_pathway2016_Final.pdf.; Hamilton, R.J. (Ed.) 2015. Tarascon Pharmacopoeia 2016 Professional Desk Reference Edition. Burlington, MA: Jones & Bartlett Learning

all patients improve on antibiotic therapy and many need either hospitalization or further antimicrobial treatment to address the infection (Rui & Kang, 2014). The pathogens most frequently associated with exacerbations of COPD are *Haemophilus influenzae* (observed in as many as 50% of cases), *Streptococcus pneumoniae* (up to 20%), and *Moraxella catarrhalis* (up to 20%). Antimicrobial pharmacology is discussed in Chapter 16.

Smoking Cessation

Because smoking is the primary cause of COPD, smoking cessation is an essential part of treatment. The highly addictive nature of nicotine means that most patients are unable to quit without assistance of some kind, even though they know that smoking is endangering their lives and preventing them from breathing easily. Physiological cravings for nicotine are typically reinforced by psychosocial habits related to smoking. In many cases, these habits cannot be successfully altered until the cravings have been quashed. Thus, smoking-cessation therapies are adjunct medical treatments for patients with COPD (these are addressed in the later section on smoking cessation).

Mucus Reduction

Another therapeutic intervention is the use of mucoactive medications to reduce mucus hypersecretion associated with COPD in some patients, particularly those with chronic bronchitis (Decramer & Janssens, 2010). One commonly used drug, *N-acetylcysteine*, is available in inhaled or nebulized form. Clinical trials found that in addition to its effects on mucus in moderate to severe COPD, *N-acetylcysteine* reduces disulfide bonds in mucoproteins (a component of mucus), causing the mucus to have decreased viscosity (Sadowska, 2012). This drug modifies small airways, limiting the restrictive aspect of the disease (Stav & Raz, 2009; Tse et al., 2013). Note that this drug should not be mixed with other drugs if used in a nebulizer, as there is no information on what the chemical admixture might do in the body.

Smoking-Cessation Therapy

It is well known that smoking is a major cause of many serious respiratory diseases, including COPD and lung cancer. In addition, for many patients with asthma, cigarette smoke is a trigger for asthma symptoms. For any patient with chronic lung disease, eliminating smoking—the patient's own, a partner's, or a parent's—is a key factor in easing symptoms and slowing progression of disease. Thus a chapter on treating respiratory disorders is incomplete if it does not address smoking cessation therapies, given that smoking cessation is a key intervention to improve respiratory dysfunction.

Oral Medications for Smoking Cessation
Antidepressants

A number of antidepressant drugs have been tested for the treatment of smoking. In theory they may be effective because they alter the chemistry in the brain that is associated with the reward/craving cycle of nicotine use (most notably dopamine and norepinephrine) and prevent depressive symptoms associated with its withdrawal (Shoaib & Buhidma, 2017). Only one of these drugs, bupropion, is approved by the Food and Drug Administration (FDA) for helping with smoking cessation. However, on rare occasions bupropion may be associated with seizures, and a patient who takes other drugs that lower the seizure threshold, including other antidepressants, antipsychotics, systemic corticosteroids, theophylline, or tramadol, should use this medication with caution. A history of seizure or bipolar disorder is a contraindication to this medication, as is pregnancy or breastfeeding.

Bupropion centrally inhibits norepinephrine and dopamine reuptake; it also is a competitive $\alpha_3\beta_4$ nicotinic acetylcholine receptor (nAChR) antagonist (see the following discussion), which makes the drug appealing for countering the neurochemistry of addiction.

Of the other antidepressants that have been tested for smoking cessation, which include **moclobemide**, **sertraline**, **venlafaxine**, **fluoxetine**, and **nortriptyline**, only **nortriptyline** had a positive impact on smoking cessation (Hughes, Stead, & Lancaster, 2007); selective serotonin-reuptake inhibitors are generally ineffective. **Nortriptyline** is less effective than **bupropion** and is not indicated for this use (Zwar, Mendelsohn, & Richmond, 2014) but is sometimes prescribed off-label for those patients who cannot tolerate approved medications.

Nicotinic-Receptor Agonists

A relatively new class of oral medications is the nicotinic-receptor agonists, which, as their name suggests, act by binding to the receptor normally stimulated by nicotine. In so doing, these agents simultaneously stimulate the receptor (thus maintaining the neurochemical effects of nicotine) and block nicotine itself from binding the same receptors (thus aiding withdrawal).

Nicotinic acetylcholine receptors are found in the CNS, muscle, and other tissues, and utilize signaling via acetylcholine. The system is quite complex, consisting of receptors composed of many variations of subunits, forming receptor pores, in various areas of the body. Two receptor subtypes important for nicotine's effects are the $\alpha_3\beta_4$ and $\alpha_4\beta_2$ receptors. *Agonists* of these receptors include acetylcholine and nicotine, among others. Nicotine binds both $\alpha_3\beta_4$ and $\alpha_4\beta_2$ receptors, causing stimulation. One path to control nicotine addiction is believed to be through affecting these receptors, and their resultant downstream effects. By blocking agonism caused by nicotine in this case, the resulting neuronal excitation normally caused by nicotine is decreased.

Although there are several medications in this class, the only drug approved for marketing in the United States is **varenicline**, an $\alpha_4\beta_2$ neuronal nicotinic acetylcholine receptor agonist that shows both fine selectivity and high affinity for its receptor site. Nicotine acts through the $\alpha_4\beta_2$ receptor to ultimately stimulate the central nervous mesolimbic dopamine system, which is thought to be tantamount to the reinforcement and reward cycle that smokers experience. By increasing the dose of **varenicline** over time, with the intention of replacing nicotine effects with **varenicline** effects, many patients are able to interrupt their physiological, addiction-based urge to smoke for a prolonged enough period of time that they are able to free themselves of the psychosocial habits that reinforce smoking.

A review of the literature (Cahill, Stead, & Lancaster, 2012) found that more patients successfully quit smoking with **varenicline** than with **bupropion**. Unfortunately, **varenicline** has a more serious side-effect profile than **bupropion**, including a potential increased risk of cardiac events in patients with a history of cardiovascular disease (Haber, Boomershine, & Raney, 2014). Given that smoking and cardiovascular disease have a strong association, it is worth taking this factor into consideration when selecting a smoking-cessation regimen with a patient.

Nursing Notes

Patients should undergo a cardiac health assessment before being offered **varenicline**, due to the potential for increased risk of cardiac events. Treatment with **varenicline** is typically targeted for 12 to 24 weeks, with the potential to repeat cycles if relapse occurs. As with any smoking-cessation attempt, patients should receive information regarding smoking cessation, advice regarding administration, and available support programs. Two dosing schedules are suggested for patients. The first schedule requires the patient to set a target "stop date," when smoking is scheduled to stop. **Varenicline** therapy should be initiated 1 week prior to the stop date. The second schedule features the concomitant use of **varenicline** and smoking, targeting complete replacement of nicotine (smoking) with **varenicline** between 8 and 35 days after initiation of treatment. To maximize the effectiveness of **varenicline**, patients should be advised to take the medication after eating, and with a full glass of water.

Nicotine Replacement Therapies

Some forms of smoking-cessation therapy focus upon breaking the psychosocial habits associated with smoking first, and use various delivery mechanisms to provide the substance of addiction—nicotine—to the patient while habit reform is undertaken. FDA-approved forms include nicotine patches, gums, nasal sprays, inhalers, and lozenges. Many of these therapies can be obtained on an over-the-counter basis; nicotine inhalers are the only drug dosage-form that requires a prescription.

It is important to note that nicotine-replacement therapy (NRT) is effective in leading to abstinence from smoking regardless of social or psychological support provided to or obtained by the patient (Stead et al., 2012); however, combining NRT with psychosocial support or therapy is more likely to help with long-term smoking cessation. Indeed, one study found that individuals who combined pharmaceutical intervention (both NRT and other medications) with behavioral support had three times the likelihood of success as those who simply purchased over-the-counter NRT (Kotz, Brown, & West, 2013).

One delivery method that has not been approved for use, and that currently lacks safety oversight and dose regulation, is e-cigarettes (electronic nicotine atomizers), which are sold online and shipped from overseas. Unlike true nicotine-replacement systems, these devices do not provide low-dose nicotine replacement, and more importantly they do not support habit reform—they merely provide for continuation of the same habits (as well as ongoing nicotine addiction) without the associated inhalation of smoke and particulate matter. Thus, e-cigarettes should not be considered a form of NRT. Patients who indicate that they currently use (or are considering using) e-cigarettes to help them quit smoking should be advised that there are significant safety concerns related to these products. Notably, substances such as diethylene glycol (a component of antifreeze) and nitrosamines (carcinogens) have been found in e-cigarette cartridges (FDA, 2017). Moreover, because they are not low-dose products, e-cigarettes may actually *increase* nicotine addiction rather than aid withdrawal.

Nursing Notes

Patients who express interest in the use of NRTs for smoking cessation should be encouraged to pursue such treatments in conjunction with social or psychological support. Support groups online or in person are widely available, or if appropriate, a referral to clinical counseling should be provided. The nurse should assist the patient in determining which method is most appropriate based on likelihood of consistent, correct use. Note that patients with unhealthy cholesterol levels associated with smoking (e.g., low high-density lipoprotein) will see no improvement until NRT is finished. Use of nicotine replacement has not been proved safe in pregnant women, although it is considered likely to be less *unsafe* than cigarette smoking.

Best Practices

Patients who indicate that they currently use (or are considering using) e-cigarettes to help them quit smoking should be advised that there are significant safety concerns related to these products.

CHAPTER SUMMARY

Respiratory disorders generally occur in one of two forms: obstructive disorders, where a patient is unable to exhale due to airway obstruction (whether that manifests in the form of inflammation or excessive mucus or both) and restrictive disorders, in which the capacity of the lung oxygen transfer is limited. Asthma is an extremely common example of an obstructive disorder. Some disorders, such as COPD, contain elements of both obstructive and restrictive disorders. Most chronic respiratory diseases can be controlled with oral and inhaled medications that suppress underlying inflammatory processes.

Acute exacerbations ("attacks") can be addressed by fast-acting "rescue" medications, although hospitalization may be required in some situations. It is important that patients learn how to accurately self-administer preventive and rescue medications, particularly those administered via MDI or DPI devices. Rescue medications utilize β_2 and muscarinic cholinergic agonism to affect responses.

Where excess mucus contributes to obstruction, the likelihood of infection increases, and patients may need mucus-thinning medications to reduce mucus (by thinning it with *N-acetylcysteine*) and antibiotics to address bacterial infections.

Many respiratory diseases, most notably COPD, occur in relation to smoking behavior. If the patient smokes, smoking cessation therapy should be offered and supported. If the patient's partner or other household members smoke, helping the patient to avoid secondhand exposure is essential to health; smoking cessation through therapeutic intervention and support should be encouraged in patients' household members. Nurses should emphasize the effects of smoking, whether primary or secondhand, in the disease process to underscore the importance of smoking cessation in treatment of respiratory diseases, particularly COPD.

Critical Thinking Questions

1. What distinguishes an obstructive airway disease from a restrictive airway disease?

2. How are the patient populations with asthma and COPD distinct from one another? How are they similar?

3. Which medications used in asthma might also be used in COPD? Why might some medications be *less* useful in COPD?

4. What are the benefits of inhaled medications versus oral medications? What are the drawbacks? What pharmacologic pathways are utilized with these drugs?

5. Which medications are used for prevention of symptoms? Which medications are "rescue" medications?

6. Describe patients for whom use of a spacer might be beneficial and explain why it should be considered.

CASE STUDIES

Case Scenario 1

Mrs. H. is a 44-year-old immigrant from the Dominican Republic who works from 6 p.m. to 2 a.m. for a company that cleans offices in many downtown high-rise buildings. She uses many different aerosol sprays as she cleans the offices. Recently, Mrs. H. has started to have some trouble with her breathing, and she occasionally finds herself audibly wheezing. She is a nonsmoker, but both her husband and her teenage son smoke cigarettes at home. Until recently, Mrs. H. had no insurance, so she was relying on herbal preparations and over-the-counter inhalers to manage her troubling symptoms. She is an enthusiastic person who embraces learning. She has been studying English at the classes offered at the local library and is becoming fluent in English. She hopes to be able to further her education, so she no longer will have to work cleaning offices.

Mrs. H. has just become eligible for health insurance through her work and has a visit scheduled with her new primary care practitioner.

Case Questions

1. Which suggestions would you make regarding removal of irritants in Mrs. H.'s environment? Be realistic and consider economic and cultural issues that might affect your answer.

2. What would a standard medication profile look like for Mrs. H.? Can you suggest a profile that would both meet her medical needs and promote adherence to the medication regimen?

3. Which medication teaching would you emphasize and why? What are the cultural and/or health literacy issues that you should consider as you develop your teaching plan?

CASE STUDIES

Case Scenario 2

Mr. N. is a 63-year-old man who has recently retired due to disability related to his COPD, a diagnosis he received 7 years previously. He lives with his wife and adult son in his own home in an urban neighborhood. Mr. N. and his wife were both heavy smokers for more than 40 years, but both have quit smoking in the past 6 months. Mr. N. has an air conditioning and filtration system in his home and is able to maintain a low-allergen, temperature/humidity-controlled environment. Despite these efforts, he is now oxygen dependent on 2 liters/min by nasal cannula. He also has a home nebulizer setup that he can use in addition to the MDIs on an as-needed basis. His baseline PF is 150 cc.

Mr. N. has an acute onset of breathlessness that does not resolve by the usual interventions at home. He is admitted to the medical unit for an acute exacerbation of his COPD. His PF is 60 cc on admission. Not only is he anxious, but he is angry that all his hard work in quitting smoking and cleaning up his environment has not worked. He is also discouraged about having to give up his job.

Case Questions

1. Which medications do you expect to be administered in the hospital? How will you determine if Mr. N.'s response to his medications is adequate?

2. What is the best way to approach this anxious, angry, and despondent patient to ensure that he will cooperate with taking his medications?

3. Upon discharge, which suggestions can you make to ensure that Mr. N. will adhere to his medication regimen? Are there any lifestyle suggestions you could make to help him cope with his chronic illness?

SUGGESTED READINGS

Beauchesne, M.F., Julien, M., Julien, L.A., Piquette, D., Forget, A., Labrecque, M., & Blais, L. (2008). Antibiotics used in the ambulatory management of acute COPD exacerbations. *International Journal of Chronic Obstructive Pulmonary Disease*, *3*(2), 319–322.

Buchman, A.L. (2001). Side effects of corticosteroid therapy. *Journal of Clinical Gastroenterology*, *33*(4), 289–294.

Dolovich, M.A., MacIntyre, N.R., Anderson, P.J., Camargo, C.A., Chew, N., Cole, C.H., . . . Smaldone, G. C. (2000). Consensus statement: Aerosols and delivery devices. American Association for Respiratory Care. *Respiratory Care*, *45*(6), 589.

Tang, H., Song, Y., Chen, J., Chen, J.Q., & Wang, P. (2005). Upregulation of phosphodiesterase-4 in the lung of allergic rats. *American Journal of Respiratory Critical Care Medicine*, *171*(8), 823–828.

REFERENCES

Aydemir, Y. (2015). Assessment of the factors affecting the failure to use inhaler devices before and after training. *Respiratory Medicine*, *109*(4), 451–458.

Berger, A. (1999). What are leukotrienes, and how do they work in asthma? *British Medical Journal*, *319*, 90.1.

Cahill, K., Stead, L.F., & Lancaster, T. (2012, April 18). Nicotine receptor partial agonists for smoking cessation. *Cochrane Database of Systematic Reviews*, *4*, CD006103.

Caughey, G.E., Preiss, A.K., Vitry, A.I., Gilbert, A.L., & Roughead, E.E. (2013). Comorbid diabetes and COPD: Impact of corticosteroid use on diabetes complications. *Diabetes Care*, *36*(10), 3009–3014.

Decramer, M., & Janssens, W. (2010). Mucoactive therapy in COPD. *European Respiratory Review*, *19*(116), 134–140.

Food and Drug Administration (FDA). (2017). FDA warns of health risks posed by e-cigarettes. *FDA Consumer Updates*. Retrieved from https://www .blacknote.com/wp-content/uploads/2017/11 /ecigarettes_0709.pdf

Haber, S.L., Boomershine, V., & Raney, E. (2014). Safety of varenicline in patients with cardiovascular disease. *Journal of Pharmacy Practice*, *27*(1), 65–70.

Hassett, D.J., Borchers, M.T., & Panos, R.J. (2014). Chronic obstructive pulmonary disease (COPD): Evaluation from clinical, immunological and bacterial pathogenesis perspectives. *Journal of Microbiology, 52*(3), 211–226. doi: 10.1007/s12275-014-4068-2

Hughes, J.R., Stead, L.F., & Lancaster, T. (2007, January 24). Antidepressants for smoking cessation. *Cochrane Database of Systematic Reviews, 1*, CD000031.

The Inhaler Steering Committee, Price, D., Bosnic-Anticevich, S., Briggs, A., Chrystyn, H., . . . Bousquet, J. (2013). Inhaler competence in asthma: Common errors, barriers to use and recommended solutions. *Respiratory Medicine, 107*(1), 37–46.

Kiser, T.H., Sevransky, J.E., Krishnan, J.A., Tonascia, J., Wise, R.A., Checkley, W., . . . for the DECIDE Investigators. (2017). A survey of corticosteroid dosing for exacerbations of chronic obstructive pulmonary disease requiring assisted ventilation. *Chronic Obstructive Pulmonary Diseases: Journal of the COPD Foundation, 4*(3), 186–193. doi: 10.15326/jcopdf.4.3.2016.0168

Kotz, D., Brown, J., & West, R. (2013, December 20). "Real-world" effectiveness of smoking cessation treatments: A population study. *Addiction, 109*(3), 491–499. doi: 10.1111/add.12429

Leuppi, J.D., Schuetz, P., Bingisser, R., Bodmer, M., Briel, M., Drescher, T., . . . Rutishauser, J. (2013). Short-term vs conventional glucocorticoid therapy in acute exacerbations of chronic obstructive pulmonary disease. The REDUCE Randomized Clinical Trial. *JAMA, 309*(21), 2223–2231. doi:10.1001/jama.2013.5023

Ouanes, I., Ouanes-Besbes, L., Abdallah, S.B., Dachraoui, F., & Abroug, F. (2015). Trends in use and impact on outcome of empiric antibiotic therapy and noninvasive ventilation in COPD patients with acute exacerbation. *Annals of Intensive Care, 5*(30). doi: 10.1186/s13613-015-0072-x

Rui, P., & Kang, K. (2014). National Hospital Ambulatory Medical Care Survey: 2014 "Emergency Department Summary Tables". http://www.cdc.gov/nchs/data/ahcd/nhamcs_emergency/2014_ed_web_tables.pdf Accessed 1.15.18

Sadowska, A.M. (2012). N-Acetylcysteine mucolysis in the management of chronic obstructive pulmonary disease. *Therapy Advances in Respiratory Disease, 6*(3), 127–135.

Scow, D.T., Luttermoser, G.K., & Dickerson, K.S. (2007). Leukotriene inhibitors in the treatment of allergy and asthma. *American Family Physician, 75*(1), 65–70.

Shoaib, M., & Buhidma, Y. (2017). Why are antidepressant drugs effective smoking cessation aids? *Current Neuropharmacology.* Advance online publication. doi: 10.2174/1570159X15666170915142122

Siddiqi, A., & Sethi, S. (2008). Optimizing antibiotic selection in treating COPD exacerbations. *International Journal of Chronic Obstructive Pulmonary Disease, 3*(1), 31–44.

Stav, D., & Raz, M. (2009). Effect of *N*-acetylcysteine on air trapping in COPD: A randomized placebo-controlled study. *Chest, 136*(2), 381–386.

Stead, L.F., Perera, R., Bullen, C., Mant, D., Hartmann-Boyce, J., Cahill, K., & Lancaster, T. (2012, November 14). Nicotine replacement therapy for smoking cessation. *Cochrane Database of Systematic Reviews, 11*, CD000146. doi: 10.1002/14651858. CD000146. pub4

Tse, H.N., Raiteri, L., Wong, K.Y., Yee, K.S., Ng, L.Y., Wai, K.Y., . . . Chan, M.H. (2013). High-dose *N*-acetylcysteine in stable COPD: The 1-year, double-blind, randomized, placebo-controlled HIACE study. *Chest, 144*(1), 106–118.

Woods, J.A., Wheeler, J.S., Finch, C.K., & Pinner, N.A. (2014). Corticosteroids in the treatment of acute exacerbations of chronic obstructive pulmonary disease. *International Journal of Chronic Obstructive Pulmonary Disease, 9*, 421–430. doi: 10.2147/COPD.S51012

Yawn, B.P., Colice, G.L., & Hodder, R. (2012). Practical aspects of inhaler use in the management of chronic obstructive pulmonary disease in the primary care setting. *International Journal of Chronic Obstructive Pulmonary Disease, 7*, 495–502.

Zuo, L., He, F., Sergakis, G.G., Koozehchian, M.S., Stimpfl, J.N., Rong, Y., . . . Best, T. M. (2014). Interrelated role of cigarette smoking, oxidative stress, and immune response in COPD and corresponding treatments. *American Journal of Physiology, 307*(3), 205–218.

Zwar, N.A., Mendelsohn, C.P., & Richmond, R. L. (2014). Supporting smoking cessation. *BMJ, 348*, f7535. doi: 10.1136/bmj.f7535 Best Practices

CHAPTER 8

Pharmacology of the Gastrointestinal Tract

Jacqueline Rosenjack Burchum and Hoi Sing Chung

KEY TERMS

5-HT$_3$ receptor antagonists
5-HT$_4$ receptor
Acid reflux disease
Aminosalicylates
Antacids
Antiemetic agents
Antihistamines
Butyrophenones
Cannabinoids
Chloride-channel activators
Cholelithiasis

Cholinergic mimetic agents
Dopamine-receptor
  antagonists
Dyspepsia
Emesis
Eructation
Gallstones
Gastritis
Gastroesophageal reflux
  disease (GERD)
Gastroparesis

Gastroprokinetic drugs
Histamine
Histamine-2 (H$_2$) receptor
  antagonists
Inflammatory bowel disease
  (IBD)
Irritable bowel syndrome
  (IBS)
Laxatives
Melena
Motility

Mucosal-protective agents
Muscarinic M$_3$ antagonists
Neurotonin-1 receptor
  antagonists
Parietal cells
Peptic ulcer disease
Phenothiazines
Proton-pump inhibitors (PPIs)
Serotonin
Serotonin 5-HT receptor
Substituted benzamides

CHAPTER OBJECTIVES

At the end of the chapter, the student will be able to:

1. Identify the major classes of medications used to control common gastrointestinal (GI) conditions or problems.

2. Describe the nurse's role in the pharmacologic and non-pharmacologic management of each GI problem.

3. Explain the mechanism(s) of drug action, primary indications, contraindications, significant drug interactions, and important adverse effects for each drug class described.

4. Use the nursing process to care for patients receiving drug therapy to treat common GI problems.

Introduction

The GI tract is often misconceived as being merely a tube for processing food and eliminating waste. In reality, it has considerably more functions than simply extracting nutrients from food. It has been referred to as "the second brain," and indeed a great many biochemical messages affecting different body systems come from, or are routed through, the enteric nervous system of the digestive tract. The GI tract produces neurotransmitters such as serotonin that affect mood and well-being (Hadhazy, 2010). It is also a key component in the body's immune defenses, being a significant interface with toxic substances, bacteria, fungi, and other potential pathogens. And, of course, the GI tract is responsible for the transfer of nutrients to the body, so that in the presence of GI disorders, a patient may suffer from nutritional deficits. Given these many functions, disease or dysfunction affecting the digestive tract can have a broad range of systemic impacts that should not be taken lightly.

Because the digestive tract is composed of multiple organs and glands (**FIGURE 8-1**), it stands to reason that there is a great variety of functions that can go wrong and cause problems. Treatments for GI disorders run the gamut from short-term approaches—for instance, control of minor gastric acidity, management of nausea and vomiting, or resolution of diarrhea or constipation—to therapy for chronic GI dysfunction, such as poor (or excessive) GI **motility**, **irritable bowel syndrome (IBS)**, **inflammatory bowel disease (IBD)**, and **gallstones**. While every condition known to affect the gut cannot be addressed in this text—drugs that treat GI cancers, for instance, are better discussed in the context of oncology medications, as they are not typical conditions seen in nonspecialist nursing practice—this chapter at least addresses the most common disorders treated with medical therapy: gastric acidity, disorders of GI motility, diarrhea, constipation, IBS, nausea and vomiting, IBD, and gallstones.

An important topic for consideration with the use of any of these drug classes is pregnancy. GI distress is a well-known, common side effect of pregnancy in healthy women, and it usually does not require medical intervention. However, in some women, the GI disturbances of pregnancy are extreme (e.g., hyperemesis gravidarum) and potentially threaten maternal and fetal well-being. While pregnancy-related health issues are not the topic of discussion here, the medications in this chapter are sometimes used to address such concerns. Also, in women with preexisting GI conditions, pregnancy can raise questions about whether the therapies they have been using might affect the fetus. **BOX 8-1** discusses the updated Federal Drug Agency (FDA) pregnancy categories into which all medications—including the major groups of GI-directed medications—are classified so that the potential for fetal toxicity can be considered in the context of both treating

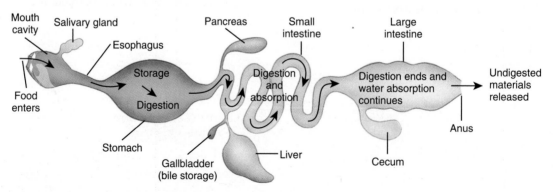

FIGURE 8-1 The gastrointestinal system's functions.

Chiras, D. (2011). *Human biology* (7th ed.). Sudbury, MA: Jones & Bartlett Learning.

BOX 8-1 Pregnancy Safety Categories Related to Pharmacology and the Gastrointestinal Tract

In 2014, the FDA replaced its existing pregnancy letter categories with a new system intended to help consumers make better informed choices and to enhance patient counseling. The previous system assigned entire drug classes to a specific category, as follows:

Category A: Studies indicate no risk to the human fetus.

Category B: Studies indicate no risk to the animal fetus; information for humans is not available.

Category C: Adverse effects reported in the animal fetus; information for humans is not available.

Category D: Possible fetal risk in humans has been reported; however, in selected cases consideration of the potential benefit versus risk may warrant use of these drugs in pregnant women.

Category X: Fetal abnormalities have been reported; and positive evidence of fetal risk in humans is available from animal and/or human studies. These drugs are not to be used in pregnant women.

The new system (effective June 30, 2015) is known simply as the Pregnancy and Lactation Labeling Rule (PLLR). Drug labeling must include a pregnancy risk summary, indicating whether the drug is systemically absorbed, if it is contraindicated in pregnancy, and risk statements based on both animal data and human data.

GI disturbances arising from pregnancy and managing existing GI disturbances during pregnancy.

The Nursing Care Process

For nurses managing patients with GI disorders, there are several key management issues to consider. First and foremost is assessing the patient's well-being; nurses are tasked with identifying any supportive measures that need to be taken and ensuring that the patient has access to them. In a patient who is experiencing mild, temporary discomfort (e.g., nausea related to a viral infection), the measures may be simple: reminding the patient to drink plenty of fluids and get rest, offering appropriate therapy (medical or otherwise) to relieve symptoms, and ensuring that social support and/or a caretaker is available should the patient's symptoms fail to improve quickly. In patients with acute or chronic GI disease, additional measures are required. If the patient is experiencing significant pain, for example, steps should be taken to rule out the possibility of acute conditions requiring surgical intervention, such as bowel obstruction, torsion, or appendicitis.

Even where pain is not present, and the patient's complaints are limited to vague, chronic discomfort ("upset stomach"), nurses should be alert to signs suggesting the complaint may have greater significance. Is the patient losing weight despite eating well? Does he or she notice symptoms are exacerbated by certain foods? If so, the patient may need assessment for a malabsorption disorder, food allergy, or celiac disease. (Most such disorders are treated by dietary changes or nutritional supplementation as appropriate, but medical therapy may also be used to alleviate lingering symptoms until lifestyle and dietary alterations are completed.)

Chronic GI complaints can be fairly burdensome for patients, particularly in older adults, in whom such complaints are relatively common. Dysfunction in the GI tract is often associated with depression, anxiety, and other affective disorders (Foster & McVey Neufeld, 2013). Thus, a second aspect of nursing care is to assess for and manage mental health concerns that arise alongside (or in response to) chronic GI issues. Does the patient seem discouraged about therapy, claiming "It doesn't work," or insisting "It won't work," when a new therapy is proposed? Does the patient appear listless, disinterested, or present a negative affect when talking about his or her GI complaint? If so, then additional measures may be required to support the patient's emotional well-being both in general and in relation to the disease process. It is important to note that the connection between the enteric nervous system and the central nervous system is profound: Stress is a precipitant of GI disease (particularly conditions such as peptic ulcer disease [PUD] and IBS), but the presence of GI disease can precipitate or exacerbate stress as well.

Finally, it is important to recognize that medications that affect the GI tract alter the behavior of a key body system in ways that are not confined to that system. Nearly all classes of GI medications are subject to significant interactions with other drugs, particularly insofar as they alter how both nutrients and other medications may be absorbed. Patient education on the potential interactions between GI medications and other substances, whether prescribed or purchased as over-the-counter (OTC) products, should be comprehensive and targeted.

Drugs to Control Gastric Acidity

Gastric acid has an important role in several physiological processes. It aids in the digestion of proteins and promotes absorption of minerals such as calcium, iron, and vitamin B_{12}. Because gastric acid is lethal to many microorganisms, it also has a role in the prevention of some enteric infections (Vakil, 2017). Unfortunately, gastric acidity can complicate a number of medical conditions. One such condition is **peptic ulcer disease**, in which infection with a microbe, *Helicobacter pylori*, promotes harmful overproduction of gastric acid and lesions on the stomach lining. Treatment of the infection with antibiotics often is not sufficient to resolve the acid levels; indeed, protocols for *H. pylori* eradication require dual antibiotic therapy to prevent resistant organisms from remaining in the gut. If left unchecked, chronic acid reflux—also known as **gastroesophageal reflux disease (GERD)**—can

contribute to remodeling of the esophagus and, potentially, more serious conditions such as esophagitis, chronic obstructive pulmonary disease (COPD), and esophageal cancer (Story, 2018).

When gastric acid creates a problem, several drugs can be used to manage or control gastric acidity. These medications include **antacids, histamine-2 (H_2) receptor antagonists**, and **proton-pump inhibitors (PPIs)**. Additionally, **mucosal-protective agents** serve to prevent the gastric acid from causing damage to the stomach and duodenum. **FIGURE 8-2** presents a schematic model of the physiological control of hydrogen ion secretion and the mechanism of actions by antacids, H_2-receptor antagonists, and PPIs.

Antacids

Antacids are the oldest drugs used to control gastric acidity. Examples of antacids include **sodium bicarbonate**, **calcium carbonate**, and formulations containing **aluminum** and/or **magnesium hydroxide**. Most of these medications are available without a prescription, and they are commonly used by the general public. For the nurse, it is important to ask about use of antacids specifically when doing a workup for a patient with GI complaints, as many patients may omit mention of these medications.

Gastric acid typically has a very low pH, in the range of 1.5 to 3.5. Antacids are weak bases that neutralize gastric acid. When a base reacts chemically with an acid, the result of the reaction is the formation of a salt and water or, in the case of **sodium bicarbonate**, a salt and carbon dioxide. As a result of this reaction, the gastric pH is increased to greater than 3.5.

Because carbon dioxide, a gas, is a product of the reaction of gastric acid and either **sodium bicarbonate** or **calcium carbonate**, **eructation** (belching) may occur when these products are taken. This does not occur with products in which the active ingredient is either **aluminum** or **magnesium hydroxide**.

Aluminum hydroxide can cause constipation. Conversely, **magnesium hydroxide**

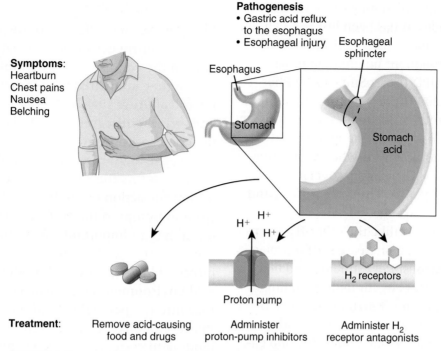

Pathogenesis
- Gastric acid reflux to the esophagus
- Esophageal injury

Symptoms:
Heartburn
Chest pains
Nausea
Belching

Esophagus

Esophageal sphincter

Stomach

Stomach acid

H^+ H^+ H^+

Proton pump

H_2 receptors

Treatment: Remove acid-causing food and drugs   Administer proton-pump inhibitors   Administer H_2 receptor antagonists

FIGURE 8-2 Treatment of gastroesophageal reflux disease (GERD).

can cause osmotic diarrhea due to unabsorbed salts. Usually, these drugs are combined to prevent these problems, but this is not always the case. For example, **magnesium hydroxide** is the active ingredient in a popular OTC medication that is sometimes given to relieve constipation.

Excessive intake of antacids could result in metabolic alkalosis. Because **magnesium** and **aluminum** are excreted by the kidneys, they should be used cautiously in patients who have renal insufficiency. In addition, excessive antacid intake may lead to exacerbation of cardiac or renal disease, as well as fluid electrolyte imbalance. Therefore, baseline values for serum chemistry, including serum ALP, ALT, AST levels, serum creatinine, and blood urea nitrogen (BUN) levels, should be obtained and recorded before antacid treatment is initiated in renally compromised patients.

Drug–Drug Interactions

Antacids can affect the absorption of most drugs by either binding to the drug, or altering the drug's solubility as a result of increasing intragastric pH value. To avoid this interaction, antacids should not be administered within one to two hours of other drugs.

Histamine 2 (H_2) Receptor Antagonists

Histamine binds to H_1, H_2 and H_3 histamine receptors throughout the body. The H_2 subtype is of importance to altering the function of the gastrointestinal tract. The stomach contains specialized cells, called **parietal cells**, that produce gastric acid in response to stimulation by **histamine**, acetylcholine, and gastrin receptors released from the surrounding antral G cells, and enterochromaffin-like (ECL) cells. H_2-receptor antagonists decrease gastric acidity by blocking H_2 receptors, thereby decreasing gastric acid production. Examples of H_2-receptor antagonists (also known as H_2 blockers) include **cimetidine**, **famotidine**, **nizatidine**, and **ranitidine**. All of these medications are sold in OTC as well as prescription formulations.

Because H_2-receptor antagonists decrease gastric acidity, their use may be associated with an increase in bacterial growth

Best Practices

To avoid drug–drug interactions, antacids should not be administered within one to two hours of other drugs.

in the stomach, which may cause GI discomfort. This condition has been linked to an increased risk of bacterial colonization in the lungs and subsequent pneumonia in patients with COPD (GlaxoSmithKline Pharmaceuticals, 2009). Intravenous infusion of H_2-receptor antagonists may cause confusion and other mental status changes; however, these effects do not occur when such drugs are taken orally. Otherwise, adverse effects are rare with **famotidine**, **nizatidine**, and **ranitidine**.

Cimetidine, unlike the other H_2-receptor antagonists, may increase serum prolactin, decrease metabolism of estradiol, and block androgen receptors by inhibiting binding of dihydrotestosterone (Katzung, Masters, & Trevor, 2011). As a result, adverse endocrine effects may occur: Women may develop galactorrhea, while men may develop gynecomastia. This drug may also cause sexual dysfunction.

Pregnant patients considering H_2-receptor antagonists should be counseled according to the PLLR. In older adults, especially those with renal or hepatic dysfunction, intravenous administration of H_2-receptor antagonists may cause mental status changes such as confusion and depression, though the mechanism through which these changes occur remains unclear (Tawadrous et al., 2014).

Drug–Drug Interactions

Cimetidine has a number of significant interactions related to its effect on several cytochrome P450 enzymes. When taken concomitantly with **cimetidine**, certain drugs metabolized by the same P450 pathways may cause toxicity. Examples of drugs that are particularly dangerous when taken concomitantly with **cimetidine** include **warfarin**, **phenytoin**, **theophylline**, and **lidocaine**. If both antacids and H_2-receptor antagonists are prescribed concomitantly, the drugs should be administered one hour apart to prevent the disturbance of absorption caused by antacids.

Best Practices

Use caution in administering PPIs with other drugs that use the CYP 2C19 and CYP 3A4 metabolic pathways.

Proton-Pump Inhibitors

PPIs are the most effective of the drugs used to control gastric acidity, particularly in the context of *H. pylori* infection, where they are paired with targeted antimicrobial drugs such as **clarithromycin** and **amoxicillin** (see BOX 8-2). Examples include **esomeprazole**, **lansoprazole**, **omeprazole**, **pantoprazole**, and **rabeprazole**. As their name implies, PPIs inhibit the action of the H^+, K^+-ATPase (proton pump) in the stomach. This proton pump has an important role in the production of gastric acid, so inhibiting its action directly blocks gastric acid production. In an acid environment PPIs are activated, and diffuse into the parietal cells of the stomach. PPIs accumulate in the secretory canaliculi, binding to cysteine groups on the ATPase, inactivating the proton pumps for one to two days, until new ATPases are made, replacing those that were inactivated. To prevent their degradation in the acidic stomach environment, PPIs are either enteric coated (allowing dissolution in alkaline pH), or combined with sodium bicarbonate (to neutralize stomach pH), allowing PPIs to accumulate at their sites of action *before* being activated.

As with H_2-receptor antagonists, decreased gastric acidity may contribute to an increase in bacterial growth in the stomach. Abdominal discomfort and diarrhea may occur in a percentage of patients. Adverse effects are uncommon when over-the-counter PPIs are taken as recommended; however, when high-dose, prescription-strength PPI therapy is continued for a year or more, atrophic gastritis (AstraZeneca Pharmaceuticals, 2012a, 2012b), osteoporosis-related bone fractures at multiple sites (Wang et al., 2017), and a rare but potentially serious magnesium deficiency (American Academy of Family Physicians, 2011) may occur, although the mechanisms for these effects are unknown.

PPIs were previously classified as pregnancy risk Category B; pregnant patients should be counseled per the PLLR. Older patients with liver impairment may require

BOX 8-2 Primary Treatment of *H. pylori* Infection

Members of the American College of Gastroenterology published the following evidence-based recommendations for clinicians in North America. All patients should first be asked about penicillin allergies and previous macrolide exposure. Based on patient response, the following first-line treatments are recommended.

If no penicillin allergy and no macrolide exposure:

- **Bismuth quadruple**: PPI (standard dose) – BID, bismuth subcitrate (120–300 mg) or subsalicylate (300 mg) – QID, tetracycline 500 mg – QID, metronidazole (250–500 mg) – QID (250mg). Treatment for 10–14 days.
- **Clarithromycin triple**: PPI (standard or double dose) – BID, clarithromycin 500 mg, amoxicillin (1 g). Treatment for 14 days.
- **Concomitant**: PPI (standard dose) – BID, clarithromycin (500 mg), amoxicillin (1 g), nitroimidazole (500 mg). Treatment for 10–14 days.

If no penicillin allergy, but macrolide exposure:

- **Bismuth quadruple**
- **Levofloxacin triple**: PPI (standard dose) – BID, levofloxacin (500 mg) – QD, Amox (1 g) – BID. Treatment for 10–14 days.
- **Levofloxacin sequential**: PPI (standard or double dose) + Amox (1 g) – BID. Treatment for 5–7 days. Followed by PPI, Amox, levofloxacin (500 mg QD), nitroimidazole (500 mg) – BID. Treatment for 5–7 days.

If penicillin allergy, but no macrolide exposure:

- **Clarithromycin triple** (substitute metronidazole 500 mg – TID for amoxicillin)
- **Bismuth quadruple**

If penicillin allergy, and macrolide exposure:

- **Bismuth quadruple**

Data from Chey, W. D., Leontiadis, G. I., Howden, C. W., & Moss, S. F. (2017). Treatment of Helicobacter pylori infection. *Am J Gastroenterol.* 112: 212–238; doi:10.1038/ajg.2016.563; published online 10 January 2017.

lower doses of these drugs due to the patients' impaired metabolic function and the drugs' prolonged half-life.

Drug–Drug Interactions

PPIs may decrease the bioavailability of drugs that require a low pH for optimal absorption. These drugs include certain antifungal drugs such as ketoconazole, and antiviral drugs such as atazanavir (Katzung et al., 2011). PPIs are extensively metabolized via two cytochrome P450 pathways, CYP 2C19 and CYP 3A4; therefore, giving a PPI along with other drugs metabolized via these pathways may affect drug metabolism. For example, patients taking warfarin and omeprazole or esomeprazole may have an increased risk of bleeding (though not with pantoprazole, as it is not a blanket drug–drug interaction) (AstraZeneca Pharmaceuticals, 2016a, 2016b; Takeda Pharmaceuticals, 2012).

Mucosal Protectants

Mucosal-protective agents do not affect gastric acid secretion; however, they play an important role in managing ulcers and similar problems caused or worsened by gastric acid. Examples include sucralfate, a local agent; bismuth subsalicylate, a bismuth compound with mucosal-protective properties; and misoprostol, a prostaglandin analog. Mucosal protectants shield the gastric mucosa from harmful effects of gastric acid via a variety of mechanisms (Wallace, 2008).

Sucralfate is an agent with limited solubility that becomes thick and sticky in acid solutions to create a protective layer on the surface of gastric mucosa. Less than 3% of the intact drug is absorbed from the intestinal tract. In the stomach, this medication is believed to utilize negative charges

Best Practices

Bismuth subsalicylate should not be given to children, especially following vaccinations for influenza and varicella, because salicylate is implicated as a causative agent of Reye syndrome.

to adhere to gastric erosions (which contain positively charged proteins) to protect gastric mucosa from further damage and promote healing (Arora Bisen & Budhiraja, 2012).

Bismuth subsalicylate coats stomach lesions, protecting them from the erosive effects of gastric secretions. This agent also has the ability to bind to microbes, providing additional protectant effects. However, the precise mechanisms by which **sucralfate** and **bismuth subsalicylate** exert their protective effects are not clear.

In contrast, **misoprostol** protects the gastric mucosa by activating prostaglandin E_1 receptors on gastric parietal cells; its protective effects are mainly due to its inhibition of gastric acid secretion via G-protein–coupled receptor-mediated inhibition of adenylate cyclase, which decreases intracellular cyclic adenosine monophosphate and proton pump activity. **Misoprostol** is typically administered with nonsteroidal anti-inflammatory drugs (NSAIDs) to prevent GI erosions due to decreased prostaglandin synthesis caused by NSAIDs.

Both **sucralfate** and **bismuth subsalicylate** have few adverse effects when taken as recommended. **Bismuth subsalicylate** commonly causes dark brown–black stools that may be mistaken for the **melena** that occurs with GI bleeding. Prolonged or excessive use of **bismuth subsalicylate** can cause constipation and may result in salicylate toxicity. The most common adverse effect of **misoprostol** is abdominal discomfort, which may occur with or without diarrhea. Other GI side effects such as nausea and vomiting, flatulence, and dyspepsia occur, but have been reported in fewer than 3% of those patients taking the drug. **Bismuth subsalicylate** should not be given to children under three, especially following vaccinations for influenza and varicella, because **salicylate** has been implicated as a causative agent of Reye syndrome. Previously, **sucralfate** was classified as pregnancy risk Category B, **bismuth subsalicylate** in pregnancy risk Category C, and **misoprostol**

in pregnancy risk Category X. Due to their varied effects, patient counseling per the PLLR is important to enhance patient education.

Drug–Drug Interactions

Sucralfate should not be given with other drugs because it may bind to them and prevent their absorption. There are no significant drug interactions with **misoprostol**.

Bismuth subsalicylate interacts with a number of drugs due to its weak acidity; patients should be advised of this potential and cautioned not to use this agent with certain medications. Notably, **bismuth subsalicylate** reacts chemically with both tetracyclines and quinolone antibiotics, resulting in decreased antibiotic absorption. It may increase the hypoglycemic effects of insulin and other drugs given for diabetes through unknown mechanisms. It may also increase the bleeding risk in patients taking **warfarin** by synergistic actions on platelet aggregation. Conversely, it may decrease the antigout effectiveness of **probenecid** and **sulfinpyrazone**. The use of **bismuth subsalicylate** is best avoided if the patient is taking other salicylates, such as **aspirin**.

Drugs to Stimulate Gastrointestinal Motility

The class of drugs used for stimulating motility is also called **gastroprokinetic drugs**. These medications act by increasing the frequency of contractions in the small intestine without disrupting their rhythm, ultimately resulting in enhanced GI motility. Such agents have been commonly used to treat a number of GI disorders, such as IBS, **acid reflux disease**, **gastroparesis**, **gastritis**, and functional **dyspepsia**. Therefore, related GI symptoms, including abdominal discomfort, bloating, constipation, heartburn, nausea, and vomiting, may be relieved by these drugs. Drugs commonly used to stimulate GI motility include cholinergic mimetic agents and dopamine (D_2) receptor antagonists (Gumaste & Baum, 2008), although researchers continue to look for additional agents (Auteri, Zizzo, & Serio, 2015; Kusano et al., 2014).

Cholinergic Mimetic Agents

Cholinergic mimetic agents (muscarinic receptor agonists, Table 5-2) have been commonly used for stimulating GI motility, accelerating gastric emptying, and improving gastroduodenal coordination. Examples of these agents include bethanechol. Such medications work by stimulating muscarinic receptors similarly to acetylcholine, only with prolonged duration of action, due to their resistance to acetylcholinesterase. Increased muscarinic receptor stimulation increases GI peristalsis, which further increases pressure on the lower esophageal sphincter, resulting in enhanced GI motility (Gumaste & Baum, 2008).

There are two different ways to increase cholinergic effects. The first approach is to agonize ("stimulate") the M_1 receptor, mimicking acetylcholine effects. The second approach is to inhibit the enzyme acetylcholinesterase, which normally metabolizes acetylcholine, and other cholinergics, including drugs; by doing so, less acetylcholine is broken down, so more is available. In addition, cholinergic mimetic drugs may stimulate muscarinic M_3 receptors on muscle cells and at myenteric plexus synapses; M_3 stimulation causes generalized vasodilation, which may lead to some of the drugs' side effects.

Cholinergic mimetic drugs are associated with a variety of side effects, including abdominal discomfort, diarrhea, hypotension and reflex tachycardia, lacrimation, miosis, salivation, and urinary urgency. Due to the multiple cholinergic effects mentioned previously, and the development of less toxic agents, bethanechol is now seldom used.

As a part of nursing concerns, cholinergic mimetic drugs should never be administered by intramuscular or intravenous injection: The fast absorption from these routes may lead to heart block or severe hypotension, due to the anticholinergic effects of the drug in the wrong location. In addition, these drugs should not be used if there is any mechanical obstruction in the gastric or urinary tracts due to their effects of increasing GI peristalsis (Gumaste & Baum, 2008).

Dopamine (D_2) Receptor Blockers

Blocking the dopamine D_2 receptor has many effects (see, in part, TABLE 5-2), including suppression of acetylcholine from myenteric motor neurons. Dopamine normally blocks acetylcholine release, negatively affecting gastrointestinal motility. By blocking the inhibitory effects of dopamine, D_2 blockers stimulate gastrointestinal motility. Although dopamine D_2-receptor blockers are most often used as antidiarrheal drugs (and will be discussed further in that section), some of these drugs are also used to stimulate GI motility. The utility of this type of drug derives from the fact that it can stimulate the GI tract without increasing gastric secretions. A good example of a dopamine D_2-receptor blocker that is prescribed for this purpose is metoclopramide.

The most common adverse effects caused by dopaminergic D_2-receptor blockers involve the central nervous system. Side effects such as Parkinson-like symptoms, tardive dyskinesia, and acute dystonia, as well as drowsiness and confusion, may occur especially in the elderly and those treated for a prolonged period. Elevated prolactin levels caused by dopamine D_2-receptor blockers can cause galactorrhea, gynecomastia, impotence, and menstrual disorders (Gumaste & Baum, 2008).

Drug–Drug Interactions

For dopaminergic D_2-receptor blockers, drug–drug interactions have been well documented with alcohol, tranquilizers, sleep medications,

Best Practices

Bismuth subsalicylate interacts with a number of drugs; patients should be advised not to use this agent with certain medications.

Best Practices

Cholinergic mimetic drugs should never be administered by intramuscular or intravenous injection: The fast absorption from these routes may lead to heart block or severe hypotension.

and narcotics. The possible mechanisms involved in these interactions are mainly due to the drugs' inhibitory effects on the central nervous system. In addition, caution is needed when administering dopaminergic D_2-receptor blockers in hypertensive patients (Hasler, 2011).

Drugs to Control Diarrhea

Diarrhea is an abnormal increase in the frequency and fluidity of bowel movements. It may be not only a type of body defense, but also a nonspecific symptom of an underlying condition or disease. The common etiologies of diarrhea include viral and bacterial infection, adverse effects of medications, GI tract inflammatory diseases, certain food allergies, and malabsorption. Therefore, the symptoms of diarrhea should be treated only after the etiologic conditions or diseases have been identified. The most commonly prescribed antidiarrheal agents include opioid agonists, bismuth compounds, and **octreotide**.

Opioid Agonists

Opioid agonists are the most effective—and most commonly prescribed—medications for the symptomatic treatment of diarrhea. As monotherapy, they are represented by **loperamide**. In addition, opioid agonists are formulated in combinations with anticholinergic drugs such as **atropine**. Examples include **diphenoxylate plus atropine** and **difenoxin plus atropine** (Kent & Banks, 2010).

Loperamide, as a nonprescription opioid agonist, does not cross the blood–brain barrier and has no analgesic properties or potential for addiction, whereas **diphenoxylate** is a prescribed opioid agonist and has analgesic properties, albeit only at nonstandard higher doses. **Loperamide** and **diphenoxylate** can act directly on the intestine to slow peristalsis dramatically and allow more fluid and electrolyte absorption in the colon. In addition, the anticholinergic properties of **atropine** in commercial preparations may contribute to the antidiarrheal action.

Opioids generally cause central nervous system depression, so they are suggested only for short-term therapy of diarrhea, due to the potential for adverse effects and dependence, especially with **diphenoxylate**. In addition, large amounts of **loperamide** may cause dry mouth, abdominal pain, tachycardia, and blurred vision, which are **atropinic** effects. All opioid agonists for the treatment of diarrhea must be taken with adequate fluid to prevent potential constipation. Opioids have a variety of adverse effects that are described in detail elsewhere. If diarrhea continues, or other symptoms such as fever, abdominal pain, or bloody stool occur, patients should be instructed to contact the prescriber quickly. Dehydration and electrolyte imbalance are more commonly encountered with use of these drugs in elderly patients (Kent & Banks, 2010).

Drug–Drug Interactions

When concurrently used with other central nervous system depressants and/or alcohol, opioid agonists can cause additive sedation. Hypertensive crisis may occur when these medications are taken in combination with monoamine oxidase inhibitors (MAOIs) due to the fact that both MAOIs and opioids increase synaptic 5-hydroxytryptamine (5-HT), which can prove toxic (Stahl & Felker, 2008). Before administration of antidiarrheal opioid agonists, it is important to rule out infectious diarrhea, including *Clostridium difficile* infection.

Bismuth Compounds

In addition to the protective use on gastric mucosal erosions discussed previously, bismuth compounds are approved as OTC drugs for diarrhea. The prototype of this class is **bismuth subsalicylate**. Although its precise mechanism of antidiarrheal drug action is unclear, **bismuth subsalicylate** can act directly by binding and adsorbing toxins and inhibiting intestinal prostaglandin and chloride secretion. These effects then contribute to reduction of diarrheal symptoms.

The earlier gastric mucosal-protective agents section discussed the adverse effects associated with bismuth compounds.

Octreotide

Octreotide can prevent diarrhea through the following mechanisms: (1) by preventing the secretion of numerous hormones and transmitters, including gastrin, serotonin, and other active peptides that promote diarrhea; (2) by directly inhibiting intestinal and pancreatic secretion and enhancing absorption; and (3) by slowing GI motility. As a drug chemically related to endogenous somatostatin, octreotide is approved to treat severe diarrhea in a wide variety of conditions and diseases, including cancers, vagotomy, dumping syndrome, short bowel syndrome, and AIDS.

The most frequent adverse effects with octreotide are GI related, such as nausea, abdominal pain, flatulence, and diarrhea. Impaired pancreatic secretion may cause steatorrhea, leading to fat-soluble vitamin deficiency. In addition, long-term use of octreotide can cause acute cholecystitis (gallstones), hyperglycemia, hypothyroidism, and bradycardia.

Drugs to Relieve Constipation

Constipation is an abnormal decrease in the frequency of bowel movements. However, the normal frequency of bowel movements varies from two to three per day to as few as one per week. Constipation can be one of the manifestations of a variety of underlying conditions or diseases, including different aspects of dietary and lifestyle causes, GI disorders, neurogenic disorders, metabolic disorders, and pregnancy, as well as adverse effects of some medications. Drugs to control constipation are classified as laxatives, of which subcategories include bulk-forming laxatives, stimulant laxatives, stool softeners/surfactants, osmotic laxatives, and miscellaneous laxatives (Singh & Rao, 2010).

Many of these medications are ineffective if fluid intake is not concomitantly increased.

Overuse of laxatives has the potential for electrolyte imbalance (Roerig, Steffen, Mitchell, & Zunker, 2010) and paradoxically to cause fecal impaction, particularly in elderly patients (Obokhare, 2012). Thus, for patients complaining of constipation, a detailed history of laxative use must be elicited before prescribing additional therapy, and those patients with acute complaints of pain should be assessed for impaction. Even where laxative therapy is appropriate, emphasis should be placed on the need for adequate fiber and fluid intake.

Obtaining from the patient a description of how the stool presents may prove challenging. There is no way around it: People are embarrassed to talk about their feces. Use of the Bristol Stool Chart (FIGURE 8-3) may be useful in obtaining information about the condition of the patient's bowel movement.

Bulk-Forming Laxatives

Bulk-forming laxatives are indigestible, hydrophilic colloids used to increase the frequency and quality of bowel movements. Examples of bulk-forming laxatives include calcium polycarbophil and psyllium mucilloid. These medications work by absorbing water to form a bulky emollient gel that distends the colon and promotes peristalsis. Bulk-forming laxatives are the safest class of laxatives, and are often used to treat chronic constipation with few adverse effects. They generally produce less abdominal cramping but may lead to more bloating and flatulence than other laxatives. As a part of nursing assessment, a basic abdominal and bowel pattern should be elicited, and the relevant history should always be taken. Bulk-forming laxatives should be administered orally after the powder form has been completely dissolved into 8 ounces of liquid.

Drug–Drug Interactions

Bulk-forming laxatives may decrease the absorption of warfarin, digoxin, nitrofurantoin, antibiotics, and salicylates.

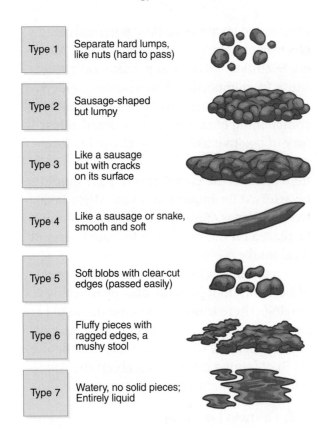

Type 1	Separate hard lumps, like nuts (hard to pass)	
Type 2	Sausage-shaped but lumpy	
Type 3	Like a sausage but with cracks on its surface	
Type 4	Like a sausage or snake, smooth and soft	
Type 5	Soft blobs with clear-cut edges (passed easily)	
Type 6	Fluffy pieces with ragged edges, a mushy stool	
Type 7	Watery, no solid pieces; Entirely liquid	

FIGURE 8-3 The Bristol Stool Chart.

Story, L. (2018). *Pathophysiology: A practical approach* (2nd ed.). Burlington, MA: Jones & Bartlett Learning.

Stimulant Laxatives

Stimulant laxatives induce bowel movement by irritating the GI tract. These agents are often used as "bowel prep" prior to bowel procedures, examinations, or surgeries. They should not be used routinely because they may cause laxative dependence. The commonly administered stimulant laxatives include **bisacodyl** and **castor oil**. Previously, **bisacodyl** was classified as pregnancy Category C, whereas **castor oil** was classified as pregnancy Category X. Under the new PLLR, patients should be informed of the risks and benefits of castor oil and would be counseled not to use it during pregnancy. The risks and benefits of **bisacodyl** should be explained to pregnant patients.

Stimulant laxatives can activate bowel movement by irritating the mucosa and enteric nervous system in the colon and altering intestinal electrolyte and fluid absorption. However, their precise mechanism of action remains poorly understood. Stimulant laxatives may cause more abdominal cramping and depletion of fluid and electrolytes, which bulk-forming laxatives do not. There has been concern about long-term use of stimulant laxatives leading to dependence and destruction of the myenteric plexus. More recent research suggests that long-term use probably is safe in most patients.

Drug–Drug Interactions

Milk or other dairy products should not be given with **bisacodyl**, as these products can dissolve the enteric coating and cause dyspepsia. In addition, **bisacodyl** should not be taken within an hour of ingesting antacids or milk; rather, it should be taken on an empty stomach for faster action and to avoid decreased absorption of other drugs.

Stool Softeners/Surfactants

Stool softeners/surfactants can soften stool materials by absorbing water and lipids. These agents are most often used to prevent constipation in high-risk populations, including patients who have recently experienced surgery, traumatic injury, or myocardial infarction (MI). The commonly used stool softener/surfactant is **docusate**. It is recommended that these agents be taken with six to eight ounces of fluid to aid in stool softening.

The most common adverse effects of stool softeners/surfactants are abdominal cramping and diarrhea. However, these are usually mild. **Docusate** was previously classified as pregnancy Category C; pregnant patients should be counseled of the risks and benefits per the PLLR. **Docusate** and other stool softeners should be used cautiously in the elderly, as these medications can produce nutritional deficits when used on a long-term basis; older adults may already be prone to such deficiencies.

Drug–Drug Interactions

Docusate should not be used in sodium-restricted patients. It should not be given concurrently with mineral oil, because this combination increases the systemic absorption of **docusate**. Long-term use may impair absorption of the fat-soluble vitamins A, D,

E, and K, because docusate will decrease the digestive tract's physical contact time with those vitamins.

Osmotic Laxatives

Osmotic laxatives can promote bowel movement in a rapid and highly effective manner. These do so by attracting water and creating more fluid stools. In other words, osmotic laxatives exert their therapeutic effects by causing a concentration gradient. They are often used for colonoscopy preparation and for purging toxins from the body. Commonly used osmotic laxatives include magnesium hydroxide, polyethylene glycol, and sodium biphosphate. Magnesium hydroxide possesses very potent activity and should be used only in certain situations, such as fecal impaction where bowel obstruction has been ruled out (Obokhare, 2012). If the patient's bowel is obstructed, *all* of these medications are contraindicated.

The most common adverse effects of osmotic laxatives are abdominal cramping and diarrhea. Osmotic laxatives should be used with caution or avoided in elderly patients due to the potential for dehydration and electrolyte imbalance. Hypermagnesemia is a concern when magnesium hydroxide is taken by patients with renal impairment due to decreased ability for magnesium elimination. Therefore, baseline electrolyte levels are important to assess and monitor.

Drug–Drug Interactions

Magnesium hydroxide may decrease the absorption of the following medications: histamine H_2-receptor antagonists, iron salts, phenytoin, digoxin, and tetracyclines.

Drugs to Treat Irritable Bowel Syndrome

IBS is one of the most common functional GI disorders, characterized by unexplained abdominal pain, discomfort, and bloating in association with altered bowel habits. The pathophysiology of IBS is still not well understood but is most likely multifactorial. For example, motor and sensory dysfunction, neuroimmune mechanisms, psychological factors (specifically, the brain–gut axis), a possible genetic component (Makker, Chilimuri, & Bella, 2015), and changes in the intraluminal milieu all may play a role in the development of this disorder (Bajor, Tornblom, Rudling, Ung, & Simren, 2014; Grundman & Yoon, 2010; Pimentel, Cash, Lembo, & Schoenfeld, 2012). To manage symptoms of IBS, medication may be prescribed along with lifestyle changes to eliminate the most troublesome symptoms such as diarrhea, constipation, or abdominal (moderate to severe) pain and to improve bowel function. Although antidiarrheal agents and laxatives have been introduced in detail in the preceding sections, three categories of medications will be added specifically for this section: anticholinergics, serotonin 5-HT receptor antagonists or agonists, and chloride-channel activators (Camilleri, 2010; De Ponti, 2013). However, no single medication has been found to be completely effective in relieving IBS over the long term.

Anticholinergics

Nonspecific or specific antimuscarinic anticholinergic agents have been used to reduce bowel motility and prevent painful cramping spasms in the intestines. Two commonly used antimuscarinics include dicyclomine, a muscarinic M_1 receptor blocker, and hyoscyamine, a nonspecific muscarinic receptor antagonist. More recently, newer selective muscarinic M_3 antagonists (which affect gastrointestinal smooth muscle contraction; see TABLE 5-2) have been developed to decrease the nonspecific anticholinergic adverse effects seen with the antimuscarinics. Such medications have shown promising results in clinical trials (Katzung et al., 2011).

Anticholinergics may exert their effect of relieving painful cramping spasms by binding to muscarinic receptors in the GI mucosa, which results in relaxation of intestinal spasms (Camilleri, 2010). They are often considered "smooth muscle relaxant drugs," although their efficacy has not been convincingly demonstrated. In addition, anticholinergics may inhibit intestinal gland secretion, thereby helping prevent severe diarrhea.

Of course, these medications can also exhibit significant undesired anticholinergic effects, such as visual disturbance, dry mouth, urinary retention, and constipation–especially those that are nonspecific muscarinic blockers. Given this side-effect profile, anticholinergics are rarely used to treat IBS, although they are recommended for some patients; efficacy may be related to ethnical differences in lifestyle, eating habits, genetics, and gut microbiota (Fukudo et al., 2015).

Serotonin 5-HT Receptor Agonists and Antagonists

Serotonin, also known as 5-hydroxytryptamine, or 5-HT, is an important neurotransmitter of the GI tract. There are at least seven known serotonin receptor subtypes, with subdivisions within some of the subtypes. The serotonin receptors involved in those GI functions consist of serotonin 5-HT_3, 5-HT_4, and 5-HT_7 receptors. 5-HT_3 receptors in the GI mediate by both central and peripheral inhibition of serotonin activity, and some, colonic transit, via vagal action in the gut and regions of the CNS where emesis is regulated. 5-HT_4 receptors are located in enteric cholinergic neurons, and are thought to help regulate (positively) peristalsis. 5-HT_7 receptors play a role in smooth muscle relaxation peripherally, and in the GI tract. **Alosetron** was the first **5-HT_3 receptor antagonist** to be approved for the treatment of women with severe IBS with predominant diarrhea who have failed to respond to conventional therapy (De Ponti, 2013). **Ondansetron** has shown efficacy in relieving loose stools, frequency, and urgency in IBS with predominant diarrhea (Garsed et al., 2013; Zheng et al., 2017), while the efficacies of three other 5-HT_3 antagonists (**graisetron**, **dolasetron**, and **palonosetron**) have not been determined in the treatment of IBS. In contrast, a partial

agonist of the **5-HT_4 receptor**, **tegaserod**, a GI motility stimulant, was approved in 2002 but later voluntarily removed from the market in 2007 due to an increased number of cardiovascular deaths. It was subsequently reintroduced only for emergency situations, and only for women younger than 55 years of age. The FDA retains the right to deny authorization for use of **tegaserod**, even in life-threatening situations, if the evidence does not support that **tegaserod**, would be effective for its intended use or if its use would put patients at additional risk (FDA, 2016b).

Alosetron is a highly potent and selective 5-HT_3 *antagonist*, whereas **tegaserod** is a serotonin 5-HT_4 receptor *partial agonist*. **Alosetron** has a much longer duration of effect, which may be due to its high affinity for and slow dissociation from 5-HT_3 receptors (Katzung et al., 2011).

The most frequently seen adverse effect of **alosetron** is constipation, which has been reported in 20% to 30% of patients. Rare episodes of ischemic colitis (approximately 3 per 1,000 patients), including some fatal cases, have occurred; hence **alosetron** is strictly restricted to women with diarrhea-predominant IBS who have not responded to conventional therapies and who have been educated about the risks and benefits (Grundman & Yoon, 2010; United States Food and Drug Administration [FDA], 2016a). More seriously, a list of severe adverse effects—including angina, heart attacks, and stroke—has been associated with the use of **tegaserod**, leading to its removal from the market except in emergency situations.

As part of the nursing process, additional assessment and evaluation of any cardiac disease and adverse effects of **alosetron** and **tegaserod** are very important to ensure patient safety. For instance, patient complaints of chest pain and lightheadedness should be aggressively investigated. In addition, more frequent vital signs and neurologic assessment may be advisable. Because both **alosetron** and **tegaserod** are subject to use under strict guidelines, patients must take these drugs exactly as prescribed and for a maximum duration of only four to six weeks. Patients are encouraged to keep a daily journal to confirm the effectiveness of therapy. Although there are no data showing specific concerns regarding **alosetron** administration in pregnant women, **tegaserod** was previously categorized as a pregnancy Category B drug (Grundman & Yoon, 2010). Understanding the risks and benefits of taking these drugs will be important to counseling pregnant women.

Drug–Drug Interactions

Significant drug interactions have not been observed clinically with serotonin 5-HT receptor agonists and antagonists, even though **alosetron** is metabolized by a number of CYP enzymes (Grundman & Yoon, 2010). However, both **alosetron** and **tegaserod** should be administered strictly as ordered and taken on an empty stomach before a meal to prevent drug–food interactions.

Chloride-Channel Activators

The type 2 volume-regulated chloride channel has been found in gastric parietal cells as well as in small intestinal and colonic epithelia. Intestinal chloride secretion is critical for intestinal fluid and electrolyte transport. **Lubiprostone** is a type 2 chloride-channel activator that has been approved by the FDA. It was introduced for the treatment of women with IBS who experience constipation as their predominant symptom (De Ponti, 2013).

Lubiprostone is a prostanoic acid derivative from a metabolite of prostaglandin E_1. It activates selective type 2 volume-regulated chloride channels, thereby decreasing small bowel and colon transit times and increasing secretion of fluid and electrolytes. Several clinical trials have demonstrated this agent's positive effects on improved spontaneous bowel movement, quality–of-life measures, stool consistency, frequency, and straining (Camilleri, 2010; Wilson & Schey, 2015).

Adverse effects of **lubiprostone** include diarrhea and nausea, which are usually mild, transient, and not associated with alteration of gastric function (Mayer, 2008).

Clinical trials have shown it to be free of serious adverse effects (Wilson & Schey, 2015). However, **lubiprostone** should not be used for any known or suspected bowel obstruction. After a healthy mother gave birth to a bilateral clubfoot infant following the drug trial (Lembo et al., 2011), **lubiprostone** was listed as Category C for pregnancy under the prior FDA guidelines. Appropriate counseling is required under PLLR and its use should be avoided in women of childbearing age (Katzung et al., 2011).

Drug–Drug Interactions

There have been no drug–drug interactions found with **lubiprostone** to date.

Drugs to Control Nausea and Vomiting

Nausea and vomiting are manifestations of a wide variety of medical conditions, including diverse diseases, systemic and GI infections, pregnancy, motion sickness, adverse effects of medications, radiotherapy, and procedures such as anesthesia and surgery (Andrews & Horn, 2006). Nausea and vomiting occur when the vomiting center in the medulla is stimulated by sensory signal input received from the digestive tract, the inner ear, or the chemoreceptor trigger zone (CTZ) located in the area postrema (Feyer & Jordan, 2011). When large amounts of fluids are vomited, dehydration, electrolyte imbalance, and acid–base imbalance may occur. Severe loss of fluid and electrolytes may cause vascular collapse and death in pediatric patients.

At least six different classes of **antiemetic agents** are available to prevent and treat nausea and vomiting, including 5-HT_3 receptor antagonists, corticosteroids, **neurotonin-1 receptor antagonists**, **dopamine-receptor antagonists**, **antihistamines/anticholinergics**, and **cannabinoids** (Adams & Urban, 2012; Feyer & Jordan, 2011; Katzung et al., 2011). In addition, combinations of antiemetic regimens have been the standard of care for the control of severe chemotherapy-induced nausea and vomiting.

5-HT₃ Receptor Antagonists

Antagonists that inhibit the actions of serotonin have been widely used for the management of chemotherapy- and radiotherapy-induced nausea and vomiting over the past decades. Examples of 5-HT$_3$ receptor antagonists include **ondansetron**, **granisetron**, **dolasetron**, and **palonosetron**.

Exposure to cytotoxic drugs or radiation may cause release of serotonin (5-HT) from enterochromaffin cells in the GI mucosa, which in turn stimulates 5-HT$_3$ receptors located on sensory nerve terminals peripherally (Sanger & Andrews, 2006). This process may initiate **emesis** (vomiting) or sensitize the sensory nervous system to promote emesis. Selective 5-HT$_3$ receptor antagonists elicit antiemetic actions through their selective antagonism at the peripheral 5-HT$_3$ receptors (Sanger & Andrews, 2006).

In general, 5-HT$_3$ antagonists are well tolerated and exhibit few side effects. Those side effects that are observed include mild headache, dizziness, constipation, and diarrhea, as well as transient elevations of hepatic aminotransferase levels (Geling & Eichler, 2005).

Drug–Drug Interactions

No significant drug–drug interactions have been observed with 5-HT$_3$ receptor antagonists, although all four agents undergo some metabolism by CYP 450 (Katzung et al., 2011).

Corticosteroids

Corticosteroids have shown impressive efficacy in treating chemotherapy-induced and postoperative nausea and vomiting. Furthermore, corticosteroids, in combination with other antiemetics, especially 5-HT$_3$ and neurokinin-1 (NK$_1$) receptor antagonists, are widely used to prevent and treat nausea and vomiting. NK$_1$ receptors are found in both the central and peripheral nervous systems, and are understood to participate in pain signals and smooth muscle contraction. NK$_1$ receptors, binding substance P, appear to be involved in delayed emesis after chemotherapy, via vasodilation and gut contractility (see the following discussion). Examples of corticosteroids used for these purposes include **dexamethasone** and **methylprednisolone.**

The general antiemetic mechanisms of corticosteroids are unclear. However, these agents' well-known effects on eicosanoid metabolism, inflammation, and edema are likely part of the explanation.

Corticosteroids used systemically have a variety of significant side effects. Long-term corticosteroid therapy carries with it a significant risk for type 2 diabetes, as well as hypertension, osteoporosis, hyperadrenalism or hypoadrenalism, and a variety of other conditions that are serious—even potentially life threatening. In patients who are already insulin resistant or diabetic, even short-term therapy with corticosteroids should be avoided because of concerns that the drugs will aggravate hyperglycemia. Due to these concerns regarding their potential adverse effects, corticosteroids are usually reserved for acute antiemetic therapy in patients for whom the benefits significantly outweigh the risks—generally, patients who experience chemotherapy-induced nausea and vomiting (CINV). For such patients, corticosteroids are highly effective (Van Ryckeghem, 2016). A study of patients taking **dexamethasone** for the prevention of delayed emesis induced by chemotherapy revealed adverse events including insomnia, indigestion/epigastric discomfort, agitation, increased appetite, weight gain, and acne (Grunberg, 2007).

Neurokinin-1 (NK₁) Receptor Antagonists

A new class of antiemetic agents, Neurokinin-1 (NK$_1$) receptor antagonists, is now available. An example is **aprepitant**, which was approved in 2003 for use in conjunction with **dexamethasone** and/or **ondansetron** for the treatment of acute and delayed emesis induced by chemotherapy. Several other investigational NK$_1$-receptor antagonists have shown clinical promise, and currently **aprepitant**, **netupitant**, and **rolapitant** are available in the United States.

During the past two decades, multiple studies have shown that substance P is a neuropeptide that acts as a neurotransmitter or neuromodulator, by preferentially binding to the NK_1 receptor involved in the emesis reflex. Neurokinin-1 receptor antagonists exert their antiemetic action through the inhibition of substance P involved in the emesis reflex both centrally and peripherally.

The most common adverse events with these drugs include fatigue, headache, anorexia, diarrhea, hiccups, and mild transaminase elevation. Very interestingly, the incidence of adverse effects reported with the three-drug combination of aprepitant, dexamethasone, and ondansetron is similar to that observed with dexamethasone and ondansetron alone. There are no reports on use of aprepitant, netupitant, and rolapitant in pregnant patients; however, administration of these drug in pregnant patients should be avoided unless other medications prove ineffective (Rapoport & Smit, 2017).

Drug–Drug Interactions

Aprepitant has been shown to induce CYP 3A4 and CYP 2C9. As dexamethasone is a substrate of CYP 3A4, aprepitant and dexamethasone often interact. In recognition of this fact, dexamethasone doses should be reduced by about 50% when it is used in combination with aprepitant. In addition, clinicians should be aware of the potential for interactions of aprepitant with warfarin, phenytoin, itraconazole, terfenadine, and oral contraceptives due to the synergistic effects on the same CYP 450 subtype systems.

Dopamine-Receptor Antagonists

Dopamine- (D_2-) receptor antagonists were traditionally used for antiemetic therapy before the introduction of $5\text{-}HT_3$ receptor antagonists. They can be categorized as phenothiazines, butyrophenones, and substituted benzamides. Among these three classes of agents, phenothiazines and butyrophenones are also useful

as antipsychotic agents (Chapter 14). The phenothiazines that are most commonly used as antiemetics are promethazine, prochlorperazine, and thiethylperazine, whereas droperidol is the main butyrophenone used for its antiemetic properties. In addition, the major substituted benzamides include metoclopramide and trimethobenzamide.

The antiemetic properties of these dopamine-receptor antagonists are mediated through the inhibition of dopamine and muscarinic receptors. It has been suggested the selectivity of the established D_2-receptor antagonists is responsible for their effectiveness as antiemetic medications.

The principal adverse effects of these central dopamine antagonists are sedation and extrapyramidal symptoms (EPS), including restlessness, dystonias, and Parkinsonian symptoms with long-term use. In addition, hypotension and prolonged QT interval may occur with droperidol. In general, phenothiazines including promethazine, prochlorperazine, and thiethylperazine were previously listed as Category C in terms of their pregnancy risk, whereas metoclopramide is relatively safe for pregnant patients (Lee & Saha, 2011).

Drug–Drug Interactions

Phenothiazines have a synergistic effect on certain antimicrobial drugs, including streptomycin, erythromycin, oleandomycin, spectinomycin, levofloxacin, azithromycin, and amoxicillin–clavulanic acid (Chan, Ong, & Chua, 2007). Metoclopramide is contraindicated in patients taking antipsychotics, and its label carries a black-box warning about the likelihood of tardive dyskinesia with long-term use—a risk that has decreased its use in clinical practice (Ehrenpreis et al., 2013).

Antihistamines and Anticholinergics

Although the H_1 antihistamines and anticholinergics are used more extensively to treat other diseases, these drugs possess weak antiemetic activity, which can be particularly useful for the treatment and prevention of motion sickness. The most commonly used anticholinergic drug for motion sickness is **scopolamine**, administered as a transdermal patch. In addition, H_1 antihistamines including **diphenhydramine**, **dimenhydrinate**, and **meclizine** are used in conjunction with other antiemetics for the treatment of emesis induced by chemotherapy.

The mechanism of action for the motion sickness indication for these H_1 antihistamines and anticholinergics is inhibition of histamine H_1 and muscarinic cholinergic M1 receptors. The major adverse effects of these medications are dizziness, sedation, confusion, dry mouth, cycloplegia, and urinary retention. Their significant anticholinergic properties may limit the use of these agents. **Scopolamine** given as a transdermal patch has proved superior to the same drug administered by oral or parenteral routes.

The anticholinergic agent **scopolamine** was listed in the previous pregnancy Category C, while H_1 antihistamines including **diphenhydramine**, **dimenhydrinate**, and **meclizine** are relatively safe. Because these drugs are not primarily indicated for use as antiemetic agents, the details of their drug interactions are discussed elsewhere.

Cannabinoids

The major cannabinoid receptors so far identified are CB1 and CB2. CB1 receptors are primarily located in the brain, whereas CB2 receptors are primarily peripheral. CB1 receptors mediate psychoactive effects, analgesia, and effects on memory. CB2 receptors mediate several inflammatory and immune responses. An isomer of the major psychoactive ingredient in marijuana, tetrahydrocannabinol (THC), **dronabinol** takes advantage of the CB1 receptors, and is used medically as an appetite stimulant and as an antiemetic. **Nabilone**, a chemically related analog to **dronabinol**, has also been approved for the treatment of chemotherapy-induced emesis. In addition, in some states it is legal to prescribe the raw form of cannabis for patients as "medical marijuana." Although some *state laws* may allow clinicians to prescribe medical marijuana, federal law still categorizes marijuana as a Schedule I substance; which in all states is *illegal*. Although these cannabinoids are able to produce psychotropic effects via the binding and activation of the cannabinoid CB_1 receptors, the mechanism for their antiemetic actions is less well defined. However, it may be explained by their potential to modulate 5-HT_3 receptor activation in the nodose ganglion as well as substance P release in the spinal cord.

The main adverse effects of these cannabinoids include euphoria, dysphoria, sedation, hallucinations, dry mouth, and increased appetite, along with tachycardia, conjunctival injection, and orthostatic hypotension. Use of marijuana cigarettes should be discouraged in patients who have any form of respiratory disorder (e.g., asthma or COPD); contrary to the claims made by medical marijuana advocates, use of the drug in smoked form is not without risks and may promote or exacerbate obstructive airway disease (Joshi, Joshi, & Bartter, 2013). In addition, heavy or long-term use carries with it physical health risks that are currently poorly understood, both in the published medical literature and in the popular media (Gordon, Conley, & Gordon, 2013). Patients seeking to use raw cannabis for relief of nausea or pain should be counseled about the risks and benefits of smoking versus taking oral cannabinoid medications, as considerable bias (both pro and con) is present in the information that is publicly available on the topic of medical marijuana.

Drug–Drug Interactions

There are no drug–drug interactions known, but cannabinoids may potentiate the effects of other psychoactive agents.

Drugs to Treat Inflammatory Bowel Disease

IBD includes ulcerative colitis and Crohn's disease. Because the etiology and the pathogenesis of IBD remain unclear, the pharmacologic management of IBD is varied and complex. The emphasis of IBD treatment is to use a combination of drugs and nutritional support to maintain patients during long periods of remission, while controlling drug toxicity and complications. Three main groups of drugs are used in the management of IBD: **aminosalicylates**, corticosteroids, and drugs that affect the immune system, such as immunosuppressants, purine analogs, methotrexate, monoclonal antibodies, antitumor necrosis factor agents, and anti-integrin agents (Katzung et al., 2011).

Aminosalicylates

Several aminosalicylates containing 5-aminosalicylic acid (5-ASA or mesalamine) have been licensed and successfully used in the treatment of IBD. These drugs include various azo compounds and different formulations of mesalamine. For instance, sulfasalazine, balsalazide, and olsalazine are listed in the category of azo compounds, while pentasa, asacol, apriso, lialda, rowasa, and canasa are part of the class of 5-ASA formulations.

It has been well documented that the active ingredient of all aminosalicylates is 5-ASA. The primary action of salicylate and other NSAIDs is due to blockade of prostaglandin synthesis by inhibition of cyclooxygenase. However, the exact mechanism of action of 5-ASA is not understood. In recognition of the fact that 80% of aqueous 5-ASA is easily absorbed from the small intestine, several derivatives and formulations of 5-ASA have been developed to optimize the amount of 5-ASA released in specific sites of the body, ideally in areas of diseased distal small bowel or colon. The potential mechanisms that may be involved include (1) the modulation of inflammatory mediators derived from the cyclooxygenase and lipoxygenase pathways, (2) interference with the production of inflammatory cytokines, (3) the inhibitory effects on nuclear factor-κB, and (4) other inhibitory effects on NK cells, mucosal lymphocytes, and macrophages.

Most aminosalicylate formulations are well tolerated. The most common adverse effects reported with olsalazine use include secretory diarrhea, subtle renal tubular changes, rare cases of interstitial nephritis, and rare hypersensitivity reactions. In contrast, sulfasalazine is associated with a higher incidence of adverse effects, most likely due to the systemic effects of the sulfapyridine molecule. The problems most commonly reported with this drug include nausea, GI upset, headache, malaise, arthralgias, myalgias, and bone marrow suppression. In addition, hypersensitivity reactions to sulfapyridine may cause fever, exfoliative dermatitis, pancreatitis, pneumonitis, hemolytic anemia, pericarditis, or hepatitis. All aminosalicylates are considered safe for use in pregnancy.

Drug–Drug Interactions

There are no significant drug–drug interactions documented with aminosalicylates. However, sulfasalazine may interfere with folic acid absorption and processing. Therefore, dietary supplementation with 1 mg/day folic acid is needed to prevent folic acid deficiency.

Glucocorticoids

Glucocorticoids are commonly used for the treatment of patients with active IBD. Prednisone and prednisolone are the oral glucocorticoids most commonly used for this indication. In addition, topical hydrocortisone formulations are used to maximize colonic tissue effects and minimize systemic absorption. Furthermore, a potent synthetic analog of prednisolone, budesonide, is available in a controlled-release oral formulation that increases the drug concentration remaining in contact with the inflamed mucosa.

The mechanisms of action of glucocorticoids in the treatment of IBD are unclear. However, these drugs are known to inhibit production of inflammatory cytokines and chemokines such as tumor necrosis factor alpha (TNF-α), interleukin 1 (IL-1), and interleukin 8 (IL-8). Other anti-inflammatory effects of glucocorticoids include reduction of expression of adhesion molecules and inhibition of gene transcription of nitric oxide synthesis, phospholipase A_2, cyclooxygenase-2, and NF-κB.

Adverse effects and drug interactions associated with glucocorticoids are discussed elsewhere in this chapter.

Purine Analogs

In addition to their anticancer and immunosuppressive properties, purine analogs, including azathioprine and 6-mercaptopurine (6-MP), known as purine antimetabolites, are used in patients with IBD who are unresponsive to aminosalicylates or glucocorticoids, or who relapse when glucocorticoids are withdrawn. Azithioprine is a prodrug that is metabolized to 6-MP by liver. The mechanism of action of these drugs in IBD is not clear, but both drugs are metabolized to the nucleotides 6-thioinosinic acid, thioguanylic acid, and 6-methylmercaptopurine ribotide. These metabolites are thought to inhibit purine ribonucleotide synthesis, which then impedes DNA synthesis and thus inhibits proliferation of cells, especially fast-growing cells—mainly T and B lymphocytes.

Dose-dependent adverse effects caused by azathioprine and 6-MP include nausea, vomiting, bone marrow suppression, and hepatic toxicity. Therefore, routine complete blood counts and hepatic function tests are important for all patients who receive these medications. In addition, hypersensitivity reactions to azathioprine and 6-MP, occurring in 5% of patients, include fever, rash, pancreatitis, diarrhea, and hepatitis.

Drug–Drug Interactions

In the quest to achieve remission in patients with active IBD, the utilization of purine analogs may allow lower dosing or elimination of glucocorticoids to control active disease. Allopurinol significantly reduces xanthine oxide catabolism of purine analogs, potentially increasing active 6-thioguanine nucleotides, which may lead to severe leukopenia. Allopurinol—a drug commonly used for gout—can inhibit xanthine oxidase, which

breaks down 6-MP. Allopurinol should not be given to patients taking 6-MP or azathioprine except in carefully monitored situations.

Purine analogs cross the placenta, but the risk of teratogenicity appears to be small. These medications may therefore be used in pregnant women with caution, if other medications prove ineffective and no other contraindications exist.

Methotrexate

Like other immunosuppressants, methotrexate has beneficial effects in patients with Crohn's disease, being able to induce and maintain remission of this condition. However, its efficacy in ulcerative colitis is uncertain.

The main mechanism of action of methotrexate is inhibition of dihydrofolate reductase, which participates in tetrahydrofolate synthesis and, therefore, inhibits the production of thymidine and purines. At the low doses used in the treatment of IBD, methotrexate may interfere with inflammatory actions of IL-1, stimulate release of adenosine, and induce apoptosis (programmed cell death) of activated T lymphocytes.

The dose of methotrexate used to treat IBD may not cause the severe adverse effects—such as bone marrow suppression, megaloblastic anemia, alopecia, and mucositis—commonly seen with the higher doses used for chemotherapy. Folic acid supplementation reduces the incidence of adverse effects. In addition, the risk of hepatic damage caused by methotrexate is low.

Methotrexate is known to interact with foods containing caffeine (e.g., coffee, tea, chocolate, cola) in such a way that the effectiveness of the drug is reduced if taken in conjunction with caffeine-containing foods. Also, liver dysfunction can develop in patients who use alcohol while taking the drug. A significant number of drugs interact with methotrexate, including some commonly found in OTC medications (e.g., various NSAIDs) that increase the blood levels of methotrexate. Consequently, patients should be cautioned against using OTC medications without first consulting their prescriber and be encouraged to report any adverse effects immediately.

Anti-Tumor Necrosis Factor Therapy

Three agents—**infliximab**, **adalimumab**, and **certolizumab pegol**—have been approved for acute and chronic treatment of patients with IBD who have shown an inadequate response to conventional treatment (Loftus, 2011). These are all tumor necrosis factor (TNF) blocking antibodies, which, by blocking the binding of TNF to its receptor, reduce inflammatory cell migration and adhesion, resulting in reduced inflammation. After six weeks of induction therapy to attain remission, approximately 60% to 70% of patients have a clinical response and 30% to 40% of patients achieve a clinical remission. However, one-third of patients eventually develop drug resistance due to the development of antibodies to TNF antibody (ATA) or non-ATA mechanisms (Altwegg & Thierry, 2014).

TNF is one of the most important pro-inflammatory cytokines in the pathogenesis of IBD. All three anti-TNF agents bind to soluble and membrane-bound TNF. Their high affinity binding prevents TNF from binding to its TNF receptors (TNFr) present on the helper T cell type 1 (TH_1) and on some, other innate immune and nonimmune cells. In addition, the binding of anti-TNF to membrane-bound TNF induces reverse signaling, which suppresses cytokine release.

The most important adverse effect of anti-TNF drugs is infection due to suppression of the TH_1 inflammatory response. This immunosuppression may allow serious infections to flourish, including bacterial sepsis, tuberculosis, invasive fungal organisms, reactivation of hepatitis B, listeriosis, and opportunistic infections. Before starting anti-TNF therapy, all patients should have tuberculin skin tests or interferon-gamma release assays to ensure that they will not experience possible reactivation of latent tuberculosis. For patients with positive test results, prophylactic therapy for tuberculosis is warranted before anti-TNF therapy begins.

In addition to resistance to drug effects, ATA development increases the likelihood of acute or delayed infusion or injection reactions. Those adverse reactions may include fever, headache, dizziness, urticaria, and mild cardiopulmonary symptoms. Delayed reactions consisting of myalgia, arthralgia, jaw tightness, rash, and edema may occur one to two weeks after anti-TNF therapy is initiated in a small proportion of patients. Moreover, anti-TNF therapy may increase the risk of lymphoma in patients with IBD.

Anti-Integrin Therapy

Natalizumab, an anti-integrin antibody, was approved by the FDA in 2008 for patients with moderate to severe Crohn's disease who have failed to respond to other therapies. This drug is administered through a carefully restricted program.

Integrins have been found to play an important role in the pathogenesis of IBD. Integrins are adhesion molecules located on the surface of leukocytes, which interact with selectins on the surface of the vascular endothelial cells, thereby allowing circulating leukocytes to adhere to the vascular endothelium and then move through the blood vessel wall into the tissue. **Natalizumab** is a humanized IgG_4 monoclonal antibody targeted against the alpha-4 subunit of integrins. It blocks interaction of integrins with selectin, thereby preventing leukocyte migration into surrounding tissue; in turn, this effect prevents IBD progression in the chronic disease process.

In initial clinical trials involving patients with Crohn's disease, **natalizumab** was found to induce progressive multifocal leukoencephalopathy (PML) due to reactivation of a human polyomavirus in three patients receiving other immunomodulators on a concomitant basis (Yousry et al., 2006). After withdrawal from the market based on risk of PML, natalizumab was reintroduced in 2008 under a restricted distribution program. Under this program, patients with refractory Crohn's disease may consider natalizumab a valuable alternative treatment (Chen, Kularatna, Stone, Gutierrez, & Dassopoulos, 2013). Other adverse effects may include acute infusion reactions and a small risk of opportunistic infections.

Drug–Drug Interactions

There are no known drug–drug interactions associated with anti-integrin therapy.

Bile Acid Therapy for Gallstones

Cholelithiasis, also known as obstruction by gallstone formation, is one of the most common disorders in the gallbladder. Although laparoscopic surgery has been widely performed soon after diagnosis of this condition in recent years, medical management of cholelithiasis continues to be utilized in patients who refuse cholecystectomy or who are poor surgical candidates. There is one oral bile acid dissolution agent available in this category: ursodiol (Portincasa, Di Ciaula, Bonfrate, & Wang, 2012).

After the discontinuation of the first oral gallstone dissolution therapy, chenodiol, due to the risks of liver toxicity and cardiovascular disease, ursodiol became employed as an oral bile acid dissolution agent. The mechanism involved in ursodiol-induced dissolution of cholesterol stones is quite complicated. As this drug is a naturally existing bile acid, the long-term daily administration of ursodiol expands the bile acid pool by 30% to 50%. However, the principal mechanism of action of ursodiol is to decrease the cholesterol content of bile by reducing hepatic cholesterol secretion, and to stabilize hepatocyte canalicular membranes.

In general, ursodiol is clinically free of severe adverse effects. Potential side effects include abdominal pain, dyspepsia, nausea, headache, and viral infection. In addition, bile salt–induced diarrhea is the most common adverse effect.

Drug–Drug Interactions

Some aluminum-based antacids decrease the absorption of many medications; thus, ursodiol's effectiveness decreases when it is given with those antacids. Furthermore, estrogen and clofibrate negate the effects of ursodiol, as these medications increase hepatic secretion of cholesterol (Felicilda-Reynaldo, 2012).

CHAPTER SUMMARY

This chapter discussed the medications indicated for a variety of GI conditions and disorders:

- To control gastric acidity, antacids, histamine H_2-receptor antagonists, PPIs, and mucosal-protective agents are prescribed.
- For stimulation of GI motility, cholinergic mimetic agents and dopamine D_2-receptor blockers are used.
- Opioid agonists, bismuth compounds, and octreotide are administered for treatment of diarrhea.
- A total of five classes of medications are used to manage constipation: bulk-forming laxatives, stimulant laxatives, stool softeners/surfactants, osmotic laxatives, and miscellaneous laxatives. Three categories of medications—anticholinergics, serotonin 5-HT receptor antagonists or agonists, and chloride-channel activators—are used for management of IBS.
- 5-HT_3 receptor antagonists, corticosteroids, neurokinin-1 receptor antagonists, dopamine-receptor antagonists, antihistamines/anticholinergics, and cannabinoids are used to manage nausea and vomiting resulting from different causes.
- Aminosalicylates, corticosteroids, and immunosuppressants are used for treatment of IBD.
- Ursodiol is the only bile acid dissolution agent given for treatment of gallstones.

Critical Thinking Questions

1. Which classes of medications are useful for treating acid reflux by reducing acid secretion?

2. Why would you discourage a patient from taking antacids with ranitidine first thing in the morning?

3. Which class of motility-stimulating drugs might be a poor choice for a patient with Parkinson disease? Why?

4. Which medication class is contraindicated in individuals with insulin resistance or diabetes? Why?

5. What supportive care is needed for patients with *either* diarrhea or constipation?

CASE STUDIES

Case Scenario 1

Mrs. S. is a 48-year-old middle school teacher who has recently been waking up in the middle of the night with abdominal pain. This happens a few nights a week. Mrs. S. just divorced her husband and has three children, aged 8 to 17 years. After a history and physical examination were concluded, Mrs. S. was scheduled for endoscopy and diagnosed with PUD. The analysis of a tissue sample taken from the site further demonstrated the presence of *Helicobacter pylori* infection. Mrs. S. was prescribed omeprazole, clarithromycin, and amoxicillin. The doctor also instructed her to schedule an appointment for another endoscopy procedure in six months.

Need to Know

1. What are the main risk factors associated with the incidence of PUD in Mrs. S.?
2. What is the rationale to concurrently administer two antibiotics and an acid-reducing drug?
3. Why is it important for Mrs. S. to complete the full course of antibiotics?

Case Questions

1. Mrs. S. was diagnosed with PUD caused by *H. pylori* infection. Which prescriptions best fit her situation?
   a. Omeprazole and clarithromycin
   b. Omeprazole and amoxicillin
   c. Omeprazole, clarithromycin, and amoxicillin
   d. Omeprazole, ranitidine, and amoxicillin

2. After teaching the patient regarding her diagnosis and medications for PUD and *H. pylori*, which statement demonstrates that further instruction is needed?
   a. I have to take all my antibiotics and antiulcer drug.
   b. I have to live a less stressful life with my diseases.
   c. I know my two diseases are related to each other.
   d. I can stop my antibiotics only when I have no heartburn.

3. A nurse preceptor wishes to explain the necessity of the combination of two antibiotics with a PPI to treat PUD and *H. pylori*. Which statement is most appropriate?
   a. A PPI is for PUD and antibiotics are for *H. pylori*.
   b. Eradiation of *H. pylori* with antibiotics is important to allow for PUD healing with the PPI.
   c. Antibiotics are for PUD and the PPI is for *H. pylori*.
   d. The combination of antibiotics helps decrease antibiotic resistance.

CASE STUDIES

Case Scenario 2

Mr. J. is an 85-year-old retired policeman. He arrives at his primary physician's office with complaint of being "backed up" and claims he is having less than one bowel movement per week. During the assessment, the nurse finds he has medical history of mild dementia, depression, and osteoarthritis of the fingers, knee, and lower back. Mr. J. takes a cholinergic drug for dementia, OTC NSAID medications and oxycodone for osteoarthritis, bisphosphonates with calcium for osteoporosis, and a selective serotonin-reuptake inhibitor (SSRI) for depression. He has been living independently since his wife died three years ago. His daughter visits him once a month.

Need to Know

1. What are the most relevant factors possibly contributing to Mr. J.'s constipation?
2. What are some nonpharmacologic treatments to help his constipation?
3. What is the best choice among the various OTC laxatives the nurse might suggest?

Case Questions

1. What are the potential factors contributing to constipation? (Select all that apply.)
   a. Aging
   b. Dementia
   c. Renal insufficiency
   d. Depression
   e. Aluminum-containing antacids
2. What are the nonpharmacologic methods to help relieve constipation? (Select all that apply.)
   a. Increasing fiber intake
   b. Decreasing fiber intake
   c. Increasing fluid intake
   d. Increasing iron intake
   e. Increasing exercise

REFERENCES

Adams, M.P., & Urban, C.Q. (2012). *Pharmacology connections to nursing practice* (2nd ed.). Upper Saddle River, NJ: Pearson.

Altwegg, R., & Thierry, V. (2014). TNF blocking therapies and immunomonitoring in patients with inflammatory bowel disease. *Mediators of Inflammation, (2014)*. doi: 10.1155/2014/172821

American Academy of Family Physicians. (2011). *Hypomagnesemia linked to PPIs can cause serious adverse effects*. Retrieved from http://www.mdmag.com/medical -news/hypomagnesemia-linked-to-ppis-can-cause -serious-adverse-effects

Andrews, P.L., & Horn, C.C. (2006). Signals for nausea and emesis: Implications for models of upper gastrointestinal diseases. *Autonomic Neuroscience: Basic and Clinical, 125*, 100–115.

Arora, S., Bisen, G., & Budhiraja, R.D. (2012). Mucoadhesive and muco-penetrating delivery systems for eradication of *Helicobacter pylori. Asian J Pharm, 6*:18-30.

AstraZeneca Pharmaceuticals. (2016a). *Prescribing information: Nexium*. Retrieved from https://www.azpi central.com/nexium/nexium.pdf#page=1

AstraZeneca Pharmaceuticals. (2016b). *Prescribing information: Prilosec*. Retrieved from https://www.azpi central.com/prilosec/prilosec.pdf#page=1

Auteri, M., Zizzo, M.G., & Serio, R. (2015). GABA and GABA receptors in the gastrointestinal tract: From motility to inflammation. *Pharmacological Research, 93*, 11–21.

Bajor, A., Tornblom, H., Rudling, M., Ung, K., & Simren, M. (2014). Authors' response: Bile acids are important in the pathophysiology of IBS. *Gut, 64*(5).

Camilleri, M. (2010). Review article: New receptor targets for medical therapy in irritable bowel syndrome. *Alimentary Pharmacology and Therapeutics, 31,* 35–46.

Chan, Y.Y., Ong, Y.M., & Chua, K.L. (2007). Synergistic interaction between phenothiazines and antimicrobial agents against *Burkholderia pseudomallei*. *Antimicrobial Agents and Chemotherapy, 51*(2), 623–630.

Chen, C.-H., Kularatna, G., Stone, C.D., Gutierrez, A.M., & Dassopoulos, T. (2013). Clinical experience of natalizumab in Crohn's disease patients in a restricted distribution program. *Annals of Gastroenterology: Quarterly Publication of the Hellenic Society of Gastroenterology, 26*(3), 233–238.

Chey, W.D., Leontiadis, G.I., Howden, C.W., & Moss, S.F. (2017). Treatment of *Helicobacter pylori* infection. *American Journal of Gastroenterology, 112,* 212–238. doi: 10.1038/ajg.2016.563.

De Ponti, F. (2013). Drug development for the irritable bowel syndrome: Current challenge and future perspectives. *Frontiers in Pharmacology, 4,* 1–12.

Ehrenpreis, E.D., Deepak, P., Sifuentes, H., Devi, R., Du, H., & Leikin, J.B. (2013). The metoclopramide black box warning for tardive dyskinesia: Effect on clinical practice, adverse event reporting, and prescription drug lawsuits. *American Journal of Gastroenterology, 108*(6), 866–872.

Felicilda-Reynaldo, R.F.D. (2012). Oral gallstone dissolution therapies. *Medsurg Nursing, 21,* 41–48.

Feyer, P., & Jordan, K. (2011). Update and new trends in antiemetic therapy: The continuing need for novel therapies. *Annals of Oncology, 22,* 30–38.

Foster, J.A., & McVey Neufeld, K-A. (2013). Gut-brain axis: How the microbiome influences anxiety and depression. *Trends in Neurosciences, 36*(5), 305–312.

Fukudo, S., Kaneko, H., Akiho, H., Inamori, M., Endo, Y., Okumura, T., . . . Shimosegawa, T. (2015). Evidence-based clinical practice guidelines for irritable bowel syndrome. *Journal of Gastroenterology, 50*(1), 11–30.

Garsed, K., Chernova, J., Hastings, M., Lam, C., Marciani, L., Singh, G., . . . Spiller, R. (2013). A randomised trial of ondansetron for the treatment of irritable bowel syndrome with diarrhoea. *Neurogastroenterology, 63*(10), 1617–1625.

Geling, O., & Eichler, H. (2005). Should 5-hydroxytraptamine-3 receptor antagonists be administered beyond 24 hours after chemotherapy to prevent delayed emesis? Systematic re-evaluation of clinical evidence and drug cost implications. *Journal of Clinical Oncology, 23,* 1289–1294.

GlaxoSmithKline Pharmaceuticals. (2009). *Tagamet product information.* Retrieved from https://www .gsk.com.au/resources.ashx/prescriptionmedicines productschilddataproinfo/1460/FileName/38A75 2DE5597F251F19E3B4A0F58AE3D/Tagamet _Tablets_Injection_PI.pdf

Gordon, A.J., Conley, J.W., & Gordon, J.M. (2013). Medical consequences of marijuana use: A review of current literature. *Current Psychiatry Reports, 15*(12), 419.

Grunberg, S.M. (2007). Antiemetic activity of corticosteroids in patients receiving cancer chemotherapy: Dosing, efficacy, and tolerability analysis. *Annals of Oncology, 18*(2), 233–240.

Grundman, O., & Yoon, S.L. (2010). Irritable bowel syndrome: Epidemiology, diagnosis and treatment: An update for health-care practitioners. *Journal of Gastroenterology and Hepatology, 25,* 691–699.

Gumaste, V., & Baum, J. (2008). Treatment of gastroparesis: An update. *Digestion, 78,* 173–179.

Hadhazy, A. (2010). Think twice: How the gut's "second brain" influences mood and well-being. *Scientific American.* Retrieved from http://www.scientifi camerican.com/article.cfm?id=gut-second-brain

Hasler, W.L. (2011). Gastroparesis: Pathogenesis, diagnosis and management. *Nature Reviews Gastroenterology and Hepatology, 8,* 438–453.

Joshi, M., Joshi, A., & Bartter, T. (2014). Marijuana and lung diseases. *Current Opinion in Pulmonary Medicine, 20*(2), 173–179.

Katzung, B., Masters, S., & Trevor, A. (2011). *Basic and clinical pharmacology* (12th ed.). New York, NY: McGraw-Hill/Lange.

Kent, A.J., & Banks, M.R. (2010). Pharmacological management of diarrhea. *Gastroenterology Clinics of North America, 39,* 495–507.

Kusano, M., Hosaka, H., Kawada, A., Kuribayashi, S., Shimoyama, Y., Zai, H. . . . Yamada, M. (2014). Gastrointestinal motility and functional gastrointestinal diseases. *Current Pharmaceutical Design, 20*(16), 2775–2782.

Lee, N.M., & Saha, S. (2011). Nausea and vomiting of pregnancy. *Gastroenterology Clinics of North America, 40*(2), 309–336.

Lembo, A.J., Johanson, F.F., Parkman, H.P., Rao, S.S., Miner, P.B. Jr., & Ueno, R. (2011). Long-term safety and effectiveness of lubiprostone, a chloride channel (CIC-2) activator, in patients with chronic idiopathic constipation. *Digestive Diseases and Sciences, 56,* 2639–2645.

Loftus, E. V. (2011). Progress in the diagnosis and treatment of inflammatory bowel disease. *Gastroenterology & Hepatology, 7*(2 Suppl. 3), 3–16.

Makker, J., Chilimuri, S., & Bella, J.N. (2015). Genetic epidemiology of irritable bowel syndrome. *World Journal of Gastroenterology: WJG, 21*(40), 11353–11361. doi: 10.3748/wjg.v21.i40.11353

Mayer, E.A. (2008). Clinical practice: Irritable bowel syndrome. *New England Journal of Medicine, 358,* 1692–1699.

Obokhare, I. (2012). Fecal impaction: A cause for concern? *Clinics in Colon and Rectal Surgery, 25*(1), 53–58. http://doi.org/10.1055/s-0032-1301760.

Pimentel, M., Cash, B.D., Lembo, A., & Schoenfeld, P. (2012). Irritable bowel syndrome: Pathophysiology and goals of therapy. *The Medical Roundtable General Medicine Edition, 1*(3), 248–256.

Portincasa, P., Di Ciaula, A., Bonfrate, L., & Wang, D.Q.H. (2012). Therapy of gallstone disease: What it was, what it is, what it will be. *World Journal of Gastrointestinal Pharmacology and Therapeutics, 3*, 7–20.

Rapoport, B., & Smit, T. (2017). Clinical pharmacology of neurokinin-1 receptor antagonists for the treatment of nausea and vomiting associated with chemotherapy. *Expert Opinion on Drug Safety, 16*(6), 697–710.

Roerig, J.L., Steffen, K.J., Mitchell, J.E., & Zunker, C. (2010). Laxative abuse: Epidemiology, diagnosis, and management. *Drugs, 70*(12), 1487–1503. doi: 10.2165/11898640-000000000-00000

Sanger, G.J., & Andrews, P.L.R. (2006). Treatment of nausea and vomiting: Gaps in our knowledge. *Autonomic Neuroscience: Basic and Clinical, 129*, 3–16.

Singh, S., & Rao, S.S.C. (2010). Pharmacologic management of chronic constipation. *Gastroenterology Clinics of North America, 39*, 509–527.

Stahl, S.M., & Felker, A. (2008). Monoamine oxidase inhibitors: A modern guide to an unrequited class of antidepressants. *CNS Spectrum, 13*(10), 855–870.

Story, L. (2018). *Pathophysiology: A practical approach.* Burlington, MA: Jones & Bartlett Learning.

Takeda Pharmaceuticals. (2012). *Prescribing information: Prevacid.* Retrieved from http://general.takedapharm .com/content/file/pi.pdf?applicationcode=66b0b94 2e82b-46ad-886a-f4aa59f5f33c&filetypecode=PREV ACIDPI

Tawadrous, D., Dixon, S., Shariff, S.Z., Fleet, J., Gandhi, S., Jain, A.K.,... & Garg, A.X. (2014). Altered mental status in older adults with histamine2-receptor antagonists: A population-based study. *European Journal of Internal Medicine, 25*(8), 701–709.

United States Food and Drug Administration (2016a). *Lotronex (alosetron hydrochloride) information.* Retrieved from https://www.fda.gov/Drugs/DrugSafety /PostmarketDrugSafetyInformationforPatients andProviders/ucm110450.htm

United States Food and Drug Administration (2016b). *Zelnorm (tegaserod maleate) information.* Retrieved from https://www.fda.gov/Drugs/DrugSafety/ucm103223 .htm.

Vakil, N.B. (2017). Physiology of gastric acid secretion. In S. Grover (Ed.), *UpToDate.* Retrieved from http:// www.uptodate.com/contents/physiology-of-gastric -acid-secretion

Van Ryckeghem, F. (2016). Corticosteroids, the oldest agent in the prevention of chemotherapy-induced nausea and vomiting: What about the guidelines? *Journal of Translational Internal Medicine, 4*(1), 46–51. doi: 10.1515/jtim-2016-0010

Wallace, J.L. (2008). Prostaglandins, NSAIDs, and gastric mucosal protection: Why doesn't the stomach just digest itself? *Physiology Review, 88*, 1547–1565.

Wang, L., Li, M., Cao, Y., Han, Z., Wang, X., Atkinson, E.J., . . . Amin, S. (2017). Proton pump inhibitors and the risk for fracture at specific sites: data mining of the FDA adverse event reporting system. *Scientific Reports, 7*, 5527. doi:10.1038/s41598-017-0552-1

Wilson, N., & Schey, R. (2015). Lubiprostone in constipation: Clinical evidence and place in therapy. *Therapeutic Advances in Chronic Disease, 6*(2), 40–50. doi: 10.1177/2040622314567678

Yousry, T.A., Major, E.O., Ryschkewitsch, C., Fahle, G., Fischer, S., Hou, J., . . . Clifford, D.B. (2006). Evaluation of patients treated with natalizumab for progressive multifocal leukoencephalopathy. *The New England Journal of Medicine, 354*(9), 924–933. doi: 10.1056/NEJMoa054693

Zheng, Y., Yu, T., Tang, Y., Xiong, W., Shen, X., Jiang, L., & Lin, L. (2017). Efficacy and safety of 5-hydroxytryptamine 3 receptor antagonists in irritable bowel syndrome: A systematic review and meta-analysis of randomized controlled trials. *PLOS one, 12*(3), e0172846. doi: 10.1371/journal.pone.0172846

CHAPTER 9

Endocrine System Drugs

Karen Crowley, Cathi Bodine, Linda Tenofsky,
Ashley Pratt, and Sarah Nadarajah

KEY TERMS

Adrenal cortex
Adrenal glands
Aldosterone
Aldosterone antagonists
Biguanides
Calcitonin
Cortisol
Diabetes mellitus
Endocrine system
Estrogen

Feedback loop
Follicle-stimulating
  hormone (FSH)
Glands
Glucagon
Homeostasis
Hormone
Hypothalamic–pituitary–
  adrenal axis
Insulin

Luteinizing hormone (LH)
Meglitinides
Ovaries
Pancreas
Parathyroid
Parathyroid hormone
  (PTH)
Pineal body
Pituitary
Progesterone

Sulfonylureas
Testes
Thiazolidinediones
Thymosin
Thymus
Thyroid
Thyroid-stimulating
  hormone (TSH)

CHAPTER OBJECTIVES

At the end of the chapter, the student will be able to:

1. Identify six primary glands in the endocrine system.

2. Describe four common conditions resulting from endocrine disorders.

3. Identify medications used to treat endocrine disorders.

4. Identify pharmacodynamics and pharmacokinetics of medications used in treating endocrine disorders.

5. Identify appropriate nursing interventions in caring for individuals with endocrine disorders.

Introduction

The **endocrine system** is a complex body system composed of **hormone**-secreting **glands** including the hypothalamus, anterior and posterior **pituitary**, **pineal body**, **thyroid**, **parathyroid**, **thymus**, **adrenal glands**, **pancreas**, and reproductive glands (**ovaries** or **testes**). Hormones are chemical messengers that are released into the blood and travel to target tissues and organs, regulating many bodily functions including growth, metabolism, and sexual reproduction. The purpose of many of these hormones is maintaining **homeostasis** by means of an array of negative and positive **feedback loops**, and direct stimulation or inhibition of the endocrine glands (FIGURE 9-1). An example of a negative feedback loop is glucose regulation. After a person eats, blood glucose rises, signaling beta cells in the pancreas to secrete the hormone insulin. Insulin enhances the conversion of glucose to glycogen, a form that may be absorbed into cells, and blood glucose decreases. After blood glucose levels reach a normal range, the pancreas halts production of insulin.

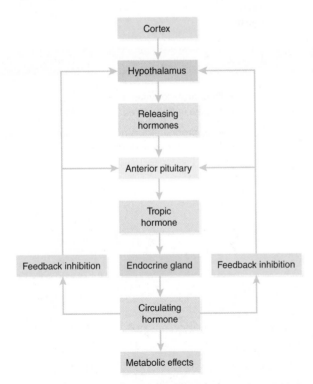

FIGURE 9-1 Normal mechanisms controlling elaboration of tropic hormones by the pituitary gland.

Disorders of the endocrine system arise when there is a disruption in one of these feedback loops, or overproduction or suppression of a hormone. Medications used to treat endocrine disorders are typically synthetic versions of innate hormones; hormones from human, animal, or plant sources; or medications that suppress or increase release of hormones.

This chapter reviews the principal glands of the endocrine system, the hormones secreted by them, and some of the medications commonly administered for endocrine disorders.

Endocrine Glands and Their Hormones

No single gland in the endocrine system is "most important" or "key"—but certainly some hormonal dysfunctions are easier to treat than others (BOX 9-1). As an example, consider the hormones insulin, which is secreted by the pancreas, and L-thyroxine (T_4), which is produced in the thyroid. Both insulin and T_4 are essential to cellular metabolism, and the absence of either in the body would lead to death of the patient. Autoimmune diseases attacking the two glands that produce these hormones are relatively common. Autoimmune hypothyroidism (Hashimoto's thyroiditis) can be treated by simply taking a tablet each day. In contrast, autoimmune diabetes (type 1 diabetes mellitus) requires an often complicated and difficult regimen of injecting two types of insulin or the use of an insulin pump, along with lifestyle changes to reduce the likelihood of short- or long-term complications. Does this mean a person with type 1 diabetes is sicker than a person with Hashimoto's thyroiditis? Not at all. Both disorders are dangerous, even life threatening.

Because there is no obvious way to prioritize the glands and hormones by importance, necessity, or other ranking, the different glands and their hormones will be described anatomically from a "head-to-toe fashion," that is, starting with the glands in the brain and moving downward (FIGURE 9-2).

BOX 9-1 Hormones of the Hypothalamus

- Thyrotropin-releasing hormone (TRH): Acts on the anterior pituitary to trigger release of thyroid-stimulating hormone (TSH) and prolactin.
- Gonadotropin-releasing hormone (GnRH): Acts on the anterior pituitary and reproductive organs to stimulate release of follicle-stimulating hormone (FSH) and luteinizing hormone (LH).
- Growth hormone-releasing hormone (GHRH): Acts on the anterior pituitary to stimulate release of growth hormone (GH).
- Corticotropin-releasing hormone (CRH): Acts on the anterior pituitary to stimulate release of adrenocorticotropic hormone (ACTH).

- Somatostatin: Acts on the anterior pituitary to inhibit release of GH and TSH (is also secreted in the pancreas and intestine).
- Dopamine: Acts on the anterior pituitary to inhibit release of prolactin.

Two other hormones—vasopressin and oxytocin—are synthesized in the hypothalamus but travel to the posterior pituitary and are released from there. Vasopressin is a key hormone regulating water reabsorption in the kidney's collecting ducts and, therefore, is responsible for regulating water loss and blood volume (hence its alternate name, antidiuretic hormone [ADH]). Oxytocin is a smooth muscle stimulant that promotes uterine contraction in childbirth and is also a contributor to emotional bonding.

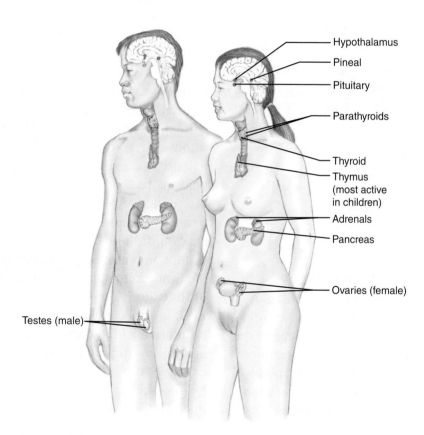

FIGURE 9-2 Human endocrine system.

Hypothalamus

The hypothalamus is located in the brain above the pituitary gland and produces hormones that start and stop the production of other hormones. The **hypothalamic–pituitary–adrenal axis** regulates almost every endocrine function in the body (**FIGURE 9-3**). Thus, dysfunction in the ability of the hypothalamus to secrete the hormones that activate other glands can have significant systemic effects.

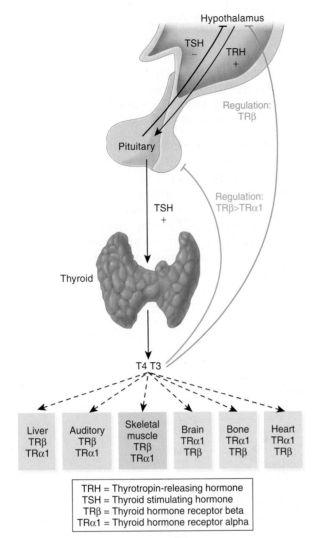

TRH = Thyrotropin-releasing hormone
TSH = Thyroid stimulating hormone
TRβ = Thyroid hormone receptor beta
TRα1 = Thyroid hormone receptor alpha

FIGURE 9-3 Hypothalamic–Pituitary–Thyroid (HPT) Axis.

Activity in other glands triggers the release of hormones by the hypothalamus. Conditions affecting hypothalamic hormone release—whether directly, via damage to the hypothalamus in such a way that it cannot or does not release one or more hormones, or indirectly, via failure of the feedback loop to signal the hypothalamus that these triggering hormones are needed—can result in a cascade of physiological problems downstream from the hypothalamus.

Pituitary

There is a popular conception of the pituitary gland as the "master gland," but that is a bit misleading, given how much of its function is controlled by the hypothalamus. Even so, the pituitary does have significant involvement in multiple endocrine functions (FIGURE 9-4).

The pituitary gland releases stimulating hormones, which affect endocrine glands throughout the body, regulating many hormone processes.

- Anterior pituitary: Secretes hormones that stimulate the adrenal glands (ACTH), thyroid (TSH), and gonads (FSH and LH). Also produces GH and prolactin.
- Posterior pituitary: Stores and releases hormones created in the hypothalamus (vasopressin and oxytocin).

Pituitary dysfunction can manifest as benign tumors or cysts that cause the gland to produce either too much or too little of one or more hormones. Inflammatory disease, autoimmune disease, or malignancy may also be sources of pituitary dysfunction. Treatment of tumors is usually surgical, especially if a tumor's presence threatens the optic nerve; in some instances, medications are used to shrink the tumor prior to surgery. Removal of tumors can lead to a permanent hormone imbalance that is then treated with hormone replacement; similarly, autoimmune and other disorders that reduce hormone levels are treated with hormone replacement. When excess hormone is produced by a tumor that cannot be removed, treatment consists of medications to suppress hormone release or function.

It is important to recognize that excess pituitary hormones can contribute to an array of dysfunctions. Excess GH, for example, can lead to hypertension, diabetes, heart or kidney failure, or heart enlargement if left untreated.

Pineal Gland

Also called the pineal body, the small pineal gland is located above and behind the pituitary gland. It secretes melatonin in response to darkness and light, and helps regulate the body's daily biological clock (circadian rhythm) and sleep/wake cycles (McDowell,

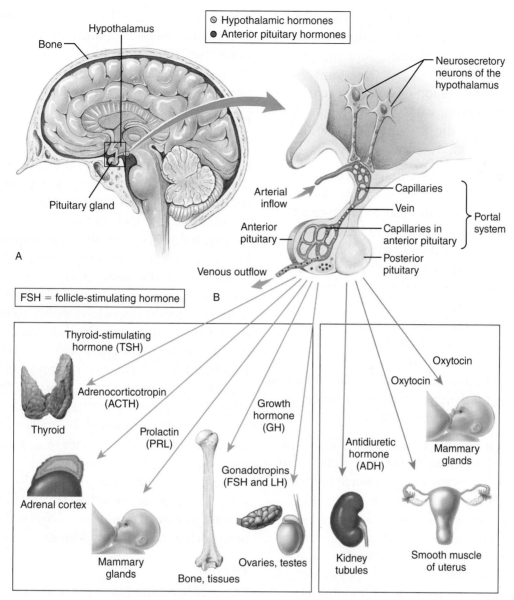

FIGURE 9-4 The pituitary gland. (A) A cross-section of the brain showing the location of the pituitary and hypothalamus. (B) The structure of the pituitary gland. Releasing and inhibiting hormones travel via the portal system from the hypothalamus to the anterior pituitary, where they affect hormone secretion.

2011). The effects of this hormone on other systems are unclear, but it appears to have an inhibitory effect on reproductive hormones such as FSH and LH, as well as a variety of effects on mood regulation.

Thyroid

The thyroid gland is a butterfly-shaped gland located in the front, lower part of the neck. It releases the hormones L-triiodothyronine (T_3) and L-thyroxine (T_4), which affect all organs, cellular metabolism, and assist in controlling functions such as heart rate, blood pressure, and muscle tone (Kemp, n.d.). Release of T_3 and T_4 is controlled by **thyroid-stimulating hormone (TSH)** through a negative feedback loop to the anterior pituitary gland. T_3 is the most metabolically active form of thyroid hormone, and T_4 is most often a precursor to it that is changed into T_3 by the activity of any of three deiodinase enzymes (enzymes that remove an iodine from T_4). The thyroid also produces **calcitonin** to inhibit osteoclast activity and formation, thus suppressing resorption of bone.

The most common disorder of the thyroid is hypothyroidism, which generally manifests as a decrease in the amount of circulating T_4. Causes of hypothyroidism include:

- Inability of the hypothalamus to produce thyrotropin-releasing hormone (TRH)
- Inability of the pituitary to produce adequate TSH in response to TRH
- Inability of the thyroid to produce T_4 in response to TSH, which itself can result from:
  - Lack of iodide in the diet (nutritional deficiency)
  - Autoimmune attack on the thyroid (Hashimoto's thyroiditis)
  - Congenital disease
  - Iatrogenic causes (e.g., medications that suppress thyroid function or interfere with feedback mechanisms)

It is less common for hypothyroidism to result from a lack of T_3, but occasionally this does occur; T_3 is generally produced outside the thyroid by the interaction of T_4 with deiodinase enzymes, which can become suppressed in instances of selenium deficiency (Pedersen et al., 2013). Selenium is a component of the amino acid selenocysteine, which is part of each of the T_4 diodinases. Medication protocols for hypothyroidism vary depending on the cause of this imbalance. In nutritional syndromes, the obvious therapeutic intervention is supplemental nutrients or dietary changes to include foods containing the needed elements (e.g., iodide, selenium). For most other causes localized to the thyroid gland, the treatment is thyroid replacement therapy with synthetic thyroxine (**levothyroxine**). If the cause of the defect is upstream from the thyroid in either the pituitary or the hypothalamus, treatment involves addressing the source of the excess or inadequacy in the triggering hormones.

Much less common is hyperthyroidism due to Graves' disease, an autoimmune disease in which the thyroid is stimulated by autoantibodies to produce excess thyroid hormones. Hyperthyroidism is treated with thyroid-suppressing medications, or complete or partial surgical removal of the thyroid gland.

Parathyroid

The parathyroid gland comprises two small pairs of glands embedded in the back of the thyroid gland. They secrete **parathyroid hormone (PTH)**, which helps regulate calcium absorption and release in the blood and bones (Kemp, n.d.). PTH is produced in response to low calcium levels; thus, excessive production of PTH (hyperparathyroidism) may be harmful to bones, as calcium is drawn from bone (and teeth) stores in response to the elevated levels. Hyperparathyroidism may also play a role in cardiac conditions, as PTH has known inhibitory effects on certain calcium channels in heart muscle (Schlüter & Piper, 1998). The opposite condition, hypoparathyroidism, is less common and usually occurs due to nutritional deficiencies (e.g., low blood magnesium levels), metabolic alkalosis, injury to the parathyroid gland (occasionally due to surgery or radioactive iodine treatment for Graves' disease), or unusual congenital conditions such as DiGeorge syndrome.

Thymus

The thymus gland is located in the upper chest behind the sternum and plays a role in immune function. It produces the hormone **thymosin** and is most active during childhood; it atrophies after adolescence. Lymphocytes passing through the thymus are stimulated by thymosin to become T lymphocytes or T-cells (Blakemore & Jennett, 2001). Disorders affecting the thymus, therefore, relate to the ability of the body to cope with disease via cell-mediated immunity (e.g., activation of pathogen-destroying phagocytes and natural killer cells).

Pancreas

The pancreas is located behind the stomach and has both endocrine and exocrine functions. For its endocrine functions, this gland secretes hormones directly into the blood. Examples include the hormones **insulin** and **glucagon**, which help regulate blood glucose. For its exocrine functions, the pancreas uses a duct system to secrete hormones, which are used outside, or on the surface of, the body (sweat and salivary glands are examples). Additional exocrine function includes secretion of enzymes that aid in digestion.

One of the most common endocrine diseases in the developed world—with fast-rising incidence in developing countries—is **diabetes mellitus**, which is a disorder of glucose metabolism (**FIGURE 9-5**). Insulin is produced by the beta cells in the pancreas in response to elevated blood glucose; the body cannot use glucose without insulin. Insulin binds to cell-surface receptors and creates a pathway for glucose transporter proteins to move glucose from the bloodstream into the cell. Insulin also enhances the conversion of glucose to glycogen in the liver and decreases the rate of protein to glucose conversion, all to decrease hyperglycemia.

Although several types of diabetes exist (see **BOX 9-2**), there are only two physiological processes that lead to diabetes: (1) poor or

nonexistent function in the pancreatic beta cells that secrete insulin, in such a way that insufficient insulin circulates to meet the body's needs, or (2) cellular resistance to insulin, so that cells' ability to utilize insulin for glucose transfer is impaired even when adequate insulin is available. The underlying causes of these two problems can vary widely. In both circumstances, blood glucose levels rise above normal levels (hyperglycemia), which can result in both short- and long-term health complications. Treatment of diabetes depends on which of the two issues is causing hyperglycemia (discussed later in this chapter).

Adrenal Glands

The adrenal glands sit atop each kidney. Each adrenal gland has two parts: the **adrenal cortex** (outer part) and the adrenal medulla (inner part). The adrenal cortex releases corticosteroids (glucocorticoids and mineralocorticoids), which help regulate metabolism, immune function, sexual function, and the balance of sodium and water. The adrenal medulla releases catecholamines (epinephrine and norepinephrine), which increase heart rate and blood pressure in response to physical and emotional cues. Dysfunction in adrenal hormone production can create catastrophic metabolic imbalances, including hypercortisolism (Cushing disease), hyperaldosteronism (Conn disease), and hypoadrenalism (adrenal insufficiency or Addison's disease). In cases of excess adrenal hormone production, these conditions are often related to a tumor on the adrenal glands that produces exogenous hormones (e.g., **cortisol** or **aldosterone**) or a tumor in the pituitary that produces excess ACTH, stimulating the adrenal glands to produce excess cortisol, resulting in hypercortisolism. In cases of inadequate adrenal hormone production, the cause is usually related to an injury or infection affecting the adrenal glands or, more commonly, the pituitary. Treatment depends on the type of dysfunction and the source of the deficiency or excess.

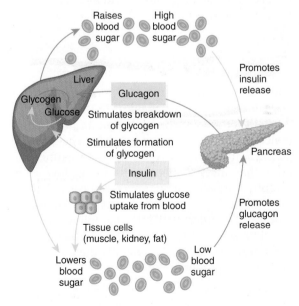

FIGURE 9-5 Glucose metabolism.

BOX 9-2   Types of Diabetes Mellitus

Type 1 Diabetes

Cause: Reduction or absence of insulin secretion in the pancreas.

Type 1 diabetes mellitus (T1DM) is usually caused by autoimmune attack against the pancreatic beta cells but can also be caused by injury to the pancreas, or failure of beta cells. It is unknown what triggers the autoimmune attack, although many patients have relatives with other autoimmune diseases (e.g., autoimmune thyroiditis or rheumatoid arthritis). The sole method of treating T1DM is insulin replacement therapy.

Type 2 Diabetes

Cause: Insensitivity of cells to insulin signaling.

Type 2 diabetes mellitus (T2DM) is the most common manifestation form of diabetes, with 90% or more of all patients with diabetes falling into this category. Except in cases where there is a known causative factor—diabetes related to other endocrine disorders such as Cushing disease or polycystic ovary syndrome (PCOS), or due to medications such as corticosteroids—T2DM is a disease that develops from the interplay of genetic predisposition with long-term environmental factors, specifically sedentary lifestyle and being overweight/obese. T2DM is treated with combinations of lifestyle therapies (e.g., exercise and dietary changes to promote weight loss and improve insulin sensitivity), medications (hypoglycemic agents), hormone therapy (insulin), and, in some instances, bariatric surgery, which has been shown to both rapidly reduce weight in obese individuals and significantly alter insulin metabolism.

Gestational Diabetes

Cause: Insensitivity of cells to insulin signaling during pregnancy.

Gestational diabetes (GDM) occurs when the normal insulin resistance that occurs in pregnancy becomes excessive and leads to hyperglycemia in the mother, and if uncontrolled, rapid growth and high birth weight in the infant. Both mother and infant are at risk of developing T2DM later in life if GDM develops and is not controlled; in addition, both are at risk of complications during pregnancy and

birth as a result of excess glucose availability. Typical treatment includes blood glucose monitoring, dietary changes, exercise (unless contraindicated), weight gain limitations, and, if indicated, cesarean delivery to prevent complications at birth. Insulin is used if other strategies are inadequate. There is a growing body of data that supports oral hypoglycemic medications (metformin and glyburide) as suitable alternatives to insulin within specific parameters (e.g., women past the first trimester who refuse—or cannot use—insulin and have not achieved satisfactory glycemic control after a trial of medical nutrition therapy) (Kalra, Gupta, Singla, & Kalra, 2015).

Latent Autoimmune Diabetes in Adults

Cause: Autoimmune attack on beta cells leading to reduction in insulin production.

Latent autoimmune diabetes in adults (LADA) involves a similar disease process as T1DM. Instead of the rapid onset that frequently characterizes T1DM, however, this variant develops relatively slowly, with patients maintaining at least some endogenous insulin production for a period of months, years, or even decades. Because the disorder is poorly understood and frequently misdiagnosed (usually as T2DM), treatment protocols for LADA have not been established; one recommendation includes combining immunomodulatory therapy to preserve beta-cell function and hypoglycemic medications to reduce blood sugar levels (Cernea, Buzzetti, & Pozzilli, 2009).

Monogenic Diabetes

Cause: Genetic mutation that causes beta cells to fail to produce insulin.

There are two main forms of this rare condition: neonatal diabetes mellitus (NDM) and maturity-onset diabetes of the young (MODY), which is usually identified in adolescence or young adulthood. In some cases, no treatment other than lifestyle modifications (e.g., low-carbohydrate diet, regular exercise) is needed to avoid hyperglycemia. In others, the patient requires a regimen similar to that followed by individuals with T1DM or LADA. Correct diagnosis of the condition is generally the greatest obstacle to appropriate therapy.

Reproductive Glands

The reproductive glands produce sex hormones that influence the development of male and female characteristics and reproductive function. In females, there are two ovaries located in the pelvis on either side of the uterus. Two hormones collectively referred to as gonadotropins, **follicle-stimulating hormone (FSH)** and **luteinizing hormone (LH)**, are released from the anterior pituitary. In women, these hormones stimulate the ovaries to produce and secrete **estrogen** and **progesterone**, which regulate the menstrual cycle, egg production, functions of pregnancy, and breast growth. In men, the testes are stimulated by FSH and LH to secrete androgens (e.g., testosterone), which influences production of sperm (Pardue et al., 2017) and signs of reproductive maturation, such as facial and pubic hair (Rey, Campo, Ropelato, & Bergadá, 2016).

Many conditions of the reproductive glands are caused by inappropriate levels of gonadotropins, many of which relate to sexual maturation in adolescence or fertility. Some of these conditions are congenital (e.g., Turner syndrome) and relatively uncommon. Others, such as PCOS (polycystic ovary syndrome) and symptomatic menopause, occur frequently, although their causes are not known. With PCOS, a suite of other endocrine abnormalities often co-occur—most notably, insulin resistance and diabetes. With menopause, the decrease in reproductive hormones is a normal part of a woman's life cycle, but the presence and severity of associated symptoms depends on a variety of genetic, physiological, and lifestyle factors. Treatment varies depending on the condition and cause of the problem, with hormone replacement being used for some deficiency syndromes and other therapies are applied as needed (e.g., **metformin** therapy in PCOS).

Treating Endocrine Conditions

The general strategy for dealing with hormone excess or deficiency is one of two obvious actions: (1) in case of excess, eliminate the source of the overproduction (often through surgery or a medication that suppresses the gland's activity), or (2) in case of deficiency, administer synthetic or natural hormones to replace what is missing. That said, some endocrine conditions are common, complicated, or both, warranting a closer look:

- Diabetes mellitus, which is a relatively widespread condition affecting millions of people that results from a dysfunction of insulin production or metabolism
- Thyroid disorders, which are likewise fairly common and involve dysfunctions of thyroid hormone production
- PCOS, a common disorder in women that is caused by excess androgens
- Adrenal dysfunction, which is somewhat less common but which has significant implications for the patient's long-term well-being, and, as noted earlier, is often related to neoplasms

Diabetes Mellitus

Diabetes mellitus occurs when the pancreas does not secrete insulin (type 1, LADA, or monogenetic types), or when cells are insulin resistant and unable to utilize circulating insulin (type 2 or GDM). Treatment may include oral or injectable hypoglycemic drugs (including **insulin**), or both. Oral hypoglycemic medications and **insulin** are available as many preparations and brands, all with the goal of normalizing blood glucose levels in people with diabetes. All patients will need to take certain steps to guard against hypoglycemia or hyperglycemia (see **BOX 9-3**).

Insulin

Until the last century there was no effective treatment for diabetes, particularly T1DM, which was inevitably fatal. The identification of insulin in 1921 led to the development of synthetic **insulins** used as the primary treatment of T1DM and as an adjunct therapy in some patients with T2DM and GDM.

BOX 9-3 Nursing Interventions in Diabetes

- Teach patients how to test blood sugar levels and urine for ketones.
- Teach appropriate insulin administration (timing, injection site rotation).
- Instruct patients on signs and symptoms of hypoglycemia.
- Instruct patients to carry a source of sugar in case of hypoglycemic events.
- Instruct patients on the need for medical alert identification.

Best Practices

At present, regular insulin is the only form of insulin that can be delivered intravenously.

Insulin comes in many formulations with differing durations of action; it may be ultra-short acting, short-acting, intermediate-acting, or long-acting, and patients may use one or a combination of forms. How quickly and for how long a type of insulin will work depends on the arrangement of amino acids in the molecule of the particular formulation.

The search continues for alternative methods of insulin delivery. Gastrointestinal (GI) enzymes destroy insulin, making an oral dosage form impractical. In 2006, the Food and Drug Administration (FDA) approved an inhaled formulation of insulin, but it was removed from the market a year later because it was not popular with patients or care providers, and there was concern about possible links to lung problems. Although research has sought a more convenient form of administration for insulin, with oral or nasal spray forms being the methods investigated most intensely, at present insulin can be delivered only by subcutaneous injection or intravenously.

Lack of insulin leads to a fairly predictable set of metabolic derangements culminating in diabetic ketoacidosis (FIGURE 9-6), which, if not treated promptly, can lead to coma and death. Patients with diabetes who no longer produce endogenous insulin, as well as those who are severely insulin resistant, require insulin or risk developing severe complications from this life-threatening condition; however, insulin needs change from day to day depending on activity levels, dietary intake, diet composition, and other factors such as

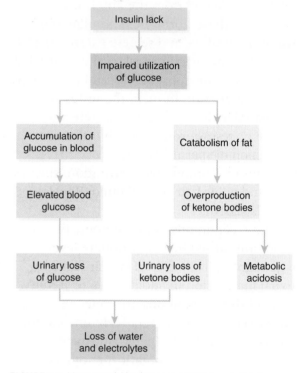

FIGURE 9-6 Major metabolic derangements in type 1 diabetes mellitus.

growth spurts (in children) or pregnancy (in adult women). Therefore, *intravenous* delivery is used only in emergencies, when the patient develops a hyperglycemic crisis or ketoacidosis. Otherwise, insulin is self-delivered, either by intermittent subcutaneous injection or by continuous infusion pump. Nurses should note that ketoacidosis may occur in patients with T2DM, albeit less frequently than T1DM.

Nursing Process

Assess

An HbA$_{1c}$ test is performed at intervals of 3 months or more to assess blood glucose control. Test results are given as a percentage of glycosylated hemoglobin, representing a measure of average blood glucose over the past 3 months (TABLE 9-1). In adult patients, an HbA$_{1c}$ result of 5.5–6.0 is ideal. In children younger than 10 years with T1DM, the desired level may be somewhat higher for two reasons: (1) pediatric patients have frequent influxes of GH, which promotes insulin resistance and therefore elevates overall blood glucose levels; and (2) target ranges (particularly in very young patients) tend to be set higher to alleviate concerns about hypoglycemia impacting brain development. A large, randomized trial of "tight control" in patients with T1DM found that those whose HbA$_{1c}$ results were consistently greater than 8% were at risk of long-term complications, such as neuropathy, kidney failure, and cardiovascular disease, while patients with better glycemic control were at much lower risk for these complications but at higher risk of hypoglycemic events (Skyler, 2004).

Patients who complain of symptoms consistent with diabetic ketoacidosis, or who present with a significant infection, should be tested for ketones with urinalysis first, followed by blood tests, and referred for *immediate* treatment if positive (see BOX 9-4). Individuals at the greatest risk include those with T1DM who use an insulin pump, because pump failures can contribute to the lack of insulin flow.

Dosing and frequency of insulin administration are usually based on blood glucose test results, diet, and expected exercise. Most patients with diabetes are instructed by a specialist or a certified diabetes educator (CDE) in how to check

Best Practices

The idea that ketoacidosis occurs only in patients with T1DM is not accurate. Patients with T2DM may present with this condition, albeit less frequently. All patients with very high blood glucose and symptoms consistent with ketoacidosis should be assessed for this life-threatening condition.

TABLE 9-1	HbA$_{1c}$ Reading Correlated to Average Blood Glucose Level for the Prior Three Months	
HbA$_{1c}$ Reading	Average Blood Glucose, Prior Three Months	In Comparison to Normal Levels (Nursing Action)
4.5	83	Subnormal (Assess for frequent hypoglycemic events and hypoglycemia unawareness; consider reducing insulin dosage.)
5.0	101	Low end of normal range (Assess for hypoglycemic events and hypoglycemia unawareness; consider adjusting insulin dosage.)
5.5	118	Normal (Provide patient with positive reinforcement: "Keep doing what you're doing!")
6.0	136	Normal (Provide patient with positive reinforcement: "Keep doing what you're doing!")
6.5	154	High end of normal (Provide patient with positive reinforcement but suggest strategies to avoid high blood glucose levels and set goals for slight reduction in HbA$_{1c}$ level.)
7.0	172	High (Assess for patterns of hyperglycemia and suggest strategies for avoiding high blood glucose levels; consider adjusting insulin regimen.)
7.5	190	High (Assess for patterns of hyperglycemia and suggest strategies for avoiding high blood glucose levels; consider adjusting insulin regimen.)
8.0–10	207–279	Excessive (Assess for patterns of hyperglycemia; suggest strategies for reducing high blood glucose levels; initiate more frequent blood glucose testing; consider adjusting insulin regimen; consider nutritional counseling and low-carbohydrate diet.)
>10	>279	Critical (Usually seen in the context of new diagnosis; counsel patient on strategies for blood glucose control. In established patient with levels greater than 10, counseling with a CDE or LICSW with expertise in diabetes issues may be required. Assess for mental health status and social issues preventing access to supplies or medication.)

Conversion: HbA$_{1c}$ = (Plasma blood glucose + 77.3)/35.6

Plasma blood glucose = (HbA$_{1c}$ × 35.6) − 77.3

Data from Rohlfing, C.L., Wiedmeyer, H.M., Little, R.R., England, J.D., Tennill, A., & Goldstein, D.E. (2002). Defining the relationship between plasma glucose and HbA1c: Analysis of glucose profiles and HbA1c in the Diabetes Control and Complications Trial. *Diabetes Care, 25,* 275–278.

BOX 9-4 Diabetic Ketoacidosis

Common Symptoms

- Decreased alertness
- Deep, rapid breathing
- Dry skin and mouth
- Flushed face
- Frequent urination or thirst that lasts for a day or more
- Fruity-smelling breath
- Headache
- Muscle stiffness or aches
- Nausea and vomiting
- Stomach pain

Exams and Tests

Ketone testing of urine or blood may be used in type 1 diabetes to screen for early ketoacidosis. Ketone testing is usually done:

- If an initial urine test is positive for ketones

- Blood test then measures beta-hydroxybutyrate

Other tests for ketoacidosis include:

- Arterial blood gas
- Basic metabolic panel
- Blood glucose test
- Blood pressure measurement

Ketoacidosis may affect the results of the following tests:

- CO_2
- Magnesium blood test
- Phosphorus blood test
- Sodium blood test
- Urine pH

Reproduced from National Institutes of Health/MedLine Plus. (2013). Diabetic ketoacidosis. Available at http://www.nlm.nih.gov/medlineplus/ency/article/000320.htm (accessed December 18, 2017).

Best Practices

Adolescent patients on insulin, particularly females, may be noncompliant with their regimen in an attempt to lose weight. Elevated HbA$_{1c}$ and body image issues in adolescents suggest a possible eating disorder (bulimia) and require follow-up.

their own blood sugar levels and how to adjust their insulin dose, to avoid hypoglycemia or hyperglycemia. Assessment should include a review of the patient's blood glucose logs to identify patterns of hypoglycemia or hyperglycemia that might warrant follow-up with a specialist or CDE.

Nurses should ask how frequently patients are testing glucose levels and whether there are any obstacles to obtaining needed supplies such as test strips, insulin, or syringes/pump supplies. Insurance limitations may restrict some patients (usually those with T2DM) to a small number (two or fewer) of test strips per day, which may hinder the patient's ability to perform adequate testing to manage blood glucose. Resources for obtaining free or reduced-cost supplies are available through the American Diabetes Association, Juvenile Diabetes Research Foundation, Diabetes Hands Foundation, Children with Diabetes, and many other organizations geared toward educating and assisting people with diabetes.

Patient Education

Patients may need education regarding the pharmacodynamics of their specific insulin brand(s). Onset time, peak effect, and duration of action can all affect how the patient responds, particularly when using more than one type of insulin. Meals, exercise, and blood glucose monitoring must be coordinated with insulin administration to avoid adverse effects. For example, a patient who typically goes for a walk in the mornings after breakfast must be educated to either eat more food or use less insulin, should he or she decide to take up jogging, as the added exertion will increase the efficiency of glucose transfer in the body, which means the insulin will clear more glucose out of the blood and into the cells. Particularly for patients with T2DM, the understanding of how exercise affects insulin metabolism can be critical toward improving their effective use of the medication (and potentially enabling them to avoid the need to use it). Teaching the value of weight loss for improving blood glucose control is important for overweight or obese patients with T2DM who use insulin, but understand that weight loss for patients with diabetes is frequently a source of emotional distress and frustration particularly because insulin use often leads to weight gain at first. Initially, it may be more helpful to stress exercise and healthy eating for blood glucose control, and provide positive reinforcement and additional education on weight loss when it occurs (as it will, in compliant patients who exercise and eat a healthy diet).

Regardless of which type of diabetes the patient has, it is important to teach patients who are using insulin about which factors put them at risk for hypoglycemia and how to watch for signs and symptoms of hypoglycemia (see BOX 9-5). Early intervention can help prevent serious adverse outcomes. Patients at risk of ketoacidosis (those with T1DM, pregnant patients, and patients with T2DM combined with severe insulin resistance or who present with an infection) should be advised of the warning signs of ketoacidosis and of the need to go to an emergency department for treatment with intravenous insulin and fluids promptly if this imbalance is suspected.

Another important teaching point for patients with diabetes of any type is the effects of corticosteroid drugs on blood glucose levels. Particularly in patients with co-occurring conditions such as asthma or severe allergies who may use corticosteroids such as prednisone on a repeated basis, it is essential to make them aware that hyperglycemia, often severe, is a side effect of such medications. It is not unusual for blood glucose levels to rise to in excess of 350 mg/dL in response to a dose of prednisone, and the insulin resistance that accompanies the drug can defeat efforts to reduce blood glucose levels, even with high doses of insulin, until the drug is discontinued. Most physicians hesitate to prescribe such drugs to patients with diabetes—and with good reason—but in some situations, there are no appropriate alternatives. Ideally, doses of insulin and/or hypoglycemic medications will be temporarily adjusted to compensate for the duration of the steroid use.

Oral and Injectable Hypoglycemic Medications

Hypoglycemic medications may be used when the pancreas secretes some insulin, but not enough to meet the body's needs (often the case in LADA or MODY), or when the body is unable to utilize the insulin that is present due to insulin resistance. Almost all such medications are used as single agents in combination with diet and exercise when treating diabetes, and it has been suggested that more aggressive intervention can prove beneficial if combinations of medications are tailored to the patient (Inzucchi et al., 2012; Moon et al., 2017). There are several categories of hypoglycemic drugs: insulin secretagogues, insulin sensitizers, α-glucosidase inhibitors, and glucagon-like peptide (GLP-1) agonists. Most are well absorbed through the GI tract and are administered in oral form, although some are given by injection.

BOX 9-5 Hypoglycemia Basics

Signs and symptoms of hypoglycemia may include the following:

- Confusion
- Double or blurred vision
- Shakiness
- Weakness
- Dizziness
- Sweating
- Hunger

Risk factors for hypoglycemia include the following:

- Too much medicine (insulin or oral hypoglycemic)
- Not enough food
- Too much exercise/activity/stress

Insulin Secretagogues

Insulin secretagogues are drugs that stimulate the beta cells in the pancreas to make more insulin, effectively enabling it to overpower cellular insulin resistance. The pancreas must have functioning beta cells for secretagogues to be effective, so these agents are used primarily in T2DM and LADA, but not in T1DM. Some of these drugs may also be used in GDM if they do not cross the placental barrier; those that do cross this barrier carry the risk of stimulating harmful insulin production in the developing fetus. Common adverse effects are related to hypoglycemia, which is usually the effect of too much medication or inadequate carbohydrate intake.

This class of drugs is primarily composed of sulfonylureas and meglitinides. **Meglitinides** include **nateglinide** and **repaglinide**. **Sulfonylureas** were some of the first oral medications used

to treat T2DM; first-generation sulfonylurea medications include **tolbutamide**, **chlorpropamide**, and **tolazamide**, while newer drugs in this class include **glipizide**, which is shorter acting; and **glyburide**, **glibenclamide**, and **gimepride**, which are longer acting. Both sulfonylureas and meglitinides inhibit adenosine triphosphate-sensitive potassium channels of the beta cell membrane (see FIGURE 9-7), thereby increasing intracellular calcium levels and promoting release of insulin's precursor to raise insulin levels (Coustan, 2007; Landgraf, 2000). Secondary effects include suppression of glucose release and insulin clearance in the liver and decrease in lipolysis. Of these drugs, only **glyburide** has been conclusively shown to cross the placental barrier to a small extent or not at all; the others either cross the placental barrier to a degree that has the potential to harm the fetus

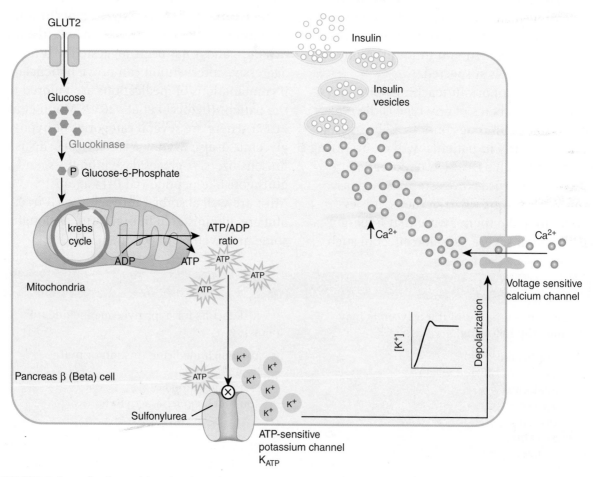

FIGURE 9-7 How sulfonylureas and meglitinides inhibit potassium channels of the beta cell membrane.

(Shepherd, Brook, Chakera, & Hattersley, 2017) or data are unclear about placental transfer (Simmons, 2015).

Insulin Sensitizers

Insulin-sensitizing agents do exactly what their name implies: They cause the body to need less insulin and to use available insulin more effectively in patients who are insulin resistant. **Biguanides** are currently represented by one drug, **metformin**, and **thiazolidinediones** by **pioglitazone**. A second thiazolidinedione, **rosiglitazone**, has limited exposure due to FDA concerns about associated cardiovascular risks (Hiatt, Kaul, & Smith, 2013). These two hypoglycemic subgroups act differently from sulfonylureas in that instead of causing more insulin to be released, they block glucose from entering the blood by decreasing glucose production from the liver and reducing glucose absorption in the intestines. They also increase insulin sensitivity, allowing for improved glucose uptake. This lowers basal and postprandial blood glucose levels in patients with T2DM. Because insulin sensitizers do not increase insulin levels within the body, patients taking such medications have a lower risk of hypoglycemia than patients taking sulfonylureas. Both biguanides and thiazolidinediones are effective in controlling blood glucose, but **metformin** has a superior safety profile; for this reason, **metformin** formulations are frequently part of the first-line treatment of T2DM, along with diet and exercise, while **pioglitazone** is used in those patients who do not respond well to **metformin**.

α-Glucosidase Inhibitors

α-Glucosidase is an enzyme necessary for glycogen-to-glucose degradation. α-Glucosidase inhibitors, like insulin sensitizers, block absorption of glucose in the digestive tract by reversibly binding to pancreatic α-amylase and intestinal α-glucosidase to reduce insulin requirements. The two medications in this class that are currently available in the United States are **acarbose** and **miglitol**. They are taken with meals to limit postprandial glycemic rises and as a result can be used for both T1DM and T2DM in patients in whom hyperglycemia is the primary concern. Use of these medications can reduce insulin usage in patients administering **insulin** and, more importantly, limit glycosylation of hemoglobin. Therefore, HbA_{1c} levels are reduced (Bischoff, 1994). These medications should not be used in individuals who are prone to hypoglycemia.

Incretin Mimetics

Incretins are hormones secreted by the intestine in response to food passing through that part of the GI tract. The two main incretins are glucagon-like peptide-1 (GLP-1) and glucose-dependent insulinotropic polypeptide (GIP). Glucagon-like peptide-1 (GLP-1) functions in a way that is beneficial for patients with diabetes: It promotes insulin release in the pancreas, slows glucose absorption in the gut, and suppresses release of *glucagon*, a pancreatic hormone that elevates the release of glucose by the liver. A synthetic incretin, **exenatide**, mimics natural GLP-1 to produce these actions, resulting in lower overall glucose levels, particularly the postprandial blood glucose peaks. This agent is also an appetite suppressant, which helps patients achieve weight loss. However, the drug is available only in injectable form and must be injected 1 hour before eating; both the delivery form and the inconvenient timing are factors that may discourage some patients from using **exenatide**. It carries a risk of hypoglycemia due to its dual activity in promoting insulin secretion while reducing glucose uptake.

Nursing Process

Assess

Patients should be assessed for contraindications to hypoglycemic drug use. In patients with T1DM and patients who are prone to hypoglycemia, agents that are associated with hypoglycemia as a side effect should not be used. In the case of **metformin**, contraindications include renal or hepatic impairment or any condition with increased risk of lactic acid production (liver disease, severe infection, excessive alcohol intake, shock, and hypoxemia).

Pregnancy, whether in a patient previously diagnosed with T1DM/T2DM or a patient who is at significant risk of GDM, is typically regarded as a contraindication to most hypoglycemic medications unless there are significant overriding factors. This is because many of the newer drugs lack information concerning their effects on a developing fetus, and most are considered to carry some risk. There is no evidence of fetal toxicity in either animal or human studies regarding metformin use. Although the drug's long-term impact on the fetus is unknown, there is no convincing evidence of fetal malformation when taken in early pregnancy (Lindsay & Loeken, 2017). Several controlled studies in human pregnancies in women with PCOS—a group prone to insulin resistance and diabetes—have found that metformin offered no benefit in preventing GDM or in reducing glucose levels during pregnancy (Legro, 2010). Glyburide is generally, if cautiously, regarded as safe during pregnancy despite conflicting data on the risks and benefits of treating pregnant women with GDM (Kimber-Trojnar et al., 2014), with some data pointing to increased risk of neonatal hypoglycemia (Song et al., 2017; Zeng et al., 2014).

Patient Education

The most significant obstacle to adequate diabetes care with hypoglycemic drugs is patient compliance. Providers must recognize that patient compliance is due to a number of factors at the system, medication, and patient levels (American Diabetes Association [ADA], 2016), or based on nonpatient factors, patient demographics, patient beliefs about medications, and perceived patient burden (Polonsky & Henry, 2016). The American Diabetes Association recommends employing a patient-centered communication style,

aligning care with the Chronic Care Model, and supporting team-based care with community involvement (ADA, 2016).

Education of patients regarding medication actions and effects is crucial. It is especially important to inform patients that most of these medications—but particularly those that block glucose absorption—must be taken in conjunction with a meal and to offer advice on the importance of timing the medication correctly. Failure to eat after a dose of any such medication carries a risk of hypoglycemia, which can be traumatic to the patient even if no actual lasting harm occurs.

As with patients who use insulin, the signs and symptoms of hypoglycemia and, where applicable, ketoacidosis should be reviewed with patients taking hypoglycemic drugs. Likewise, the effects of corticosteroid medications should be reviewed with those patients likely to require or use such medications, particularly patients newly diagnosed with diabetes who have a history of using such medications.

Thyroid Disorders

As noted earlier, there are two basic types of thyroid disorder: excessive production of thyroid hormones (hyperthyroidism) and inadequate production of thyroid hormones (hypothyroidism). The latter is more common and is most often caused by chronic lymphocytic thyroiditis or Hashimoto's thyroiditis (an autoimmune disorder). Hypothyroidism may also be a side effect of the treatment of hyperactive thyroid disease. Regardless of the cause, hypothyroidism is almost universally treated with hormone replacement therapy.

Graves' disease, which is also autoimmune in nature, is the most common cause of hyperthyroidism, the result of an overactive or overstimulated thyroid gland. Treatments include blocking the stimulus to the thyroid gland with medication, or deactivating the thyroid gland with radioactive iodine so that it no longer produces thyroid hormones.

Thyroid Hormone Replacement

Identification of the underlying cause of hypothyroidism is important in choosing the correct thyroid therapy. Lack of dietary iodine can lead to hypothyroidism (three atoms of iodine are needed to make T_3, and four iodine atoms for T_4). Dietary supplementation would be adequate treatment in such cases, so increasing the availability of iodine-rich foods such as seafood, eggs, or dried seaweed used for sushi, or even switching to an iodized table salt, could be all that is required. Pituitary disorders—usually benign tumors that suppress the production of TSH—can also lead to hypothyroidism; these conditions need to be treated at the source. Hypothyroidism may also be a secondary effect of adrenal dysfunction, specifically hypercortisolism (Arnaldi et al., 2003), as high cortisol levels tend to suppress thyroid precursor hormones (TRH and TSH). However, hypercortisolism also unmasks existing autoimmune hypothyroidism, so while treating hypercortisolism might resolve hypothyroidism, patients should be monitored to ensure this is the case.

In hypothyroidism that results from dysfunction in the thyroid itself (congenital or acquired hypothyroidism), **levothyroxine sodium**, a synthetic T_4 hormone, is indicated as replacement or supplementation of T_4. This medication may also be used as treatment for, or to prevent, euthyroid goiters.

Synthetic T_4 has a mechanism of action identical to naturally occurring thyroid hormone, although the mechanism of thyroid hormones' action in cells is not well understood. Synthetic thyroid hormone increases oxygen consumption in most tissues and stimulates the basal metabolic rate, heat production (thermogenesis), and the metabolism of carbohydrates, lipids, and proteins. Common adverse reactions of thyroid replacement therapy are related to symptoms of hyperthyroidism resulting from the increased metabolic rate actions of T_4 and T_3, which include tachypnea, tachycardia, weight loss, fever, and anxiety. Side effects may occur in any system of the body because of the wide-ranging effects of thyroid hormones.

Nursing Process

Assess

Patients should be assessed for the likelihood of dietary causes for hypothyroidism prior to starting **levothyroxine** therapy. Patients should also be assessed for potential contraindications to thyroid replacement therapy, including any of the following conditions:

- Untreated subclinical or overt thyrotoxicosis, which would be significantly worsened by use of **levothyroxine**
- Acute myocardial infarction, because use of **levothyroxine** may increase oxygen consumption in cells
- Uncontrolled adrenal insufficiency (correcting adrenal insufficiency may correct hypothyroidism)
- Known hypersensitivity to the medication (although this is very rare)

Thyroid medications are available in a series of graduated doses. For most patients, **levothyroxine** replacement dose is related to body mass; a daily dose of about 1.6 mcg **levothyroxine**/kg body mass is adequate replacement for most adults. This is equivalent to 100 mcg daily or 125 mcg daily for an average-size woman or man, respectively (Vaidya & Pearce, 2008). In otherwise healthy patients, this dose may be used as initial therapy; however, in frail or elderly patients, particularly those with cardiac comorbidities (discussed later), it is prudent to start at a lower dose of about 25 mcg and gradually increase to one that is well tolerated. In either case, the patient's TSH and T_4 levels should be rechecked at least six weeks post initiation to determine whether the dose is adequate. The dose may thereafter be adjusted upward in increments of 12.5–25 mcg until serum TSH reaches a normal range (e.g., 0.5–4.0) and clinical symptoms have subsided. In patients with autoimmune hypothyroidism, it is not uncommon for the dose to gradually increase over time as the damage done by the autoimmune disease process expands. Patients should have thyroid hormone levels checked at least yearly, and more often if symptomatic or if optimal dosing has not yet been established.

In patients with established disease, blood work should be performed to check the TSH level and, if the patient's prior levels have been unstable, the free T_4 level. Free T_3 rarely needs to be checked unless the clinician has reasons to suspect an alternative diagnosis.

A number of special considerations arise when using thyroid hormones to treat hypothyroidism. Patients with diabetes who are put on thyroid replacement therapy may require increased doses of **insulin**/oral hypoglycemic medications, because thyroid hormones increase glucose absorption, utilization, and production. Patients taking anticoagulants may require a lower dose of the anticoagulant after their thyroid levels and metabolic rate are normalized. In patients with hypothyroidism prior to pregnancy, thyroid levels decrease as early as the fifth week of gestation, so the dose should be increased early in gestation to avoid cognitive impairment in the fetus (Alexander et al., 2004). **Levothyroxine** is considered safe for use in pregnant women. Patients who begin taking calcium supplements may experience recurrence of hypothyroid symptoms if taken at the same time as their thyroid replacement hormone (see the "Patient Education" section).

Patient Education

Hypothyroidism is an easy disorder to treat, *if patients are compliant with their medication regimen and testing protocol*. However, many patients lack understanding of the importance of the thyroid to overall health, so they may not take the need for compliant use of medication seriously. It is important to educate patients that daily use of the medication and communication of hypothyroid signs and symptoms to healthcare providers is crucial to maintain long-term health. Patients also need to understand that finding the level at which they have no hypothyroid symptoms may take some time, particularly if they have been suffering from undiagnosed subclinical hypothyroidism for a prolonged time. Patients need to understand that treatment for this disease process is a lifelong treatment plan and even if they begin to feel better on the medication, they need to continue their daily doses.

Levothyroxine is best taken daily on an empty stomach, at whichever time the patient finds to be both most convenient and most likely to promote compliance with the need to take the medication (1) daily *and* (2) in a fasting state.

Calcium carbonate supplements have a known suppressive effect on **levothyroxine** therapy. Studies suggest that taking these supplements within four hours of taking **levothyroxine** can cause the **levothyroxine** to adsorb to the **calcium carbonate** and thus reduce its bioavailability, but if the timing of the drug and the supplement are appropriately spaced, there should be no interaction (Mazokopakis, Giannakopoulos, & Starakis, 2011). Patients who are already taking a calcium supplement, such as **calcium carbonate** when initiating **levothyroxine** therapy or who use dairy products as a means of supplementing their calcium intake should be advised to take the supplements/dairy foods in the afternoon or evening if they take **levothyroxine** in the morning (or vice versa). In general, if calcium intake is separated from **levothyroxine** dosing by at least four hours, there should be no interaction.

Because iatrogenic hyperthyroidism is a risk in patients with hypothyroidism, they should be educated about the symptoms of both hypothyroidism and hyperthyroidism as well as the health ramifications should either condition be undertreated.

Thyroid Hormone Suppression

Hyperthyroidism occurs when patients have excessive output of thyroid hormones. The impact of this condition on body functions may be dramatic, as it represents a "revving of the engine" in multiple organ systems. Hyperthyroidism causes the overall metabolic rate to increase, resulting in rapid heart-beat/palpitations, hypertension, weight loss, nervousness/anxiety, abnormal liver function, and, in some cases, hypercortisolism with associated hyperglycemia.

Patients with untreated hyperthyroidism are at risk of a condition referred to as thyrotoxicosis, or *thyroid storm*. This condition is also a risk factor in patients treated for hyperthyroidism with partial rather than total thyroidectomy. It is triggered by exposure to a physiological stressor, such as trauma or infection. The symptoms of thyroid storm include agitation, altered mental state, confusion, diarrhea, fever, tachycardia, shaking/shivering, sweating, high blood pressure (especially systolic), and respiratory symptoms consistent with congestive heart failure or pulmonary edema.

In patients in whom this condition is related to pituitary or hypothalamic dysfunction (excess output of precursor hormones), treatment includes removal of any neoplasms that may be producing exogenous TSH or TRH to stimulate excess T_4 production. However, in other situations, the cause is endemic to the thyroid itself. The most common cause of hyperthyroidism is Graves' disease, an autoimmune condition that causes thyroid hyperplasia. In such instances, there are a number of options for treating the dysfunction: (1) removal of part or all of the thyroid gland (often followed by **levothyroxine** therapy); (2) ablation of the thyroid with radioactive iodine; or (3) medications to decrease the production of TSH, which in turn decreases the amount of thyroid

hormone produced by the thyroid gland. **Methimazole** and **propylthiouracil (PTU)** are the drugs most commonly used for treating hyperthyroidism.

Many medications interact with **methimazole** and **PTU**. For example, a patient with hyperthyroidism will have increased metabolism of **theophylline**, a medication used in the treatment of respiratory disorders. As medical treatment for hyperthyroid becomes effective (which may take weeks to months, due to the thyroid's ability to store large amounts of hormone), serum **theophylline** levels may increase due to the reduction in the rate of metabolism. Careful monitoring of all medications is important during the first few months of hyperthyroid treatment.

Methimazole and **PTU** both pose a risk of teratogenicity; thus, women who are of childbearing age should use birth control to prevent pregnancy when taking these medications. If already pregnant when the condition develops, a consultation with a maternal/fetal specialist (perinatologist) is warranted, as hyperthyroidism creates a number of risks to the pregnancy. Despite the potential for birth defects, the benefits of treatment outweigh the increased risk of pre-eclampsia, premature labor, and miscarriage. For treating hyperthyroidism during pregnancy, **PTU** is preferred during the first trimester, as the risk of congenital anomaly is thought to be lower. **Methimazole** is preferred in the second and third trimesters.

Nursing Process

Assess

In newly diagnosed patients who are initiating medical therapy, baseline vital signs are obtained with the goal of identifying current metabolic status. Comprehensive assessment of the patient's cardiac status to identify potential cardiac complications includes blood pressure measurements (prone, seated, standing), electrocardiogram (rate, rhythm, presence of dysrhythmias), and heart rate. Oxygenation and respiratory rate are other key observations, as are mental status, weight, and sleep patterns. The goal of therapy is to bring all elevated processes into a more normal, well-regulated state; by measuring baseline values at time of diagnosis, the nurse can gain an appreciation for whether the therapy is working over time. It is important to recognize that medical therapy does not work for all patients; only 20% to 30% of patients with hyperthyroidism achieve remission after 12 to 18 months of medical therapy (Iagaru & MacDougall, 2007).

Nurses should be aware that the patient's condition affects his or her response to surroundings and take steps to alleviate discomfort. Reduce the exam room's temperature or, if that is not possible, provide cool compresses to a patient who feels overheated. If possible, offer the patient privacy in a quiet room to reduce anxiety and nervousness. Offer eye shades or eyedrops to patients who demonstrate or complain of photosensitivity or dry eyes.

Watch for signs of agranulocytosis (decrease in white blood cell count), such as sudden onset of fever and sore throat, during treatment with either **PTU** or **methimazole**.

In patients who have been previously treated, the assessment should include signs of treatment failure—such as lack of stabilization of weight (continued weight loss), presence of tremula, anxiety, tachycardia, heat intolerance, or exophthalmos. Patients who have previously been treated with partial thyroidectomy should be assessed for the possibility of thyrotoxicosis if symptomatic.

Patient Education

Patients suffering from hyperthyroidism are "stuck on high"; it is therefore important to teach them to avoid environmental triggers that impact their metabolic rate until their therapy successfully brings them into a euthyroid state. Teach patients to avoid stimulants such as coffee, sweets, tea, soft drinks, energy bars, and cigarette smoking. The patient's diet should be high in calories and protein; suggest protein shakes as between-meal snacks to supplement intake. Stress-reduction techniques such as meditation, cognitive-behavioral therapy, yoga, and other relaxation modalities should be recommended.

Polycystic Ovary Syndrome (PCOS)

PCOS is a complex endocrine disorder in women that disrupts a number of body functions: reproductive, cardiovascular, glucose transport, and often other key metabolic processes such as thyroid function. Its origins are poorly understood, but the common factor seems to be an imbalance in two pituitary gonadotropins—LH and FSH. Normally, LH stimulates theca cells in ovarian follicles to produce androgens; these androgens are then converted to estrogen by aromatase, which is expressed in the granulosa cells of the follicle. Meanwhile, FSH stimulates granulosa cells to produce inhibin (which suppresses FSH in a negative feedback loop) and promote oocyte development. In PCOS, for reasons that are not clear, LH is overproduced while FSH is either normal or underproduced. This imbalance leads to development of a self-reinforcing feedback loop (FIGURE 9-8) in which the excess LH leads to excess androgens, but the lack of stimulation by FSH means that the granulosa cells are unable to stimulate follicle development. However, aromatase in body tissues (especially adipocytes, which is why obesity contributes) allows some of the excess androgens to be converted to estrogen, so that the feedback loop of estrogen prompts continued release of LH.

Women with PCOS, therefore, have excess androgens and often relatively high estrogen levels but low progesterone. This combination frequently leads to menstrual irregularities and infertility, as the follicles fail to fully develop within the ovary (although this does not happen in all women

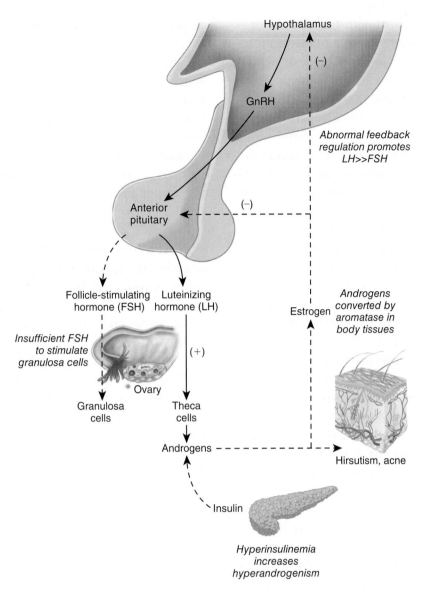

FIGURE 9-8 Hormonal Interactions in PCOS.

with PCOS). In addition, the presence of excess androgens in women is associated with insulin resistance, although determining the nature of this association has proved challenging. Otherwise-healthy women treated with testosterone, for example, are more likely to develop insulin resistance (Corbould, 2008), but whether that is an effect of the androgen increase or another, preexisting condition that is unmasked by exogenous androgen use is difficult to identify. Either way, it is clear that the elevated androgen levels exacerbate glucose intolerance in women and leave them at risk of metabolic syndrome and diabetes.

PCOS is very common, affecting as many as 15% to 20% of women to some degree (Sirmans & Pate, 2014). Most women with this condition are diagnosed in their teens or early 20s as a result of the menstrual irregularities and physical effects such as excessive body hair (hirsutism), acne, and central (abdominal) weight gain associated with the disorder, all of which can contribute to psychosocial problems such as the depression and other mental health issues commonly observed in women with PCOS (Barry, Kuczmierczyk, & Hardiman, 2011; Conte, Banting, Teede, & Stepto, 2015). PCOS is also a significant risk factor for many chronic disease states with nearly 60% of PCOS patients being obese and insulin resistant, and 40% developing T2DM, dyslipidemia, and cardiac disease (McGowan, 2011). It is important to treat this syndrome to help reduce these long-term negative health consequences.

First-line therapy for PCOS involves lifestyle changes, including nutritional counseling and exercise to help stave off the threat of diabetes by promoting weight loss and improved glucose metabolism, both of which contribute to stabilization of some of the more distressing syndromes related to the condition. When efforts at lifestyle therapy are inadequate or unsuccessful, medications are selected based on the specific metabolic disorders observed in each patient, including insulin resistance and anovulation/menstrual irregularities related to high androgen levels.

Insulin-sensitizing drugs such as metformin are frequently used in patients with insulin-resistance (see the earlier discussion of these agents in the diabetes section). To address menstrual irregularities and anovulation, a number of medications may be prescribed. Women who are not trying to become pregnant are typically prescribed hormone-based oral contraceptives to help reduce free testosterone levels. These medications are composed of ethinyl estradiol (which reduces secretion of LH and FSH in the pituitary) and a progestin (e.g., norgestimate, norethindrone, desogestrel, and particularly drospirenone, which itself has anti-androgen effects). Use of these medications establishes regular menstrual cycles, suppresses circulating androgens, and increases production of the sex-hormone–binding globulin, which binds to testosterone and estrogen and helps further decrease androgen levels.

Use of oral contraceptives may be enough to alleviate unwanted hair growth, but if not, an androgen-blocking agent, such as spironolactone may be added, with the precaution that the patient must be compliant with her oral contraceptives while using it,

as pregnancy should be avoided while using this medication. Leuprolide, a GnRh receptor suppresses secretion of LH and FSH, subsequently suppressing gonadal sex steroid production. Finasteride inhibits the type 2 isoenzyme of 5-α-reductase, which is responsible for dihydrotestosterone-to-testosterone conversion. Leuprolide and finasteride may be used to reduce hirsutism in some patients but should be prescribed only if oral contraceptives plus spironolactone do not work. Eflornithine cream is thought to inhibit the skin activity of ornithine decarboxylase, thus reducing the rate of hair growth and is sometimes used to treat facial hirsutism (Kumar, Naguib, Shi, & Cui, 2016; Vissing, Taudorf, Haak, Philipsen, & Haedersdal, 2016).

In women who *are* trying to conceive, of course, use of contraceptives will not be helpful. For these women, emphasis is placed on following lifestyle guidelines intensively for approximately 6 to 12 months; the goal is for such patients to lose weight, stabilize glucose metabolism, and reduce circulating androgens by this mechanism before making use of either the selective estrogen receptor modulator clomiphene citrate or, less frequently, the aromatase inhibitor letrozole to induce ovulation (Kamath & George, 2011). Clomiphene binds to estrogen receptors and induces ovulation by promoting release of additional gonadotropins from the pituitary. Letrozole prevents conversion of androgens to estrogen, thereby eliminating a negative feedback loop that suppresses gonadotropin release. In either case, the result is increased FSH secretion from the anterior pituitary; in many women, that effect is enough to promote ovulation. Standard therapy for clomiphene citrate is an oral dose timed to the woman's menstrual cycle, so that she begins taking the medication on the second to fifth day after the onset of menstruation and then once per day for five consecutive days. The dose starts at 50 mg and, if ineffective, may be increased by 50 mg at each subsequent cycle until pregnancy occurs or a maximum dose of 250 mg is reached, whichever comes first. Approximately 52% of women treated with the lowest dose ovulate in their first cycle post treatment; of the remaining 48%, all but 2% will ovulate at a higher dose (Practice Committee for Reproductive Medicine, 2013). Triggering ovulation does not, of course, automatically mean pregnancy will be achieved; only 40% to 45% of infertile women treated with clomiphene become pregnant (Kamath & George, 2011).

Nursing Process

Assess

Women presenting with PCOS should first be assessed for understanding the relationship among diet, exercise, and relief of PCOS symptoms. It has been shown repeatedly in clinical practice that diet and exercise are the first-line therapy for PCOS (Ravn, Haugen, & Glintborg, 2013), and even where medications are used, they should be regarded as adjunct treatments.

The patient's blood pressure and fasting blood glucose should be measured, and a lipid panel drawn to assess for elevated cholesterol. Dietary counseling to identify ways to reduce caloric intake and avoid sources of cholesterol should be provided. Before starting any therapy intended to address PCOS-related symptoms, a negative pregnancy test must be obtained; while PCOS frequently renders women infertile, some can and do get pregnant, and use of oral contraceptives and certain other medications is not recommended in pregnant women.

Once pregnancy has been ruled out, discuss the patient's wishes for future childbearing. Does she desire children? If so, is she ready to begin the process of trying to conceive, or is having children something she wants to do in the future? The answers to these questions help identify whether a particular therapy (e.g., oral contraceptives and/or spironolactone) may or may not be appropriate.

Patient Education

Educating the patient on combining lifestyle therapy with medication is a critical component of successful therapy for PCOS. It may be difficult for patients to recognize that the prescription they have been given is merely an adjunct, and that the dietary and exercise regimen recommended to them is the real "cure" that they seek. For women seeking relief of infertility, identifying a two-part goal of (1) being able to *get* pregnant and (2) being able to have a *healthy* pregnancy via preconception weight loss and insulin resensitization may be extremely valuable.

For women who wish to undertake clomiphene citrate therapy to induce ovulation, strong encouragement to lose weight prior to attempting the regimen may help in its success. When therapy is initiated, the timing and dosing of the five-day cycle should be carefully outlined (in writing as well as verbally). Referral to a reproductive endocrinologist may be needed if clomiphene citrate therapy does not result in ovulation or pregnancy.

In women not seeking pregnancy, education for the correct use of oral contraceptives is necessary, particularly if spironolactone is prescribed for reduction of hirsutism. Because oral contraceptives are associated with a risk of blood clots and stroke, patients who use tobacco should be counseled about smoking cessation. Patients should be educated on the signs and symptoms associated with blood clots and stroke, such as severe headache, abdominal pain, chest pain, visual changes, and leg pain.

Adrenal Disorders

As with thyroid disease, there are two forms of adrenal dysfunction: inadequate production of the two key adrenal hormones cortisol and aldosterone (adrenal insufficiency [Addison disease]) and excess production of these hormones (hyperaldosteronism [Conn disease] and hypercortisolism [Cushing disease]), which are nearly always due to an adenomatous tumor in either the pituitary or

> **Best Practices**
>
> In PCOS, the medication prescription the patient has been given is merely an adjunct; the dietary and exercise regimen recommended to her is the real "cure" that she seeks.

the adrenal gland that produces either exogenous aldosterone/cortisol or exogenous precursor hormones (ACTH or vasopressin).

Adrenal Insufficiency

Primary adrenal insufficiency (Addison disease) results when the cortex of the adrenal glands does not produce any, or enough, adrenocortical hormones—that is, corticosteroids. Secondary adrenal insufficiency occurs when the adrenal glands do not receive ACTH, which is secreted by the pituitary. Normally, ACTH binds to receptors in the adrenal cortex to stimulate the production of cortisol; thus, if the pituitary is not secreting enough ACTH, the body lacks an adequate supply of cortisol. The solution in either case is to replace the missing hormone(s).

Two commonly used medications mimic the key effects of cortisol and aldosterone and, therefore, are administered as hormone replacement. Prednisone (to replace cortisol) and fludrocortisone (to replace aldosterone) are corticosteroids used to treat adrenal insufficiency. Prednisone is metabolized by the liver into prednisolone, which then inhibits leukocyte infiltration, reducing inflammation and the humoral immune response. Fludrocortisone acts on the renal distal tubules, affecting sodium/potassium balance and helping to maintain blood volume and pressure. Side effects are dependent on the dose and duration of use. For treatment of Addison disease, the dose is smaller, replacing the naturally occurring amount of hormone, and not higher doses as indicated for an anti-inflammatory effect; therefore, side effects are minimal.

Nursing Process

Assess

In a patient presenting with symptoms and history suspicious for adrenal insufficiency, there are a number of ways to assess the likelihood of this rare condition. Ask the patient the following questions:

1. Do you have a history of recent infection, steroid use, or adrenal or pituitary surgery?
2. Do you have a history of poor tolerance for stress, weakness, fatigue, and intolerance for strenuous or moderate exercise?
3. Do you experience cravings for salty foods?
4. Have you recently experienced menstrual alterations or alterations in sexual function?
5. Have you recently experienced appetite disturbances, weight loss, anorexia, diarrhea, or nausea?
6. Have you recently experienced greater-than-normal loss of hair on your head or hair loss on your body?
7. Do you experience greater levels of fatigue or weakness at certain times of the day?

Positive answers to these questions, and a pattern of symptoms that are worse in the morning and improved in the evening, are suggestive of adrenal insufficiency.

In a patient with suspected adrenal insufficiency, assess for fever or elevated temperature and orthostatic hypotension. Patients' skin should be inspected for typical alterations in melanin characterized by "bronzing" of lighter skin areas such as scars, skin folds, or genitals. In addition, look for bluish-black discoloration in the oral and mucous membranes, and assess whether the membranes seem dry.

A key component to adrenal insufficiency is reduction of fluid volume and dehydration related to aldosterone deficiency. Thus, assessment of patients presenting with known or suspected adrenal insufficiency includes reviewing signs and symptoms such as condition of the mucosa, skin turgor, tachycardia, and blood pressure, with a goal of identifying and treating dehydration and limiting cardiac stress as quickly as possible. Electrolytes should be monitored, as hyperkalemia is common. Blood work to assess thyroid levels should be performed to obtain a baseline, as adrenal insufficiency may produce or unmask hypothyroidism; if the latter, the thyroid condition will require treatment after the adrenal insufficiency is resolved.

Patient Education

Patients should be counseled in the appropriate use of medications and likely side effects. The National Institutes of Health's patient education publication on adrenal insufficiency provides appropriate guidance for most patients. Patients with a history of adrenal insufficiency or new-onset diagnosis should be referred for psychosocial assessment, as emotional stress is frequently a trigger of adrenal crisis. Instruction on symptoms of adrenal insufficiency and when to notify a clinician of renewed symptoms should be provided.

Hypercortisolism (Cushing Disease)

Hypercortisolism is caused either by excess ACTH secretion or by autonomous cortisol release from the adrenal cortex and results, in general, from one of two causes: the presence of a cortisol- or ACTH-producing adenoma (usually in either the pituitary gland or the adrenal gland, although occasionally such tumors occur elsewhere) or long-term use of corticosteroids. In the latter case, the solution is to withdraw the causative drug under a clinician's care. In the former, surgery or radiotherapy to remove the adenoma is usually, but not always, the solution.

When surgery or radiation proves ineffective, medications may be used to suppress the synthesis and secretion of cortisol or its precursor, ACTH, or to block the effects of either one. Medication use is chronic, because while the drugs can halt the effects of the disorder, they do not actually alter the underlying pathology. For this reason, medical treatment is used in only patients who have a contraindication for surgery, who refuse surgery, in whom no adenoma can be located, who are waiting for radiation to take effect, or as part of a multifaceted approach when the pituitary tumor turns out to be cancerous (Castinetti, Morange, Conte-Devolx, & Brue, 2012). These medications include three established therapies—ketoconazole, mitotane, and metyrapone—and two more recent medications—mifepristone and pasireotide diaspartate.

The three older drugs all block cortisol production, but their main disadvantage is that none of these drugs is FDA approved for this use, nor are these medications normally administered at the doses needed to achieve the cortisol-blocking effect (DeSimone, Morales, & Vetter, 2010). When using ketoconazole, mitotane, or metyrapone, clinicians must pay close attention to side effects.

Mifepristone and pasireotide are both FDA approved for use in Cushing disease, but their mechanisms of reducing cortisol levels differ. Mifepristone is a competitive antagonist of glucocorticoid receptors, and binds to glucocorticoid receptors to prevent cortisol binding (Johanssen & Allolio, 2007); pasireotide binds to somatostatin receptors (subtypes 1, 2, 3, and 5) that are critical in triggering ACTH secretion (Colao et al., 2012). For mifepristone, cortisol cannot act upon the body, which reduces the effects of hypercortisolism; for pasireotide, cortisol's precursor hormone, ACTH, is suppressed, which is helpful in instances where ACTH overproduction is the cause of the condition (Colao et al., 2012).

Ketoconazole was previously a first-line choice for many clinicians due to its safety profile (DeSimone et al., 2010) until the approval of mifepristone and pasireotide. Although ketoconazole is actually an antifungal agent, its therapeutic drug action is attributed to one of its *side effect*s: it inhibits 17α-hydroxylase, an enzyme needed for cortisol production (Gross, Mindea, Pick, Chandler, & Batjer, 2007); therefore, use of ketoconazole reduces cortisol levels. However, the dose needs to be titrated up to therapeutic levels, so achieving relief of associated symptoms may take time. On average, ketoconazole has been found to induce remission in approximately 70% of patients using doses of 400–800 mg/day; its most common serious side effect, liver toxicity, occurs in 12% of patients according to one study (Gross et al., 2007), although overall risk of liver injury remains unclear (Greenblatt & Greenblatt, 2014). Another problem with this medication is its high level of drug–drug interactions with other medications due to its effects on CYP enzymes, which alters the body's ability to metabolize a great many common medication classes (e.g., benzodiazepines, some calcium-channel blockers, **theophylline**, **warfarin**, various medications for erectile dysfunction and some statin drugs). In addition, medications such as **phenytoin**, H_2-recepter blockers, and proton-pump inhibitors may decrease **ketoconazole** concentration in the bloodstream. **Ketoconazole** is a teratogen and pregnant patients should be counseled accordingly.

Mitotane is an anticancer drug that, like **ketoconazole**, inhibits several hydroxylase enzymes needed for cortisol synthesis—albeit different ones than **ketoconazole** (Gross et al., 2007). Like **ketoconazole**, **mitotane** must be titrated up to a therapeutic (high) dose of 4–12 g/day. In this dose range, the drug destroys cells in the adrenal cortex. Its most common side effects of nausea and hypercholesterolemia limit its use and make it the second-line choice after **ketoconazole**. **Mitotane** is also poses risk of teratogenicity, and pregnancy should not be attempted for at least two years after discontinuing the drug due to its long retention in the body (Castinetti et al., 2012).

Metyrapone works by blocking 11β-hydroxylase to halt cortisol production. This drug can be used as monotherapy, but it is most often used as adjunctive therapy with radiation or in combination with **mitotane** or **aminoglutethimide**. It must be titrated upward, usually starting at doses of 0.5–1 g and increasing to a maximum dose of 6 g (Gross et al., 2007). It is less effective than other agents and is not readily available, making it a less desirable option.

Mifepristone is better known for its FDA-approved use as the controversial abortifacient RU-486 and thus, its use is contraindicated in pregnancy (Patil & Edelman, 2015). Unlike the earlier-generation enzyme-blocking medications, **mifepristone** is a competitive antagonist, i.e., it blocks cortisol by binding directly to glucocorticoid receptors and, therefore, acts comparatively rapidly in addressing Cushing symptoms (Castinetti, Conte-Devolx, & Brue, 2010), including rapidly lowering elevated blood pressure and blood glucose levels. Its main drawback is that too high a dose can cause the patient to

acquire adrenal insufficiency, despite the patient having (as a result of the blockade of receptors) elevated ACTH and cortisol concentration; the only way to gauge if this is happening is to watch for clinical signs of adrenal insufficiency, including hypotension, hypoglycemia, and rapid weight loss. The high cortisol levels associated with too-high dosing also place the patient at significant risk of hypokalemia. Thus, patients using this medication need close monitoring to ensure maintenance of therapeutic levels.

Pasireotide was approved by the FDA in 2012 for treatment of Cushing disease due to corticotrophic (ACTH- or cortisol-producing) adenomas. It has a high affinity for somatostatin receptors, one of which (SSTR-5) is often overexpressed in pituitary adenomas. By binding to these receptors, **pasireotide** reduces the ability of these receptors to be activated and, therefore, dampens production of ACTH. However, while it is useful in decreasing cortisol concentration, it frequently does not normalize it (Arnaldi & Boscaro, 2010) and can cause worsening hyperglycemia in as many as one-third of patients taking it (Castinetti et al., 2012; Colao et al., 2014).

Nursing Process

Assess

Hypercortisolism brings with it risk of diabetes, hypertension, and cardiac dysfunction, including cardiac arrest. Patients should have a full workup for markers of these disorders at initial diagnosis; potassium and blood glucose levels should be monitored during treatment for all patients, but especially those on **mifepristone** or **metyrapone** (which cause hypokalemia) and **pasireotide** (which can cause hyperglycemia). Patients should be asked about symptoms of liver dysfunction, and follow-up testing may be required as some medications (**ketoconazole**) can be toxic to the liver. Active or past hepatitis, alcoholism, or other liver disease should be assessed. Liver function tests should be obtained if there is any reason for concern.

At each follow-up visit, patients should have their weight, blood pressure, blood glucose, and potassium levels measured. Particularly in patients on **mifepristone**, clinical signs consistent with adrenal insufficiency should be noted as a potential indicator of overtreatment.

Patient Education

Patients whose hypercortisolism is due to an adenoma that failed to respond to prior treatment or are unsuited to surgical or radiation treatment must be educated regarding the need for compliance with the medical regimen on a long-term basis. Medical therapy is not curative in the way that surgery or radiation can be; thus, patients who are not candidates for surgery or radiotherapy will likely require medication for the duration of their lives. The consequences of hypercortisolism are significant, so an understanding of the symptoms associated with diabetes, hypertensive crisis, cardiac issues, and so forth should be reviewed. Use of stimulants such as caffeine and nicotine should be discussed and discouraged, because they exacerbate the systemic stress that excess cortisol places on the body. Similarly, high-intensity exercise can be harmful in patients whose cortisol levels are abnormally high, even if they are not currently suffering from clinical symptoms of Cushing syndrome. Patients should be advised to choose lower-intensity exercise, including tai chi, walking, yoga, swimming, and other types of exercise that work the body without markedly raising heart rate or blood pressure.

Patients whose hypercortisolism is due to use of corticosteroid drugs will likely need to be switched to another, nonsteroid medication. Corticosteroids should not be stopped abruptly, but rather tapered over time, so that the adrenal glands (which reduce cortisol production in the presence of the drug) can increase production. Patients should be instructed how to gradually reduce corticosteroid doses in manners consistent with good practice, and informed of symptoms that could indicate too-rapid decrease, including severe fatigue, weakness, body aches, and joint pain. The time to fully withdraw from corticosteroids such as **prednisone** varies depending on the dose the patient took and for how long; tapering can take a week to several months.

Hyperaldosteronism (Conn Disease)

Hyperaldosteronism, like hypercortisolism, is a disease process in which the adrenal glands produce excess aldosterone. Aldosterone acts on the kidneys to regulate water, sodium, and potassium levels in the body, so excessive amounts lead to hypernatremia, hypokalemia, and fluid retention. Two types of primary hyperaldosteronism exist: Approximately 40% of cases result from an aldosterone-producing adenoma (APA; sometimes called an aldosteroma), while the remainder are due to idiopathic adrenal hyperplasia (IAH) in which both adrenal glands undergo thickening. There are also several forms of familial aldosteronism that are rare, accounting for fewer than 1% of cases (Chrousos & Sertedaki, 2012). Secondary hyperaldosteronism is usually the product of a disease process such as hypertension, heart failure, cirrhosis of the liver, or kidney disease (nephrotic syndrome). The discussion here focuses on treatment of primary hyperaldosteronism.

As is true of hypercortisolism, the preferred treatment for APA-related hyperaldosteronism is to remove the tumor responsible for the excess hormone secretion and treat any hormone deficiencies with replacement therapy. When this is not possible, medical therapy to suppress the effects of aldosterone is used. In IAH, surgical removal of one or both of the adrenal glands (IAH is rarely unilateral) can be enough to restore one in five patients to normal blood pressure levels, but most will also need suppression therapy. For this reason, patients with IAH-related primary aldosteronism are usually treated with medical therapy using **aldosterone antagonists** such as **spironolactone** or **eplerenone**, which inhibit sodium resorption through the renal nephron collecting ducts. If those drugs cannot be used, potassium-sparing diuretics such as **amiloride** are employed. The therapeutic regimen of choice is **spironolactone** combined with antihypertensive drugs, as some studies have shown this to be the most effective way of managing hypertension in these patients (Bloch & Basile, 2011). However, **spironolactone** does carry a higher risk of adverse effects than **eplerenone**, which is a more selective medication. Of these problems, the most serious potential side effect is hyperkalemia, which is significantly more likely in patients on **spironolactone** than in those taking **eplerenone** (Bloch & Basile, 2011).

Even with the aldosterone antagonists currently in use, many patients still suffer from some degree of high blood pressure. Numerous classes of drugs are used to treat hypertension; they will not be discussed here. The focus of this discussion is on medical treatment of the underlying disease process, and exploring the multitude of ways that clinicians tackle high blood pressure is the subject of other parts of this text (see Chapter 6). However, nurses should be aware that most, if not all, patients being treated for this disorder will be taking blood pressure medications, possibly from more than one class (e.g., angiotensin-converting enzyme inhibitors, calcium-channel blockers, thiazide diuretics), along with their aldosterone-suppression therapy. Such combinations may be challenging to manage. Blood pressure measurements should be taken with every visit, and some patients may need at-home blood pressure monitoring.

Critical Thinking Questions

1. Describe negative and positive feedback loops. Which alterations in feedback contribute to Cushing syndrome? To PCOS?

2. How are T1DM and T2DM different? What makes them similar? Which type is most similar to GDM, and why?

3. Which mental health effects would you expect to see in patients who have hypothyroidism? How do these differ from the effects of hyperthyroidism?

4. Name the hormones produced in the adrenal cortex and briefly describe their functions.

5. In a patient with very low TSH values, what would you expect to find if you measured free T_4? What might contribute to such findings in a patient being treated for hypothyroidism?

CASE STUDIES

Case Scenario 1

MG is a 61-year-old African American female who is a new patient to the primary care clinic where you are working as a nurse. Her chief complaint is fatigue that has been increasing over the past year. She also complains of hoarseness, and her friends have told her that her voice has deepened. She has gained weight over the last 6 months and has noticed some loss of muscle strength and difficulty getting around. Upon further questioning, she admits that she has to wear a sweater most of the time, even if others in the room are comfortable in light clothing. She takes one prescription and two OTC medications (noted in the following medication list). She started taking a multivitamin last month hoping that it would give her more energy, and she has been using an OTC stool softener daily for the last few months due to increasing problems with constipation. Her past medical history includes primary hypertension, diagnosed 10 years ago, that is well controlled with HCTZ. She denies diabetes or high cholesterol; she is post-menopausal. Her parents are deceased; her older sister has "thyroid trouble," but she knows of no other health problems in her family. She does not use any tobacco products, nor does she drink alcohol or use recreational drugs. She wears a step-counter and tries to walk at least 5,000 steps daily. She tries to follow the DASH diet recommendations. She is single, has two grown children, and is employed full-time as a librarian.

Medication list:
HCTZ 12.5 mg once daily
OTC calcium carbonate 500 mg BID
Multivitamin once daily
OTC docusate sodium 100 mg once daily
Allergies: NKDA
Vital signs: BP: 120/70; P: 60/minute, regular; Respirations: 12/minute, regular; Oral temperature: 97.0°F. Weight: 164#; Ht: 63"; BMI: 29.

During the history-taking part of the visit, you notice that MG has a deep voice and moves rather slowly. You also notice that her hair is sparse and coarse, and her skin is cool and dry.

The healthcare provider performs a thorough physical exam. She agrees with your observation that MG's skin is cool, dry, and coarse; her hair is sparse; and her eyebrows do not extend to the outer canthus. She also notes that MG has an enlarged tongue and a moderately enlarged thyroid gland without nodules. Her lung sounds are clear over all fields, and her heart is in regular sinus rhythm with no ectopic beats. Her abdomen is soft and non-tender, but stool is palpable in the left lower quadrant. Her deep tendon reflexes are slowed to 1+/4+ bilaterally, and she has 1+/4+ non-pitting dependent edema in both lower extremities.

Lab values from today's visit (normal values in parentheses): Free T4: 0.4 ng/dL (0.8–2.8 ng/dL); TSH: 12.4 IU/L (0.4–4.0 IU/L); Antithyroglobulin antibodies: positive (none detected). CBC, lipid panel, and CMP are within normal range.

The provider determines that MG has primary hypothyroidism due to autoimmune thyroiditis (also called Hashimoto disease). MG is to start taking levothyroxine 50 mcg once daily and return to check TSH in four to six weeks. The dosage may be titrated up after the next visit. You are to instruct MG about primary hypothyroidism, management with levothyroxine, and any relevant information regarding side effects or drug–drug interactions with this medication.

Case Questions

1. Based on data collected during history-taking and physical exam, you identify several areas where MG has needs that should be addressed. Write a nursing diagnosis that addresses one of these needs.

2. What is the half-life ($t_{1/2}$) for levothyroxine? How does the $t_{1/2}$ of levothyroxine relate to the timing for rechecking TSH? Why should the TSH be checked in four to six weeks rather than in one to two weeks?

3. MG asks you, "How did I get Hashimoto disease? Is it contagious?" How will you respond to her questions?

4. What do you need to know about the multivitamin she is taking? Are there any potential drug interactions between the levothyroxine and her other medications?

5. What important information should you provide for MG regarding taking her other medications and the levothyroxine? What time of day do you suggest MG takes the levothyroxine?

6. Write one short-term goal that can be met today regarding the nursing diagnosis you identified in question What intervention can you implement during the visit to meet this goal?

7. How might MG know that the levothyroxine is having its desired effect? What symptoms might indicate she needs to contact her provider to be seen sooner than four to six weeks?

8. MG asks about how long she will need to take levothyroxine. She is hoping that the medication will "take care of the problem" so she can get back to her "normal life." How will you respond to this question?

9. Outline one strategy to help MG be adherent to taking levothyroxine for the remainder of her life.

CASE STUDIES

Case Scenario 2

AV is a 46-year-old Hispanic male who presents to your primary care clinic for his six-month appointment "to check my blood pressure and cholesterol." Although this is a follow-up appointment, he admits to a chief complaint of nocturia three to four times each night that disrupts his quality of sleep. He also complains of increased thirst, fatigue, and mild blurred vision necessitating the use of reading glasses. He admits daytime urine frequency but relates it to drinking a lot of water and sugared caffeinated soda while working. He drinks one cup of coffee each morning. He has gained about 15 pounds over the last six months and admits to eating more between-meal high calorie snacks due to an irregular work schedule. He denies chest pain/pressure, palpitations, shortness of breath, cough, dysuria, difficulty starting urine stream, or incomplete bladder emptying. His past medical history includes primary hypertension diagnosed five years ago and well-controlled; dyslipidemia, diagnosed three years ago; and prediabetes diagnosed two years ago. He takes two prescription medications: one for HTN and one for high cholesterol. He denies OTC medications or herbal preparations. His parents live in a Central American country; both have diabetes, and his father recently had a myocardial infarction at age 66. His brothers both have high blood pressure, and one sister has diabetes. He knows of no other health problems in the family. He does not use any tobacco products or recreational drugs/substances; he drinks beer with his friends most weekends. He works in construction, so he reports he is physically active on his job. He knows about the DASH diet, but he does not follow it. He is married and has three children. He is literate in both Spanish and English.

Medication list:
Enalapril/HCTZ 10/25 mg one tab each morning
Atorvastatin 40 mg one tab daily at bedtime
Allergies: NKDA
Vital signs: BP: 134/78; P: 82/minute, regular; Respirations: 12/minute, regular; Oral temperature: 98.0°F. Weight: 230#; Ht: 69"; BMI: 34.

The healthcare provider performs a thorough physical exam. His fundoscopic exam shows no retinopathy. His lung sounds are clear over all fields, and his heart is in regular sinus rhythm with no ectopic beats. His abdomen is soft, non-tender, with no organomegaly. There is no suprapubic nor costovertebral angle tenderness. AV has no lower extremity edema and a normal response to monofilament fiber test of bilateral feet showing 10/10 sensation.

Lab values from today's visit (normal values in parentheses): Fasting plasma glucose: 210 mg/dL (<100 mg/dL); Hemoglobin A1c: 8.5% (5.7–6.4%: prediabetes; ≥ 6.5% diabetes); Urine glucose: 2+ (absent); Spot urine microalbumin/creatinine ratio: 45 mcg/mg (<30 mcg/mg); Serum creatinine: 0.98 (0.5–1.2 mg/dL).

The provider determines that AV has type 2 diabetes mellitus (T2DM) based on a fasting blood glucose >200 and hemoglobin A1c ≥ 6.5%. He also has mild microalbuminuria. He is to begin taking metformin 1,000 mg every 12 hours and insulin glargine 10 unit daily at bedtime. AV will be referred to the clinic diabetes nurse educator for diabetes self-management education; however, he will not be able to see this person until later this week. The glargine will not be titrated up until after AV sees the diabetes nurse educator. The provider asks you to teach AV about how to take his new medications and how to test his blood glucose. You are also to encourage AV to make at least one change in his dietary patterns before his next clinic visit. He is to be scheduled for a follow-up visit with the provider in one month.

Case Questions

1. Based on data collected during history-taking, physical exam, and lab results, you identify several areas where AV has a need that should be addressed. Choose two needs you assessed, and write nursing diagnoses that address these needs.

2. AV is going to start taking the biguanide metformin for the first time. Should you advise him to start with the full 1,000 mg dose twice daily? Why or why not?

(continues)

CASE STUDIES (CONTINUED)

3. Is it safe for AV to take his evening dose of metformin at the same time as he takes his insulin? Why or why not?

4. AV is your last patient of the day, and your clinic has some samples of insulin glargine in a prefilled pen of 100 units/ml. You decide to supervise his first injection of 10 units. Explain the steps he needs to follow to self-inject 10 units subcutaneously.

5. What important information should you provide for AV regarding expected side effects and adverse effects of both metformin and the basal insulin glargine?

6. What should AV do if he forgets to take a dose of his metformin? What should he do if he forgets to take his evening insulin dose?

7. You teach AV how to perform a finger stick to check his blood glucose, and he demonstrates correct technique. How often/when should he check his blood glucose during the first two to three days until he meets with the diabetes nurse educator?

8. Write one short-term goal that can be met today as you encourage AV to make at least one change in his dietary patterns before the next appointment. What intervention can you implement during today's visit to meet this goal?

9. Using the SMART goal format, write one long-term goal for AV directed toward adherence to his medication regimen.

10. Outline one strategy AV could use to promote medication adherence.

REFERENCES

Alexander, E.K., Marqusee, E., Lawrence, J., Jarolim, P., Fischer, G.A., & Larsen, P.R. (2004). Timing and magnitude of increases in levothyroxine requirements during pregnancy in women with hypothyroidism. *New England Journal of Medicine, 351,* 241–249.

American Diabetes Association (ADA). (2016). Standards of medical care in diabetes – 2016 abridged for primary care providers. *Clinical Diabetes, 34*(1), 3–21.

Arnaldi, G., Angeli, A., Atkinson, A.B., Bertangna, X., Cavagnini, F., Chrousos, G. P., . . . Boscaro, M. (2003). Diagnosis and complications of Cushing's syndrome: A consensus statement. *Journal of Clinical Endocrinology & Metabolism, 88*(12), 5593–5602.

Arnaldi, G., & Boscaro, M., (2010). Pasireotide for the treatment of Cushing's disease. *Expert Opinion on Investigational Drugs,* (7), 889–898.

Barry, J., Kuczmierczyk, A., & Hardiman, P.J. (2011). Anxiety and depression in polycystic ovary syndrome: A systematic review and meta-analysis. *Human Reproduction, 26,* 2442–2451.

Bischoff, H. (1994). Pharmacology of alpha-glucosidase inhibition. *European Journal of Clinical Investigation, 24*(Suppl. 3), 3–10.

Blakemore, C., & Jennett, S. (2001). Thymus. *Encyclpedia.com.* Retrieved from http://www.encyclopedia.com/topic/thymus_gland.aspx

Bloch, M.J., & Basile, J.N. (2011). Spironolactone is more effective than eplerenone at lowering blood pressure in patients with primary aldosteronism. *Journal of Clinical Hypertension, 13*(8), 629–631.

Castinetti, F., Conte-Devolx, B., & Brue, T. (2010). Medical treatment of Cushing's syndrome: Glucocorticoid receptor antagonists and mifepristone. *Neuroendocrinology, 92*(Suppl. 1), 125–130.

Castinetti, F., Morange, I., Conte-Devolx, B., & Brue, T. (2012). Cushing's disease. *Orphanet Journal of Rare Diseases, 7,* 41. Retrieved from http://www.ncbi.nlm.nih.gov/pmc/articles/PMC3458990/

Cernea, S., Buzzetti, R., & Pozzilli, P. (2009). β-cell protection and therapy for latent autoimmune diabetes in adults. *Diabetes Care, 32*(Suppl. 2), S246–S252.

Chrousos, G.P., & Sertedaki, A. (2012). Hyperaldosteronism. *Medscape Reference.* Retrieved from http://emedicine.medscape.com/article/920713-overview

Colao, A., De Block, C., Gaztambide, M.S., Kumar, S., Seufert, J., & Casanueva, F.F. (2014). Managing hyperglycemia in patients with Cushing's disease treated with pasireotide: Medical expert recommendations. *Pituitary, 17,* 180. doi: 10.1007/s11102-013-0483-3

Colao, A., Petersenn, S., Newell-Price, J., Finding, J.W., Gu, F., Maldonado, M., . . . Biller, B.M. (2012). A 12-month phase 3 study of pasireotide in Cushing's disease. *New England Journal of Medicine, 366*(10), 914–924.

Conte, F., Banting, L., Teede, H.J., & Stepto, N.K. (2015). Mental health and physical activity in women with polycystic ovary syndrome: A brief review. *Sports Medicine, 45,* 497. doi: 10.1007/s40279-014-0291-6

Corbould, A. (2008). Effects of androgens on insulin action in women: Is androgen excess a component of female metabolic syndrome? *Diabetes and Metabolic Research Review, 24*(7), 520–532.

Coustan, D.R. (2007). Pharmacological management of gestational diabetes: An overview. *Diabetes Care, 30*(Suppl. 2), S206–S208.

DeSimone, E.M., Morales, P.C., & Vetter, J.M. (2010). Management of Cushing's syndrome. *US Pharmacist, 35*(6), 25. Retrieved from http://www.uspharmacist.com/content/d/feature/i/1120/c/21057/

Greenblatt, H.K., & Greenblatt, D.J. (2014). Liver injury associated with ketoconazole: Review of the published evidence. *The Journal of Clinical Pharmacology, 54*(12), 1321–1329.

Gross, B.A., Mindea, S.A., Pick, A.J., Chandler, J.P., & Batjer, H.H. (2007). Medical management of Cushing disease. *Neurosurgical Focus, 23*(3), E10. Retrieved from http://www.medscape.com/viewarticle/566310_2

Hiatt, W.R., Kaul, S., & Smith, R.J. (2013). The cardiovascular safety of diabetes drugs – Insights from the rosiglitazone experience. *New England Journal of Medicine, 369*, 1285–1287.

Iagaru, A., & MacDougall, I.R. (2007). Treatment of thyrotoxicosis. *Journal of Nuclear Medicine, 48*(3), 379–389.

Inzucchi, S.E., Bergenstal, R.M., Buse, J.B., Diamant, M., Ferrannini, E., Nauck, M., . . . Matthews, D.R. (2012). Management of hyperglycemia in type 2 diabetes: A patient-centered approach: Position statement of the American Diabetes Association (ADA) and the European Association for the Study of Diabetes (EASD). *Diabetes Care, 35*(6), 1364–1379. doi: 10.2337/dc12-0413

Johanssen, S., & Allolio, B. (2007). Mifepristone (RU 486) in Cushing's syndrome. *European Journal of Endocrinology, 157*(5), 561–569.

Kalra, B., Gupta, Y., Singla, R., & Kalra, S. (2015). Use of oral anti-diabetic agents in pregnancy: A pragmatic approach. *North American Journal of Medical Sciences, 7*(1), 6–12. doi: 10.4103/1947-2714.150081

Kamath, M.S., & George, K. (2011). Letrozole or clomiphene citrate as first line for anovulatory infertility: A debate. *Reproductive and Biologic Endocrinology, 9*, 86. Retrieved from http://www.ncbi.nlm.nih.gov/pmc/articles/PMC3148573/

Kemp, S. (n.d.). Anatomy of the endocrine system. Retrieved from http://www.emedicinehealth.com/anatomy_of_the_endocrine_system/article_em.htm

Kimber-Trojnar, Z., Marciniak, B., Patro-Malysza, J., Skorzynska-Dziduszko, K., Ponjedzialek-Czaikowska, E., . . . Oleszczuk, J. (2014). Is glyburide safe in pregnancy? *Current Pharmaceutical Biotechnology, 15*(1), 100–112.

Kumar, A., Naguib, Y.W., Shi, Y., & Cui, Z. (2016). A method to improve the efficacy of topical eflornithine hydrochloride cream. *Drug Delivery, 23*(5), 1495–1501.

Landgraf, R. (2000). Meglitinide analogues in the treatment of type 2 diabetes mellitus. *Drugs and Aging, 17*(5), 411–425.

Legro, R.S. (2010). Metformin during pregnancy in polycystic ovary syndrome: Another vitamin bites the dust. *Journal of Clinical Endocrinology & Metabolism, 95*(12), 5199–5202.

Lindsay, R.S., & Loeken, M.R. (2017). Metformin use in pregnancy: Promises and uncertainties. *Diabetologia, 60*(9), 1612–1619. doi: 10.1007/s00125-017-4351-y

Mazokopakis, E.E., Giannakopoulos, T.G., & Starakis, I.K. (2011). Interaction between levothyroxine and calcium carbonate. *Canadian Family Physician, 54*(1), 39.

McDowell, J. (2011). *Encyclopedia of human body systems* (Vol. 1, pp. 151–206). Santa Barbara, CA: ABC-CLIO.

McGowan, M.P. (2011). Polycystic ovary syndrome: A common endocrine disorder and risk factor for vascular disease. *Current Treatment Options in Cardiovascular Medicine, 13*(4), 289–301.

Moon, M.K., Hur, K.-Y., Ko, S.-H., Park, S.-O., Lee, B.-W., Kim, J.H., . . . Committee of Clinical Practice Guidelines of the Korean Diabetes Association. (2017). Combination therapy of oral hypoglycemic agents in patients with type 2 diabetes mellitus. *Diabetes & Metabolism Journal, 41*(5), 357–366. doi: 10.4093/dmj.2017.41.5.357

Pardue, A., Dvoretz, I., Wright, C., Custard, A., Barbara, E., & Langat, D. (2017). Follicle stimulating hormone and reproductive aging. *The FASEB Journal, 31*(1), 935.3.

Patil, E., & Edelman, A. (2015). Medical abortion: Use of mifepristone and misoprostol in first and second trimesters of pregnancy. *Current Obstetrics and Gynecology Reports, 4*(1), 69–78.

Pedersen, I., Knudsen, N., Carlé, A., Schomburg, L., Köhrle, J., Jørgensen, T., . . . Laurberg, P. (2013). Serum selenium is low in newly diagnosed Graves' disease. *Clinical Endocrinology, 79*(4), 584–590.

Polonsky, W.H., & Henry, R.R. (2016). Poor medication adherence in type 2 diabetes: Recognizing the scope of the problem and its key contributors. *Patient Preference and Adherence, 10*, 1299–1307. doi: 10.2147/PPA.S106821

Practice Committee for Reproductive Medicine. (2013). Use of clomiphene citrate in infertile women: A committee opinion. *Fertility and Sterility, 100*, 341–348.

Ravn, P., Haugen, A.G., & Glintborg, D. (2013). Overweight in polycystic ovary syndrome: An update on evidence based advice on diet, exercise and metformin use for weight loss. *Minerva Endocrinologica, 38*(1), 59–76.

Rey, R.A., Campo, S.M., Ropelato, M.G., & Bergadá, I. (2016). Hormonal changes in childhood and puberty. In P. Kumanov & A. Agarwal (Eds.), *Puberty: Physiology and abnormalities* (pp. 23–37). Cham, Switzerland: Springer.

Rohlfing, C.L., Wiedmeyer, H.M., Little, R.R., England, J.D., Tennill, A., & Goldstein, D.E. (2002). Defining the relationship between plasma glucose and HbA$_{1c}$: Analysis of glucose profiles and HbA$_{1c}$ in the Diabetes Control and Complications Trial. *Diabetes Care, 25*, 275–278.

Schlüter, K.D., & Piper, H.M. (1998). Cardiovascular actions of parathyroid hormone and parathyroid hormone-related peptide. *Cardiovascular Research, 37*(1), 34–41.

Shepherd, M., Brook, A.J., Chakera, A.J., & Hattersley, A.T. (2017). Management of sulfonylurea-treated monogenic diabetes in pregnancy: Implications of placental glibenclamide transfer. *Diabetic Medicine, 34*, 1332–1339.

Simmons, D. (2015). Safety considerations with pharmacological treatment of gestational diabetes mellitus. *Drug Safety, 38*, 65. doi: 10.1007/s40264-014-0253-9

Sirmans, S.M., & Pate, K.A. (2014). Epidemiology, diagnosis, and management of polycystic ovary syndrome. *Clinical Epidemiology, 6*, 1–13. doi: 10.2147/CLEP.S37559

Skyler, J.S. (2004). DCCT: The study that forever changed the nature of treatment of type 1 diabetes. *British Journal of Diabetes and Vascular Disease, 4*(1), 29–32.

Song, R., Chen, L., Chen, Y., Si, X., Liu, Y., . . .Feng, W. (2017). Comparison of glyburide and insulin in the management of gestational diabetes: a meta-analysis. *PLoS One, 12*(8), e0182488. doi: 10.1371/journal.pone.0182488

Vaidya, B., & Pearce, S.H.S. (2008). Management of hypothyroidism in adults. *British Medical Journal, 337*, a801.

Vissing, A.C., Taudorf, E.H., Haak, C.S., Philipsen, P.A., & Haedersdal, M. (2016). Adjuvant eflornithine to maintain IPL-induced hair reduction in women with facial hirsutism: A randomized controlled trail. *Journal of the European Academy of Dermatology and Venereology, 30*(2), 314–319.

Zeng, Y.C., Li, M.J., Chen, Y., Jiang, L., Wang, S.M., Mo, X.L., & Li, B.Y. (2014). The use of glyburide in the management of gestational diabetes mellitus: A meta-analysis. *Advances in Medical Sciences, 59*(1), 95–101.

CHAPTER 10

Medications for Eye and Ear Disorders

Tara Kavanaugh

KEY TERMS

KEY TERMS

Acute otitis media (AOM)
Angle-closure glaucoma
Anterior chamber
Blood–retinal barrier
Carbonic anhydrase Cerumen
Ciliary muscle
Conjunctivitis
Cornea
Glaucoma
Impaction

Intraocular pressure (IOP)
Intravitreal
Iris
Iris sphincter
Iritis
Keratoconjunctivitis sicca
Lacrimation
Low- or normal-tension
    glaucoma
Middle ear

Miosis
Mucosal membranes
Open-angle glaucoma
Ophthalmic
Optic nerve
Otalgia
Otic
Otitis externa
Otitis media with
    effusion (OME)

Otorrhea
Peripheral vision
Periocular
Pupil
Retina
Tympanic membrane
Uveitis

CHAPTER OBJECTIVES

At the end of the chapter, the reader will be able to:

1. Demonstrate correct techniques for instillation of topical ophthalmic (eye) medications.

2. Identify the classes of medications used for treating glaucoma.

3. Identify the classes of medications used for treating dry eye disorders.

4. Describe appropriate use of ophthalmic antibiotic and steroid preparations.

5. Identify the classes of medications used in treating otic (ear) disorders.

6. Discuss nursing considerations for managing patients using medications to treat vision and otic/auditory dysfunction.

Introduction

Illnesses affecting the senses can be very disturbing to patients, but none affects day-to-day life like the loss of sight or hearing, whether temporary (e.g., in the case of an infection that obstructs vision or impairs hearing) or permanent. Any condition that impairs the ability to see or hear may have a profound effect on the patient's sense of well-being. When treating conditions that affect the eyes and ears, nurses should always be conscious of the likely impact of the problem on the patient's daily life and provide supportive care as needed. In this chapter, the medications used to treat a variety of illnesses of the eyes and ears are reviewed and discussed from a pharmacologic standpoint, with special attention paid to the impact of the illness and the medication on patient well-being.

Medications for Ophthalmic Disorders

The human eye is a complex and delicate organ, and in some respects it is difficult to treat when diseased or dysfunctional because of its anatomic configuration (**FIGURE 10-1**). Unlike most other areas of the body, the eye lacks a layer of skin for subcutaneous injection, and muscles and blood vessels are made relatively inaccessible by the bony socket surrounding each eye. While it *is* possible to inject medication directly into the eye via either **periocular** or **intravitreal** injection, these routes are uncomfortable to patients and require specialized training; moreover, with intravitreal injections, the distribution of drugs is often not uniform (Aldrich et al., 2013), making these routes useful in only a limited number of situations. Systemic administration via the intravenous or parenteral route presents the challenge of passing medication across the **blood–retinal barrier**, as blood that feeds the **retina** (including any medication molecules) must pass through this barrier before entering the eye (Aldrich et al., 2013). Only certain sizes of molecules can pass through the blood–retinal barrier, so medications delivered systemically by the oral route may be unable to penetrate into the eye even though the drug arrives intact near its intended site of action. Thus, medications used to treat diseases, injuries, or disorders in the eye are usually administered in one of three ways: (1) by topical administration on the **cornea** or **mucosal membranes** of the affected eye, (2) via the oral systemic route, or (3) a combination of both methods.

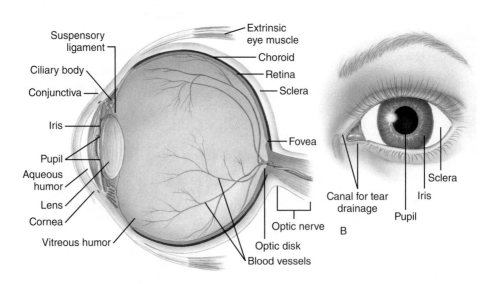

FIGURE 10-1 Anatomy of the eye.

Proper Instillation of Topical Ophthalmic Medication

Topical administration of medication into the eye (either by the patient *or* the nurse) can be tricky because of the innate reflexes that protect the eye from infiltration by foreign bodies and irritants, such as blinking and watering of the eyes (**lacrimation**). Eye tissue is quite sensitive, particularly when injured or infected, so opening the eyelids wide to receive a medication may be painful. Furthermore, if a patient has not previously received **ophthalmic** medication, he or she may flinch away from a clinician attempting to treat an ophthalmic disorder, making it difficult to ensure that the medication reaches the places where it will do the most good. For this reason, it will be useful to discuss how such medications are properly administered before discussing the variety of liquid or ointment medications that are intended for use directly on the eye.

Drops

Many medications are available in the form of aqueous solutions, usually a combination of saline with or without preservatives and buffers to protect the eye from irritation. Administration may be done either by a nurse or by the patient, although most commonly eyedrops are offered so that patients may self-administer the medication. Nurses should, however, make sure patients are aware of proper technique for eyedrop instillation (see the "Eye Medication Administration, Step-by-Step" box). These medications are convenient and inexpensive, but their key drawback is that they do not have extended contact-time with the cornea because they are diluted and eliminated by tears produced in response to the introduction of the foreign substance (Goodolf, 2014).

While drops are convenient because most patients are capable of self-administering them, patients should be assessed for their capacity to do so, as certain circumstances may make an ointment more advantageous. Small children, for example, are less likely to receive the full benefit of any medication given in eyedrop form, even with a parent doing the actual administration, because they simply cannot sit still and exert control of their eye to the extent needed for successful instillation. Adults with tremula or poor hand–eye coordination would also likely benefit from an ointment rather than drops, if this formulation is available for the medication in question. Some patients may experience allergic responses to the buffers or preservatives used in standard formulations, even if the medication is one that previously has been used systemically without incident; if this occurs, a compounding pharmacist may be able a formulate a dosage form that does not include these ingredients (Goodolf, 2014).

Ointments

Ointments used in the eye are generally composed of medication compounded into a gel-like base of inactive matrix, such as paraffin (a wax), mineral oil, or petrolatum. Applying such preparations generally requires less coordination than using drops (see the "Eye Medication Administration, Step-by-Step" box), but the base frequently leaves a film on the cornea that causes blurred vision and minor, short-term discomfort to the patient. Some patients also may experience allergic responses to the base, just as with drops. However, advantages of ointments, aside from ease of use, include that they allow for a higher concentration of medication to be placed in the eye than eyedrops, and longer retention as well, because the base is usually water insoluble and is not washed away by tear production (Aldrich et al., 2013). Particularly when treating an infection, these properties make ointments more attractive than drops as a delivery vehicle.

> **Best Practices**
>
> Some patients may experience allergic responses to the buffers or preservatives used in standard ophthalmic formulations; if this occurs, some sterile compounding pharmacies may be able to compound drops that eliminate these ingredients.

Glaucoma

Glaucoma is not a single disease, as the name implies, but rather a group of diseases that

Procedure for Administration of Eye Medications

Eyedrops

1. Wash hands thoroughly with soap and water.
2. Gently tilt the patient's head back and provide support. Alternatively, have the patient lie down.
3. Shake the medication bottle thoroughly (if formulated as a suspension).
4. Don gloves if mandated by clinic protocols.
5. Gently depress the patient's lower eyelid and ask them to "look up."
6. Squeeze the dropper to release one drop at a time into the eye.
7. Use caution, as the dropper tip must remain sterile and not touch the patient's eye.
8. Have the patient rest for 1-2 minutes, with eyes closed, before administering remaining drops.
9. Use a clean tissue to wipe away any excess medication from areas around the eye.
10. Wait at least 15 minutes before administering another eye medication, if multiple medications are prescribed.

Eye Ointment

1. Wash hands thoroughly with soap and water.
2. Gently tilt the patient's head back and provide support. Alternatively, have the patient lie down.
3. Don gloves if mandated by clinic protocols.
4. Warm the tube of ointment between your hands for 1-2 seconds.
5. Gently depress the patient's lower eyelid to create a "pocket."
6. Squeeze one-quarter inch of the ointment into the "pocket."
7. Use caution, as the tip of the tube must remain sterile and not touch the patient's eye.
8. Have the patient rest with eyes closed for 1-2 minutes.
9. Use a clean tissue to wipe away any excess medication from areas around the eye.
10. Inform patient that Inform patient that their vision may be blurry for up to 30 minutes following ointment administration.

damage the **optic nerve** because of elevated **intraocular pressure (IOP)**, which can result in vision loss and blindness. With early detection and treatment, vision loss can be prevented. In the United States, glaucoma is the leading cause of blindness in African Americans and the third leading cause of blindness in people of European descent (Moroi & Lichter, 1996). The risk of developing **open-angle glaucoma** increases in all races after the age of 60, but it is highest in African Americans older than age 40, Mexican Americans, and people with a family history of glaucoma (National Eye Institute [NEI], 2015). Additional risk factors for development of open-angle glaucoma include high eye pressure, thinness of cornea, and abnormal optic nerve anatomy (Acott et al., 2014).

Eye pressure is a major risk factor for optic nerve damage. In front of the eye is a space known as the **anterior chamber** from which clear fluid flows in and out, to nourish the nearby tissues (NEI, 2015). The fluid leaves the chamber at the open angle where the cornea and the **iris** meet. When the fluid reaches that angle, it flows through a spongy meshwork, like a drain, to leave the eye (**FIGURE 10-2**).

In open-angle glaucoma, despite the angle being open, the fluid passes too slowly through the drain, causing the fluid to build up and increase pressure in the eye to the point that the optic nerve may be damaged. When the optic nerve is damaged from increased pressure in the eye, vision loss may result (NEI, 2015). Another major risk factor for optic nerve damage is elevated blood pressure or **hypertension** (NEI, 2015). Thus, the principal goal of treatment is to reduce pressure in the eye, generally by increasing drainage of fluid out of the eye.

Not every person with increased eye pressure will develop glaucoma. Whether or not

Normal flow of aqueous humor

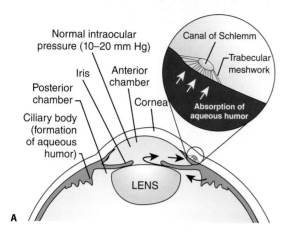

A

Chronic (open-angle) glaucoma

Degeneration and obstruction of trabecular meshwork and canal of Schlemm decreases absorption of aqueous humor

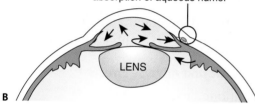

B

Acute (narrow or closed-angle) glaucoma

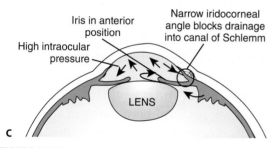

C

FIGURE 10-2 Intraocular pressure in (A) the normal eye, (B) an eye with open-angle glaucoma, and (C) an eye with acute-angle glaucoma.

a person develops glaucoma depends on the level of eye pressure that the optic nerve can tolerate without being damaged; this varies from person to person (NEI, 2015). It is also possible to develop glaucoma without any increased intraocular pressure. This condition is known as **low- or normal-tension glaucoma** (NEI, 2015).

If open-angle glaucoma is untreated, slow loss of **peripheral vision** will result,

causing people to miss objects to the side and out of the "corners" of their eyes, as if they are looking through a tunnel (NEI, 2015). Over time, straight-ahead or central vision may continue to decrease until vision is completely lost (NEI, 2015). In low-tension or normal-tension glaucoma, the optic nerve is damaged, resulting in narrow side vision in people who have normal eye pressure (NEI, 2015).

Angle-closure glaucoma is a medical emergency. In this condition, the fluid at the front of the eye, in the anterior chamber, cannot drain through the angle where the cornea and iris meet, and the angle gets blocked off by part of the iris, causing a sudden increase in eye pressure (NEI, 2015). Symptoms typically include pain, nausea, redness of the eye, and blurred vision. Immediate evaluation is necessary to restore the flow of fluid in the eye to prevent blindness.

Anti-glaucoma medications are divided into the following categories: topical beta blockers, adrenergic agonists, miotics, carbonic anhydrase inhibitors, sympathomimetics, and prostaglandin analogs. The pharmacokinetics and duration of activity of medications in each of these classes are summarized in TABLE 10-1.

Beta Blockers

Beta blockers are a class of medications with many therapeutic uses (Chapter 6). Although more typically associated with their use in cardiac conditions such as hypertension, topically applied (ophthalmic administration) beta-adrenergic antagonists (beta blockers) reduce intraocular pressure in patients with elevated or normal intraocular pressure by decreasing ciliary body production of aqueous humor (Noecker, 2006; Wójcik-Gryciuk, Skup, & Waleszczykb, 2016). Visual acuity, pupil size and accommodation remain unaffected by ophthalmic beta blockers.

Best Practices

Though increased intraocular pressure in only one of the major glaucoma risk factors, the principal goal of glaucoma treatment is to reduce pressure in the eye, generally by increasing drainage of fluid out of the eye.

TABLE 10-1	Pharmacokinetics: Topical Anti-glaucoma Agents	
Generic Name	Class	Duration
Acetazolamide	Carbonic anhydrase inhibitor	8–12 hours
Apraclonidine	Alpha-adrenergic agonist	7–12 hours
Betaxolol	Beta blocker	12 hours
Brimonidine	Alpha-adrenergic agonist	12 hours
Brinzolamide	Carbonic anhydrase inhibitor	N/A
Carbachol	Miotic	6–8 hours
Carteolol	Beta blocker	12 hours
Dipivefrin	Sympathomimetic	12 hours
Dorzolamide	Carbonic anhydrase inhibitor	About 8 hours
Echothiophate	Miotic	Days/weeks
Epinephrine	Sympathomimetic	12 hours
Latanoprost	Prostaglandin analog	24 hours
Levobunolol	Beta blocker	12–24 hours
Methazolamide	Carbonic anhydrase inhibitor	10–18 hours
Metipranolol	Beta blocker	12–24 hours
Pilocarpine	Miotic	4–8 hours
Tafluprost	Prostaglandin analog	24 hours
Timolol	Beta-blocker	12–24 hours
Unoprostone	Prostaglandin analog	24 hours

Data from Wynne, A.L., Woo, T.M., & Millard, M. (2002). *Pharmacotherapeutics for nurse practitioner prescribers*. Philadelphia, PA: F. A. Davis.

TABLE 10-2	Topical Beta Blockers Used for Glaucoma	
Generic	Type	Notes
Timolol	Nonselective (blocks both β_1 and β_2 receptors)	All brands come in 0.25% and 0.5% concentrations
Levobunolol	Nonselective (blocks both β_1 and β_2 receptors)	0.25% and 0.5% concentrations
Carteolol	Nonselective (blocks both β_1 and β_2 receptors)	1% concentration
Metipranolol	Nonselective (blocks both β_1 and β_2 receptors)	0.3% concentration
Betaxolol	Selective (blocks only β_1 receptors)	0.25% and 0.5% concentrations

The pharmacokinetics of beta blockers, insofar as they are used for therapy of glaucoma, remains unknown. Clinical observation determines the pharmacodynamic responses. Topical application of ophthalmic beta blockers can lead to systemic absorption through conjunctiva and lacrimal drainage system, causing side effects on the cardiac and pulmonary systems (Noecker, 2006). Onset, peak, and duration of action vary widely among these products (Wilson, Shannon, & Shields, 2012; Wynne, Woo, & Millard, 2002). Beta blockers are metabolized in the liver and excreted in the urine, bile, and feces. Topical beta blockers that are available for glaucoma treatment are sold as drops rather than

ointments and include the medications described in TABLE 10-2 (Sambhara & Aref, 2014).

Therapeutic and Adverse Effects

As mentioned earlier, ophthalmic anti-glaucoma agents can be absorbed into the systemic circulation and reach concentrations that can cause systemic effects. When this occurs, it can cause complications in patients with chronic medical conditions such as sinus bradycardia, cardiogenic shock, atrioventricular (AV) heart block, heart failure, asthma, and chronic obstructive pulmonary disease (COPD), because blockade of β_1 and β_2 receptors can depress cardiac and pulmonary function (Lee et al., 2014; Wilson et al., 2012). All beta-blocking medications, but especially cardioselective β_1 antagonists (e.g., atenolol, esmolol, and metoprolol), should be used only with caution in patients with COPD, coronary artery disease, and asthma. Studies of patients with glaucoma and cardiac or pulmonary comorbidities revealed that these patients were more likely to need hospitalization or emergency room care (Sambhara & Aref, 2014). In particular, those patients treated with nonselective beta blockers (the majority of available ophthalmic beta blockers fall into this category) were nearly twice as likely as those treated with selective agents to need such care (Sambhara & Aref, 2014). Clinicians should consider the systemic effects, carefully weigh the potential risks, and coordinate care with a cardiac or pulmonary specialist as needed.

Caution should also be exercised when prescribing beta-adrenergic blockers to pregnant women, children, and geriatric patients, because of the cardioselective β_1-receptor blocking and risk for heart failure in geriatric populations. In these populations, close monitoring is required. Beta-adrenergic blockers should not be given to patients with known hypersensitivity reactions, heart block, congestive heart failure, or cardiogenic shock because of the β_1-selective adrenergic receptor blocking properties of these drugs. Caution should also be used in patients with hyperthyroidism, as beta-adrenergic blockers can precipitate thyroid storm (Wilson et al., 2012). Potential adverse effects of beta-blockers are discussed in Chapters Five and Six.

Drug Interactions

Antihypertensives

Beta-adrenergic blockers should be prescribed with caution for glaucoma in patients undergoing treatment for hypertension, AV block, cardiogenic shock, and heart failure, as well as certain types of pulmonary diseases including asthma and COPD, because of the likelihood of drug interactions or synergisms. Oral beta blockers prescribed for hypertension can result in compounded antihypertensive effects when given with ophthalmic beta blockers (see Table 10-2) so care should be taken to monitor patients' blood pressure and pulse.

Antiarrhythmics

Medications used to treat irregular or rapid heartbeats, such as **diltiazem**, **verapamil**, **amiodarone**, and **digoxin**, can cause significant effects on the AV node and may cause complete heart block; thus, they should be used with caution and patients should be monitored carefully. **Verapamil** (a calcium channel blocker) coadministration can cause bradycardia and asystole; consequently, this medication should not be used concurrently with ophthalmic beta blockers (NPPR, 2012; Wynne et al., 2002).

Asthma and COPD Medications

Beta-*antagonists* used for glaucoma may reduce the effects of β_2 *agonists* used to treat obstructive pulmonary disease. While this is primarily an issue with systemic, long-acting medications taken *orally* (e.g., **salbutamol** and **terbutaline**), this interaction may also occur with inhaled formulations, whether short or long acting. Individuals taking beta-agonist bronchodilators should avoid using beta blockers when possible (Lee et al., 2014; NPPR, 2012).

Miotics

Miotics (**TABLE 10-3**) are medications that produce two effects in the eye: (1) **miosis**—that

TABLE 10-3	Topical Miotics Used for Glaucoma	
Generic	Type	Notes
Carbachol (carbamylcholine)	Muscarinic receptor agonist	Contraindicated in patients with asthma, coronary insufficiency, gastroduodenal ulcers, and incontinence due to potential for exacerbation of symptoms.
Demecarium	Acetylcholinesterase inhibitor	Use with caution in patients undergoing concurrent systemic therapy with cholinesterase inhibitors (e.g., in Alzheimer disease or myasthenia gravis).
Echothiophate	Acetylcholinesterase inhibitor	Medication's action on acetylcholinesterase is irreversible. Contraindicated with succinylcholine and other cholinesterinase inhibitors.
Pilocarpine	Muscarinic receptor agonist	Available in both eyedrop and gel forms. Use with caution in patients with asthma or other existing eye problems (e.g., dry eye, which is sometimes treated with the same class of medication via the oral route).

is, constriction of the **pupil** secondary to the contraction of the **iris sphincter**, and (2) contraction of the **ciliary muscle** (Lehne, 2013; Wójcik-Gryciuk et al., 2016). As the ciliary muscle contracts, the trabecular meshwork through which fluid must pass opens, allowing more rapid outflow of fluid and, consequently, reduced eye pressure. Miotic agents further reduce outflow resistance by causing the iris sphincter to contract (Tamm, Braunger, & Fuchshofer, 2015). For all practical purposes, it is not unlike turning a knob to open a vent—a purely mechanical response. However, one drawback to such agents is that pupillary constriction can limit night vision, and their application may also be accompanied by a burning sensation in the eye and a headache (Sambhara & Aref, 2014).

Therapeutic and Adverse Effects

Various miotics may possess differing mechanisms of action. Some bind to the muscarinic acetylcholine receptor to stimulate it directly (muscarinic receptor agonists). Others inhibit the enzyme acetylcholinesterase, which breaks down acetylcholine, thereby increasing the amount of acetylcholine needed to stimulate the receptors. In either case, the end result is the same: The receptors are stimulated and the *outflow of fluid increases* so as to lower intraocular pressure. Both types of medications are usually supplied as eyedrops.

These agents are contraindicated in patients with ocular inflammation and in disorders where constriction of the pupil is not desirable (e.g., **uveitis**, **iritis**, and some forms of secondary glaucoma). In such instances, dilation of the pupil is preferable to prevent scarring of the pupil, because it can no longer react appropriately as a result of the inflammation present from such conditions (Wilson et al., 2012; Wynne et al., 2002).

Miotics can cause blurred vision, photophobia, myopia, angle-closure glaucoma, corneal clouding, ciliary spasm, and headache because of stimulation of the cholinergic receptors in the eye. If systemically absorbed, these medications may cause headache, hypertension, salivation, sweating, nausea, vomiting, and iris cysts (Glaucoma Research Foundation [GRF], 2012; NPPR, 2012; Wynne et al., 2002).

Carbonic Anhydrase Inhibitors

Carbonic anhydrase (CA) is an enzyme that is found in many tissues in the body, including the eye, that assists in converting carbon dioxide to carbonic acid and bicarbonate ions. As their name makes clear, carbonic anhydrase inhibitors prevent the production of this enzyme. When CA is inhibited in the ciliary body, bicarbonate ion formation is slowed, with subsequent reduction in sodium and fluid transport (Tamm et al., 2015). This decreases the secretion of aqueous humor in the eye, diminishing the amount of fluid available to exert pressure; thus, intraocular pressure decreases.

At present, only two such drugs are available for topical application—**brinzolamide** and **dorzolamide**, both of which are supplied as drops. Two other medications—**acetazolamide** and **methazolamide**—are available in oral formulas for systemic administration; however, these medications, which are sulfonamide derivatives, are associated with significant adverse effects, so they are not generally considered first-line agents (Sambhara & Aref, 2014).

Therapeutic and Adverse Effects

Carbonic anhydrase inhibitors should be used with caution in pregnant and breastfeeding women. These drugs are categorized as sulfonamide drugs, meaning that they can induce allergic reactivity in patients with sulfonamide allergies; in patients with known sensitivity to such drugs, they should not be used.

Carbonic anhydrase inhibitors can cause stinging, burning, or other eye discomfort (GRF, 2012) and bitter taste and superficial punctate keratitis (NPPR, 2012; Wynne et al., 2002). Side effects of the tablet form (systemic) of **methazolamide** may include tingling or loss of strength in the hands and feet, upset stomach, lack of mental clarity, memory problems, depression, kidney stones, and frequent urination (GRF, 2012).

Drug Interactions

Metabolic Competitors

Acetazolamide, when taken with barbiturates, **aspirin**, or **lithium**, interacts with these agents in such a way that both drugs are metabolized more quickly, which may lead to decreased effectiveness of interacting drugs. In contrast, if taken with amphetamines, **quinidine**, **procainamide**, or tricyclic antidepressants, **acetazolamide** can cause decreased excretion, leading to toxicity of both the interacting drugs (NPPR, 2012; Wynne et al., 2002). **Brinzolamide** has no known drug interactions. **Dorzolamide** interacts with oral carbonic anhydrase inhibitors causing potential additive effects, so concurrent use of these medications is not recommended. **Methazolamide** interacts with **diflunisal**, causing significant decreases in intraocular pressure, and should be avoided with administration of other carbonic anhydrase inhibitors. Concurrent use with salicylates (**aspirin**) may cause accumulation of **methazolamide** that can result in central nervous system (CNS) depression and metabolic acidosis, and should be avoided. **Topiramate** use concurrent with use of carbonic anhydrase inhibitors increases the risk of renal calculi and should be avoided.

Basic-pH Drugs

Medications with a basic pH effect on circulation (i.e., pH > 7), when combined with carbonic anhydrase inhibitors, inhibit renal excretion. Thus, the coadministration of basic drugs with the following agents should be avoided: **atropine**, **diazepam**, **amoxicillin**, **epinephrine**, **methyldopa**, **metoprolol**, **nicotine**, **norepinephrine**, **pilocarpine**, and other carbonic anhydrase inhibitors.

Acidic-pH Drugs

Potassium should be closely monitored when patients are taking other medications that have an acidic pH effect on circulation (i.e., pH < 7), such as **amoxicillin**, **acetazolamide**, **ampicillin**, **aspirin**, **furosemide**, **ibuprofen**, **levodopa**, **methyldopa**, **theophylline**, and **warfarin**. Carbonic anhydrase inhibitors generally promote excretion of acidic drugs. Corticosteroids as well as potassium-depleting diuretics also cause hypokalemia, and potassium should be closely monitored (NPPR, 2012; Wynne et al., 2002).

Alpha-Adrenergic Agonists

Alpha-adrenergic receptors play key roles in two functions affecting the eye's fluid balance: vasoconstriction and pupillary constriction. Both α_1 and α_2 receptors contribute to vasoconstriction, but α_2 receptors, in particular, are specific to the eye. Constriction of the blood vessels in the ciliary body slows the production of aqueous humor, thereby reducing fluid levels and, consequently, pressure (Sambhara & Aref, 2014; Wójcik-Gryciuk et al, 2016). Thus, stimulating the alpha receptors, but most of all the α_2 receptors, to promote vasoconstriction in the eye offers valuable therapeutic effects for glaucoma.

Alpha-adrenergic agonists are medications that bind to the alpha-adrenergic receptors in tissues (Chapter 5). They are, in essence, mimetics for the hormones **epinephrine** and norepinephrine, which are produced under certain physiological circumstances. In fact, until some of the newer, more selective alpha-adrenergic agonists were introduced, **epinephrine** itself was an option for treating glaucoma; however, because it is nonselective and has multiple, potentially undesirable systemic effects, this medication is now used only rarely for this indication. Instead, medications that are selective for the α_2 receptor have been developed (Arthur & Cantor, 2011). Aside from **epinephrine**, one nonselective alpha-adrenergic receptor agonist is used for glaucoma treatment—**dipivefrin hydrochloride** 0.1%; two α_2-selective agonists—**apraclonidine hydrochloride** 1% and **brimonidine** 0.1%, 0.15%, and 0.2%—are also used as glaucoma therapies. The medication of choice is **brimonidine**, which is better tolerated by patients and equally or more effective than other drugs in this class. **Apraclonidine** is rarely used for glaucoma today because a high rate of follicular **conjunctivitis** has been associated with its use. Moreover, in combination with **timolol**, a non-selective (β_1 and β_2) antagonist, **brimonidine** has been found to offer a potential neuroprotective effect (Arthur & Cantor, 2011), although this is offset, somewhat, by the potential risk of bradycardia that the combination appears to induce (Sambhara & Aref, 2014).

Therapeutic and Adverse Effects

Alpha-adrenergic agonists can cause foreign body sensation (the sensation that something is irritating the eye) in 10% to 39% of patients. Also, ocular pain (Tamm et al., 2015; NPPR, 2012), burning or stinging upon instillation of the eyedrop, fatigue, headache, drowsiness, dry mouth, and dry nose occur as the result of α_2-adrenergic agonist activity (GRF, 2012). Alpha-2 agonists can protect neurons from injury caused by ischemia (Lehne, 2013).

These agents are contraindicated in nursing mothers and in children (Tamm et al., 2015; Wilson et al., 2012). They should be used cautiously in patients with cardiac, renal, or liver disease. **Brimonidine** should not be used with contact lenses in place. Patients should wait approximately 15 minutes before inserting contact lenses after instillation of the solution because **brimonidine** can be absorbed on soft contact lenses (Tamm et al., 2015; Wilson et al., 2012). If systemically absorbed, side effects may include headache, hypertension, tachycardia, and cardiac arrhythmias (Tamm et al., 2015; NPPR, 2012). **Apraclonidine** is contraindicated in patients with **clonidine** hypersensitivity, while **dipivefrin** is contraindicated in narrow-angle glaucoma and in aphakic patients who are missing the lens of their eye either congenitally or as the result of surgery or trauma (Tamm et al., 2015; Wilson et al., 2012).

Drug Interactions

Cardiovascular Drugs

Alpha-adrenergic agonists—**apraclonidine** in particular—may interact with cardiovascular agents, including beta blockers/thiazide diuretic combination drugs, cardiac glycosides, and beta blocker monotherapies, in ways that may lead to reduction in pulse and blood pressure. Consequently, care should be used with their concurrent administration, to include careful monitoring of blood pressure and pulse.

Psychotropic Medications

Monoamine oxidase inhibitors (MAOIs) interact with **apraclonidine**, and concurrent use of these therapies is contraindicated (NPPR, 2012). **Brimonidine** interacts with CNS depressants including alcohol, barbiturates, opiates, sedatives, and anesthetics, causing an additive CNS depression; it should be used with caution for ophthalmic indication if the patient is taking any medications with CNS depressive effects, and patients should be cautioned against use of alcohol or nonprescribed/over-the-counter depressant drugs. In patients taking tricyclic antidepressants concomitantly with alpha-adrenergic agonists, intraocular pressure should be monitored because this combination of drugs can lower circulating amines and reduce pressure excessively.

Other Precautions

Epinephrine can interact with anesthetics such as **cyclopropane** and halogenated hydrocarbons, potentially causing cardiac arrhythmias; thus, it should be discontinued several days prior to surgery (three to seven days depending on the duration of action of the drug) (NPPR, 2012; Wynne et al., 2002). **Dipivefrin** does not have any known drug interactions.

Prostaglandin Analogs

Prostaglandins are lipid compounds derived from arachidonic acid that act as chemical messengers throughout the body. Although they have systemwide effects as key mediators of inflammation (Ricciotti & FitzGerald, 2011), these agents are important in glaucoma therapy because they help to increase uveoscleral outflow (Wynne et al., 2002; Wójcik-Gryciuk et al., 2016). How they accomplish this is not fully understood, but potential mechanisms include relaxation of the ciliary muscle and remodeling of extracellular matrix tissue within the ciliary body. A variety of drugs are analogs to prostaglandins and, therefore, produce similar effects (TABLE 10-4).

Therapeutic and Adverse Effects

Of the various classes of medications used in glaucoma, prostaglandin analogs are usually the first-line choice. Most of the medications available in this class are highly effective, offering a reduction in intraocular pressure of approximately 30%, which can translate into a decrease in pressure of 6.5–8.4 mm Hg at trough and peak time points (Sambhara & Aref, 2014). Another significant benefit is that prostaglandin analogs are consistent in their activity overnight, keeping intraocular pressure reduced while patients sleep, in contrast to other medications that have less consistency in their overnight activity profiles. Prostaglandin analogs are generally well tolerated and have few side effects, some of which are strictly cosmetic in nature—

darkening and thickening of eyelashes and darkening of the iris, for example. Other side effects include stinging, blurred vision, eye redness, itching, and burning due to topical administration of the prostaglandin agonist drug (GRF, 2012; NPPR, 2012; Wynne et al., 2002). Very rarely, patients may experience a systemic reaction consisting of flu-like symptoms, muscle/joint pain, and allergic skin reaction (Sambhara & Aref, 2014).

Prostaglandin analogs should be used with caution in pregnant women, in patients with intraocular inflammation or iritis, and aphakic patients (Wilson et al., 2012; Wynne et al., 2002). The medications should not be administered while contact lenses are in place, and they are contraindicated in lactating women and in children.

Adverse Drug Reactions

Almost no drug interactions are known with prostaglandin analogs. Multiple medications from this class should not be used simultaneously, however.

Chronic Dry or Bloodshot Eyes

At one point or another, everyone experiences dry and/or bloodshot eyes. Not enough sleep, poor hydration, hormonal changes related to the menstrual cycle or menopause, irritants such as smoke or fumes, keeping contact lenses in too long, prolonged exposure to wind or sun—all of these factors can contribute to dryness in the eyes. Dryness itself is sometimes the cause of swelling of the blood vessels in the sclera, which leads to the reddened "bloodshot" eyes that sometimes accompany it, but often this condition is separate, related to inflammation within the eye. This can be due to allergy, infiltration by particulate matter, or microbial infection.

Chronic dry eye (**keratoconjunctivitis sicca**) is a condition in which the problem is not temporary, but persists due to an underlying condition affecting tear production in tear ducts. The cause may be simple aging or age-related hormonal changes, but a number of chronic diseases also affect the quantity

TABLE 10-4	Prostaglandin Analogs Used in Glaucoma
Generic	Notes
Bimatoprost	Used once daily. One of three agents with equivalent efficacy.
Latanoprost	Used once daily. One of three agents with equivalent efficacy.
Tafluprost	Used once daily. Less well studied than other drugs in its class because it was introduced fairly recently.
Travoprost	Used once daily. One of three agents with equivalent efficacy.
Unoprostone	Used twice daily. Efficacy found to be somewhat lower than other agents in this class.

or composition of tears, leading to dry eye; diabetes, thyroid disease, and rheumatoid arthritis, for example, can all have this effect (American Optometric Association [AOA], 2018). In addition, certain autoimmune conditions affect mucous membranes throughout the body, including the eyes, such as Sjögren syndrome. Finally, use of certain medications to treat unrelated conditions, such as oral antihistamines, decongestants, blood pressure medications, and certain antidepressants, can lead to lower tear production and drying of the mucous membranes, resulting in chronic dry eyes that are often painful and itchy (AOA, 2018).

While treatment protocols vary depending on the cause of the condition, a number of medications are used to relieve the symptoms of dry or bloodshot eyes resulting from multiple causes. This section describes these medications and indicates how they are used.

Ocular Lubricants

In the majority of cases, the first line of defense against dryness in the eyes is adequate sleep and water intake. Most often, if given sleep and hydration, the body can produce adequate tears to meet its needs—although admittedly this capacity is lessened by aging. Where sleep and hydration fail to resolve the problem, artificial tears can supplement natural tears and provide tear-like lubrication for dry eyes. These ocular lubricants are solutions that contain a balance of salts to maintain ocular tonicity, buffers to adjust pH, viscosity-enhancing agents to prolong the duration of the lubricant's retention on the eye, and preservatives (Tamm et al., 2015). Ocular lubricants are not absorbed systemically, so they lack appreciable pharmacokinetic properties.

Therapeutic and Adverse Effects

There are no known contraindications for ocular lubricants. The main problem with their use is that relief is usually only temporary, which is problematic for patients suffering from chronic dryness of the eyes.

Some ocular lubricants contain benzalkonium chloride and should not be used in patients who wear soft contact lenses because the released benzalkonium concentration that remains on soft contact lenses is beyond the upper limits for safe wear (Chapman, Cheeks, & Green, 1990).

Ocular lubricants may cause transient stinging and blurred vision due to the preservatives contained in the lubricant.

Drug Interactions

There are no known drug interactions with ocular lubricants, although patient use in conjunction with medications for glaucoma is probably ill advised, because use of artificial tears could reduce the efficacy of the glaucoma medication.

Ophthalmic Vasoconstrictors

Ophthalmic vasoconstrictors are sympathomimetic agents with activity similar to epinephrine and norepinephrine that constrict the conjunctival blood vessels and act minimally on the ocular tissue itself (Duzman et al., 1983). They are used to provide temporary relief from eye redness due to ocular irritants. Many are sold as over-the-counter products; the agents approved for this purpose comprise the following medications (Food and Drug Administration [FDA], 2013):

- Naphazoline hydrochloride, 0.01–0.03%
- Phenylephrine hydrochloride, 0.08–0.2%
- Tetrahydrozoline hydrochloride, 0.01–0.05%
- Oxymetazoline 0.025%

Little is known about the pharmacokinetics of ophthalmic vasoconstrictors. The duration of action for **naphazoline** is three to four hours, that for **oxymetazoline** is four to six hours, and that for **tetrahydrozoline** is one to four hours.

Therapeutic and Adverse Effects

Ophthalmic vasoconstrictors should be used with caution in pregnant women, but this is primarily because their safety for use during pregnancy remains unknown and unstudied. In a study in rabbits, oxymetazoline was absorbed slowly into the eye: Only 0.006% of the original drug concentration was found in the aqueous humor 30 minutes after instillation, with the balance remaining primarily in the extraocular tissues (99. 004%) (Duzman et al., 1983). Safety indicators including blood pressure, heart rate, intraocular pressure, pupil size, and visual acuity did not change significantly from baseline after administration of ocular vasoconstrictors (Duzman et al., 1983).

Ophthalmic vasoconstrictors are contraindicated in patients with a known hypersensitivity to the components of the products and in patients with narrow-angle or angle-closure glaucoma because of the vasoconstriction that occurs within the vascular system of the conjunctiva (Bausch & Lomb, 2010; Duzman et al., 1983). Use in pediatric patients, especially infants, may result in CNS depression leading to coma and marked reduction in body temperature (Bausch & Lomb, 2010).

The most serious adverse reaction is increased intraocular pressure due to constriction of the vascular system of the conjunctiva (Bausch & Lomb, 2010). This effect is likely due to the drug's direct stimulation action on the alpha-adrenergic receptors in the arterioles of the conjunctiva, which results in decreased conjunctival congestion (Bausch & Lomb, 2010). Ocular vasoconstrictors may cause transient ocular stinging and burning upon instillation of the solution, as well as blurred vision, mydriasis, increased lacrimation, irritation, and discomfort. Rebound congestion and eye redness may occur with prolonged use greater than three days (NPPR, 2012; Wynne et al., 2002).

Drug Interactions

Naphazoline interacts with tricyclic antidepressants and maprotiline, which act, in part, by inhibiting presynaptic norepinephrine reuptake, causing increased pressor effects. Patients currently receiving MAOIs may experience a severe hypertensive crisis if given a sympathomimetic drug (Bausch & Lomb, 2010). MAOIs may cause exaggerated adrenergic effects and should not be used within 21 days of naphazoline. Systemic effects are more likely if these agents are used in combination with beta-adrenergic blockers (NPPR, 2012; Wynne et al., 2002). There are no known drug interactions with oxymetazoline and tetrahydrozoline.

Corticosteroids

Corticosteroids have well-known anti-inflammatory properties. When used judiciously, they can be helpful in reducing the red, inflamed appearance that comes with injury or infection to the eye. These agents are sometimes used to address inflammation after cataract surgery as well. However, ocular preparations of these medications (TABLE 10-5) have a variety of known adverse effects, both local and systemic.

Therapeutic and Adverse Effects

Corticosteroids have well-known systemic effects. In the eye, these effects consist of quelling of the inflammatory response via inhibition of multiple inflammatory cytokine effects. Unfortunately, the potential impacts of these medications go beyond simply reducing inflammation. Just as they do when used systemically, topical corticosteroids can induce hypertension; increased intraocular pressure and glaucoma are significant risks of local corticosteroid administration, due to glucocorticoid effects on vasculature. Another risk is suppression of immune responses in the eye. Posterior subcapsular cataracts can develop as soon as four months after initiating topical corticosteroid use. Using topical corticosteroids carries other risks as well, including ptosis (drooping eyelid) and reduction in ocular movement, as well as slower wound healing in surgical patients or those with eye injuries.

Corticosteroid drops or ointments should not be used in patients with glaucoma, as these medications may increase intraocular pressure.

TABLE 10-5	Ophthalmic Corticosteroids
Generic	**Form**
Dexamethasone	Drops: 0.1% suspension
Dexamethasone + neomycin	Drops: Suspension of dexamethasone 0.1% + neomycin equivalent to 3.5 mg/mL
Dexamethasone + neomycin + polymyxin B	Drops: Suspension of neomycin equivalent to 3.5 mg/mL, polymyxin B 10,000 units, dexamethasone 0.1%
Dexamethasone + tobramycin	Drops: Suspension of tobramycin 0.3% + dexamethasone 0.1%
Difluprednate	Drops: Emulsion, ophthalmic 0.05%
Fluorometholone	Drops: 0.1% and 0.25% suspension Ointment: 0.1%
Loteprednol	Drops: 0.2% and 0.5% suspension Ointment: 0.5% Gel: 0.5%
Prednisolone	Drops: Solution, ophthalmic, as sodium phosphate: 1% Suspension, ophthalmic, as acetate: 0.12%, 1%
Prednisolone + gentamicin	Drops: Gentamicin sulfate equivalent to 0.3% gentamicin base; prednisolone acetate (microfine suspension) 1.0%
Prednisolone + polymyxin B + neomycin	Drops: Prednisolone acetate (microfine suspension) 0.5%, neomycin sulfate equivalent to 0.35% neomycin base, polymyxin B sulfate 10,000 units/mL
Prednisolone + sulfacetamide	Drops: Suspension of sulfacetamide sodium 10% + prednisolone acetate 0.2%

Drug Interactions

Potential drug–drug interactions with corticosteroids are mainly those with other locally applied ophthalmic preparations.

Ophthalmic Antibiotics

It is not uncommon for redness, itching, and dryness to be the result of microbial infections introduced into the eyes. Indeed, given how often people unconsciously rub dirty fingers into and around the eyes, not to mention the proximity of the eyes to the rich source of microbes that the mouth and nose jointly represent, the miracle is that infections of the eye are not more common!

Patients who present with redness and dryness that have not responded to either over-the-counter lubricants or vasoconstrictors, or both, most likely are experiencing either an allergic response to a substance they have encountered or a viral or bacterial infection. These three conditions can be distinguished from one another by the exudate produced, which is usually watery and mucus-like for a viral infection, yellow-green and thick for a bacterial infection, and absent in an allergic response (Story, 2012).

The most common presentation of an ocular infection of this kind is conjunctivitis, in which the eye appears bright red, swollen, and painful. Infectious conjunctivitis is highly contagious, and patients should be encouraged to avoid touching their eyes or face, to wash hands frequently, and to limit face-to-face contact with others for the duration of the infection—particularly if only one eye is infected, as hygienic measures can prevent infection of the contralateral eye.

Best Practices

Patients with glaucoma should not use corticosteroid medications.

Best Practices

Patients should be told that skipping or delaying doses of topical antibiotics for eye infections could prolong the infection.

Unfortunately, while these steps are often enough to resolve an infection in an adult, they are virtually impossible to enforce in a small child, who will likely need medication.

Treatment of conjunctivitis may involve use of a variety of agents, most of which are intended to reduce inflammation and relieve soreness and swelling. If the underlying cause is bacterial and the infection is particularly severe (and therefore unlikely to resolve on its own), a number of antibiotic ophthalmic agents are available for use (TABLE 10-6). Note that some options are superior to others when dealing with conjunctivitis in an infant; pediatric limitations are included alongside all ophthalmic antibiotic preparations listed.

The key concern with using ocular antibiotics is the potential for developing resistance. Some bacterial causes of eye infections are gram-positive bacterial pathogens, such as *Staphylococcus aureus*, *Staphylococcus epidermis*, and *Streptococcus pneumoniae* (Haas, Gearinger, Usner, Decory, & Morris, 2011), but others are gram-negative organisms (*Haemophilus influenzae*), many of which have developed resistance to oral antibiotics as a result of overly frequent use. Thus, proper dosing and use of a broad-spectrum agent are key factors in resolving the infection and preventing recurrence due to resistance. The patient should be informed that skipping or delaying doses could promote resistance and lead to prolonged infection and discomfort.

Chronic conjunctivitis that responds poorly to therapy with antibiotics and corticosteroids could indicate undiagnosed glaucoma and should be assessed by an ophthalmologist. Clinicians should also recognize that conjunctivitis is sometimes a product, rather than a precursor, of glaucoma treatment. The preservatives used in a variety of glaucoma medications, particularly the preservative known as benzalkonium chloride (BAK), can be toxic to the conjunctiva if used for extended periods (Rasmussen, Kaufman, & Kiland, 2014). A patient using glaucoma medications who presents with repeated bouts of conjunctivitis

TABLE 10-6	Ophthalmic Topical Antibiotics		
Generic	Antibiotic Class	Preparation	Pediatric
Azithromycin	Macrolide antibiotic	1% solution	Children 1 year and older
Bacitracin	Polypeptide antibiotic	500 U/g unguent	Not used in pediatric patients
Besifloxacin	Fluoroquinolone	0.6% suspension	Children 1 year and older
Ciprofloxacin	Fluoroquinolone	0.3% solution or unguent	Children 1 year and older
Erythromycin	Macrolide antibiotic	0.5% unguent	Children 2 months and older
Gatifloxacin	Fluoroquinolone	0.3% solution	Children 1 year and older
Gentamycin	Aminoglycoside	0.3% solution or unguent	Not used in pediatric patients
Levofloxacin	Fluoroquinolone	1.5% solution	Children 6 years and older
Moxifloxacin	Fluoroquinolone	0.5% solution	Children 1 year and older
Ofloxacin	Fluoroquinolone	0.3% solution	Children 1 year and older
Polymyxin B + bacitracin	Antibiotic combination	Unguent	Not used in pediatric patients
Polymyxin B + neomycin + gramicidin	Antibiotic combination	Solution or unguent	Not used in pediatric patients
Polymyxin B + trimethoprim	Antibiotic combination	Solution	Children 2 months and older
Tobramycin	Aminoglycoside	0.3% solution or unguent	Children 2 months and older

may need alternative medications that lack preservatives, or surgical therapy.

Therapeutic and Adverse Effects

The therapeutic effect of ocular antibiotics is primarily achieved through regular and correct use of the medication. Thus, patients must be instructed on the appropriate way to instill the medication as well as given a schedule of use.

Most antibiotics have few adverse effects, particularly when used in topical form, but patients' history of antibiotic use should be taken to identify the possibility that they might have encountered a resistant bacterium. In a survey of clinical studies at multiple sites (Haas et al., 2011), a significant level of antibiotic resistance to ciprofloxacin was noted in *Staphylococcus* and *Streptococcus* isolates, so changing agents may be advisable in patients who show no response to ciprofloxacin or who have extensive past oral antibiotic use.

Drug Interactions

Few drug interactions are known with topical ophthalmic antibiotics. Systemic absorption is unlikely. Patients who are concurrently using other eye preparations for dry eye, glaucoma, or similar conditions should avoid using these medications at the same time, as they may dilute the efficacy of one another.

Drugs Used in Treating Otic Disorders

The most common medical therapies for otic use treat one of three basic problems: (1) ear wax buildup leading to hearing loss; (2) infection of the ear, either bacterial or fungal; or (3) pain associated with such an infection. Because infections of the ear are common in children and a frequent source of visits to medical clinics, the majority of this section addresses the medications used to treat these illnesses.

There are three types of ear infections that occur in different parts of the ear (FIGURE 10-3). **Acute otitis media (AOM)** is a type of ear infection that is usually painful and can have other symptoms such as redness of the **tympanic membrane** (eardrum), pus in the ear, fever, pulling or tugging on the affected

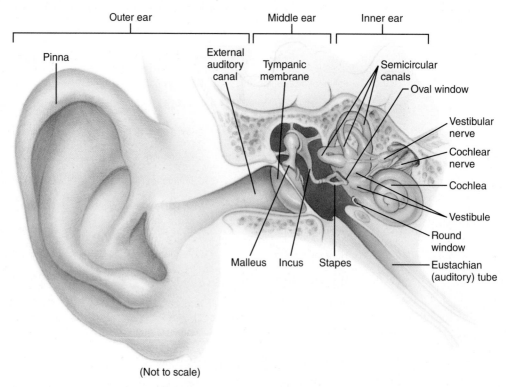

FIGURE 10-3 The structure of the ear.

ear (in children), and irritability (Centers for Disease Control and Prevention [CDC], 2012). **Otitis media with effusion (OME)** is the buildup of fluid in the **middle ear** without the signs and symptoms of pain, redness of the eardrum, pus, or fever; it may be caused by viral upper respiratory infections, allergies, or exposure to irritants, including cigarette smoke (CDC, 2012). The fluid does not usually cause any pain and goes away on its own, so it does not require any treatment with antibacterial agents. The final type of ear infection is **otitis externa**, more commonly known as "swimmer's ear," which is an infection of the inner ear and the outer ear canal. It can cause the ear to itch or become red and swollen to the point that touching it or even applying pressure to the ear is quite painful. Pus may also drain from the ear (CDC, 2012). Antibiotics are usually needed to treat otitis externa.

In addition, when pain from ear infections is significant (although these illnesses are sometimes painless and go unnoticed), analgesics may be needed. Use of analgesia in small children, especially, can present a concern for parents, who should be advised regarding which medications are safest, how much and how often to dose, and which symptoms of toxicity to watch for.

Prevention Begins at Birth

Preventing AOM and reducing the risk of otic complications in children can be done in several ways, but many of the most useful strategies must be initiated in infancy, preferably at birth. Mothers of newborns and expectant mothers should be advised on strategies for limiting their child's exposures to ear infections, including the following measures (CDC, 2012; Giebink, 1994):

- Breastfeeding exclusively for at least the first six months of an infant's life reduces AOM in infancy and early childhood.
- If breastfeeding is not possible, avoid supine bottle-feeding; infants should be fed in an upright position.
- Avoid childcare centers when respiratory illnesses are prevalent.
- Eliminate exposure to tobacco smoke, both firsthand and secondhand, as well as air pollution; use of a high-efficiency particulate absorption (HEPA) filter in the infant's room can assist with limiting exposure to pollutants.
- Avoid pacifier use, or reduce pacifier use after six months of age.
- Preventing and treating influenza produces a modest reduction in the incidence of AOM, but only during influenza season.
- Vaccinating against pneumococcal infection can reduce the risk of AOM slightly.

Acute Otitis Media

Pain in the ear (**otalgia**) has many causes, not all of which are related to infection. To correctly diagnose AOM, the clinician must not only note otalgia, often characterized by a child tugging at or holding the ear, but other symptoms of AOM, including fever, vomiting,

A Word About Wax

Many pathogens are introduced into the ear by well-meaning individuals seeking to clear their ears of wax. While excessive accumulation of **cerumen** (ear wax) leads to conductive hearing loss, impaction, and an environment conducive for the development of otitis externa (Wynne et al., 2002), manual removal of cerumen merely exacerbates the problem. Yet it is nonetheless necessary to clear excess wax to prevent the problem of **impaction**, in which cerumen dries and hardens to form a plug in the external ear canal, which is difficult and painful to remove. Treatment of excess cerumen or impacted cerumen includes instillation of mineral oil or carbamide peroxide. When instilled in the ear canal, this combination softens the cerumen and allows for removal by irrigation with warm water or saline (van Wyk, 2017). If the external ear canal is excoriated, treatment with antibiotic or steroid otic preparations will prevent development of otitis externa.

irritability, impaired hearing, sleeplessness, and **otorrhea** (fluid drainage) or purulent discharge from the ear (Lehne, 2013). AOM can be caused by bacterial or viral infection, or both (TABLE 10-7) and is characterized by fluid, either purulent or nonpurulent, behind the tympanic membrane. When fluid is behind the tympanic membrane, the membrane can bulge outward, causing pain and possible perforation of the tympanic membrane, and resulting in otorrhea. In children with viral or nonbacterial AOM, the tympanic membrane usually does not bulge outward. There is always the possibility of co-infection with bacteria and viruses, and sometimes a pathogenic *bacterium* cannot be isolated. These instances are reflected in the percentages shown in Table 10-7.

AOM develops when a microbial infection (which can be either viral or bacterial, but is usually viral) in the nasopharynx causes blockage of the Eustachian tube, causing negative pressure in the middle ear (Lehne, 2013). When the Eustachian tube finally does open to equalize the pressure in the ear, bacteria and viruses can enter the middle ear as the result of an inefficient mucociliary action, making the transport of pathogens back to the nasopharynx impossible, and resulting in the colonization of bacteria or virally infected cells in the middle ear mucosa. Bacteria are present in 70% to 90% of children with middle-ear fluid, and viruses are present in about 50% of children with middle ear fluid.

TABLE 10-7	Pathogens Most Commonly Associated with Acute Otitis Media
Streptococcus pneumoniae	40–50%
Haemophilus influenzae	20–25%
Moraxella catarrhalis	10–15%
No bacteria found	20–30%
Respiratory viruses with or without bacteria	48%

Data from Lehne, R.A. (2013). Pharmacology for Nursing Care, 8th ed. St. Louis, MO: Elsevier, pp.1346–51; CDC, 2012

The viruses that are most commonly associated with AOM include respiratory syncytial virus (RSV), rhinovirus, influenza virus, and adenoviruses (CDC, 2012). The bacteria most commonly associated with AOM include *Streptococcus pneumoniae*, *Haemophilus influenzae*, and *Moraxella catarrhalis* (Table 10-7) (CDC, 2012).

Choosing an Antibacterial Agent

AOM is the most common infection for which antibacterial agents are prescribed for children in the United States (American Academy of Pediatrics [AAP], 2004; Lieberthal et al., 2013). Recently, there has been much discussion about the necessity of the antibacterial therapy for treatment of AOM. Making this diagnosis requires (1) a history of acute onset of signs and symptoms, (2) the presence of middle ear effusion, and (3) signs and symptoms of middle-ear inflammation (AAP, 2004; Lieberthal et al., 2013). Children with AOM usually present with a history of rapid onset of signs and symptoms of AOM such as otalgia (pulling on the ear in an infant), otorrhea, and fever (AAP, 2004; Lieberthal et al., 2013). These findings are nonspecific for otalgia, however, and can also represent upper respiratory infections. The infection must also disrupt sleep or daily activities to warrant an AOM diagnosis (CDC, 2012).

In 2013, the AAP and the American Academy of Family Physicians released new guidelines for treating children with AOM. They recommend basing treatment on three factors: age, illness severity, and the degree of diagnostic certainty (AAP, 2004; Lieberthal et al., 2013). The guidelines also include the important new option of observation, defined as management of symptoms alone for a period of 48 to 72 hours, allowing time for AOM to resolve on its own, which happens in most cases (AAP, 2004; Lieberthal et al., 2013). If the symptoms persist past this time period, then antibiotic therapy is warranted and initiated. One important point with the observation option is that it is appropriate only if follow-up can be ensured with the child's healthcare provider. The following statements should be considered for the recommendation of observation:

- Most episodes of AOM resolve spontaneously without any antibiotic treatment.
- Immediate antibacterial therapy is only marginally superior to observation at resolving AOM and is *no* better at resolving pain and/or distress.
- Parents find the observation approach an acceptable treatment plan for their child.

Delaying the initiation of antibacterial therapy does not significantly increase the risk for mastoiditis, which occurs when bacteria invade the mastoid bone (Lehne, 2013).

The AAP and American Academy of Family Practice recommend the following criteria:

- Diagnosing AOM by confirming a history of acute onset of the signs of middle ear effusion (MEE) and evaluating for the presence of signs and symptoms of middle ear inflammation
- Identifying pain and treating it
- Observation for children who have the assurance of follow-up based on diagnostic certainty, age (greater than 2 years), and illness severity
- If antibacterial agents are necessary, starting with amoxicillin 80–90 mg/kg per day based on the anticipated clinical response and the microbiologic flora likely to be present (AAP, 2004; Lieberthal et al., 2013)

If the patient fails to respond to the initial management of AOM with amoxicillin 80–90 mg/kg per day within the first 48 to 72 hours and the symptoms persist, then either another disease is present or the antibacterial therapy was inadequate and should be based on the likely pathogens present (see Table 10-7) and the clinical experience.

The criteria for choosing observation versus initiating antibiotic therapy are detailed in Table 10-8 and are based on the patient's age, the severity of the illness/symptoms, and the certainty of the diagnosis (AAP, 2004; Lieberthal et al., 2013). Any child who is younger than six months of age, regardless of the certainty of the diagnosis or the severity of the symptoms, should receive antibiotic therapy, whereas children who are six months to two years old should receive antibiotics only with diagnostic certainty of AOM. If the diagnosis is uncertain, antibiotics should be reserved only for severe illness or severe symptoms. For children more than two years old, antibiotics are reserved for those whose diagnosis is certain and whose symptoms are severe (AAP, 2004; Lieberthal et al., 2013).

What About Decongestants?

Many parents, when confronted with a child who has a cold and who complains or shows signs of ear pain, reach for over-the-counter decongestants to help relieve the child's symptoms. These medications are not recommended, according to the AAP, because there are too few data supporting their use and, more importantly, no clear understanding of their risks. Manufacturers voluntarily discontinued over-the-counter medications intended for children younger than two years in 2008 and relabeled medications for older children as unsuited for those younger than the age of four as a result of these concerns (FDA, 2011).

The Food and Drug Administration's (FDA) recommendations for treating children under four with cough and cold symptoms are as follows:

- A cool mist humidifier helps nasal passages shrink and allows for easier breathing. (Do not use warm mist humidifiers, as they can cause nasal passages to swell and make breathing more difficult.)
- Saline nose drops or spray keeps nasal passages moist and helps avoid stuffiness.

- Nasal suctioning with a bulb syringe, either with or without saline nose drops, works especially well for infants less than one year old. Older children often resist its use.
- Acetaminophen or ibuprofen can be used to reduce fever, aches, and pains. Acetaminophen is preferred for infants and children younger than age two. Parents should carefully read and follow the product's instructions for use label.
- Drinking plenty of liquids will help the child stay well hydrated.

In short, the best evidence available suggests that decongestants and cough suppressants should be left on the shelf when it comes to pediatric patients. Nurses should offer parents information based on the FDA's recommendations for managing their child's upper respiratory symptoms and treat any associated ear infection, if present, according to standard protocols.

When antibacterial therapy is warranted, high-dose **amoxicillin** (40–45 mg/kg twice daily) is the first-line treatment. The benefits include efficacy, safety, low cost, pleasing taste, and narrow microbiologic spectrum (AAP, 2004; Lieberthal et al., 2013). If the infection persists after 48 to 72 hours of treatment, however, the patient should be reexamined, and a second-line agent, such as **amoxicillin/clavulanate**, should be used as appropriate (Harmes et al., 2013). For patients who have a **penicillin allergy**, the treatment depends on the severity of the reaction. If the allergy is not severe (severe Type 1 hypersensitivity reaction), a cephalosporin may be used (e.g., **cefdinir**, **cefuroxime**, or **cefpodoxime**). If the allergy is severe (Type 1 hypersensitivity that causes urticaria or other immediate-type anaphylactic symptoms), a cephalosporin should be avoided because of the possible cross-reactivity (Lehne, 2013). **Azithromycin** or

clarithromycin, both of which are macrolide antibiotics, should be the first-line treatment options in these instances.

Although many instances of AOM occur secondary to upper respiratory infections, the use of decongestants or nasal steroids does not aid in resolving the ear infection and their use is not recommended (Harmes et al., 2013).

Treatment for Antibiotic-Resistant AOM

Antibiotic resistance is defined by the persistence of symptoms including fever, otalgia, otorrhea, and a red bulging tympanic membrane despite 48 to 72 hours of antibiotic therapy (AAP, 2004; Lieberthal et al., 2013). Major risk factors for antibiotic resistance (Lehne, 2013) include the following:

- Attending day care
- Age less than two years old
- Exposure to antibiotics in the previous one to three months
- Winter and spring seasons

The United States has seen an increase in the incidence of antibiotic resistance because of the overuse of antibiotics, leading to the development of resistant pathogens. Often, strains of *H. influenzae* and *M. catarrhalis* are resistant to beta-lactam antibiotics because they have evolved the ability to produce beta lactamase, an enzyme that inactivates **amoxicillin** and certain other beta-lactam antibiotics. *S. pneumoniae* can be resistant to multiple antibiotics, including **erythromycin**, **trimethoprim/sulfamethoxazole**, **amoxicillin**, and other beta-lactam antibiotics (Lehne, 2013). The resistance to **amoxicillin** is not the result of beta-lactamase production, but rather reflects synthesis of altered penicillin-binding proteins (PBPs) that have an affinity for **amoxicillin**, which has a much lower PBP than **penicillin**.

Pharmacodynamics

The medications used to treat otitis externa include combination products that contain

Best Practices

FDA recommendations for treating children under age four with cough and cold symptoms focus on supportive care. Evidence suggests forgoing decongestants and cough suppressants for pediatric patients. Nurses should offer parents information based on FDA recommendations for managing their child's upper respiratory symptoms and treat any associated ear infection, if present, according to standard protocols.

corticosteroids and antibiotics or antibiotics alone. The exact mechanism of action for corticosteroids such as hydrocortisone in this indication remains unknown, but it is thought that they act by the induction of phospholipase A_2 inhibitory proteins that control inflammatory mediators such as prostaglandins and leukotrienes (Wynne et al., 2002). Neomycin is active against *Staphylococcus aureus* and *Proteus* and *Enterobacter* species. Polymyxin B is active against gram-negative bacteria (including *P. aeruginosa, E. coli,* and *H. influenzae*), while gentamicin is a broad-spectrum aminoglycoside that is active against *P. aeruginosa, Staphylococcus,* S. *pneumoniae,* beta-hemolytic streptococci, and *Enterobacter* species. The fluoroquinolones (ciprofloxacin and ofloxacin) are active against *Staphylococcus,* S. *pneumoniae, Proteus* and *Enterobacter* species, and *P. aeruginosa.* Acid and alcohol solutions contain 2% acetic acid; they reduce inflammation and exert their antibacterial and antifungal effects by decreasing pH in the ear (Wynne et al., 2002).

Therapeutic and Adverse Effects

Hypersensitivity to any of the components in an otic medication is a contraindication to its use. Ciprofloxacin and combination antibiotic and cortisone-like solutions are contraindicated in tympanic membrane perforation because they possess ototoxicity characteristics, and they carry a risk of sensorineural hearing loss due to cochlear damage, mainly destruction of the hair cells in the organ of Corti (Howard, 2012; JHP Pharmaceuticals, 2008). However, neomycin/polymyxin B/hydrocortisone otic suspension may be used with tympanic membrane perforation. Superinfection and overgrowth of nonsusceptible organisms and fungi can result from prolonged use of topical antibiotics (Wynne et al., 2002).

Contact dermatitis, local reactions, and superinfections from prolonged use can result from use of topical otic preparations.

Ofloxacin otic medications may cause taste alterations as well as dizziness, vertigo, and paresthesia in patients with ruptured tympanic membranes due to the systemic absorption of the medication (NPPR, 2012; Wynne et al., 2002). Ototoxicity may occur with prolonged use of combination antibiotic and cortisone-like solutions (NPPR, 2012; Wynne et al., 2002).

Drug Interactions

There are no significant drug interactions for topical otic preparations.

Otitis Media with Effusion

OME is a painful condition characterized by fluid in the middle ear that does not have any evidence of local or systemic illness, such as the fever, vomiting, irritability, or otorrhea observed with AOM (AAP, 2004; Lieberthal et al., 2013). OME patients may have some associated hearing loss, but there is rarely pain associated with the condition. The presence of fluid may persist for weeks to months after the AOM infection has resolved, rendering antibiotics useless in treating this condition. Therefore, antibiotics should not be recommended or used to treat OME.

Otitis Externa and Its Management

Otitis externa (OE) is an acute, painful inflammation of the external auditory canal that is usually caused by a bacterial infection, but rarely can be caused by a fungal infection. Occasionally the infection may spread to the surrounding tissues and cause serious, even life-threatening, complications in immunocompromised and diabetic individuals (Wynne et al., 2002). The majority of cases of OE respond to topical treatment. The most common pathogens implicated in OE are *Pseudomonas aeruginosa* and *Staphylococcus aureus,* but other potential causative bacteria/pathogens include *Staphylococcus epidermidis* and *Microbacterium otitidis.*

Symptoms of acute otitis externa include otalgia and otorrhea, impaired hearing, purulent discharge, and pronounced tenderness of the auricle with manipulation such as during chewing (Sander, 2001). Otitis externa occurs because of abrasion in the ear canal and/or excess moisture, both of which facilitate bacterial colonization with *P. aeruginosa* and *S. aureus* (Bojrab, Bruderly, & Abdulrazzak, 1996; Clark, Brook, Bianki, & Thompson, 1997; Dibb, 1991; Hajioff & MacKeith, 2015; Nichols, 1999). The abrasion creates a site for bacteria to enter the epithelium, while excess moisture washes away the protective cerumen, thereby creating an environment that supports the growth of bacteria (Wynne et al., 2002). Otitis externa abrasions can be caused by the use of cotton-tipped swabs or inserting fingers, toothpicks, pencils, ear syringing, hearing aids, or earplugs into the ear. Other causes can include the presence of excess moisture resulting from swimming, bathing, perspiration, or high humidity (Sander, 2001). Occasionally, otitis externa can be caused by chronic dermatologic diseases such as eczema, psoriasis, seborrheic dermatitis, or acne (Hajioff & MacKeith, 2015; Sander, 2001).

Acute bacterial otitis externa is characterized by scant to thick white mucus. In contrast, fungal otitis externa is characterized by a fluffy, white to off-white discharge, with small black or white conidiophores on white hyphae (associated with *Aspergillus*) (Sander, 2001).

Prevention

The best way to prevent OE is to maintain good hygiene and promote the natural defenses that the body has against OE. The patient should not put anything in the ear canal, including cotton-tipped applicators, fingers, toothpicks, pencils, or other objects that could damage or abrade the ear canal and remove the protective cerumen layer. The patient should dry the ear canal after swimming, bathing, and showering by thoroughly drying the ear with a towel and promoting drainage of excess water by tipping the head to the side. The patient should not remove cerumen and should not use earplugs, except for swimming.

Treatment

Treatment with systemic antimicrobials should be initiated for initial therapy only if there is involvement outside the ear canal, or specific patient-based reasons (such as immunocompromised patients) exist. Otherwise, treatment with topical preparations should be instituted (Rosenfeld et al., 2014). The treatment goals for otitis externa are to reduce pain and eliminate the pathogen. For most patients, this involves treating pain with analgesics and administering topical antibiotics or acetic acid solutions. Rarely, oral antibiotics may be necessary, if the infection is extensive. The ear should be kept as dry as possible for 7 to 10 days until the treatment course is completed.

Topical Medications

The external auditory canal should be cleansed as thoroughly as possible and a wick, made of cotton usually, should be inserted to assist with draining and swelling. In addition, topical antibacterial therapy should be initiated (Sander, 2001). Simple acidification with 2% acetic acid is usually the best choice. However, topical antibiotic agents can be placed in direct contact with the bacteria and are the next choice for treatment of otitis externa (Sander, 2001). Table 10-9 provides more information on the various treatment options.

Steroids added to otic drops may be used to decrease inflammation and edema of the external ear canal, and can help resolve symptoms more quickly, but not all studies reveal a benefit from this treatment. In addition, topical steroids can be sensitizers that can cause hypersensitivity reactions to antigens through repeated exposure (Bojrab et al., 1996; "Diagnosis and Treatment of Acute Otitis Externa," 1999; Sander, 2001).

While treatments vary slightly, it is most commonly recommended that otic drops be given for 3 to 5 days beyond the cessation of symptoms. This usually results in a total 5- to 7-day course of treatment with topical agents (Sander, 2001). In the case of severe infections, 10 to 14 days of treatment may be warranted. Follow-up is not required unless the symptoms are not improving (Clark et al., 1997). Typically, three or four drops of the topical antibiotic preparation are placed in the affected area four times daily, whereas fluoroquinolones are applied in the affected area twice daily ("Diagnosis and Treatment of Acute Otitis Externa," 1999; Jones, Milazzo, & Seidlin, 1998; Simpson & Markham, 1999).

To minimize the dizziness associated with instillation of otic drops, it is recommended that the bottle be warmed by gently rubbing it between the hands for several minutes prior to administration of the drops. A small cotton plug that is moistened with the antibiotic drops can also be used to help retain the drops in the ear if the patient cannot lie still long enough to allow adequate absorption (Sander, 2001). Manipulating the tragus of the affected ear can assist with sufficient distribution throughout the external auditory canal (Sander, 2001). If the patient has an ear wick, the drops should be applied more often while the patient is awake—every three to four hours. Additionally, with a wick, the ear should be examined more often and cleansed more frequently to decrease the edema. The wick should be removed when it is no longer necessary (Bojrab et al., 1996).

Systemic Treatment

Rarely, systemic antibiotics may be required for treatment of acute otitis externa that is not responding to topical treatments. Systemic antibiotics should be used with concurrent AOM or if local or systemic spread has occurred or is suspected (Halpern, Palmer, & Seidlin, 1999). This treatment

should be reserved for patients who have temperatures higher than 38.3°C (101.0°F), severe pain, and regional lymphadenopathy of the preauricular or anterior or posterior cervical chains (Sander, 2001). Additionally, otitis media should be considered as a concomitant diagnosis when the patient has an upper respiratory infection or is younger than two years of age, as otitis externa is considered uncommon in these populations (Sander, 2001). Furthermore, systemic antibiotics should be used in patients with early signs of necrotizing otitis externa, and in those whose immunity may be compromised, such as individuals with diabetes, those taking systemic corticosteroids, or those with an underlying chronic dermatitis ("Diagnosis and Treatment of Acute Otitis Externa," 1999; Jones et al., 1998; Nichols, 1999; Sander, 2001; Selesnick, 1994).

Fungal Otitis Externa (Otomycosis)

Approximately 10% of otitis externa is caused by fungi and not bacteria, with the two most common fungal pathogens being *Aspergillus* (causing 80% to 90% of otitis externa) and *Candida* (causing 10% to 20% of otitis externa) (Bojrab et al., 1996; Boustred, 1999; Dibb, 1991; Sander, 2001). Fungi are usually the primary pathogen in otitis externa when there is excessive moisture and heat (Sander, 2001). Often fungal otitis externa is asymptomatic, with diagnosis made through observation of the unique discharge from the external auditory canal (Sander, 2001). When symptoms are present, discomfort is the most common complaint, followed by pruritus that is quite intense. The pruritus causes further scratching and damage to the epidermis. Patients may also describe a feeling of fullness in the ear (Sander, 2001).

Treatment

Cleansing the ear canal by suctioning is the first treatment, as well as administration of acidifying drops, such as 2% **acetic acid** (Sander, 2001). The patient should be evaluated at the end of the treatment for resolution of symptoms because the infection can persist asymptomatically (Sander, 2001). If the infection persists, over-the-counter **clotrimazole** 1% solution should be used; if tympanic membrane perforation is suspected, however, **tolnaftate** 1% solution should be used to prevent ototoxicity associated with **clotrimazole** (Lucente, 1993; Sander, 2001). *Aspergillus* infections may be resistant to **clotrimazole** and may require the use of oral **itraconazole** (Sander, 2001).

Analgesics

Ear infections are frequently accompanied by pain. Treating this pain with systemic analgesics can be problematic for parents, particularly when the patient is an infant. Nonsteroidal anti-inflammatory drugs (NSAIDs) are associated with upper gastrointestinal tract complications (Bianciotto et al., 2013), particularly if combined with salicylates (which are generally not advised for use in young children due to the association with Reye syndrome). Use of **acetaminophen** in 10–15 mg/kg doses has been found to be effective as a fever reducer (Temple, Temple, & Kuffner, 2013), and this agent is a reasonably effective analgesic.

Topical anesthetics, typically **benzocaine**, can also be used to treat the pain associated with otitis media until systemic antibiotics are able to take effect (Wynne et al., 2002). **Benzocaine** may be combined with glycerin, a hygroscopic agent that helps coat the ear canal more easily (Wynne et al., 2002).

CHAPTER SUMMARY

- Eye and ear diseases are uniquely distressing to the patient. They are frequently addressed with topical and local interventions rather than systemic medications.
- Eye diseases stem from a variety of problems but can be treated with solutions or unguents containing appropriate medications.
- Glaucoma, in particular, is treated with a variety of medication classes that are applied directly to the eyes.
- Proper technique in using ophthalmic medications must be taught to patients to ensure optimal results.

- Bacterial infections of the eyes and ears are not automatically treated with antibiotic therapy due to concerns about antibiotic resistance, but persistent or severe infections may be addressed with appropriate medications.
- Otic infections are treated, depending on whether they are AOM or external, with antimicrobials, but following age-based guidelines. External ear infections should be treated with topical agents unless circumstances warrant broad-spectrum systemic antimicrobials. Pain associated with most otic infections should usually be treated with NSAIDs.

Critical Thinking Questions

1. The nurse is caring for a patient with a known history of glaucoma. The patient complains of blurred vision, severe headache, and severe pain. What is the priority action for the nurse?
   a. Notify the physician immediately.
   b. Administer a narcotic analgesic.
   c. Document the findings because these are expected symptoms.
   d. Place the patient in a darkened room.

2. What is the mechanism of action of the prostaglandin analogs used to treat glaucoma?
   a. Decreased aqueous humor formation
   b. Increased aqueous humor outflow
   c. Dilated pupils
   d. Decreased production of vitreous humor

3. The patient should be aware of the possible side effects of beta blockers used in the treatment of glaucoma. The nurse should include which of the following in the treatment plan?
   a. Brown pigmentation of the iris and eyelid
   b. Loss of eyelashes
   c. Bradycardia
   d. Tachycardia

4. From the following list of signs and symptoms, identify which are associated with AOM. Select all that apply.
   a. Fever
   b. Ear pain
   c. Somnolence
   d. Otorrhea

5. From the following signs and symptoms, identify which are associated with OME.
   a. Fever
   b. Vomiting
   c. Irritability
   d. Fluid in the middle ear

CASE STUDIES

Case Scenario 1

A two-year-old child presents to the clinician's office with her mother. The mother states that her daughter has been sick for five days. The child has a runny nose with "green" discharge, has a temperature of 99.9°F, and has been tugging at her left ear for the last two days. She does not have any history of "ear problems" according to the mother. There are no smokers in the household. The only medication that the girl is taking at this time is fluoride, according to the mother (sodium fluoride drops 0.5 mg, 0.5 mL daily). The mother notes that she had to speak louder to her daughter over these last several days in order for her daughter to understand her.

The girl does not appear in any acute distress. She is well developed and well nourished. Physical exam findings are as follows:
- Vital signs: temperature 99.2°F, blood pressure 90/55, pulse 100, respirations 20.
- Eyes: sclera injected with clear discharge leaking from eyes.
- Ears: external ear canal with yellow-brown earwax present.
- External pinna: no lesions or masses.
- Left tympanic membrane: bulging, translucent, pink, intact, clear fluid noted behind tympanic membrane; light reflex diffuse; unable to visualize all of the bony landmarks.
- Right tympanic membrane: translucent, intact, no fluid visualized; light reflex sharp; able to visualize all bony landmarks.
- Nares: clear discharge from nares bilaterally.
- Lymph nodes: small anterior and posterior cervical nodes palpated on left side, no pre-auricular nodes palpated.
- Throat: pink, moist, tonsils not enlarged, clear postnasal drainage present in the posterior pharynx.
- Heart: regular rate; S_1 and S_2 heart sounds present.
- Lungs: clear to auscultation bilaterally anterior and posterior.

Case Questions
1. Based on the exam findings, what are the possible reasons for the girl's ear pain?
2. How should the nurse educate the mother on the exam findings and potential treatment plan?
3. What are the signs and symptoms for AOM and OME?

CASE STUDIES

Case Scenario 2

Sophie is a four-year-old Hispanic female with a complaint of bilateral "eye drainage" who is routed to the fast-track clinic of the ED where you work. Sophie's mother tells you that Sophie's eye drainage started yesterday in one eye, and today both her eyes were matted shut with thick, yellow secretions when she woke up. Sophie has had cloudy nasal drainage and mild, nonproductive cough for the last three days. She attends full-day pre-K, and several children have been ill with

(continues)

CASE STUDIES (CONTINUED)

similar "cold symptoms" during the last week. She denies fever, eye pain or itching, photophobia, headache, loss of vision, rash, nausea or vomiting. No other family members are currently ill. Sophie's past medical history includes uncomplicated term birth with no subsequent chronic diseases, hospitalizations, serious injuries, or surgeries. She has no history of allergic rhinitis, asthma, or atopic dermatitis. She is seen regularly by a pediatrician for her annual well-child check-ups, and her immunizations/health screenings are up to date. She was last seen by her pediatrician three months ago for her annual check-up. She takes no medications, herbal products, or supplements. Sophie's parents are both employed; she has 2 older siblings. Her immediate family have no chronic illness. Sophie is not exposed to tobacco smoke.

Medication list: None; Allergies: NKDA

Vital signs: BP: 90/50; P: 95/minute, regular; Respirations: 20/minute, regular; Oral temperature: 98.8°F. Weight: 32 lbs.; Ht: 38"; BMI: 52nd percentile (healthy weight).

The healthcare provider performs a targeted physical exam. Sophie is alert and cooperative; she is in no acute distress. Her visual acuity is 20/30 for each eye and both eyes together. Her visual fields are intact; her pupils are round, equal, and reactive to light bilaterally. The conjunctivae are injected bilaterally, and tenacious yellow-green material is present. Her lids are mildly edematous bilaterally; there is no periorbital erythema or edema. Her pharynx is clear; tympanic membranes are dull bilaterally but mobile; pre-auricular lymph nodes are nonpalpable. Her lung sounds are clear bilaterally.

The provider makes a clinical diagnosis of acute bacterial conjunctivitis based on symptomatology. He prescribes trimethoprim-polymyxin B sulfate, a topical antibiotic with-broad spectrum activity that has shown to be safe in children. He asks you to instruct the parent about instillation of the eye drops, dosing frequency, adverse effects, duration of treatment, and prevention of contamination of the medication bottle. Sophie is to follow-up with her pediatrician at her next scheduled appointment or sooner if her condition worsens or does not improve in 24–48 hours.

Case Questions

1. Sophie's mother is concerned about how to instill the eye drops in her very mobile four-year old daughter who does not like anything put into her eyes. What can you teach her about a good technique to use with small children when instilling eye drops?

2. What is the dosing frequency and duration of treatment for trimethoprim-polymyxin B sulfate?

3. What should you say if Sophie's mother asks, "Will the eye drops hurt when I put them in her eyes?"

4. How can Sophie's mother protect the sterility of the antibiotic eye drop solution?

5. Sophie's family members may be at risk for contracting the infection from her. Write a nursing diagnosis that reflects this risk.

6. Write one short-term goal (something that can be achieved today) directed toward avoiding the outcome of spread of infection to other family members.

7. What adverse effects might occur with the use of this medication? What specific information will you tell Sophie's mother about when to call the clinic for a reevaluation of her illness?

8. When can Sophie return to pre-K? Would you recommend that someone at her school instill the eye drops during school hours?

REFERENCES

AAOS. (2004). *Paramedic: Anatomy and physiology*. Sudbury, MA: Jones and Bartlett.

Acott, T.S., Kelley, M.J., Keller, K.E., Vranka, J.A., Abu-Hassan, D.W., Li, X., . . . Bradley, J.M. (2014). Intraocular pressure homeostasis: Maintaining balance in a high-pressure environment. *Journal of Ocular Pharmacology and Therapeutics, 30*(2-3), 94–101.

Aldrich, D.S., Bach, C.M., Brown, W., Chambers, W., Fleitman, J., & Tin, G.W. (2013). Ophthalmic preparations. *Pharmacopeial Forums, 39*(5), 1-21.

American Academy of Pediatrics (AAP), Subcommittee on Management of Acute Otitis Media. (2004).

Diagnosis and management of acute otitis media. *Pediatrics, 113*(5), 1451–1465.

American Optometric Association (AOA). (2018). Dry eye. Retrieved from https://www.aoa.org/patients-and-public/eye-and-vision-problems/glossary-of-eye-and-vision-conditions/dry-eye

Arthur, S., & Cantor, L.B. (2011, April 20). Update on the role of alpha-agonists in glaucoma management. *Experimental Eye Research, 93*(3), 271–283. doi: 10.1016/j.exer.2011.04.002

Bausch & Lomb. (2010). *Naphazoline hydrochloride –naphazoline hydrochloride solution/drops* [Package insert]. Tampa, FL: Author. Retrieved from http://dailymed.nlm.nih.gov/dailymed/archives/fdaDrugInfo.cfm?archiveid=20190

Bianciotto, M., Chiappini, E., Raffaldi, I., Gabiano, C., Tovo, P.A., Sollai, S., . . . Menniti-Ippolito, F.; Italian Multicenter Study Group for Drug and Vaccine Safety in Children. (2013). Drug use and upper gastrointestinal complications in children: A case-control study. *Archives of Diseases of Childhood, 98*(3), 218–221.

Bojrab, D.I., Bruderly, T., & Abdulrazzak, Y. (1996). Otitis externa. *Otolaryngology Clinics of North America, 29*, 761–782.

Boustred, N. (1999). Practical guide to otitis externa. *Australian Family Physician, 28*, 217–221.

Centers for Disease Control and Prevention (CDC). (2012). Ear infections. Retrieved from https://www.cdc.gov/antibiotic-use/community/for-patients/common-illnesses/ear-infection.html

Chapman, J.M., Cheeks, L., & Green, K. (1990). Interactions of benzalkonium chloride with soft and hard contact lenses. *Archives of Ophthalmology, 108*(2), 244–246.

Chiras, D. (2012). *Human biology* (7th ed.). Burlington, MA: Jones & Bartlett.

Clark, W.B., Brook, I., Bianki, D., & Thompson, D.H. (1997). Microbiology of otitis externa. *Otolaryngology Head and Neck Surgery, 116*, 23–25.

Diagnosis and treatment of acute otitis externa: An interdisciplinary update. (1999). *Annals of Otology Rhinology & Laryngology, 176*(Suppl.), 1–23.

Dibb, W.L. (1991). Microbial aetiology of otitis externa. *Journal of Infections, 22*, 233–239.

Duzman, E., Anderson, J., Vita, J.B., Lue, J.C., Chen, C.C., & Leopold, I.H. (1983). Topically applied oxymetazoline: Ocular vasoconstrictive activity, pharmacokinetics, and metabolism. *Archives of Ophthalmology, 101*(7), 1122–1126.

Food and Drug Administration (FDA). (2011). An important FDA reminder for parents: Do not give infants cough and cold products designed for older children. Retrieved from http://www.fda.gov/Drugs/ResourcesForYou/SpecialFeatures/ucm263948.htm

Food and Drug Administration (FDA). (2017). Ophthalmic vasoconstrictors. In *Code of Federal Regulations Title 21* (Ch.1, Part 349, Subpart B, Sec. 349.18). Retrieved from http://www.accessdata.fda.gov/scripts/cdrh/cfdocs/cfcfr/CFRSearch.cfm?fr=349.18

Giebink, G.S. (1994). Preventing otitis media. *Annals of Otology, Rhinology and Laryngology, 163*(Suppl.), 20–23.

Glaucoma Research Foundation (GRF). (2012). Cholinergic (miotic) medication guide. Retrieved from https://www.glaucoma.org/treatment/medication-guide.php#cholinergic_miotic

Goodolf, D.M. (2014). Assessment and management of patients with eye and vision disorders. In J.L. Hinkle & K. Cheever (Eds.), *Brunner & Suddarth's textbook of medical-surgical nursing.* (13th ed., pp 1850–1852). Philadelphia, PA: Lippincott Williams & Wilkins.

Haas, W., Gearinger, L.S., Usner, D.W., Decory, H.H., & Morris, T.W. (2011). Integrated analysis of three bacterial conjunctivitis trials of besifloxacin ophthalmic suspension, 0.6%: Etiology of bacterial conjunctivitis and antibacterial susceptibility profile. *Clinics in Ophthalmology, 5*, 1369–1379.

Hajioff, D., & MacKeith, S. (2015). Otitis externa. *BMJ Clinical Evidence, 2015*, 0510.

Halpern, M.T., Palmer, C.S., & Seidlin, M. (1999). Treatment patterns for otitis externa. *Journal of American Board of Family Practice, 12*(1), 1–7.

Harmes, K.M., Blackwood, R.A., Burrows, H.L., Cooke, J.M., Harrison, R.V., & Passamani, P.P. (2013). Otitis media: Diagnosis and treatment. *American Family Physician, 88*(7), 435–440.

Howard, M.L. (2010). Middle ear, tympanic membrane, perforations treatment and management. *Medscape.* Retrieved from http://emedicine.medscape.com/article/858684-treatment

JHP Pharmaceuticals. (2008). *Cortisporin-TC-colistin sulfate, neomycin sulfate, thonzonium bromide and hydrocortisone acetate suspension* [Package insert]. Rochester, MI: JHP Pharmaceuticals. Retrieved from http://dailymed.nlm.nih.gov/dailymed/archives/fdaDrugInfo.cfm?archiveid=11240

Jones, R.N., Milazzo, J., & Seidlin, M. (1998). Ofloxacin otic solution for treatment of otitis externa in children and adults. *Archives of Otolaryngology, Head and Neck Surgery, 123*, 1193–2000. [Published erratum appears in *Archives of Otolaryngology, Head and Neck Surgery, 124*, 711.]

Lee, D.S.H., Markwardt, S., McAvay, G.J., Gross, C.P., Goeres, L.M., Han, L., . . . Tinetti, M.E. (2014). Effect of β-blockers on cardiac and pulmonary events and death in older adults with cardiovascular disease and chronic obstructive pulmonary disease. *Med Care, 52*(0 3), S45–S51.

Lehne, R.A. (2013). Additional important drugs. In *Pharmacology for nursing care* (8th ed., pp. 1346–1351). St. Louis, MO: Elsevier Saunders.

Lieberthal, A.S., Carroll, A.E., Chonmaitree, T., Ganiats, T.G., Hoberman, A., Jackson, M.A., . . . Tunkel, D.E. (2013). The diagnosis and management of acute otitis media. *Pediatrics, 131*, e964–e999. doi: 10.1542/peds.2012-3488

Lucente, F.E. (1993). Fungal infections of the external ear. *Otolaryngology Clinics of North America, 26*, 995–1006.

Moroi, S.E., & Lichter, P.R. (1996). Ocular pharmacology. In A.L. Wynne, T.M. Woo, & M. Millard, *Pharmacotherapeutics for nurse practitioner prescribers* (p. 790). Philadelphia, PA: F. A. Davis.

National Eye Institute. (2015). Facts about glaucoma. Retrieved from https://www.nei.nih.gov/health/glaucoma/glaucoma_facts

Nichols, A.W. (1999). Nonorthopaedic problems in the aquatic athlete. *Clinical Sports Medicine, 18,* 395–411, viii.

Noecker, R.J. (2006). The management of glaucoma and intraocular hypertension: Current approaches and recent advances. *Therapeutics and Clinical Risk Management, 2*(2), 193–206.

Nurse practitioner prescribing reference (NPPR). (2012, Spring). New York, NY: Prescribing Reference.

Rasmussen, C.A., Kaufman, P.L., & Kiland, J.A. (2014). Benzalkonium chloride and glaucoma. *Journal of Ocular Pharmacology and Therapeutics, 30*(2–3), 163–169.

Ricciotti, E., & FitzGerald, G.A. (2011). Prostaglandins and inflammation. *Arteriosclerosis, Thrombosis, and Vascular Biology, 31*(5), 986–1000.

Rosenfeld, R.M., Schwartz, S.R., Cannon, C.R., Roland, P.S., Simon, G.R., Kumar, K.A., . . . Robertson, P.J. (2014). Clinical practice guideline: acute otitis externa. *Otolaryngology–Head and Neck Surgery, 150*(1): S1-S24.

Sambhara, D., & Aref, A.A. (2014). Glaucoma management: Relative value and place in therapy of available drug treatments. *Therapeutic Advances in Chronic Disease, 5*(1), 30–43.

Sander, R. (2001). Otitis externa: A practical guide to treatment and prevention. *American Family Physician, 63*(5), 927–937.

Selesnick, S.H. (1994). Otitis externa: Management of the recalcitrant case. *American Journal of Otology, 15,* 408–412.

Shaw, M. (2016.) How to administer eye drops and eye ointment. Nursing Standard. 30, 39, 34-36. Date of submission: February 9 2016; date of acceptance: March 8 2016. Retrieved from https://rcni.com/sites/rcn_nspace/files/ns.30.39.34.s42.pdf.

Simpson, K.L., & Markham, A. (1999). Ofloxacin otic solution: A review of its use in the management of ear infections. *Drugs, 58,* 509–531.

Story, L. (2012). *Pathophysiology: A practical approach.* Burlington, MA: Jones & Bartlett.

Tamm, E.R., Braunger, B.M., & Fuchshofer, R. (2015). Intraocular pressure and the mechanisms involved in resistance of the aqueous humor flow in the trabecular meshwork outflow pathways. *Progress in Molecular Biology and Translational Science, 134,* 301–314.

Temple, A.R., Temple, B.R., & Kuffner, E.K. (2013). Dosing and antipyretic efficacy of oral acetaminophen in children. *Clinical Therapeutics, 35*(9), 1361–1375, e1–e45.

van Wyk, F.C. (2017). Cerumen impaction removal. *Medscape.* Retrieved from https://emedicine.medscape.com/article/1413546-overview

Wilson, B.A., Shannon, M.T., & Shields, K.M. (2012). *Pearson health professional's drug guide 2011–2012.* Upper Saddle River, NJ: Pearson Education.

Wójcik-Gryciuk, A., Skup, M., & Waleszczykb, W.J. (2016). Glaucoma—State of the art and perspectives on treatment. *Restorative Neurology Neuroscience, 34*(1), 107–123.

Wynne, A.L., Woo, T.M., & Millard, M. (2002). *Pharmacotherapeutics for nurse practitioner prescribers* (pp. 782–808). Philadelphia, PA: F. A. Davis.

CHAPTER 11

Pharmacology of the Genitourinary System

Diana M. Webber

KEY TERMS

Androgens
Benign prostate hyperplasia (BPH)
Complicated UTI
Contraception
Corpus cavernosum
Cystitis
Erectile dysfunction

Gonadotropin
Gonadotropin-releasing hormone (GnRH)
Ovulation
Phosphodiesterase-5 (PDE-5) inhibitor
Progestin
Prostate

Prostatitis
Pyelonephritis
Recurrent UTI
Sexually transmitted infections (STIs)
Testosterone
Uncomplicated UTI
Urethra

Urethritis
Urinary incontinence
Urinary tract
Urinary tract infection (UTI)
Vesicoureteral reflux (VUR)

CHAPTER OBJECTIVES

At the end of the chapter, the reader will be able to:

1. Discuss the basic pharmacotherapeutic concepts in three genitourinary conditions: urinary tract infection (UTI), male erectile dysfunction (ED), and female hormonal contraception.

2. Describe the nurse's role in the pharmacologic management of UTI, ED, and hormonal contraception.

3. Explain the mechanisms by which estrogens and progestins prevent conception.

4. Describe the pharmacology for the drugs discussed in this chapter in terms of class, therapeutic indication, mechanism of action, interactions, side effects, and toxicity.

5. Identify relevant nursing considerations for medications used for management of UTI, ED, and hormonal contraception.

Introduction

The genitourinary system is an unusual convergence of two separate bodily functions: reproduction and waste elimination. It includes the entire **urinary tract** as well as the organs related to reproduction in both men and women (**FIGURE 11-1**). When treating ailments of this system, the clinician must, therefore, "wear two hats"—that is, consider disease processes (and potential outcomes) that may have origins in or impacts on more than one set of functions. For example, an ailment of the urinary tract, such as a simple infection, can have repercussions for the patient's sexual functioning, and vice versa. This association can complicate patients' understanding of disease processes, even when the illness is as straightforward (in theory) as a simple bacterial infection. Particularly when such infections may have been sexually transmitted, embarrassment or shame about the nature of the illness can provoke responses in patients that make treating them difficult.

The focus of this chapter includes male and female lower and upper UTIs (e.g., **urethritis**, bacterial cystitis, pyelonephritis), vaginitis, benign prostatic hyperplasia and male erectile dysfunction (ED), sexually transmitted infections (STIs), and female pharmacologic contraception.

Urinary Tract Infections

Although the anatomy and physiology of the male and female genitourinary tract

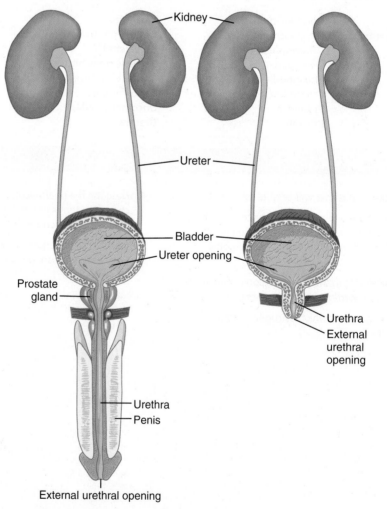

FIGURE 11-1 Anatomy of the male (left) and female (right) urinary tracts.

partially protect this system from pathogenic invasion, certain factors may contribute to increased incidence of **urinary tract infection (UTI)**. In females, these factors include a short, straight **urethra**, which facilitates bacterial access to the bladder, and hormonal influences such as postmenopausal estrogen deficiency with concomitant vaginal acidification (**FIGURE 11-2**). The acid environment of the vagina allows for bacterial colonization with subsequent ascending microbial invasion of the bladder. In fact, the lifetime risk for UTI in females is estimated to be 60.4%, and at least one-third of women in the United States are diagnosed with UTI before age 24 (Griebling, 2005a).

By contrast, males (other than prior to one year of age, when male UTI incidence exceeds that of females), have only a 13.6% lifetime risk for UTI. Most adult male UTIs are the result of obstruction of the urinary tract from benign hyperplasia of the **prostate** (BPH), typically occurring after age 50 years (**FIGURE 11-3**) (Griebling, 2005b). **Urinary incontinence**, estrogen deficiency, chronic constipation, chronic

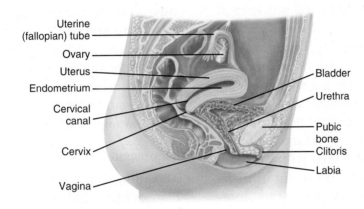

FIGURE 11-2 The female urogenital system, and anatomical relationships for UTIs.

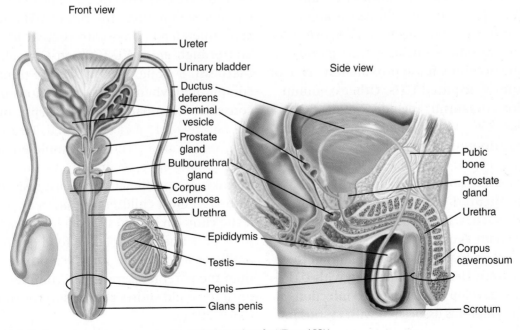

FIGURE 11-3 Urethra and prostate gland, and anatomical relationships for UTIs and BPH.

diseases such as diabetes, use of urinary catheters, and other factors contribute to increased incidence of UTI in the older adult population (Beveridge, Davey, Phillips, & McMurdo, 2011).

UTI in children is usually related to a structural or functional abnormality of the kidney, the ureters, or the vesicoureteral valves. Among these abnormalities, **vesicoureteral reflux (VUR)** is the most likely cause in pediatric patients with UTI (Koyle & Shifrin, 2012). Other risk factors for UTI in pediatric patients include chronic constipation, dysfunctional voiding patterns, and lack of circumcision in males.

UTIs are diagnosed by the presence of symptoms such as urinary urgency and frequency, pain with voiding, lower back or suprapubic pain, and dark or malodorous urine. These symptoms are similar in males and females. Fever without an obvious source is the most frequent presenting symptom for UTI among infants younger than two years. Older men with prostatic obstruction of the urethra retain urine in the bladder, and may develop asymptomatic (possibly chronic) UTI. Laboratory tests such as urinalysis, with urine culture and sensitivity (C&S), not only confirms the UTI diagnosis and identifies the causative pathogen, but also allows for appropriate antimicrobial selection. *Escherichia coli* is the most common urinary tract pathogen, and accounts for approximately 85% of community-acquired UTIs. Other common infectious organisms include *Proteus, Pseudomonas, Klebsiella*, and *Staphylococcus saprophyticus* (Hooton, 2012).

It is useful to categorize UTIs to facilitate treatment decisions: **complicated UTI** and **uncomplicated UTI**. Uncomplicated UTIs, termed **cystitis**, generally occur in healthy, nonpregnant, ambulatory females with no functional or anatomic abnormalities of the urinary tract. Healthy young men with UTI may also develop uncomplicated infection, although symptoms associated with cystitis in

men may be indicative of an underlying inflammation in the prostate (and, therefore, should be investigated further).

Complicated UTI in Adults

Complicated UTI can occur in both men and women of any age. Most clinicians agree that any UTI in males is considered complicated, especially in men older than 50 years, simply because their risk for underlying conditions is higher. UTIs associated with an immunocompromised state, a concurrent metabolic disease, an anatomic or functional abnormality that impairs urine flow, or colonization by an atypical organism such as yeast, are considered complicated. Recurrent and pediatric UTIs are also categorized as complicated. Infections in such cases have an increased risk of treatment failure and/or adverse long-term consequences and require different pharmacologic management.

Complicated UTI in Pediatric Patients

According to the American Academy of Pediatrics (AAP, 2011), uncircumcised infant males have a 1% greater risk for developing UTI even if no other risk factors are present. A systematic review of randomized controlled trials (RCTs) indicates that circumcision reduces the risk of UTI and is recommended in boys with **recurrent UTI** and/or high-grade VUR (Singh-Grewal, Macdessi, & Craig, 2005). UTIs are termed complicated when the risk for serious or fatal consequences—particularly urosepsis or renal failure—is higher than usual. Treatment in a complicated UTI, then, should employ the most effective agent with the best pharmacokinetic profile and the least resistance. Although most children can be treated orally, if the clinician believes the child appears toxic or is unable to tolerate food or fluids orally, or if adherence may be a problem, then the parenteral route is recommended until the child shows clinical improvemen (AAP, 2011).

Medications for Treatment of Uncomplicated UTI (Cystitis)

For further information about antimicrobial agents, the reader is referred to Chapter 16. First-line pharmacologic agents for uncomplicated UTI include trimethoprim-sulfamethoxazole, nitrofurantoin, and fosfomycin trometamol. In UTIs that prove resistant to these agents, fluoroquinolones and beta-lactam drugs are recommended as second-line agents.

Trimethoprim-Sulfamethoxazole

Trimethoprim-sulfamethoxazole (TMP-SMX, or SMX-TMP) is active against many Enterobacteriaceae, including *Escherichia coli*, *Klebsiella pneumoniae*, and *Proteus mirabilis*. TMP-SMX is standard therapy for uncomplicated cystitis in women unless the prevalence of local resistance to the drug is greater than 10% to 20%. Patient factors favorable to the use of TMP-SMX include no recent antimicrobial use, hospitalization, or recurrent UTI in the past year.

SMX and TMP act synergistically to inhibit bacterial folic acid synthesis. By using two agents that act on the organism via two different mechanisms that affect the same metabolic pathway, the combination drug avoids the development of bacterial resistance to either component alone (Masters, O'Bryan, Zurlo, Miller, & Joshi, 2003).

Pharmacokinetics

Both TMP and SMX are well absorbed from the gastrointestinal (GI) tract. The combination drug's half-life is 8 to 14 hours; therefore, it must be dosed twice daily. The usual dose when treating uncomplicated UTIs is 160/800 TMP-SMX mg, one tablet twice daily, for 3 days. The drug is excreted in urine, so the dose must be lowered in patients with renal insufficiency.

Nursing Considerations

The patient's human immunodeficiency virus (HIV) status should be assessed before prescribing TMP-SMX, as adverse reactions are most common in HIV-infected patients and may occur in as many as 65% of those receiving the drug. Follow-up testing of urine for pathogen eradication is not necessary in uncomplicated UTI due to the low resistance and high efficacy of this antimicrobial agent.

Some healthcare professionals may recommend phenazopyridine to help lessen the pain or discomfort caused by urinating. Phenazopyridine is a pain reliever *only*; it does *not take the place of an antibiotic* and should be taken concurrently with the prescribed antibiotic. Patients should be cautioned to use this medication for a maximum of three days, as it can mask symptoms, and be warned that it changes the color of the urine to bright orange/red and

Myth Buster

Although certain conditions and practices, such as recent change in sex partner, pregnancy, constipation, postmenopausal hormone changes, instrumentation of the urinary tract, and neurogenic bladder, have been shown to be associated with the development of UTIs, some suspected factors have not been proven to contribute to UTI risk in women with no preexisting risk factors. These unproven risk factors include perineal hygiene (not wiping from front to back), tub bathing, bubble bath, swimming, type of underwear, tampon use, precoital or postcoital voiding patterns, body mass index (BMI), and drinking carbonated sodas or juice (Hooton, 2012). It is important that nurses dispel common myths associated with the development of UTI while supporting practices shown to prevent this bothersome infectious process.

can stain clothing. Nurses should emphasize that **phenazopyridine** does not cure the infection.

Nitrofurantoin

Nitrofurantoin is a synthetic antimicrobial agent that is effective against 90% of the clinical strains of *E. coli*. Most other bacteria show resistance to **nitrofurantoin**. This drug is indicated for uncomplicated UTI due to *E. coli*.

Nitrofurantoin is enzymatically reduced by microbial nitroreductases within the bacterial cell. The reduced derivatives bind to bacterial ribosomal proteins and disrupt cell metabolism by interfering with protein and DNA synthesis (Garau, 2008).

Pharmacokinetics

Although the drug has only 40% to 50% GI absorption, this percentage can be enhanced when **nitrofurantoin** is taken with food. It is highly concentrated in urine.

Nursing Considerations

Guidelines for treatment of uncomplicated UTI do not recommend urine culture and sensitivity to identify the specific pathogen; however, **nitrofurantoin** has little activity against bacteria other than *E. coli*. Evaluation for the expected clinical outcome includes contacting the patient two to three days after he or she has started this medication to assess for subjective improvement.

Fosfomycin Trometamol

Fosfomycin trometamol is a broad-spectrum bactericidal antibiotic that is effective against beta-lactamase–producing *E. coli*, *P. mirabilis*, and *Klebsiella pneumoniae*. It is specifically labeled for treatment of uncomplicated UTI. **Fosfomycin** acts as a bacterial cell-wall inhibitor by binding to and inhibiting the enzyme (known as MurA) responsible for the synthesis of components necessary to produce the peptidoglycan layer of the bacterial cell wall. It exerts immunomodulatory effects, mainly on lymphocyte and neutrophil function, possibly due to **fosfomycin's** effects on acute inflammatory cytokine signaling (Falagasa, Vouloumanoua, Samonisd, & Vardakasa, 2016) and reduces the ability of bacteria to adhere to urinary epithelial cells (Roussos, Karageorgopoulos, Samonis, & Falagas, 2009).

Pharmacokinetics

The bioavailability of **fosfomycin** is 40% when taken orally as a 3 g single dose. Its peak distribution to the urine occurs 4 hours after administration, and it persists in the body for 48 hours. High concentrations of **fosfomycin** are present in the bladder for 36 hours.

Nursing Considerations

Assess the patient for medication adherence patterns; this antibiotic is appropriate when adherence may be low, as a single dose may be given in-clinic.

Second-Line Agents for UTI

Fluoroquinolones

Ciprofloxacin and **levofloxacin** are first- and second-generation fluoroquinolones, respectively. This antibiotic class comprises broad-spectrum antibacterial agents with activity against gram-positive and gram-negative bacteria. By selectively binding to one of the catalytic sites during the formation of negative supercoils in bacterial DNA, fluoroquinolones inhibit two types of bacterial enzymes, topoisomerase 4 and DNA gyrase, required for DNA replication, transcription, repair, and recombination (Wagenlehner, Wullt, & Perletti, 2011).

The fluoroquinolones are indicated for complicated (**levofloxacin**) and uncomplicated (**ciprofloxacin**) UTI. **Levofloxacin** is labeled only for persons older than 18 years due to the risk of tendonitis or tendon rupture. Members of this drug class are recommended only when the pathogen is penicillin resistant or macrolide resistant. The half-life of **ciprofloxacin** is much shorter than that of **levofloxacin**, necessitating twice-daily dosing with the former drug.

Pharmacokinetics

Fluoroquinolones show concentration-dependent bactericidal activity. The oral formulation is rapidly absorbed. Members of this drug class also have good tissue penetration and a high concentration in the urinary tract (especially **levofloxacin**).

Nursing Considerations

Because they chelate certain cations in the stomach and GI tract, fluoroquinolones should not be given within two hours of antacids containing aluminum, magnesium, or calcium; sucralfate; iron preparations; and multivitamin/mineral supplements containing zinc. If the patient ingests caffeine, there may be increased central nervous system (CNS) stimulation, as fluoroquinolones inhibit the CYP4501A2 enzyme that normally regulates caffeine metabolism.

Beta-Lactam Agents

Beta-lactam agents are generally less effective than other antimicrobial drugs for UTI. **Amoxicillin** is an aminopenicillin that is active against *E. coli* and *P. mirabilis,* but inactive against most other *Enterobacter* species and *Pseudomonas.* When combined with the beta-lactamase inhibitor **clavulanate**, **amoxicillin** is more stable against beta lactamase, an enzyme produced by many bacteria that inactivates the beta-lactam ring present on all beta-lactam drugs. Other beta-lactam agents (second- and third-generation cephalosporins) are active against gram-negative bacteria such as *E. coli, Klebsiella,* and *P. mirabilis.* These agents are more stable against beta-lactamase than are the penicillins.

Pharmacokinetics

Most oral beta-lactam agents have a short half-life and must be dosed two to four times daily. Some parenteral forms may be dosed once daily.

Nursing Considerations

Beta-lactam antibiotics have significant impact on GI microflora, sometimes leading to diarrhea and possibly impaired absorption of combined oral contraceptive pills (OCPs). Therefore, the nurse should assess for use of OCPs and recommend alternative contraception for the duration of treatment. The GI effects are seen more often with prolonged use of these agents.

Non-Antimicrobial Biological Mediators for Prevention of Uncomplicated Recurrent Cystitis

Cranberry Juice, Capsules, or Tablets

The current hypothesis regarding the potential effectiveness of cranberries in preventing UTIs is that cranberries contain fructose and type A proanthocyanidins (PACs), which in urine can inhibit the adherence of type 1 and P fimbriae of *E. coli* to the uroepithelial cell receptors on the bladder wall (Guay, 2009; Hooton, 2001; Raz, Chazan, & Dan, 2004). Without the ability to adhere, the *E. coli* bacteria are unable to infect the mucosal surface (Hisano, Bruschini, Nicodemo, & Srougi, 2012).

When compared to no treatment, unsweetened cranberry juice (or 500 mg capsules/tablets of cranberry juice extract) *may* be effective for prevention of recurrent UTI in premenopausal women (Singh, Guatam, & Kaur, 2016). However, there is no consistency in formulation or established dose for efficacious use of cranberry products (Guay, 2009) and larger studies are needed to confirm efficacy of cranberry in UTI prevention (Fu, Liska, Talan, & Chung, 2017). When cranberry was compared to prophylactic **TMP-SMX** in the same population, **TMP-SMX** proved *more* effective than cranberry in the prevention of recurrent UTI (Beerepoot et al., 2011).

Nursing Considerations

Many women have had word-of-mouth "information" about the use of cranberry as a prophylactic or even a "cure" for UTI. Most who act upon this information will do so by drinking sweetened cranberry juice products, thinking that this is a more "natural" or less expensive means of treating their ailment than using medication. These patients need to be provided with accurate information about how to address UTI symptoms and which forms of cranberry extract have value versus which do not. Moreover, because cranberry can interact with medications that are metabolized via the cytochrome P450 pathway, patients who take such medications and who acknowledge using cranberry juice or supplements should be assessed for the possibility of drug interactions.

Topical/Local Estrogen

American College of Obstetricians and Gynecologists (ACOG, 2016) guidelines state that randomized trials are required before conclusively recommending use of topical/local estrogen for postmenopausal women with recurrent UTI. The Society of Obstetricians and Gynaecologists of Canada (SOGC) indicates that vaginal estrogen should be offered to postmenopausal women who experience recurrent UTIs (see also Geerlings, Beerepoot, & Prins, 2014).

Vaccines and Probiotic Application

Both ACOG and SOGC found insufficient evidence to recommend the use of vaccines for recurrent UTI (ACOG, 2008). An initially promising vaccine—OM-89—was not confirmed to prevent recurrent UTI (Beerepoot & Geerlings, 2016). The use of probiotics (vaginal lactobacilli application) shows promise (specifically, oral capsules with *Lactobacillus rhamnosus* GR-1 and *Lactobacillus reuteri* RC-14 in postmenopausal women and intravaginal suppositories with *Lactobacillus crispatus* in premenopausal women) (Beerepoot & Geerlings, 2016), but as yet both ACOG and SOGC have not found enough evidence to recommend their use for recurrent UTI (ACOG, 2008).

Treatment of Complicated UTI

A complicated UTI is a urinary infection occurring in a patient with a structural or functional abnormality of the genitourinary tract. Bladder outlet obstruction due to BPH may be associated with urinary stasis and contribute to an increased risk of complicated UTI in men 50 years and older (discussed later in this chapter). Invasive diagnostic studies associated with urine obstruction also increase risk for UTI and associated prostatitis or pyelonephritis. In addition, chronic medical conditions increase the risk of developing UTI, including diabetes mellitus, renal insufficiency, immunosuppression, and kidney stones (Neal, 2008).

A wider variety of pathogens and increased drug resistance are more common among persons with complicated UTI; for this reason, fluoroquinolones are recommended as first-line drug therapy rather than **TMP-SMX**, which has an increased likelihood of microbial resistance, or **nitrofurantoin**, which has limited effectiveness against pathogens other than *E. coli*. Whenever possible, drug initiation should be delayed pending results from urine culture so that the agent can be targeted to the specific infectious organism. **Levofloxacin**, **ciprofloxacin**, and **norfloxacin** may be used as oral therapy (Nicolle, 2005), with other medications under evaluation (Giancola et al., 2017; Shah et al., 2018). Parenteral therapy is indicated if patients are unable to tolerate oral therapy, if they have impaired GI absorption, or if the infecting organism is known or suspected to be resistant to oral agents.

Fever is unusual in men with uncomplicated UTI, and its occurrence signals a complicated UTI with concomitant acute **prostatitis**, orchitis, or **pyelonephritis**. The nurse should evaluate for these conditions and for drug intolerance or nonadherence to oral antibiotics. Because of their high risk for recurrent infection, men with a complicated UTI should have a follow-up visit in 2 to 4 weeks to ensure resolution of symptoms.

Candida albicans Vaginitis (Vaginal Yeast Infection)

Infections of the vaginal mucosa are common in women of reproductive age. While some of the organisms causing vaginitis are sexually transmitted (see the "Sexually Transmitted Infections" section later in this chapter), *Candida albicans*, a yeast, generally is not. Thus, it is not necessary to treat the sexual partners of patients diagnosed with vaginal candidiasis (Schwebke, 2012).

Vaginal candidiasis is distinguished from other forms of vaginitis by the characteristic "cheesy" discharge and a positive potassium hydroxide smear. Oral antibiotic use often precedes candidiasis (Xu et al., 2008), and this type of infection is more likely to occur in immunosuppressed and diabetic women (Nyirjesy & Sobel, 2013). If possible, diagnosis should include in-office microscopic inspection of wet mount samples for hyphae to positively identify yeast.

Treatment of vaginal candidiasis can be undertaken with either oral medication (fluconazole, 150 mg single dose, which may be repeated 3 to 7 days later if indicated) or intravaginal therapy, which can consist of a cream (butoconazole or clotrimazole 2% cream 5 g × 3 days) or a vaginal suppository (miconazole 200 mg × 3 days or 1,200 mg × 1 day). Some intravaginal creams are sold as over-the-counter products (e.g., miconazole, butoconazole, clotrimazole), and patients may attempt self-treatment prior to coming to the healthcare provider for evaluation. However, many women who self-diagnose a "yeast infection" actually have vaginitis of bacterial or parasitic origin, which is why the treatment fails. On average, over-the-counter azole creams have about an 80% cure rate if used as directed (Angotti, Lambert, & Soper, 2007).

Pharmacokinetics

Fluconazole is highly bioavailable (93%) and reaches its peak plasma concentration within 3 to 4 hours after administration. This drug and is eliminated unchanged in the urine; in 48 hours, nearly 60% of an initial dose of 150 mg may be recovered in the urine (Debruyne, 1997). The half-life of fluconazole is approximately 36 hours in most

patients, which is why a single, oral dose is usually effective in treating most *Candida albicans* infections.

"Feminine Itching"

Some over-the-counter medications are advertised as relieving "intense itch" or "itching due to thrush." These products consist of combinations of anesthetics such as benzocaine or lidocaine, plus external analgesics (resorcinol) and topical corticosteroids (hydrocortisone) (Angotti et al., 2007). These products do exactly what they say they do—relieve the pruritus and irritation, without curing the underlying infection. Patients who present with symptoms of vaginitis should be advised that these products produce only symptomatic relief and not cure. Assessment for the cause of vaginitis is the best way to identify an appropriate curative therapy.

Nursing Considerations

Recurrent or persistent vaginal candidiasis infections are generally related to an underlying chronic disease (e.g., diabetes), and should prompt assessment of therapy (if previously diagnosed) or diagnostic testing. Alternatively, a patient with recurrent infections may have been colonized with a non-*albicans* species of *Candida* that is resistant to first-line therapy with fluconazole (e.g., *C. glabrata*, which is particularly prevalent in persons with diabetes [Goswami et al., 2006; Nyirjesy & Sobel, 2013]). These considerations should be taken into account when treating patients with recurrent yeast infections.

Benign Hyperplasia of the Prostate

Benign prostate hyperplasia (BPH) is very common among men older than age 50. Some studies estimate that by age 50, 50% of men have at least histologic evidence of hyperplasia; of those men, approximately 25% experience bothersome lower urinary tract symptoms such as hesitancy, urgency, frequency, difficulty starting or stopping urine flow, and feelings of incomplete bladder emptying (Roehrborn, 2012). These symptoms, classified as obstructive and/or irritative, occur because the enlarged prostate presses against the urethral canal and interferes with normal urination. Complications from long-term urinary obstruction may include chronic UTI and renal scarring. Pharmacologic treatment is primarily based on the degree of discomfort the patient experiences, as a result of these bothersome symptoms.

Published guidelines recommend several different pharmacotherapeutic agents to alleviate the symptoms caused by BPH. Currently recommended drug classes include antimuscarinic agents, alpha blockers, 5-α-reductase inhibitors, combinations of these drug categories, and the **phosphodiesterase-5 (PDE-5) inhibitor tadalafil** used for ED. The labeling of a PDE-5 inhibitor for BPH is a promising avenue for BPH treatment, as ED and BPH often co-occur.

Although their exact pharmacologic mechanisms are not well understood, some plant products have been studied sufficiently to make dietary supplement recommendations. Two such products include extracts from the berry of the saw palmetto (*Serenoa repens*) and stinging nettle (*Urtica dioica*). Some researchers postulate that saw palmetto binds to alpha-1 (α_1) adrenoceptors, muscarinic cholinoceptors in the lower urinary tract tissues (Suzuki et al., 2009). Stinging nettle appears to exert its effect on the prostate through interactions with sex hormone–binding globulin (SHBG), aromatase, epidermal growth factor, and prostate steroid membrane receptors (Chrubasik, Roufogalis, Wagner, & Chrubasik, 2007). Other dietary supplements utilized, but not subjected to rigorous study, include extracts of the African plum tree (*Pygeum africanum*), pumpkin seed (*Cucurbita pepo*), South African star grass (*Hypoxis rooperi*), and rye pollen (*Secale cereale*). Earlier studies with saw palmetto had suggested modest efficacy in treatment of lower urinary tract symptoms (LUTS); however, more vigorous studies have shown mixed results with this treatment (American Urological Association [AUA], 2014; Novaro et al., 2016).

Medications for the Treatment of BPH
Antimuscarinic Agents (Tolterodine)

Antimuscarinic agents block the neurotransmitter acetylcholine in the central and peripheral nervous system, reducing its effects on the bladder neurons through competitive inhibition. These agents have a dose-dependent effect, with higher doses producing more adverse effects such as worsening urinary retention. These agents are recommended for BPH *only under two conditions*: (1) when overactive bladder symptoms (urgency, frequency, urge incontinence) exist, but there is no indication of bladder outlet obstruction; or (2) when overactive bladder symptoms are not relieved by other BPH agents.

Nursing Considerations

Prior to initiating this drug, the patient should be evaluated for urinary retention.

Selective α_1-Adrenoreceptor Antagonists (Alfuzosin, Prazosin, Doxazosin, Tamsulosin, Terazosin)

Selective α_1-adrenoreceptor antagonists (also called α-adrenergic blockers) block postsynaptic α_1-receptors, resulting in both venous and arterial vasodilation with relaxation of vascular and other smooth muscles, including those of the urinary bladder, bladder neck, urethra, and prostate. Because there are fewer α_1-receptors in the bladder wall than in the bladder neck, these drugs are able to reduce bladder outflow obstruction without impairing bladder contractility (AUA, 2010). These agents are used to treat *urinary outlet obstruction symptoms* such as urinary hesitancy, incomplete bladder emptying, straining, and decreased force of urine stream in men with BPH.

Nursing Considerations

When considering the adverse effects of these medications, it is important to evaluate patients for reflex tachycardia and hypotension; these effects are associated more often with doxazosin and terazosin than with other agents. If the patient is taking an antihypertensive agent, the dose may need to be adjusted.

5-α-Reductase Inhibitors (Finasteride, Dutasteride)

The 5-α-reductase inhibitor class of drugs is composed of synthetic testosterone derivatives. Because the growth of the prostate depends on androgens, decreasing androgenic activity may effectively reduce prostate volume in men with BPH. The inhibition of the prostate enzyme 5-α-reductase blocks the conversion of testosterone by this enzyme to its metabolite, 5-α-dihydrotestosterone (DHT), which is an *active* metabolite. Decreasing conversion of testosterone to DHT reduces testosterone-related biological effects. The two drugs in the 5-α-reductase inhibitor category act slightly differently. Finasteride is a competitive inhibitor of the type 2 isoform of 5-α-reductase, whereas dutasteride blocks both type 1 and type 2 isoforms, resulting in more suppression of DHT synthesis. Both finasteride and dutasteride act to reduce androgen-dependent increases in prostatic volume; however, adequate symptomatic relief may require several months of therapy (AUA, 2014).

Pharmacokinetics

The half-life of 5-α-reductase inhibitors is about 8 hours; however, the level of DHT is reduced for about 24 hours.

Nursing Considerations

5-α-reductase inhibitors decrease serum prostate-specific antigen (PSA) values by approximately 50%. Any increase of serum PSA should prompt a referral for further follow-up and discussion with the patient's healthcare provider. Evaluate patients for gynecomastia, ED, and decreased libido at each follow-up visit.

PDE-5 Inhibitors (Tadalafil)

Agents in this drug class act as selective vasodilators for treatment of impotence in men with ED. This drug class has also been shown to improve LUTS in men with BPH. Further pharmacologic information is provided in the next section, "Erectile Dysfunction."

Erectile Dysfunction

Erectile dysfunction (ED) is a common condition reported by about half of men aged 40–70 years. Defined as the inability to sustain an erection adequate for sexual satisfaction (Andersson, 2011), ED typically results from a lack of blood flow through the **corpus cavernosum** of the shaft of the penis. Although ED can have other etiologies, it usually is a result of neurogenic or vascular conditions. Following the first-line recommendation to treat any underlying medical conditions and offer psychosexual counseling, the two main categories of pharmacologic agents used to treat erectile problems are PDE-5 inhibitors and alprostadil, a prostaglandin that can be either injected directly into the corpus cavernosum or inserted as a urethral suppository. In both instances, the medications act to increase the availability or activity of cyclic guanosine monophosphate (cGMP) and cyclic adenosine monophosphate (cAMP), both of which promote relaxation of vascular smooth muscle. In normal physiology, stimulation of the muscarinic receptors by acetylcholine leads to nitric oxide (NO) release. This NO, upon diffusing into the smooth muscle cells of the corpus cavernosum, stimulates cGMP activity to relax smooth muscles, increase blood flow, and produce an erection. Whether the dysfunction leading to ED is a dysfunction in this system or is unrelated, increasing cGMP or cAMP activity aids in overcoming it.

Various medications associated with chronic disease may contribute to ED. As hypertension, diabetes, dyslipidemia, and obesity are significantly associated with ED, it is likely that men seeking treatment for ED may also be taking medications that contribute to the problem. According to a systematic analysis (Baumhaken et al., 2011), antihypertensive medications associated with a higher incidence of ED include thiazide diuretics and beta blockers (except for **nebivolol**). The risk of ED associated with beta blockers is 5 per 1,000 patients (Ko et al., 2002). Additionally, **spironolactone**—a weak inhibitor of testosterone synthesis—may exert a negative effect on erectile function. Angiotensin-converting enzyme inhibitors, angiotensin-receptor blockers, loop diuretics, and calcium-channel blockers are reported to have no relevant effect on ED; therefore, members of these drug categories could be used as alternative medications for hypertensive therapy.

The mechanisms responsible for the ED effects of these medications are not always clear. Some studies suggest that sodium depletion associated with thiazide diuretics leads to increased central alpha-2 adrenergic function, which may depress erectile performance (Baumhaken et al., 2011). Other studies have suggested that diuretics exert a direct effect on vascular smooth muscle cells or decrease the response to catecholamines (Sica, 2004). Beta-blockers, especially the nonselective agents such as propranolol, may decrease levels of testosterone and, therefore, affect erectile function.

Cross-sectional studies have shown associations between lifestyle, substance-use habits and ED. Lifestyle habits studied include smoking, alcohol, and sedentary lifestyle (Reffelmann & Kloner, 2006). Other unhealthy lifestyle factors examined include obesity, a substantially increased waist circumference, and use of drugs such as amphetamine, LSD, cocaine, heroin, and other narcotics. Unfortunately, cross-sectional studies can only speculate as to a cause-and-effect relationship between lifestyle or substance-use habits and ED (Christensen, Gronbaek, Pedersen, Graugaard, & Frisch, 2011).

Medications for the Treatment of ED

PDE-5 Inhibitors (Sildenafil, Tadalafil, Vardenafil)

PDE-5 inhibitor agents are selective vasodilators indicated for the treatment of impotence in men with ED (FIGURE 11-4). **Tadalafil** has been shown to significantly improve urinary symptoms of BPH as well. The drug works by increasing the availability of cGMP, leading to muscle relaxation, vasodilation, and erection. cGMP is inactivated by PDE-5; thus, PDE-5 inhibitors decrease the breakdown of cGMP by competitively occupying the PDE-5 binding sites (Andersson, 2011).

PDE-5 inhibitors enhance the effects of NO. This increases blood flow and allows an erection, in response to sexual stimulation.

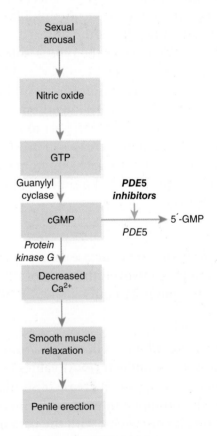

FIGURE 11-4 Biochemistry of PDE-5 inhibitors.

Pharmacokinetics

PDE-5 inhibitors are rapidly absorbed, with an onset of action 30 to 60 minutes after administration. The duration of action for **sildenafil** and **vardenafil** is 4 to 6 hours, and the duration for **tadalafil** is 36 hours.

Nursing Considerations

Patients should be evaluated for orthostatic hypotension, as PDE-5 inhibitors reduce supine blood pressure by 7–8 mm Hg. Patients' baseline blood pressure should be at least 90/60 mm Hg. Patients *must* be advised that concurrent administration of these drugs with any form of **nitroglycerine**—a vasodilating drug commonly used for angina—is absolutely contraindicated. Precaution is recommended when α-adrenoreceptor blockers are used with PDE-5 inhibitors. Evaluate patients for concurrent use of antibiotics, antifungals, and grapefruit juice, as these substances will reduce clearance of PDE-5 inhibitors by way of their CYP3A4 isoenzyme inhibition. The nurse should also evaluate patients for priapism, a persistent erection (lasting longer than four hours). Although rare, priapism is a very serious side effect of all PDE-5 inhibitors, that should be reported immediately to the healthcare provider.

Alprostadil

Alprostadil is a synthetic prostaglandin E_1, a derivative of arachidonic acid, which acts as a smooth muscle vasodilator and is indicated for treatment of impotence in men with ED. **Alprostadil** is administered by intracavernous injection or by intraurethral suppository. It stimulates the production of cAMP; this causes smooth muscle relaxation of the corpus cavernosum, thereby increasing the diameter of cavernous arteries and leading to penile erection. This drug can be used in patients who have sustained nerve injury to the penis, as it does not depend on NO, or an intact nervous system, for its pharmacological activity (Nehra, 2007).

Pharmacokinetics

Within 60 minutes of intracavernous injection, 96% of **alprostadil** is metabolized by an enzyme present in the corpus cavernosum, prostaglandin 15-hydroxydehydrogenase. Although some **alprostadil** enters the systemic circulation, its presence does not lead to changes in vital signs or other serious adverse effects.

Nursing Considerations

Intraurethral alprostadil (IUA) has a lower efficacy than the injected form; however, pain associated with injection and resistance to self-injection results in 30% patient discontinuance in favor of **IUA** after three months (Nehra, 2007).

Sexually Transmitted Infections

The genitourinary tract is a particularly welcoming environment for pathogens, and many of the bacterial, fungal, parasitic, and viral organisms that infect the genitourinary tract can be transmitted to sexual partners. Preventive measures for transmission of **sexually transmitted infections (STIs)** include abstinence and use of barriers, such as condoms (although inconsistent or incorrect use of barrier methods can reduce their effectiveness as means of STI prevention).

Unlike many other conditions described in this chapter, STIs carry a distinct stigma associated with the nature of disease transmission. This is a particularly important factor among adolescents, who may avoid being screened for or notifying partners of STIs if they view STIs as stigmatizing (Cunningham, Kerrigan, Jennings, & Ellen, 2009; Reed et al., 2015). Stigma is related to the fact that risk of contracting an STI increases in accordance with the number of sexual partners the patient has encountered in his or her past. This is particularly true for women, as historically, the key vector of STI transmission has been prostitution (East, Jackson, O'Brien, & Peters, 2012). While this is no longer necessarily true, women diagnosed with an STI are likely to express negative self-perceptions, fear of rejection, and feelings of unworthiness (East et al., 2012). In the public's (and often the patient's) perception, a person who contracts an STI is often partly responsible for the illness because it results from the patient's "choices." Such choices include (or may be perceived to include) sexual relations with multiple partners or partnering with an infected person. Nurses who encounter patients diagnosed with an STI should be aware that patients may be unusually reluctant to discuss the disorder frankly due to shame or embarrassment.

The cause of STIs run the gamut of infectious organisms: viruses, bacteria, and parasites; there are too many such infections to provide a comprehensive listing of all organisms and therapeutic regimens here. This discussion focuses on the most common types of infections and medication classes used in their treatment.

Sexually Transmitted Viral Infections

A number of STIs are caused by viral infections. These include *molluscum contagiosum*, which is usually treated surgically; genital warts, caused by human papillomavirus (HPV), some strains of which also cause cervical cancer; genital herpes, caused by herpes simplex virus 2 (HSV-2); hepatitis B virus (HBV), which is often sexually transmitted, although it can be transmitted by other routes; and HIV, a retrovirus known to cause acquired immune deficiency syndrome (AIDS). Some strains of HPV and HBV can be prevented via vaccination, but HSV-2 and HIV cannot; individuals infected with these viruses generally have a lifelong chronic infection that can flare up periodically.

HPV, Genital Warts, and Cervical Cancer

More than 40 strains of HPV are known to infect the genitourinary tract. The vast majority (90%) of these infections resolve without intervention within two years (Datta, Dunne,

Saraiya, & Markowitz, 2012), and most strains are nononcogenic (non-cancer-causing). However, some strains cause the development of genital wart lesions (HPV-6, HPV-11); others (HPV-16 and HPV-18 in particular), if *unresolved,* may cause cervical, vulvar, vaginal, penile, and anal cancers (Datta et al., 2012). Female patients diagnosed with oncogenic strains of HPV should be screened routinely for cervical cancer.

Treatment is usually considered only when genital warts arise, and is intended to remove the warts rather than eliminate the underlying infection. Therapies include **podofilox** 0.5% solution or gel, **imiquimod** 5% cream, and **sinecatechins** 15% ointment (Datta et al., 2012), which may be applied by the patient. If these therapies are ineffective, medical options such as bichloroacetic acid or podophyllin resin, applied by the clinician, are possible. These drugs act by various, unrelated mechanisms, including acting as toxins and as immunomodulators.

Herpes and HIV Infections

Neither herpes nor HIV is curable at present. Genital herpes is not life threatening, but it can be bothersome to the patient. Moreover, genital herpes represents a significant threat to the infants of women who become pregnant and give birth without treatment. In a neonate infected as it passes through the birth canal, herpes can spread to the brain and other internal organs, leading to lasting disabilities or even death (ACOG, 2007).

Herpes infections are managed depending on the severity of symptoms; antiviral medications such as acyclovir, famciclovir, and valacyclovir (nucleoside analogs, refer to Chapter 16) are used intermittently to reduce flares' duration and discomfort when flares are infrequent, or are provided daily to suppress viral activity altogether in individuals subject to frequent and/or severe flares. TABLE 11-1 provides the Centers for Disease Control and Prevention's (CDC's) recommended regimens for treating the initial clinical episode of herpes.

In the case of HIV, the long-term potential effects of the virus on the immune system are significant and potentially deadly. Therefore, antiretroviral therapy is recommended for all patients with HIV, regardless of CD4 T-lymphocyte cell count, to prevent HIV-associated mortality and morbidity (U.S. Department of Health and Human Services – AIDS Info, 2017). TABLE 11-2 lists the medications used in HIV treatment. Their mechanisms of action are discussed in Chapter 16.

Nursing Considerations

A new diagnosis of HSV-2 and especially HIV infection can be an emotionally devastating experience for the patient. Nurses should be prepared to assist these patients with referrals for counseling as well as treatment.

Many of the medications used to treat viral infections have drug–drug interactions due to their metabolism by the cytochrome P450 pathway. Consequently, vigilance is necessary when a patient taking other medications (including herbal products) begins HIV therapy.

HIV infection may coincide with other STIs. Of note is the interaction that occurs between HIV and syphilis, in which the latter causes increases in the HIV viral load and suppresses the CD4 cell count (Jarzebowski et al., 2012). Patients diagnosed with HIV should be assessed for STIs prior to initiating a treatment regimen.

Sexually Transmitted Bacterial Infections

The most commonly reported bacterial STIs are chlamydia (*Chlamydia trachomatis*) and gonorrhea (*Neisseria gonorrhoeae*). Coinfection with these two organisms is common, with chlamydia being found in as many as 40% of individuals diagnosed with gonorrhea (Zenilman, 2012). Syphilis (*Treponema pallidum*) is a less common bacterial STI, but if left untreated has significant clinical consequences, *particularly* when it occurs in concert with HIV infection. Bacterial vaginosis, which presents as vaginitis caused by an opportunistic infection of the vagina, can develop from any

TABLE 11-1	CDC Recommended Regimens for Treatment of Genital Herpes
Medication	Dose Options
Initial Clinical Episode	
Acyclovir*	400 mg orally three times a day for 7–10 days **or** 200 mg orally five times a day for 7–10 days.
Famciclovir	250 mg orally three times a day for 7–10 days.
Recurrent Episodes – Episodic Therapy	
Acyclovir*	400 mg orally three times a day for 5 days **or** 800 mg orally twice a day for 5 days **or** 800 mg orally three times a day for 2 days.
Famciclovir	125 mg orally twice daily for 5 days **or** 1 g orally twice daily for 1 day **or** 500 mg once, followed by 250 mg twice daily for 2 days.
Valacyclovir	500 mg orally twice a day for 3 days **or** 1 g orally once a day for 5 days.
Recurrent Episodes – Suppressive Therapy	
Acyclovir	400 mg orally twice a day.
Famiciclovir	250 mg orally twice a day.
Valacyclovir	500 mg orally once a day **or** 1 g orally once a day.**
Severe HSV Disease	
Acyclovir (IV) + oral therapy as per recurrent episodes	5–10 mg/kg IV every 8 hours for 2–7 days or until clinical improvement is observed, followed by oral antiviral therapy to complete at least 10 days of total therapy. Patients with HSV encephalitis require 21 days of IV therapy. Acyclovir dose adjustment is recommended for impaired renal function.

*In pregnant women, acyclovir is preferred, as safety profiles for the other drugs are not as well established (ACOG, 2007). For all medications listed, treatment can be extended if healing is incomplete after 10 days of therapy.
**For suppressive therapy of recurrent HSV, valacyclovir 500 mg once a day might be less effective than other valacyclovir or acyclovir dosing regimens in persons who have frequent recurrences (i.e., ≥10 episodes per year).
Data from Centers for Disease Control and Prevention, Sexually Transmitted Diseases Treatment Guidelines, 2015. Available at https://www.cdc.gov/std/tg2015/herpes.htm

of a variety of bacteria commonly present in the vagina. It is frequently seen in women with multiple sexual partners, as a coinfection with other STIs, and in association with the use of vaginal douches, which alter vaginal pH and/or floral balance (specifically a decrease in the presence of *Lactobacillus* species, which are protective).

Bacterial STIs are typically treated with antibiotic therapy. A key point in this approach, however, is knowing which agents

TABLE 11-2	Antiretroviral Therapies for HIV

Recommended Initial Regimens for Most People with HIV

Recommended regimens are those with demonstrated durable virologic efficacy, favorable tolerability and toxicity profiles, and ease of use.

INSTI + 2 NRTIs:

- DTG/ABC/3TC[a] (**AI**)—if HLA-B*5701 negative
- DTG + tenofovir[b]/FTC[a] (**AI** for both TAF/FTC and TDF/FTC)
- EVG/c/tenofovir[b]/FTC (**AI** for both TAF/FTC and TDF/FTC)
- RAL[c] + tenofovir[b]/FTC[a] (**AI** for TDF/FTC, **AII** for TAF/FTC)

Recommended Initial Regimens in Certain Clinical Situations

These regimens are effective and tolerable, but have some disadvantages when compared with the regimens listed above, or have less supporting data from randomized clinical trials. However, in certain clinical situations, one of these regimens may be preferred.

Boosted PI + 2 NRTIs: (In general, boosted DRV is preferred over boosted ATV)

- (DRV/c or DRV/r) + tenofovir[b]/FTC[a] (**AI** for DRV/r and AII for DRV/c)
- (ATV/c or ATV/r) + tenofovir[b]/FTC[a] (**BI**)
- (DRV/c or DRV/r) + ABC/3TC[a] – **if HLA-B*5701—negative (BII)**
- (ATV/c or ATV/r) + ABC/3TC[a]—**if HLA-B*5701—negative and HIV RNA < 100,000 copies/mL (CI** for ATV/r and **CIII** for ATV/c)

NNRTI + 2 NRTIs:

- EFV + tenofovir[b]/FTC[a] (**BI** for EFV/TDF/FTC and **BII** for EFV + TAF/FTC)
- RPV/tenofovir[b]/FTC[a] (**BI**)—**if HIV RNA < 100,000 copies/mL AND CD4 > 200 cells/mm**^{3}

INSTI + 2 NRTIs:

- RAL[c] + ABC/3TC[a] (**CII**)—**if HLA-B*5701—negative and HIV RNA < 100,000 copies/mL**

Regimens to Consider when ABC, TAF, and TDF Cannot be Used:[d]

- DRV/r + RAL (BID) (**CI**)—**if HIV RNA < 100,000 copies/mL AND CD4 > 200 cells/mm**^{3}
- LPV/r + 3TC[a] (BID)[e] (**CI**)

[a]3TC may be substituted for FTC, or vice versa, if a non-fixed dose NRTI combination is desired.
[b]TAF and TDF are two forms of tenofovir approved by the FDA. TAF has fewer bone and kidney toxicities than TDF, while TDF is associated with lower lipid levels. Safety, cost, and access are among the factors to consider when choosing between these drugs.
[c]RAL can be given as 400 mg BID or 1,200 mg (two 600 mg tablets) once daily.
[d]Several other NRTI-limiting treatment strategies are under investigation.
[e]LPV/r plus 3TC is the only boosted PI plus 3TC regimen with published 48-week data in a randomized controlled trial in ART-naïve patients. Limitations of LPV/r plus 3TC include twice-daily dosing, high pill burden, and greater rates of gastrointestinal side effects than other PIs.
Key to Acronyms: 3TC = lamivudine; ABC = abacavir; ART = antiretroviral therapy; ATV = atazanavir; ATV/c = atazanavir/cobicistat; ATV/r = atazanavir/ritonavir; BID = twice daily; CD4 = CD4 T lymphocyte; DRV = darunavir; DRV/c = darunavir/cobicistat; DRV/r = darunavir/ritonavir; DTG = dolutegravir; EFV = efavirenz; EVG = elvitegravir; EVG/c = elvitegravir/cobicistat; FDA = Food and Drug Administration; FTC = emtricitabine; HLA = human leukocyte antigen; INSTI = integrase strand transfer inhibitor; LPV/r = lopinavir/ritonavir; NNRTI = non-nucleoside reverse transcriptase inhibitor; NRTI = nucleoside reverse transcriptase inhibitor; PI = protease inhibitor; RAL = raltegravir; RPV = rilpivirine; TAF = tenofovir alafenamide; TDF = tenofovir disoproxil fumarate
Guidelines for the Use of Antiretroviral Agents in Adults and Adolescents Living with HIV: https://aidsinfo.nih.gov/guidelines

will work for which organisms, and which will not. Antibiotic resistance is an issue for gonorrhea, which has developed resistance to cephalosporin antibiotics as well as

fluoroquinolones (Centers for Disease Control and Prevention [CDC], 2013; see especially "Drug-resistant *Neisseria gonorrhoeae*," http://www.cdc.gov/drugresistance/threat -report-2013/pdf/ar-threats-2013-508.pdf# page=55). TABLE 11-3 describes antibiotic therapies for bacterial STIs.

Nursing Considerations

Patient allergy to the specific antibiotics used to treat gonorrhea and syphilis is of particular concern due to the relative lack of response these two organisms show toward other agents. In patients with a known allergy to the principal drug of choice, consultation with CDC or other infectious disease specialists may be useful to identify the optimal treatment regimen.

Any patient diagnosed with a bacterial STI is at risk of other STIs, including HIV and herpes; testing should be offered, and patients counseled on effective prevention of STIs, including HIV. In all of the infections noted previously, aside from bacterial vaginosis, partners of the infected individual will likely need treatment as well, even if asymptomatic. Legal reporting requirements and partner notification for certain diseases vary from state to state; nurses should maintain awareness of the requirements of individual states and of the CDC with respect to notifiable diseases.

Sexually Transmitted Parasitic Infections

Several parasitic organisms are transmitted via sexual contact. Two of these, the mite *Sarcoptes scabiei* (scabies) and the parasitic louse *Pthirus pubis* (crab louse), infest the external genitalia by direct skin contact between an individual with an infected partner. Note that condom use does not prevent such contact. A third parasite, *Trichomonas vaginalis*, infects the urogenital tract. Although both men and women can be infected with this pathogen, the symptoms generally differ; women may have a foul odor, vaginal itching, and/or a greenish-yellow, frothy discharge, while men generally are asymptomatic. TABLE 11-4 summarizes the treatment regimens for these STIs.

TABLE 11-3	Antibiotic Therapies for Sexually Transmitted Bacterial Infections		
Disease	Bacterium	Agent(s) Used	Notes
Gonorrhea	*Neisseria gonorrhoeae*	<u>Ceftriaxone</u> 250 mg IM plus azithromycin 1 g orally in a single dose	*N. gonorrhoeae* has developed multidrug resistance, including resistance to cefixime, as reported by CDC in 2013. Currently, ceftriaxone is the only agent known to which the bacterium lacks resistance. Different strains may be resistant to different agents. Patients must be advised of the importance of close compliance.
Syphilis	*Treponema pallidum*	Parenteral <u>benzathine penicillin G</u>*; if allergic, doxycycline may be used	2.4 million units IM in a single dose. If allergic to penicillin, 100 mg doxycycline orally twice daily for 14 days.
Chlamydia	*Chlamydia trachomatis*	<u>Doxycycline</u> 100 mg orally twice a day for 7 days Azithromycin 1 g orally in a single dose	Alternative regimens: Erythromycin base 500 mg orally four times a day for 7 days or Erythromycin ethylsuccinate 800 mg orally four times a day for 7 days **or** levofloxican 500 mg orally once daily for 7 days **or** ofloxican 300 mg orally twice a day for 7 days. Individuals who had sexual contact with the patient within 60 days before onset of symptoms should be examined, tested for urethral or cervical chlamydial infection, and treated with a chlamydia regimen
Bacterial vaginosis	Various	<u>Metronidazole</u> 500 mg oral twice daily for 7 days **or** metronidazole gel 0.75%, one full applicator (5 g) intravaginally, once a day for 5 days **or** clindamycin cream 2%, one full applicator (5 g) intravaginally at bedtime for 7 days	Cure rates of 70–80%, with recurrence common. Association with other STIs, including HIV, suggests that patients presenting with bacterial vaginosis should be tested for other STIs.

*The CDC reports that practitioners have inadvertently prescribed combination benzathine-procaine penicillin instead of the standard benzathine penicillin product; nurses should be aware of the similar names of these two products and alert to the possibility of errors in prescribing or dispensing the agent for treating syphilis. The preferred agent is indicated by underline.

Data from Centers for Disease Control and Prevention, Sexually Transmitted Diseases Treatment Guidelines, 2015. Available at https://www.cdc.gov/std/tg2015 /tg-2015-print.pdf

TABLE 11-4	Treatment Regimens for Parasitic Sexually Transmitted Infections	
Organism	Treatment	Notes
Pthirus pubis (crab louse)	Permethrin 1% cream rinse applied to affected area and washed off after 10 minutes **or** pyrethrins with piperonyl butoxide applied to the affected area and washed off after 10 minutes	Treatment must be accompanied by thorough cleansing of the patient's and partner's bedding, clothing, linens, and other potential reservoirs with hot water. Sexual abstinence for up to 2 weeks is also needed to break the cycle of reinfection. Treatment failure is usually due to poor compliance.
Sarcoptes scabiei (scabies)	Topical: permethrin 5% cream, Oral: ivermectin, 200 mcg/kg–250 mcg/kg, repeated in 2 weeks	Topical medications should be selected depending on patient needs. Combination of a topical medication with oral ivermectin has been shown to be effective in crusted scabies.
Trichomonas vaginalis	Metronidazole or tinidazole, 2 g oral single dose	Resistance to metronidazole has been noted in some strains of *T. vaginalis*. Use of tinidazole can usually overcome this issue. Failure to respond to prolonged therapy with tinidazole warrants referral to susceptibility testing.

Data from Centers for Disease Control and Prevention, Sexually Transmitted Diseases Treatment Guidelines, 2015. Available at https://www.cdc.gov/std /tg2015/tg-2015-print.pdf

Pharmacokinetics

Permethrin is the first-line agent for both scabies and crab lice because it is poorly systemically absorbed, nontoxic even in young children, and highly effective. It has no known drug interactions and is contraindicated only in persons with known sensitivity. Of note, it has a residual effect of up to 14 days when used to treat pubic lice, which helps to reduce recurrence by killing emerging insects.

Lindane is lipophilic and is absorbed poorly through the skin, albeit somewhat better than either **permethrin** or **malathion** (approximately 9%). It should be avoided in pregnant women due to its potential to be stored in placental tissue. Use of this agent with oil-based skin preparations could increase the absorption of the drug and should be avoided. **Lindane** has a long half-life (approximately 18 hours) and is metabolized in the liver.

Malathion is poorly absorbed (approximately 4%) and does not accumulate in body tissues. It is classified as a cholinesterase inhibitor, but its effects on cholinesterases in humans are very small. There are, however, only limited data regarding its use topically in humans; thus **malathion** is regarded strictly as a second-line agent for parasitic STIs at present.

Ivermectin is metabolized by the cytochrome P450 pathway, so it could be expected to interact with other drugs that use this pathway. Its elimination half-life is approximately 12 hours, but it has been observed to have antiparasitic activity lasting considerably longer, even as long as several months (González Canga et al., 2008). While it is not considered equal to **permethrin** in terms of safety and efficacy, **ivermectin** remains a viable option for patients who have difficulty in compliance with the **permethrin** regimen and/or who have a high burden of infestation.

Metronidazole for trichomoniasis has oral bioavailability approaching 100% (Lau, Lam,

Piscitelli, Wilkes, & Danziger, 1992); rapid absorption, reaching its maximum serum concentration in 1 to 2 hours if taken on an empty stomach; and a half-life of approximately 12 hours. It has a number of drug interactions that may be of concern; most notably, it increases the anticoagulant effects of **warfarin** and may produce an acute psychosis/confusional state when taken within 2 weeks of **disulfiram**. **Tinidazole** is biotransformed mainly by CYP3A4, so it carries the potential for similar significant interactions.

Nursing Considerations

Treatment of scabies and pubic lice with **permethrin** is known to be highly effective and nontoxic. The key consideration for patients is compliance with the full regimen—that is, not simply using the correct medications as directed, but also performing the needed environmental and behavioral adjustments that ensure complete eradication of the parasite. Washing of linens, bedding, and clothes; prophylactic treatment of partners (and, in the case of scabies, other residents of the household, including children); and abstinence from sexual activity for 14 days are essential components of the therapeutic regimen. Treatment failure is nearly always due to noncompliance (as no resistance to permethrin is known in these organisms), or the use of the wrong formulation (Cox, 2000), as the 1% **permethrin** cream rinse used for body lice is occasionally used by mistake instead of the 5% cream or rinse indicated for scabies and crab lice. Patients should be carefully instructed about what to use and for how long to use it.

Lindane has potential CNS toxicity; it has been banned from agricultural use, and its use in pharmaceutical indications is restricted. This drug's potential neurologic effects contraindicate its use in children, and resistance among body lice has been noted. Similar resistance has not been noted in scabies, but the concerns about its use are the same. For all these reasons, among the treatment options available, lindane is the agent of last resort.

Malathion is considered superior to lindane as a second-line agent for these parasites because of its lower toxicity; if not for the fact that its safety has not been fully investigated, it might well be considered a first-line agent (Idriss & Levitt, 2009). No animal or human studies have shown evidence of teratogenicity or increased risk of congenital malformations (Patel, Lambert, & Schwartz, 2016). The one drawback with malathion is its flammability; a potential hazard exists for patients should they approach an open flame during use or after application. Patients, particularly those who smoke, should be advised of this hazard and warned to wash hands thoroughly after use, and to limit exposure to flames from stoves or cigarettes.

Female Hormonal Contraception

Human reproduction involves a complex interaction among various hormones, glands, and organs in both males and females. Hormones secreted by the pituitary gland that stimulate the female gonads or reproductive organs are called gonadotropins. Beginning with the secretion of gonadotropin-releasing hormone (GnRH) by the hypothalamus, a hormone cascade stimulates the pituitary to release the gonadotropins follicle-stimulating hormone (FSH) and luteinizing hormone (LH) (FIGURE 11-5).

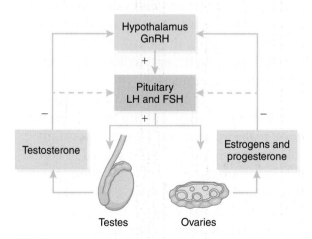

FIGURE 11-5 Gonadotropin-releasing hormones and follicle-stimulating hormones.

These hormones then stimulate the ovaries to produce three categories of gonadal steroids: estrogens (including estradiol, estrone, and estriol), progestins (most importantly, progesterone), and small amounts of androgens (such as testosterone). The menstrual cycle (FIGURE 11-6) is the most obvious result of the interactions among GnRH, FSH, and LH. The rate of production of the pituitary hormones plus the gonadal steroid hormones varies throughout the typical 28-day cycle to produce regular bleeding and shedding of the lining of the uterus (Katzung, Masters, & Trevor, 2012).

The gonadal steroid hormones are nonpolar, lipid-soluble substances that rapidly diffuse across the cell membrane following synthesis and are then transported by carrier proteins to their target organs. Gonadal steroid hormones are synthesized from the enzymatic alteration of cholesterol. Therefore, the regulation of these hormones is accomplished by controlling the enzymes that modify the steroid hormone in question (Katzung et al., 2012).

The first contraceptive—a combination of a synthetic form of estrogen that oxidized to ethinyl estradiol (EE), plus a progesterone derivative—was approved by the Food and Drug Administration (FDA) for use in the United States in 1960. An estimated 9.7 million U.S. women use oral hormonal contraceptives (Daniels, Daugherty, & Jones, 2015) and have a wide variety from which to choose (FIGURE 11-7; see also TABLE 11-5). Two main categories of hormonal preparations are available for contraception: combined estrogen and progestin, and continuous progestin therapy without estrogen. Combined estrogen/progestin preparations are further divided into monophasic (the same dose of each component daily throughout the month) or multiphasic (the dose of each component changes throughout the month to more closely reflect normal menstrual cycle fluctuations) options. The various mechanisms of action include inhibition

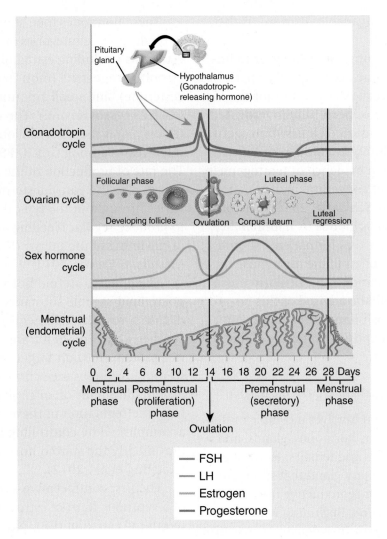

FIGURE 11-6 The menstrual cycle.

of **ovulation** by suppressing LH (estrogen), alteration of cervical mucus so as to hinder sperm transport, and modification of the endometrial lining of the uterus so as to make implantation of a fertilized ovum more difficult (progesterone).

Estrogen Analogs

Most estrogen analogs—that is, synthetic compounds with estrogenic effect—are either ethynyl estradiol (EE) or metabolize to this form. In women who have a uterus, estrogen analogs must be combined with a progestin, typically progesterone, to prevent endometrial hyperplasia and the associated increased risk of uterine cancer. The primary effect of ovarian-secreted estrogen is to promote the growth and maturation of the fallopian tubes, the uterus, and the vagina; additionally, this hormone promotes development of female secondary sex characteristics such as skeletal growth, distribution of body fat, breast development, and axillary and pubic hair patterns. Estrogens have additional actions in that they affect mood and emotions, increase synthesis of clotting factors, prevent bone reabsorption, and play an important role during childbirth. With regard to contraception, estrogen prevents ovulation largely through selectively inhibiting the release of FSH by the pituitary gland. Estrogen also causes increased production and/or thinning of the cervical mucus, and it causes the lining of the uterus to thicken or proliferate

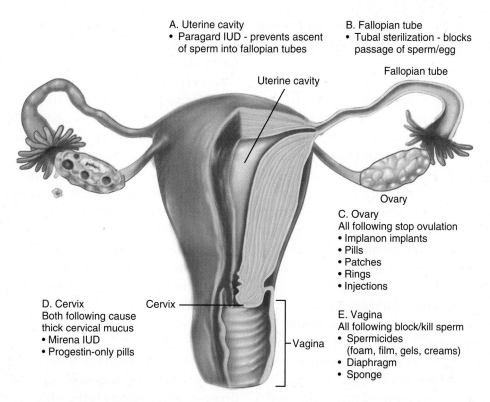

A. Uterine cavity
• Paragard IUD - prevents ascent of sperm into fallopian tubes

B. Fallopian tube
• Tubal sterilization - blocks passage of sperm/egg

Uterine cavity

Fallopian tube

Ovary

C. Ovary
All following stop ovulation
• Implanon implants
• Pills
• Patches
• Rings
• Injections

D. Cervix
Both following cause thick cervical mucus
• Mirena IUD
• Progestin-only pills

Cervix

Vagina

E. Vagina
All following block/kill sperm
• Spermicides (foam, film, gels, creams)
• Diaphragm
• Sponge

FIGURE 11-7 Preventing pregnancy with hormonal contraceptives: Contraceptive types and sites of actions.

New data from: https://www.cdc.gov/nchs/nsfg/key_statistics/c.htm#currentuse; Page last reviewed: April 18, 2017; Page last updated: April 18, 2017; Content source: CDC/National Center for Health Statistics 1600 Clifton Road Atlanta, GA 30329-4027 USA 800-CDC-INFO (800-232-4636), TTY: 888-232-6348 [Email CDC-INFO /U.S. Department of Health & Human Services/ HHS/Open/ USA.gov].

TABLE 11-5	Current Use of Contraceptive Methods

Percentage of women 15–44 years of age using specified contraception in month of interview:

	2002[1]	2006-2010[2]	2011-2015[3]
Not currently using contraception (currently pregnant, postpartum, trying to get pregnant, not having sex, etc.)	38.1%	37.8%	38.4% (0.70)
Percentage using any contraceptive method	61.9%	62.2%	61.6% (0.70)
Pill	19.2%	17.1%	15.9% (0.60)
Female sterilization	16.7%	16.5%	14.3% (0.66)
Male condom	14.7%	10.2%	9.2% (0.41)
Male sterilization	6.3%	6.2%	4.5% (0.32)
Intrauterine device (IUD)	1.3%	3.5%	6.8% (0.38)
Withdrawal	5.4%	3.2%	3.9% (0.28)
Depo-Provera™	3.3%	2.3%	2.6% (0.17)

Note: Women could be using more than one method in the month of interview. In this table, women are classified roughly according to the one most effective contraceptive method they are using. Additional methods women may be using are not shown here.

Sources:
[1]Series 23, No. 25, Table 57[PDF – 4.5 MB]
[2]NHSR No. 60, Table 1[PDF – 443 KB]
[3]Special tabulation by NCHS

(Practice Committee of the American Society for Reproductive Medicine, 2008).

Progestins

Synthetic progestin (also called progestogen) preparations, in contrast to estrogen analogs, may be given without an estrogen component; and this is advantageous when estrogen administration is not desired or is contraindicated. The primary effect of progesterone, which is synthesized in the body from cholesterol and secreted mainly by the corpus luteum, is to maintain pregnancy and prevent endometrial sloughing and miscarriage. Other effects of progesterone and other progestins are to increase basal body temperature at ovulation, increase insulin levels, increase synthesis of low-density lipoproteins, and increase sodium retention with subsequent fluid retention by the kidneys. Some synthetically produced progestins also exert androgen-like effects such as increasing body or facial hair (hirsutism) growth and increasing sebum production with associated acne. With regard to contraception, progestin suppresses ovarian and pituitary function to inhibit ovulation (but to a lesser degree than estrogen); thickens the cervical mucus, which makes sperm transport to the fallopian tubes more difficult; and causes endometrial atrophy so that implantation of a fertilized ovum cannot occur (Katzung et al., 2012).

Currently, four different forms or generations of synthetic progestins are used in hormonal contraceptives. The first-generation progestins, all of which are converted to norethindrone *in vivo*, contribute to spotting and breakthrough bleeding. The second-generation progestins, norgestrel and levonorgestrel, were developed to decrease this unexpected bleeding by increasing androgenic activity. However, this worsened the adverse effects of acne, hirsutism, and dyslipidemia. Third-generation progestins, desorgestrel and norgestimate, show decreased androgenicity; these agents also result in fewer unfavorable effects. The fourth-generation progestins, drospirenone and dienogest, are derived from spironolactone and testosterone, respectively. Spironolactone is a synthetic steroid with anti-androgenic and weak progestin activity (Practice Committee of the American Society for Reproductive Medicine, 2008). Although there is a risk of elevated serum potassium due to its potassium-sparing activity, this contraceptive has been shown to improve acne and other androgen effects associated with polycystic ovary syndrome (PCOS). As a testosterone derivative, dienogest does not possess the potassium-sparing effects of spironolactone; however, it is anti-androgenic and, therefore, effective for women with acne and/or PCOS.

Testosterone

The ovaries also produce small amounts of androgens from cholesterol. Among the androgens, testosterone is the only biologically active hormone. The physiological effects of testosterone in females are not well established, but this hormone may contribute to pubic hair growth during puberty, increased libido, and prevention of bone demineralization (Katzung et al., 2012). Most testosterone in the female is bound, along with estrogen, to a carrier protein (SHBG) and is, therefore, not biologically active. Some hormone contraceptive agents block the action of SHBG, which causes an increase in the amount of free testosterone in the body with increased androgen-like effects.

Pharmacodynamics

The major difference between the endogenous estrogen and progestins and those synthetically produced is in their oral bioavailability. The two currently available oral preparations of estrogen—EE mestranol (which is oxidized to EE)—and all of the progestins undergo significant first-pass metabolism via the CYP450 enzyme system. As estrogens and progestins are both nonpolar steroid hormones, following metabolism they easily pass through the lipid cell membrane and bind to estrogen and progesterone receptors distributed between the nucleus and the cytoplasm. Cells with estrogen and progesterone receptors are located in tissues throughout the body, including the ovaries, endometrium, pelvic structures, liver, bone, breast tissue, brain, and more; therefore, OCPs have significant systemic effects. In the absence of estrogen or progesterone, their specific receptors are inactive and have no effect on DNA. Once the hormones have bound to their respective receptors, the hormone–receptor complex travels into the nucleus and binds to DNA. This facilitates synthesis of various proteins and regulates the activity of various genes (Katzung et al., 2012), leading to the effects noted previously. Progestin-only compounds also suppress mid-cycle peaks of LH and FSH and inhibit progesterone receptor synthesis (Hibbert, Stouffer, Wolf, & Zelinski-Wooten, 1996).

Delivery System Comparison

Hormonal contraceptives are marketed in oral, transdermal, vaginal, implanted, and injected forms. Varying doses of each hormone can be selected to minimize adverse effects, to take advantage of certain beneficial effects, and to tailor menstrual bleeding to the woman's lifestyle and preferences. A Cochrane review found that combined OCPs, transdermal patches, and vaginal rings were equally efficacious, with a failure rate of 0.3 per 100 women per year with perfect use and 8.0 per 100 women per year with typical use (Lopez, Grimes, Gallo, & Schulz, 2010). According to Mosher and Jones (2010), the failure rate during the first year of use for injectable forms of contraception is similar, at 6.7 per 100 women per year.

Oral Hormonal Contraceptives

Over the last 50 years, OCPs that combine estrogen and progestin have been modified to limit the amount of active hormone, in an attempt to lessen their side effects without decreasing their efficacy in preventing pregnancy. In recent years, combined oral contraceptives (COCs) have been developed for extended-cycle patterns so that women take daily tablets but have hormone withdrawal–induced menstrual bleeding only once every 3 months or once a year. Although return to normal fertility following discontinuance of COCs with monthly cycles is immediate, women taking extended-cycle preparations may experience up to a 3-month delay in ovulation after discontinuing the medication (Practice Committee of the American Society for Reproductive Medicine, 2008).

Progestin-only oral contraceptive formulations have been developed for women who are unable to take estrogen for the following reasons: a history of, or risk for, venous thromboembolic events (VTE) or deep-vein thrombosis; immediate postpartum or lactating status; cigarette smoking status of more than one pack/day and age greater than 35 years; untreated hypertension; liver disease; diabetes with microvascular complications and/or age greater than 35 years; migraine headaches; estrogen-sensitive cancer; and prolonged immobilization or surgery of the legs (Bonnema, McNamara, & Spencer, 2010). Maintaining a consistent (same time every day) schedule for taking the tablets is more important for progestin-only pills than for COCs, as more than a three-hour delay in taking the progestin-only tablets can cause failure of contraception.

Transdermal Contraceptive System

The transdermal combined estrogen–progestin patch has been used in the United States since 2002. The patch releases EE and a progestin that metabolizes into the third-generation progestin **norgestimate**. As women using the patch are exposed to higher serum concentrations of estrogen, their risk for VTE may be up to twice that of women taking COCs.

Vaginal Rings

An ethylene vinyl acetate vaginal ring containing estrogen and progestin was approved for use in the United States in 2001.

The ring releases EE and a prodrug of the third-generation progestin **desorgestrel**. The advantage of the vaginal ring is in once-monthly self-administration rather than a daily tablet or weekly patch.

Implants

The first implantable contraceptive device was approved by the FDA in 1990; however, it was withdrawn from the market due to problems with its removal. A newer implant, approved in 2006, has demonstrated effectiveness for up to three years and contains a single nonbiodegradable rod. This device releases a metabolite of **desorgestrel**, a third-generation progestin, and does not release any estrogen. The most common adverse effect associated with this method is unpredictable breakthrough uterine bleeding.

Intrauterine Device

A **levonorgestrel (LNG)** -releasing intra-uterine device (IUD) was approved for use in the United States in 2000. The IUD may be left in place for up to five years; it has a low failure rate, decreases menstrual bleeding by 75% due to suppression of endometrial proliferation, and has a low rate of associated ectopic pregnancy. Following its removal, the woman experiences a rapid return to normal fertility. Because there is only a local (intrauterine) release of progestin, the incidence of side effects is small. As a progestin, **LNG's** suppression of ovulation is minimal; pregnancy does not occur either because the thickened cervical mucus hinders sperm motility or the atrophied endometrial lining does not allow implantation of a fertilized ovum.

Injectable Progestins

Two long-acting injectable progestins are currently approved for use in the United States. Both are formulations of **medroxyprogesterone acetate (MPA)**, and their mechanism of action is to suppress ovulation for 12 to 14 weeks. Return to normal fertility is delayed following discontinuance of this type of contraception; the median return to ovulation is 10 months, and 20% of women who discontinue **MPA** do not resume ovulation within 12 months (Practice Committee of the American Society for Reproductive Medicine, 2008).

Emergency Contraception

Hormonal early contraception (EC) refers to the use of high dose combination estrogen/progestin (not discussed here), progestin receptor modulators **ulipristal acetate**, or progestin-only (**LNG**) oral tablet formulations to prevent pregnancy following unprotected sexual intercourse or contraceptive failure. The drug *products* are also called ECPs.

LNG is most effective when used within 72 hours of unprotected intercourse, and its mechanism of action appears to result from either an inhibition or a delay of ovulation. Other possible mechanisms, still unsupported by research studies, include interference with corpus luteum function, thickening of cervical mucus, and alterations in tubal transport of the sperm, egg, or embryo (International Consortium for Emergency Contraception, 2012). **LNG** prevents pregnancy only when taken before fertilization of the ovum has occurred; studies do not show that changes occur in the endometrium that would make it unfavorable for implantation of an embryo after administration of this preparation (Shrader, Hall, Ragucci, & Rafie, 2011). In the United Sates, **LNG**-containing ECPs are available *without* a prescription and may be purchased by females (or males) regardless of age (the FDA removed age restrictions on the sale of LNG-ECPs; however, check state law as age restrictions may vary from state to state). The only FDA-approved emergency contraceptive in the United States that does *not* contain **LNG** is **ulipristal acetate**.

Ulipristal acetate is approved for EC within 120 hours of unprotected intercourse or contraceptive failure and is currently available only by prescription. This selective progesterone receptor modulator has mixed progesterone agonist and antagonist properties. After administration, it binds to the progesterone receptor and results in a delay of ovulation by at least 5 days if taken before the peak of LH at mid-cycle. Alterations in the endometrium that decrease likelihood of implantation may also occur (Shrader et al., 2011).

EC is absolutely contraindicated in confirmed pregnancy. Although EC reduces the risk of pregnancy by 75% to 88%, it should be noted that EC is still less effective at preventing pregnancy than consistent use of any other contraceptive method, and should not be used in their place (Practice Committee of the American Society for Reproductive Medicine, 2008). The most common side effects associated with ECPs, related to the drugs' mechanism of action, include nausea, vomiting, and delay in resuming menses.

Nursing Considerations

There is great deal of confusion and misconception surrounding the use of ECPs; not all ECPs are the same.

In the United States, LNG-only ECPs are sold over the counter. There are many generic equivalents of the original brand-name drug available. An LNG-only ECP drug product contains either two tablets (0.75 mg each) to be taken 12 hours apart, or a single 1.5 mg tablet (hence the one dose).

Although it is not covered here, what is known as the "morning after pill" is a hormonal-combination tablet that contains 100 mcg of estrogen and 0.5 mg of progesterone. The recommended dosing is to take one tablet, followed by a second dose 12 hours later. The incidence of side effects is much higher with the hormonal-combination tablets. Not only has the morning after pill been shown to be less effective at preventing pregnancy than the LNG-ECPs, approximately 1 in 5 women vomit after taking the morning-after pill, necessitating another dose.

Hormonal ECPs do not terminate an established pregnancy. However, a woman who has taken an ECP and has a confirmed pregnancy should contact her health care provider immediately.

The above mentioned ECPs should not be confused with what is known as the "abortion pill" (known by several different names, such as RU-486, mifepristone. It is important to note that both its indication for use and its mechanism of drug action differ dramatically from any type of emergency contraceptive; it is not an ECP nor should it be considered to be an ECP.

Urinary Incontinence

Urinary incontinence occurs in both men and women and can be a source of considerable emotional discomfort. Symptoms range from "leaking" small amounts of urine to a complete inability to restrain urine flow via maintenance of voluntary muscle control. Management depends on its cause; in many cases, urinary incontinence is related to weakness in pelvic floor muscles, which can be strengthened or supported by exercise therapy or surgical intervention. Medication is the preferred therapy only in specific situations, such as overactive bladder (McDonagh, Selover, Santa, & Thakurta, 2009). Medications used for this indication are anticholinergics, with one or two exceptions. TABLE 11-6 lists medications used in treatment of overactive bladder.

TABLE 11-6	Medications Used for Treating Overactive Bladder
Generic Names	**Drug Class**
Darifenacin	Anticholinergic
Flavoxate hydrochloride	Anticholinergic
Hyoscyamine sulfate	Anticholinergic
Oxybutynin	Anticholinergic
Oxybutynin chloride	Anticholinergic
Solifenacin	Anticholinergic
Tolterodine	Antimuscarinic
Trospium	Anticholinergic

CHAPTER SUMMARY

- Genitourinary tract issues affect not one but two aspects of patients' lives: waste elimination through urination and sexual function.
- In both instances, the presence of dysfunction can cause considerable emotional as well as physical discomfort to patients, who may be reluctant to discuss their health concerns due to shyness or embarrassment.
- Stigma is particularly relevant in the case of sexually transmitted infections, where patient beliefs about morality may affect their willingness to undergo screening and treatment.
- The impact of even minor genitourinary tract issues can be a significant mental health consideration for many patients.

Critical Thinking Questions

1. Which clinical and laboratory findings are consistent with the diagnosis of acute uncomplicated lower UTI in both males and females?

2. What is the most common urinary tract pathogen causing UTI and why?

3. Which factors differentiate complicated from uncomplicated UTI?

4. Explain the pathophysiology as to why impeded urine outflow might cause a UTI.

5. Which considerations affect the choice of agent used in treating bacterial STIs?

6. Which causative organism for vaginitis is not usually sexually transmitted?

7. Why are antiviral medications usually not indicated in treatment of HPV infection?

CASE SCENARIO 1

BW, a 23-year-old female, presents to the women's health clinic complaining of painful urination for 1 day. She also reports urinary urgency, voiding small amounts every 15 to 30 minutes, and pain over her lower abdomen. She did not sleep well the previous night due to waking up frequently to void. She denies fever, vomiting, diarrhea, constipation, vaginal discharge, urine leakage, or blood in her urine. She denies ever having similar symptoms in the past, takes no routine medications except for contraceptive vaginal ring, is a nonsmoker, has no known drug allergies, and has no history of renal calculi or urinary tract disease/abnormalities.

BW states she is sexually active with one lifetime partner; her last menstrual period ended 1 week ago, and she is 100% adherent to using the contraceptive ring as directed. She tells you that in the last 24 hours she has been drinking "a lot of cranberry juice because I heard that is supposed to cure a urine infection." She also confides that her mother told her that her symptoms were probably because BW must not be "wiping from front to back or cleaning myself well after using the toilet."

BW's vital signs are within normal range; she is afebrile. Her physical exam is unremarkable except for suprapubic tenderness to palpation; she has no organomegaly or costovertebral angle tenderness. A dipstick urinalysis is performed on a clean-catch specimen of BW's urine, which shows cloudy, yellow urine; pH 5.0; specific gravity 1.015; glucose negative; protein negative; trace blood; leukocyte esterase moderate; nitrite positive. The urine HCG test is negative for pregnancy.

The provider makes the diagnosis of acute, uncomplicated UTI and decides to prescribe TMP-SMX 160/800, one tablet twice daily for 3 days. The decision to prescribe empirically—that is, without culturing the urine to identify the bacteria causing the infection—is appropriate according to evidence-based practice guidelines (ACOG, 2008). BW is instructed to drink six to eight cups of water daily while taking the antibiotic and to discontinue drinking excessive amounts of cranberry juice.

CASE SCENARIO 1 (CONTINUED)

Case Questions

1. Why is it important to know whether BW is pregnant?
2. Should the provider have performed a urine culture to identify the pathogen causing BW's UTI?
3. Is it necessary to have BW return to the clinic after completing the course of antibiotic to confirm resolution of the infection?
4. What should the nurse tell BW regarding how the prescribed antibiotic "works"?
5. What should the nurse tell BW about the use of cranberry juice or products to prevent UTI?

CASE SCENARIO 2

JR, a 4-month-old male presents to the pediatric clinic with subjective fever for 2 days. Associated symptoms include decreased appetite, loose stools, and irritability. He is breastfeeding every 3 to 4 hours, but not as vigorously as usual; has had wet diapers four times in the last 24 hours, which is less than his usual six to eight wet diapers daily; and has experienced loose stools four times in the last 24 hours, with no blood in the stool. His past medical history is unremarkable: term birth without complications during pregnancy or delivery; no significant illnesses since birth; length, weight, and head circumference at 50th percentile for age; developmental milestones passed appropriately. JR is current with all routine immunizations, he does not take any routine medications except for supplemental vitamin D, and he does not attend a daycare program.

JR's vital signs are as follows: T 38.9°C, P 156, R 36. The physical exam is completely unremarkable for source of fever. JR is alert, interacts with the nurse, and has a nontoxic appearance. His anterior fontanelle is flat. The EENT exam is completely within normal limits. His lungs are clear; the heart rate and rhythm are regular. His abdomen is soft and nontender, and there is no organomegaly. His external genitalia indicate a Tanner 1 uncircumcised male with bilaterally descended testes. His skin is warm and dry, with moist mucous membranes and no rashes.

Urine was obtained by catheterization, and a dipstick urinalysis was performed in the clinic that was positive for nitrites and leukocyte esterase. Urinalysis showed the following: cloudy yellow urine; pH 5.5; specific gravity 1.025; glucose/protein negative; RBC: 2–3/HPF; WBC: 3–5/HPF. The urine specimen was sent to the lab for culture and sensitivity. The CBC results were as follows: WBC 9.4, hemoglobin/hematocrit 10.5/33, platelets 390,000, 51% neutrophils, 46% lymphocytes, 2% monocytes, 1% eosinophils. After 48 hours, the urine culture showed more than 100,000 CFU of *E. coli*, a bacterium that is sensitive to the beta-lactam cephalosporins ceftriaxone, cefixime, and cefotaxime, and to amoxicillin-clavulanate, nitrofurantoin, and ciprofloxacin.

JR's provider diagnoses acute febrile UTI without urosepsis and, following evidence-based guidelines, prescribes an injection of ceftriaxone 500 mg IM prior to leaving the clinic. The infant is to return the following day for reevaluation and a second ceftriaxone injection. Further oral antibiotic therapy is prescribed after receiving the culture and sensitivity report: oral cefixime two times daily for 14 days. JR is also scheduled for a renal ultrasound within the next 2 weeks; if it is abnormal, a voiding cystourethrogram will be performed to evaluate for hydronephrosis and/or VUR.

(continues)

CASE SCENARIO 2 (CONTINUED)

Case Questions

1. When is a pediatric UTI considered uncomplicated, and how does its treatment differ from that of a complicated pediatric UTI?

2. Although *E. coli* shows very low resistance to ciprofloxacin, this antibiotic is not typically prescribed to infants. Why is this so?

3. JR's mother asks you whether circumcision might prevent another episode of UTI in her son. How would you respond to her question?

4. How would you evaluate JR for therapeutic benefit from the ceftriaxone injection when he returns to the clinic the following day?

CASE SCENARIO 3

RM, a 59-year-old male, presents to his primary care provider with a complaint of painful urination of increasing intensity over the last week. Associated symptoms include subjective fever, urinary frequency, urgency, and new-onset urge incontinence resulting in inability to get to the bathroom before leaking urine. RM also describes pain over his lower abdomen and bilateral mid-back region. He reports his urine is cloudy and foul smelling, but he denies visible blood. He denies chills, diarrhea, constipation, vomiting, or previous similar symptoms; however, he admits that for several years he has had problems with urinary frequency (worse at night), a weak, interrupted stream of urine, and feeling like he cannot completely empty his bladder. He says that these symptoms are a significant bother and are worsening.

RM states that he is currently sexually active with a single partner for the last 20 years. He routinely takes daily medications for type 2 diabetes mellitus, essential hypertension, and high cholesterol; he has not taken any antibiotics in the previous 6 months. At his last routine medical visit 2 months ago, RM's blood tests indicated excellent control of these chronic conditions. A PSA blood test performed 6 months ago was also in normal range. RM denies a personal or family history of structural or functional urinary tract disorders, or bladder, prostate, or renal cancer. He is a nonsmoker. He has been drinking less fluid for the past 2 days due to worsening urinary frequency and urgency. He reports no known drug allergies.

RM's vital signs are within normal range except for a low-grade fever of 37.5°C. Upon physical exam, the provider notes suprapubic tenderness and costovertebral angle tenderness. RM is circumcised; digital rectal exam shows a mildly enlarged, nontender prostate gland without nodules. Microscopic mid-stream urinalysis shows cloudy, dark-yellow urine; pH 6.2; specific gravity 1.030; glucose negative; protein negative; RBC 8–10/HPF; WBC 18–20/HPF; nitrite positive. A urine culture, performed and made available after 48 hours, shows more than 100,000 colonies of *Klebsiella pneumoniae*. A baseline PSA blood test is in the normal range (1.2 ng/mL).

The provider makes a diagnosis of acute, complicated UTI (pyelonephritis), likely due to lower urinary tract obstruction and subsequent urinary stasis resulting from BPH. RM is given a prescription for levofloxacin 750 mg once daily for 5 days. As RM is nontoxic, outpatient treatment is an acceptable option. The provider schedules an appointment for 2 weeks to follow up for resolution of the UTI and to discuss treatment of BPH.

CASE SCENARIO 3 (CONTINUED)

Case Questions

1. Which contributing factors may have predisposed RM to pyelonephritis?
2. With a complicated UTI, why is a fluoroquinolone antibiotic recommended rather than TMP-SMX or nitrofurantoin?
3. When would IV antibiotics be preferred over the oral route in treatment of complicated UTI?
4. What is an alternative fluoroquinolone antibiotic that could have been prescribed to this patient?
5. For which therapeutic outcome should the nurse evaluate this patient?

CASE SCENARIO 4

JS is a 58-year-old man who presents to his primary care provider for a routine check-up. During the medication review, he mentions that he is having significant ED that has been worsening over the last year. This is very distressing to him and to his wife, and JS wonders if any of his medications might be causing the problem. He is obese, and he has been treated for hypertension and type 2 diabetes mellitus (T2DM) for the last 8 to 10 years. His current medications include a thiazide diuretic, hydrochlorothiazide, and a beta blocker (metoprolol) for blood pressure. JS is taking metformin twice daily for T2DM. He denies significant urinary frequency, hesitancy, urgency, dribbling, incontinence, or weak stream. He reports no morning erections, nocturnal erections, or spontaneous erections adequate for sexual satisfaction. He does not exercise regularly, and he has a 20-pack/year cigarette smoking history.

JS's vital signs are BP 152/92, P 84/min, and R 20; his BMI is 34. His physical exam is unremarkable with a normal cardiac exam including peripheral pulses, normal male genitalia, normal prostate exam, and no abdominal tenderness or organomegaly.

The metabolic panel shows normal renal and liver function, but JS has an elevated fasting blood sugar of 160 mg/dL. JS's lipid panel shows elevated triglycerides, elevated low-density lipoprotein, and low high-density lipoprotein.

The provider decides to change JS's antihypertensive regimen to a combination angiotensin II receptor type-1 blocker and calcium-channel blocker. He also increases the metformin dose to the maximum daily dose, and he adds a statin drug for JS's dyslipidemia. Because JS is not taking nitrates or alpha-blocking drugs for hypertension, a PDE-5 inhibitor is initiated to improve his ED. The provider also stresses smoking cessation and the importance of daily physical activity with JS as factors shown to improve ED. JS is referred to a nutritionist for education about low-fat food choices and to initiate a weight-loss program.

Case Questions

1. In JS's initial drug regimen, which medications may have contributed to his ED, and how might this be occurring?
2. Which antihypertensive drugs do not seem to contribute to ED?
3. From JS's medical history, which factors not directly related to medications may be contributing to his ED?
4. What is an appropriate plan for discussing adverse effects associated with use of PDE-5 inhibitors?

REFERENCES

American Academy of Pediatrics (AAP). (2011). Urinary tract infection: Clinical practice guideline for the diagnosis and management of initial UTI in febrile infants and children 2–24 months. *Pediatrics, 128*(3), 595–610.

American College of Obstetricians and Gynecologists (ACOG). (2007). ACOG Practice Bulletin, No. 82: Management of herpes in pregnancy. *Obstetrics & Gynecology, 109*(6), 1489–1498.

American College of Obstetricians and Gynecologists (ACOG). (2016). ACOG Practice Bulletin, No. 91: Treatment of urinary tract infections in non-pregnant women. *Obstetrics & Gynecology, 111*(3), 785–794. doi: 10.1097/AOG.0b013e318169f6ef

American Urological Association (AUA). (2014). American Urological Association guideline: Management of benign prostatic hyperplasia. Retrieved from http://www.auanet.org/benign-prostatic-hyperplasia-(2010-reviewed-and-validity-confirmed-2014)

Andersson, K.E. (2011). Mechanisms of penile erection and basis for pharmacological treatment of erectile dysfunction. *Pharmacological Reviews, 63*(4), 811–859.

Angotti, L.B., Lambert, L.C., & Soper, D.E. (2007). Vaginitis: Making sense of over-the-counter treatment products. *Infectious Diseases in Obstetrics and Gynecology*, 974424. doi: 10.1155/2007/97424

Baumhaken, M., Schlimmer, N., Kratz, M., Gacket, G., Jackson, G., & Bohm, M. (2011). Cardiovascular risk, drugs and erectile function: A systematic analysis. *International Journal of Clinical Practice, 65*(3), 289.

Beerepoot, M., & Geerlings, S. (2016). Non-antibiotic prophylaxis for urinary tract infections. *Pathogens, 5*(2), E36. doi: 10.3390/pathogens5020036

Beerepoot, M.A., ter Riet, G., Nys, S., van der Wal, W.M., de Borgie, C.A., de Reijke, T.M., . . . Geerlings, S. E. (2011). Cranberries vs antibiotics to prevent urinary tract infections: A randomized double-blind noninferiority trial in premenopausal women. *Archives of Internal Medicine, 171*(14), 1270–1278.

Beveridge, L.A., Davey, P.G., Phillips, G., & McMurdo, M.E.T. (2011). Optimal management of urinary tract infections in older people. *Clinical Interventions in Aging, 6*, 173–180.

Bonnema, R.A., McNamara, M.C., & Spencer, A.L. (2010). Contraception choices in women with underlying medical conditions. *Am Fam Physician.* 2010 Sep 15;82(6):621–628.

Centers for Disease Control and Prevention (CDC). (2013). Antibiotic resistance threats in the United States, 2013. Retrieved from http://www.cdc.gov/drugresistance/threat-report-2013/

Christensen, B.S., Gronbaek, M., Pedersen, B.V., Graugaard, C., & Frisch, M. (2011). Associations of unhealthy lifestyle factors with sexual inactivity and sexual dysfunctions in Denmark. *Journal of Sexual Medicine, 8*(7), 1903–1916.

Chrubasik, J.E., Roufogalis, B.D., Wagner, H., & Chrubasik, S. (2007). A comprehensive review on the stinging nettle effect and efficacy profiles. Part II: Urticae radix. *Phytomedicine, 14*(7–8), 568–579.

Cox, N.H. (2000). Permethrin treatment in scabies infestation: Importance of the correct formula. *BMJ, 320*(7226), 37–38.

Cunningham, S.D., Kerrigan, D.L., Jennings, J.M., & Ellen, J.M. (2009). Relationships between perceived STD-related stigma, STD-related shame and STD screening among a household sample of adolescents. *Perspectives on Sexual and Reproductive Health, 41*(4), 225–230.

Daniels, K., Daugherty, J., & Jones, J. (2015). Current contraceptive status among women aged 15–44: United States, 2011–2013. *National Health Statistics Reports, 173*. Retrieved from http://www.cdc.gov/nchs/data/databriefs/db173.pdf

Datta, D., Dunne, E.F., Saraiya, M., & Markowitz, L. (2012). Human papillomaviruses. In J.M. Zenilman & M. Shahmanesh (Eds.), *Sexually transmitted infections: Diagnosis, management, and treatment* (pp. 43–56). Burlington, MA: Jones & Bartlett.

Debruyne, D. (1997). Clinical pharmacokinetics of fluconazole in superficial and systemic mycoses. *Clinical Pharmacokinetics, 33*(1), 52–77.

East, L., Jackson, D., O'Brien, L., & Peters, K. (2012). Stigma and stereotypes: Women and sexually transmitted infections. *Collegian, 19*(1), 15–21.

Falagasa, M.E., Vouloumanoua, E.K., Samonisd, G., & Vardakasa, K.Z. (2016). Fosfomycin. *Clinical Microbiology Reviews, 29*(2), 321–347.

Fu, Z., Liska, D., Talan, D., & Chung, M. (2017). Cranberry reduces the risk of urinary tract infection recurrence in otherwise healthy women: A systematic review and meta-analysis. *The Journal of Nutrition, 147*(12), 2282–2288. https://doi.org/10.3945/jn.117.254961

Garau, J. (2008). Other antimicrobials of interest in the era of extended-spectrum β-lactamases: Fosfomycin, nitrofurantoin and tigecycline. *Clinical Microbiology and Infection, 14*(s-1), 198–202.

Geerlings, S.E., Beerepoot, M.A.J., & Prins, J.M. (2014). Prevention of recurrent urinary tract infections in women: Antimicrobial and nonantimicrobial strategies. *Infectious Disease Clinics of North America, 28*(1), 135–147.

Giancola, S.E., Mahoney, M.V., Hogan, M.D., Raux, B.R., McCoy, C., & Hirsch, E.B. (2017). Assessment of fosfomycin for complicated or multidrug-resistant urinary tract infections: Patient characteristics and outcomes. *Chemotherapy, 62*, 100–104.

González Canga, A., Sahagún Prieto, A.M., Diez Liébana, M.J., Fernández Martínez, N., Sierra Vega, M., & García Vieitez, J.J. (2008). The pharmacokinetics and interactions of ivermectin in humans: A mini-review. *AAPS Journal, 10*(1), 42–46.

Goswami, D., Goswami, R., Banerjee, U., Dadhwal, V., Miglani, S., Lattif, A.A., & Kochupillai, N. (2006). Pattern of *Candida* species isolated from patients with diabetes mellitus and vulvovaginal candidiasis and their response to single dose oral fluconazole therapy. *Journal of Infection, 52*(2), 111–117.

Griebling, T.L. (2005a). Urologic Diseases in America project: Trends in resource use for urinary tract infections in women. *Journal of Urology, 173*(4), 1281–1287.

Griebling, T.L. (2005b). Urologic Diseases in America project: Trends in resource use for urinary tract infections in men. *Journal of Urology, 173*(4), 1288–1294.

Grönlund, J., Saari, T.I., Hagelburg, N., Neuvonen, P.J., Olkkola, K.T., & Laine, K. (2011). Miconazole oral gel increases exposure to oral oxycodone by inhibition of CYP2D6 and CYP3A4. *Antimicrobial Agents and Chemotherapeutics, 55*(3), 1063–1067.

Guay, D.R. (2009). Cranberry and urinary tract infections. *Drugs, 7*(69), 775–807.

Hibbert, M.L., Stouffer, R.L., Wolf, D.P., & Zelinski-Wooten, M.B. (1996). Midcycle administration of a progesterone synthesis inhibitor prevents ovulation in primates. *Proc. Natl. Acad. Sci. USA*, 93, 1897–1901.

Hisano, M., Bruschini, H., Nicodemo, A.C., & Srougi, M. (2012). Cranberries and lower urinary tract infection prevention. *Clinics* (Sao Paulo), *67*(6), 661–667. doi: 10.6061/clinics/2012(06)18

Hooton, T.M. (2001). Recurrent urinary tract infection in women. *International Journal of Antimicrobial Agents, 17*(4), 259–268.

Hooton, T.M. (2012). Uncomplicated urinary tract infection. *New England Journal of Medicine, 366*(11), 1028–1037.

Idriss, S., & Levitt, J. (2009). Malathion for head lice and scabies: Treatment and safety considerations. *Journal of Drugs in Dermatology, 8*(8), 715–772.

International Consortium for Emergency Contraception. (2012). Mechanism of action: how do levonorgestrel-only emergency contraceptive pills (LNG ECPS) prevent pregnancy? Retrieved from http://www.cecinfo.org/icec-publications/mechanism-action-levonorgestrel-emergency-contraceptive-pills-lng-ecps-prevent-pregnancy/

Jarzebowski, W., Caumes, E., Dupin, N., Farhi, D., Lascaux, A.S., Piketty, C., . . . Grabar, S. (2012). Effect of early syphilis infection on plasma viral load and CD4 cell count in human immunodeficiency virus-infected men. *Archives of Internal Medicine, 172*(16), 1237–1243. doi:10.1001/archinternmed.2012.2706

Katzung, B.G., Masters, S.B., & Trevor, A.J. (2012). *Basic and clinical pharmacology*. New York, NY: McGraw-Hill/Lange.

Ko, D.T., Hebert, P.R., Coffey, C.S., Sedrankya, A., Curtis, J.P., & Krumholz, H.M. (2002). Beta-blocker therapy and symptoms of depression, fatigue, and sexual dysfunction. *Journal of the American Medical Association, 288*(3), 351.

Koyle, M.A., & Shifrin, D. (2012). Issues in febrile urinary tract infection management. *Pediatric Clinics of North America, 59*(4), 909–922.

Lau, A H., Lam, N.P., Piscitelli, S.C., Wilkes, L., & Danziger, L.H. (1992). Clinical pharmacokinetics of metronidazole and other nitroimidazole anti-infectives. *Clinical Pharmacokinetics, 23*(5), 328–364.

Lopez, L.M., Grimes, D.A., Gallo, M.F., & Schulz, K.F. (2010). Skin patch and vaginal ring versus combined oral contraceptives for contraception (Review). *Cochrane Library, 3*.

Masters, P.A., O'Bryan, T.A., Zurlo, J., Miller, D Q., & Joshi, N. (2003). Trimethoprim-sulfamethoxazole revisited. *Archives of Internal Medicine, 163*(4), 402–410. Retrieved from http://archinte.jamanetwork.com/article.aspx?articleid=215162#MECHANISMOFACTION

McDonagh, M.S., Selover, D., Santa, J., & Thakurta, S. (2009). Drug class review: Agents for overactive bladder. *Drug Class Reviews, Final Report Update 4*. Retrieved from http://www.ncbi.nlm.nih.gov/books/NBK47183/

Mosher, W.D., & Jones, J. (2010). Use of contraception and use of family planning services in the United States: 1982–2008. *Advance Data from Vital and Health Statistics, 23*(29). Retrieved from http://www.cdc.gov/NCHS/data/series/sr_23/sr23_029.pdf

Neal, D.E. Jr. (2008). Complicated urinary tract infections. *Urologic Clinics of North America, 35*, 13–22. doi: 10.1016/j.ucl.2007.09.010

Nehra, A. (2007). Oral and non-oral combination therapy for erectile dysfunction. *Reviews in Urology, 9*(3), 99–105. Retrieved from http://www.ncbi.nlm.nih.gov/pmc/articles/pmc2002499/

Nicolle, L.E. (2005). Complicated urinary tract infection in adults. *Canadian Journal of Infectious Diseases and Medical Microbiology, 16*(6), 349–360. Retrieved from http://www.ncbi.nlm.nih.gov/pmc/articles/PMC2094997/

Novaro, G., Giannarini, G., Alcaraz, A., Cozar-Olmo, J-M., Descazeaud, A., Montorsi, F., & Ficarra, V. (2016). Efficacy and safety of hexanic lipididosterolic extract of *Serenoa repens* (Permixon) in the treatment of lower urinary tract symptoms due to benign prostatic hyperplasia: Systematic review and meta-analysis of randomized controlled trials. *European Urology Focus, 2*(5), 553–561.

Nyirjesy, P., & Sobel, J.D. (2013). Genital mycotic infections in patients with diabetes. *Postgraduate Medicine, 125*(3), 33–46.

Patel, V.M., Lambert, W.C., & Schwartz, R.A. (2016). Safety of topical medications for scabies and lice in pregnancy. *Indian Journal of Dermatology, 61*(6), 583–587. http://doi.org/10.4103/0019-5154.193659

Practice Committee of the American Society for Reproductive Medicine. (2008). Hormonal contraception: Recent advances and controversies. *Fertility and Sterility, 90*(5s), S103–S113.

Raz, R., Chazan, B., & Dan, M. (2004). Cranberry juice and urinary tract infection. *Clinical Infectious Diseases, 38*(10), 1413–1419. Retrieved from http://cid.oxfordjournals.org/content/38/10/1413.long

Reed, J.L., Huppert, J.S., Gillespie, G.L., Taylor, R.G., Holland, C.K., Alessandrini, E.A., & Kahn, J.A. (2015). Adolescent patient preferences surrounding partner notification and treatment for sexually transmitted infections. *Academic Emergency Medicine, 22*(1), 61–66.

Reffelmann, T., & Kloner, R.A. (2006). Sexual function in hypertensive patients receiving treatment. *Vascular Health and Risk Management, 2*(4), 447–455.

Roehrborn, C. (2012). Benign prostatic hyperplasia and lower urinary tract symptom guidelines.

Canadian Urological Association Journal, 6(5 Suppl. 2), S130–S132. Retrieved from http://www.ncbi.nlm.nih.gov/pmc/articles/PMC3481951/

Roussos, N., Karageorgopoulos, D.E., Samonis, G., & Falagas, M.E. (2009). Clinical significance of the pharmacokinetic and pharmacodynamics characteristics of fosfomycin for the treatment of patients with systemic infections. *International Journal of Antimicrobial Agents, 34*(6), 506–515.

Schwebke, J.R. (2012). Vaginitis. In J.M. Zenilman & M. Shahmanesh (Eds.), *Sexually transmitted infections: Diagnosis, management, and treatment* (pp. 57–66). Burlington, MA: Jones & Bartlett.

Shah, K.J., Cherabuddi, K., Shultz, J., Borgert, S., Ramphal, R., & Klinker, K.P. (2018). Ampicillin for the treatment of complicated urinary tract infections caused by vancomycin-resistant *Enterococcus spp.* (VRE): A single-center university hospital experience. *International Journal of Antimicrobial Agents, 51*(1), 57–61.

Shrader, S.P., Hall, L.N., Ragucci, K.R., & Rafie, S. (2011). Updates in hormonal emergency contraception. *Pharmacotherapy, 31*(9), 887–895.

Sica, D.A. (2004). Diuretic-related side effects: Development and treatment. Retrieved from http://www.medscape.com/viewarticle/489521_10

Singh, I., Gautam, L.K., & Kaur, I.R. (2016). Effect of oral cranberry extract (standardized proanthocyanidin-A) in patients with recurrent UTI by pathogenic *E. coli*: A randomized placebo-controlled clinical research study. *International Urology and Nephrology, 48*(9), 1379–1386. doi: 10.1007/s11255-016-1342-8

Singh-Grewal, D., Macdessi, J., & Craig, J. (2005). Circumcision for the prevention of urinary tract infection in boys: A systematic review of randomized trials and observational studies. *Archives of Disease in Childhood, 90*(4), 853–858.

Suzuki, M., Ito, Y., Fujino, T., Abe, M., Umegaki, K., Onoue, S., . . . Yamada, S. (2009). Pharmacological effects of saw palmetto extract in the lower urinary tract. *Acta Pharmacologica Sinica, 30*(3), 227–281.

U.S. Department of Health and Human Services – AIDS Info. (2017). Initiation of antiretroviral therapy. Guidelines for the Use of Antiretroviral Agents in Adults and Adolescents Living with HIV. Retrieved from https://aidsinfo.nih.gov/guidelines/html/1/adult-and-adolescent-arv/10/initiation-of-antiretroviral-therapy

Wagenlehner, F.M.E., Wullt, B., & Perletti, G. (2011). Antimicrobials in urogenital infections. *International Journal of Antimicrobial Agents, 38*(S), 3–10.

Xu, J., Schwartz, K., Bartoces, M., Monsur, J., Severson, R.K., & Sobel, J.D. (2008). Effect of antibiotics on vulvovaginal candidiasis: A MetroNet study. *Journal of the American Board of Family Medicine, 21*(4), 261–268.

Zenilman, J.M. (2012). In J.M. Zenilman & M. Shahmanesh (Eds.), *Sexually transmitted infections: Diagnosis, management, and treatment* (pp. 31–42). Sudbury, MA: Jones & Bartlett.

Special Conditions and Supplemental Areas

CHAPTER 12

Drugs Associated with Pregnancy, Labor and Delivery, and Lactation

Jean Nicholas

KEY TERMS

Albumin
Atony
Beta-mimetic drugs
Cytotoxic
Eclampsia
Epidural anesthesia
Fetotoxic
Gastric reflux

Gestational diabetes
Gestational hypertension
Group B streptococcal
    infection
Human placental growth hor-
    mone (hpGH)
Human placental lactogen
    (hPL)

Hyperglycemia
Hypoglycemia
Insulin resistance
Magnesium sulfate
Nonprogressing labor
Postpartum
Pre-eclampsia
Prenatal vitamins

Preterm labor
Proteinuria
Respiratory distress
    syndrome
Teratogen
Tocolytic drugs
Vasodilation

CHAPTER OBJECTIVES

At the end of the chapter, the student will be able to:

1. Describe the mechanism of action, dosages, side effects, and nursing considerations for drugs commonly used in pregnancy, labor and delivery, and postpartum.

2. Discuss physiological reasons why drug use in pregnancy and lactation is limited.

3. Explain changes to the Food and Drug Administration pregnancy categories and give an example of a teratogenic drug.

4. Identify common conditions in pregnancy that may require management with medication.

5. Compare and contrast drugs used in uterine stimulation and uterine relaxation.

6. Describe nursing care of a labor patient receiving analgesia or regional anesthesia.

Introduction

The use of any drug just prior to or during pregnancy and lactation requires close surveillance due to the unique physiological changes that occur in the body during these periods. Drug effects are often unpredictable, particularly when using newer drugs, for which less information is available about possible effects in this population. Yet because pharmaceutical companies do not test drugs on pregnant or lactating women—such testing, with no knowledge of the potential harm to the fetus, would be unethical—drug effects on the fetus or newborn are known only after they occur and are reported.

Some drugs are known to be harmful to the fetus (**fetotoxic**) due to a large number of reported cases. A classic example is **thalidomide**, a drug that was widely used in Europe during the late 1950s and early 1960s to treat severe nausea in pregnancy. This drug was prescribed and eventually marketed on an over-the-counter basis, before the discovery that it was a **teratogen**—that is, a compound that interferes with the normal developmental process in the fetus (Sachdeva, Patel, & Patel, 2009). Thousands of babies were born with malformed or missing limbs before **thalidomide** was removed from the market, and many thousands more women likely suffered miscarriage as a result of using this drug. **Thalidomide** is an extreme example—many other fetotoxic drugs have effects that are less dramatic but still noticeable, and even with **thalidomide** the effects were present in approximately half of the babies whose mothers took the drug, not all of them. Nevertheless, it makes no sense to put the fetus at any risk of malformation or health effects unless there is a clear need to do so. For this reason, the default position of most clinical practices is to use no drug unless other measures fail. Yet 9 out of 10 pregnant women take at least one medication during their pregnancy, and in the past 30 years the number of women taking four or more medications has more than doubled (Mosley, Smith, & Dezan, 2015).

FDA Pregnancy Categories

The Food and Drug Administration (FDA) is responsible for reviewing and approving medications. In 1979, as a result of experience with both **thalidomide** and another drug, **diethylstilbestrol (DES)**, which caused less dramatic but still important teratogenic effects (Mittendorf, 1995), the FDA created a categorization system for drugs used in pregnancy, derived from the *Labeling for Prescription Drugs Used in Man Regulations*. The categorizations were made on the basis of animal studies and anecdotal reports or post-hoc reviews of outcomes of patients who took the drugs.

In 2014 the FDA replaced existing pregnancy letter categories with a new system intended to help consumers make better informed choices as well as to enhance patient counseling. The previous system assigned entire drug classes to specific letter categories (A, B, C, D, and X), according to the known or reported level of risk to the human (or animal) fetus. However, patients and practitioners felt that the categories could be confusing and there was not a definitive "yes" or "no" as to what was safe for patients. Further, the categories were incorrectly viewed as a continuum of most safe (Category A) to least safe (Category X) and did not address the adverse effects of drug therapy discontinuation during pregnancy (Pernia & DeMaagd, 2016). Finally, the Centers for Disease Control and Prevention's web page on medications and pregnancy (https://www.cdc.gov/pregnancy /meds/treatingfortwo/research.html) notes, "A 2011 study of all medications approved by FDA from 1980 through 2010 found that 91% of the medications approved for use by adults in general had insufficient data to determine the risk of using the medication during pregnancy."

Labeling will now follow the process outlined in the FDA's 2014 *Content and Format of Labeling for Human Prescription Drug and Biological Products; Requirements for Pregnancy and Lactation Labeling*, more commonly referred to as the Pregnancy and Lactation Labeling Rule (PLLR). Both the content and format of information changed under the PLLR. While there remain three labeling subsections, the scope of those sections has been broadened (see TABLE 12-1).

The decision to use or not use a drug will no longer be based on the assigned FDA category, but rather on what is optimal for the patient, given the risk to her life or health, the risk of harm to the fetus, and the way the pregnant woman prioritizes those risks once informed of them. According to the PLLR, medication labels must be continually updated as new data is available (Blattner, Danesh, Safaee, & Murase, 2016). The labeling rules apply only to prescription medication; over-the-counter drug labels are not affected.

That may sound alarming to both clinician and patient. However, in practice, *most* medications *can* be given relatively safely in pregnancy to the majority of patients. That does not mean, however, that there are no risks, or that every effort should not be made to minimize risks. This is especially true when the medication being considered is **cytotoxic**—that is, toxic to cells, and is especially important for drugs that target fast-growing cells—such as most cancer drugs. Considerations that the clinician and patient should discuss when undertaking therapy include the following:

- Are there effective nonpharmacologic therapies that could be tried first?

- How significant is the risk to the mother's health versus the risk to the fetus?
- If medication must be used, are there available options that are lower in risk to the fetus?
- If no lower-risk medication is available, is using a reduced dose an option, despite the presumably reduced efficacy?
- Is delaying therapy until the fetus reaches a more advanced stage of development an option? Would doing so prove helpful to the fetus? Would doing so increase the risk of severe consequences to the mother?

> **Best Practices**
>
> In the majority of cases, medications can be given safely in pregnancy, but every effort should be made to minimize risks.

Medication Use on a Preconception Basis and in Early Pregnancy

Several circumstances may occur that introduce the possibility of medication use during pregnancy. First, a woman may be healthy, but a condition may arise during pregnancy for which medication is needed (it may or may not be related to the pregnancy). Second, the woman may have an existing undiagnosed or borderline health issue that was not being treated before she became pregnant, but that worsened or was "unmasked" due to her pregnancy. Examples would be a woman who had subclinical hypothyroidism and developed hypothyroid symptoms while pregnant because of the extra metabolic burden of pregnancy, or a woman with an undiagnosed tumor, which, responding to the pregnancy hormones, became palpable. Third, a woman who is already taking medication for a health concern may become pregnant, either intentionally or accidentally. In all of these cases, the woman's medication use (new or ongoing) needs to be assessed with regard to its effects on the fetus.

Physiological Changes in Pregnancy

Nurses should be aware that many physiological measures change during pregnancy, so

TABLE 12-1	PLLR Labeling Subsections	
Previous Labeling	New Labeling
8.1 Pregnancy	8.1 Pregnancy Labor and Delivery
8.2 Labor and Delivery	8.2 Lactation
8.3 Nursing Mothers	8.3 Females and Males of Reproductive Potential

Data from Content and Format of Labeling for Human Prescription Drug and Biological Products; Requirements for Pregnancy and Lactation Labeling (Federal Register/Vol. 79, No. 233/Thursday, December 4, 2014).

that they are not regarded as (and potentially treated as) abnormalities. The mother's blood plasma volume (and therefore cardiac output) increases approximately 50%. Increased renal flow (the glomerular filtration rate rises by about 55% during pregnancy) may lead to more rapid excretion of drugs. Oxygen consumption also increases by about 20%, which may have implications for women who require bronchodilators. After about 20 weeks, plasma lipid levels increase in the mother, with the ratio of low-density lipoprotein to high-density lipoprotein increasing (Sanghavi & Rutherford, 2014). The increased production of hormones (e.g., estrogen, progesterone, human placental lactogen, growth hormone) may alter the metabolism of drugs. Other biochemical changes include alterations in serum creatinine, urea, liver enzyme tests (alkaline phosphatase increases by as much as 400%), and thyroid function.

The physiological changes that occur during pregnancy influence the effects of drugs in both the mother and the fetus. For example, the increase in plasma volume produces a dilutional effect and lowers many drug concentrations more than would otherwise be expected. The resulting lower levels of **albumin** may decrease drug binding, thus freeing up more drug for transfer to the fetus. Such effects make it difficult to predict how a drug will work in the pregnant woman and how that same drug will affect the fetus.

Of particular note is the change that occurs in insulin utilization. During pregnancy, increases in two specific pregnancy-related hormones, **human placental lactogen (hPL)** and **human placental growth hormone (hpGH)**, cause an increased resistance to insulin (Moore, 2018). This phenomenon is a normal physiological change that ensures the growing fetus receives an adequate amount of glucose for its growth. However, **insulin resistance** can lead to inadequate glucose uptake for the mother and higher than normal circulating levels of glucose. Fats and proteins must then be broken down and used by the mother's body for energy, resulting in a negative nitrogen balance and ketosis. If diabetes develops (or is already present) in the mother, it can have significant effects on the fetus and lead to complications during birth.

Placental transfer of drugs occurs by the fifth week after conception. The fetal and maternal bloodstreams are separated by only a thin barrier, which many drugs easily penetrate. Because the fetus has low levels of albumin, drug binding is minimal. The fetal liver is immature, resulting in poor metabolism of drugs and greater effect of the medications on fetal tissue. Excretion of drugs is similarly affected due to the immaturity of the fetal kidneys.

In a woman of reproductive age who may become pregnant (i.e., one who is sexually active and not using an effective contraceptive method), the key concern is that she may ingest drugs that are potentially harmful to the fetus before she is aware she is pregnant. Although the embryo is fairly resistant to fetotoxic substances in the first week or two post conception, all of the fetal organs are formed during weeks three to eight of pregnancy (Sachdeva et al., 2009). Drugs taken during this time may cause organs to be malformed or to malfunction. Medications taken from week nine onward do not necessarily affect organ and tissue formation but may influence how well the organs develop or function during pregnancy or after birth. The fetal brain, in particular, is highly sensitive to chemical inputs and continues to develop **postpartum**; for this reason, medication use is a concern not only during pregnancy, but also for the duration of postpartum breastfeeding, in women who choose to breastfeed.

Ideally, a woman who requires a prescribed drug for an ongoing health problem will plan ahead if she wishes to become pregnant. Under such circumstances, she may be able to change the drug to one less likely to affect the fetus in the first weeks of pregnancy. Moreover, the nutritional needs of pregnant women change, making it advisable to initiate the use of **prenatal vitamins** to ensure adequate amounts of essential vitamins and minerals. Because folic acid deficiency is linked to defects in the fetal neural tube (brain and spinal cord), all women in their reproductive years are encouraged to consume at least 400 mcg of folic acid daily. Many foods are now enriched with folic acid. Iron is the only other nutritional supplement whose intake needs to be increased during pregnancy. Most women can get enough of the vitamins and minerals they need for pregnancy and lactation through a varied and balanced diet.

Only a few therapeutic drugs are known to be fetotoxic, so medications with extreme effects on fetal development can usually be avoided during pregnancy. A more difficult challenge is avoiding drugs that may have effects that are not readily observed (e.g., drugs that affect long-term brain, lung, or other tissue development) or that may alter the process of pregnancy (e.g., by stimulating early labor or reducing placental function). Drug effects are often unpredictable; a medication that has no effect in one pregnancy may do harm in another, even in the same mother. This is why so few drugs are considered truly "safe" during pregnancy. When a prescribed drug is considered critical for the mother's health, the risks to the fetus versus the benefits for the mother must be carefully weighed. The goal of drug treatment during pregnancy is to provide as much benefit as possible to the mother while minimizing impact on fetal development and well-being.

Use of Nonprescribed and Illicit Drugs

While this chapter is primarily concerned with prescribed or recommended medications during pregnancy, it is also important to mention the potential impact of nonprescribed and illicit drugs. Nonprescribed drugs may include over-the-counter medications that the pregnant woman has been accustomed to using on an occasional basis to treat minor ailments, such as sleep aids, cough and cold medications, analgesics, antacids, and so forth. Such drugs may contain ingredients that have the potential to harm the fetus or that could interact in harmful ways with prescribed medications. Nonprescribed drugs may also include herbal or nutritional products sold as supplements, teas, or beverages. These include such ingredients as chamomile, ginseng, potassium, B vitamins, glucosamine, taurine, and so forth. Many patients do not regard these "natural remedies" as "drugs" and may fail to mention them during an initial pregnancy assessment; indeed, many patients may not even realize they are ingesting these ingredients because they have been added to a beverage or tea and the patient did not carefully read the label. Yet because such products may have unexpected effects or interact with prescribed medications, it is essential that an account of *all* such substances be elicited from the patient and assessed with regard to safety. Some herbal products, such as ginseng, rosemary, and some forms of chamomile, are generally recognized as safe for women who are not pregnant but can be unsafe during pregnancy (Kennedy, Lupattelli, Koren & Nordeng, 2016; Dante, Bellei, Neri, & Facchinetti, 2014). Not enough studies have been done to measure the effects of various herbs on pregnant women or fetuses. Conflicting information on the internet regarding the use of herbal products only confounds the issue. Therefore, the best practice is to consult with a health care provider before taking *any* 'natural' medicine or herbal product during pregnancy, or, avoid the products altogether.

In addition, some pregnant women may ingest harmful nonprescribed drugs for recreational purposes, whether legal or otherwise—for example, alcohol, tobacco, narcotics, methamphetamine, and otherwise legal medications that were not prescribed for her use (e.g., psychotropics or pain medications). Particularly with respect to illegal drug use and alcohol abuse, patients may be unwilling to give an honest history of drug use or misuse for fear of legal repercussions. Nurses may also have concerns related to liability, depending on state law about reporting illicit drug use in expectant mothers; however, the position statement of the American Nurses Association (ANA, 2011) on this subject is that nurses should regard addiction or drug abuse as an illness to be treated via coordination with social services, not law enforcement. If abuse of nonprescribed/illicit drugs or alcohol is suspected, the patient should be assured of confidentiality, educated about the repercussions of drug use for her fetus, and offered assistance with withdrawing from the drugs or medications in question. In women with significant addiction issues, this withdrawal *must* take place under medical supervision to ensure the safety of both the woman and her fetus.

Patient Emotions Around Medication Use

For patients who used medications prior to becoming aware of pregnancy, reassurance that the likelihood of harm is minimal is appropriate, except in instances where the medication is absolutely contraindicated. Such occasions will probably be extremely rare, because women taking such medications (e.g., **isotretinoin**) are usually warned about the potential for harm in pregnancy and advised to use an effective birth control method. For patients who must initiate or continue use of a medication during pregnancy, a thorough discussion of the risks and potential strategies to minimize risk is required under the PLLR. Patients should be reassured that these changes will be undertaken with considerable care to limit risks to both mother and fetus.

Common Conditions Arising in Pregnancy

It is beyond the scope of this chapter to address all possible conditions that coincide with pregnancy. However, discussion of the most common conditions arising from or coinciding with pregnancy, and the best treatments for these conditions, can help the nurse gain an understanding of the factors likely to be encountered in practice.

Constipation

The increased weight of the growing uterus as well as the relaxing effects of the hormones produced in greater amounts during pregnancy can lead to decreased intestinal motility, with resulting constipation. It is preferable to treat this condition by a preventive approach—that is, by encouraging increased fluids, a diet high in fiber, and regular exercise. If medication is necessary, bulking agents such as **psyllium** are preferred because they are not absorbed by the circulatory system. Stool softeners such as **docusate** may also be prescribed. If constipation is severe, a mild osmotic laxative such as milk of magnesia (**magnesium sulfate**) can be used on occasion, but osmotic and stimulant laxatives should be used on only a short-term basis because of concerns about dehydration and electrolyte imbalances (Trottier, Erebara, & Bozzo, 2012), which can promote premature labor.

Diabetes Mellitus

Diabetes mellitus, a defect in glucose transport, is a common condition in women of childbearing age. While describing the treatment regimens for the different types of diabetes is beyond the scope of this chapter, a few general facts can be presented.

There are three basic types of diabetes mellitus: type 1, type 2, and gestational diabetes. **Gestational diabetes** is a variant of type 2 diabetes in which insensitivity to insulin signaling develops in response to some of the endocrine changes of pregnancy.

In women who already have diabetes when they become pregnant, these changes may exacerbate the existing metabolic issue, and their current treatment regimen must be adjusted to account for it. Women who use insulin to manage type 1 diabetes may, for example, find that they need to increase their insulin dosage(s) or reduce their carbohydrate intake and increase their exercise regimen to maintain good glucose control. Women who manage their type 2 diabetes with exercise and diet alone may find that adding a hypoglycemic medication becomes necessary, while those who are already taking a hypoglycemic medication may need to increase the dose or add insulin to avoid hyperglycemia. Additionally, a consideration for these women is the fact that some oral hypoglycemic medications are safer than others with respect to fetal outcomes, and they may need to change oral medications or temporarily switch to insulin out of concern for fetal well-being.

In women who develop gestational diabetes, the medication considerations are slightly different. Gestational diabetes is defined as glucose intolerance of varying severity first appearing in pregnancy. The peak time for gestational diabetes to manifest itself is at 28 weeks' gestation, when the level of the hormone hPL is greatest. All pregnant women should be screened for blood glucose levels at 28 weeks, unless their medical history and risk factors indicate a need for earlier assessment.

The goal of treatment of diabetes is to prevent both **hyperglycemia** and **hypoglycemia**, both of which are detrimental to the developing fetus as well as the mother. A mildly elevated blood glucose level may be treated with dietary changes and increased exercise, just as it is in a nonpregnant person. Frequent monitoring is needed using a glucometer. If these changes do not result in lower glucose levels, drug treatment is needed to prevent the many known complications that may result, including macrosomia (excessive birth weight), which can increase the risk of potential complications during parturition, hypoglycemia in the neonate,

jaundice, and preterm birth. Endogenous (injected) insulin is usually required, as many oral antidiabetic agents cross the placenta.

Heartburn

Heartburn is a common discomfort of pregnancy, with symptoms worsening as the uterus grows upward and displaces the stomach. Gastric contents are regurgitated into the esophagus, resulting in a burning sensation. The increased level of progesterone in pregnancy also contributes because of its relaxant effect in the gastrointestinal (GI) tract. To avoid heartburn, pregnant women should eat smaller, more frequent meals, avoid fried or fatty foods, and drink adequate amounts of fluids. Antacids can be used safely because their effect is localized to the stomach. If the heartburn is accompanied by **gastric reflux**, an antisecretory agent (H_2 blocker), such as **ranitidine**, may be prescribed. A number of studies have demonstrated the safety of this class of drugs (Gilboa, Ailes, Rai, Anderson, & Honein, 2014).

Nausea and Vomiting in Pregnancy

Women who become pregnant so commonly experience nausea and vomiting that prevalence rates in the U.S are estimated at 70% (Einarson, Piwko & Koren, 2013). While common in the first trimester for most pregnancies, nausea and vomiting for some women can last through the 22nd week of gestation or beyond. A small portion of pregnant women (1-3%) (Nuangchamnong & Niebyl, 2014; London, Grube, Sherer, & Abulafia, 2017) experience a severe form of nausea and vomiting called hyperemesis gravidarum. Signs and symptoms include severe vomiting, dehydration, weight loss, headaches, extreme fatigue, and electrolyte imbalance. Hyperemesis gravidarum is the second most common cause of hospitalization for pregnant women in the US, following preterm labor (London, Grube, Sherer, & Abulafia, 2017). Treatment is primarily supportive, with IV fluid replacement and antiemetics. While several antiemetics are available, the combination of delayed-release doxylamine succinate and pyridoxine hydrochloride is the only pharmacological treatment to receive FDA Pregnancy Category A status, under the previous FDA pregnancy categories. This means there were adequate and well-controlled studies performed with no demonstrated risk to the fetus in the first trimester of pregnancy (Nuangchamnong & Niebyl, 2014). As such, it is considered a first-line treatment for nausea and vomiting in pregnancy (Madjunkova, Maltepe, & Koren, 2014).

Hypertension in Pregnancy

Hypertension is the most common maternal complication, occurring in approximately 12% of all pregnancies. The management of this disorder varies depending on the gestational age at which it is detected, the severity, and the progression of symptoms. **Gestational hypertension** is defined as systolic blood pressure equal to or greater than 140 mm Hg and/or diastolic blood pressure equal to or greater than 90 mm Hg on at least 2 occasions, at least 6 hours apart, after the 20th week of gestation in a woman who was previously normotensive (King & Brucker, 2011). **Pre-eclampsia** is diagnosed when the gestational hypertension is accompanied by **proteinuria** (300 mg or greater in 24 hours). Severe pre-eclampsia is hypertension with systolic blood pressure greater than 160 mm Hg or diastolic blood pressure greater than 110 mm Hg. The goal of treatment is to prevent seizures (**eclampsia**). Lowering the mother's blood pressure with antihypertensive drugs is reserved for severe cases when the threat of a cerebral vascular event, such as stroke, is imminent.

Many antihypertensive drugs cause **vasodilation** (opening of blood vessels). This effect may divert vital blood supply away from the uterus. Thus, treatment with antihypertensive agents is undertaken with care in pregnant women. For mild hypertension, medications are avoided as much as possible and offered only if lifestyle therapies

such as stress management techniques, bed rest, and other supportive care interventions do not stabilize the rising blood pressure, or if hypertension onset is rapid and severe. Oral medications used for hypertension in pregnancy include **methyldopa** (first-line agent of choice), **hydralazine**, **hydrochlorothiazide**, and **nifedipine** (Mustafa, Ahmed, Gupta, & Venuto, 2012; Vest & Cho, 2012). Diuretics, such as **hydralazine** and **hydrochlorothiazide**, carry a risk of volume contraction and electrolyte disturbances, as well as hyperuricemia. Angiotensin-converting enzyme (ACE) inhibitors and angiotensin receptor antagonists are absolutely contraindicated in pregnancy (Vest & Cho, 2012). Most beta blockers are regarded as unsafe in pregnant women as well, due to the increased risk of preterm birth, small for gestational age babies, or perinatal mortality.

As pre-eclampsia becomes more severe or is progressing rapidly, the patient is hospitalized, and intravenous **magnesium sulfate**, a central nervous system depressant, is initiated. **Magnesium sulfate** may act as a vasodilator and/or protector of the blood–brain barrier from edema, although its mechanism has yet to be defined. A bolus, or loading, dose of 4–6 g is given intravenously over 30 minutes, followed by a continuous infusion of 1–2 g per hour until the patient is stabilized and no adverse effects noted (see TABLE 12-2).

Group B Streptococcal Infection

Pregnant women can become infected with any number of viruses or bacterial infections. Nurses must be especially concerned about **Group B streptococcal infection**. Approximately 30% of pregnant women are colonized with Group B strep infection in the vaginal or rectal area. Most are asymptomatic. If untreated during the birth process, Group B strep can be acquired by the infant as he or she passes through the infected genital tract; this may result in serious, even fatal, cases of pneumonia or meningitis in the newborn. All pregnant women are tested for Group B strep at about

TABLE 12-2	Pre-eclampsia Therapy in a Hospital Setting

Drug: Magnesium sulfate

Action	**Nursing Considerations**
CNS suppressant: blocks nerve transmission, decreasing the possibility of convulsion in cases of severe pre-eclampsia.	Close observation during administration.
	Hourly vital signs. Protocols may call for discontinuing magnesium sulfate if the respiratory rate falls below 12 per minute.
Because it acts as a smooth muscle relaxant, it may also lower blood pressure, although this is not the intended use.	Monitor urine output; an indwelling catheter should be inserted. Output less than 30 mL per hour is a sign of toxicity.
Dosage	
Given intravenously as an infusion.	Monitor ordered laboratory studies: serum magnesium levels, urine protein, and other kidney function tests.
Loading dose: usually 4–6 g IV over 30 minutes.	Assess deep tendon reflexes (patellar) as ordered. Loss of reflexes may indicate magnesium toxicity.
Maintenance dose: 1–2 g per hour.	
Side Effects	The antidote for magnesium toxicity is calcium gluconate. Keep an ampule readily available at the bedside.
Due to vasodilation, facial flushing, feeling of warmth, lethargy. Nausea and vomiting, visual changes (e.g., blurred vision), heart palpitations, headache.	Continuous fetal heart rate monitoring.
	After delivery of the infant, continue IV magnesium sulfate as ordered for 12–24 hours. Seizures can occur in the postpartum period.
Signs of magnesium toxicity include decreased respirations, diminished or absent reflexes, and decreased urine output. Postpartum hemorrhage can occur due to the relaxant effect on the uterine muscles.	

Data from Davidson, M., London, M., & Ladewig, P. (2012). *Maternal–newborn nursing and women's health* (9th ed.). Saddle River, NJ: Pearson.

35 weeks' gestation. If she tests positive, the woman is treated with intravenous antibiotics during labor to reduce the bacterial load present at the time of birth. **Penicillin G** is the drug of choice; **clindamycin** is an alternative in those women who are allergic to **penicillin**.

Human Immunodeficiency Virus

A woman who tests positive for human immunodeficiency virus (HIV) must be given antiretroviral therapy during pregnancy to decrease the viral load and reduce the chance of transmission to the fetus. Without treatment, the risk of maternal–fetal transmission of HIV is about 25%. Antiretroviral therapy during pregnancy can reduce this risk to about 2% (Department of Health and Human Services [HHS], 2012). If the maternal viral load of HIV RNA is less than 400 copies/mL, treatment during labor and delivery is no longer considered necessary (HHS Panel on Treatment of HIV in Pregnancy, 2012). One drug in particular, **efavirenz (EFV)**, is associated with a small increase in the risk of neurologic birth defects, especially during the first trimester of pregnancy; experts are divided on whether this drug should be avoided (Sax, 2014) or used (Ford, Calmy, & Mofenson,

2011), however, the FDA advises against its use in the first trimester of pregnancy (Department of Health and Human Services [DHHS], 2017).

Treatment for the infant is usually continued prophylactically until about 6 weeks of age. Because the infant's blood will contain the same HIV antibodies as the mother, the infant must be tested using a more specific test for disease, or monitored for up to 18 months, when the maternal antibodies would have cleared the infant's system. Because HIV can be transmitted through breastmilk, breastfeeding is not recommended for infected mothers.

Neoplastic Disease

While it is not common for women to be diagnosed with cancer while pregnant (or vice versa), it does happen. In such a scenario, therapy needs to be balanced between optimizing the fetal outcome and maintaining the therapeutic benefit for the mother. Although many women believe (wrongly) that the co-occurrence of pregnancy and cancer automatically means choosing between the life of the fetus and the life or health of the mother, either short or long term, advances in cancer therapy have allowed many women to successfully combat certain types of cancer (particularly breast cancer) without needing to resort to pregnancy termination.

Chemotherapy drugs for the most part target fast-dividing cells, which is problematic for fetal growth. It has been generally determined that such drugs are most dangerous to the fetus in the first trimester. However, use of these medications can be undertaken with caution in the second and third trimesters.

Because of the great variety of drugs used in cancer treatment, and the development of more targeted medications that address specific types of neoplasms, the discussion of individual medications is too extensive for this chapter. However, information on treating cancer during pregnancy is available from a wide range of sources, including the American Cancer Society, the American Society of Clinical Oncologists, and the National Cancer Institute.

Drugs Used During Labor

A variety of medications may be used in relation to labor and delivery. Some are used to prevent, halt, or delay premature onset of labor (**preterm labor**); some are used to induce or speed up an overdue or **nonprogressing labor**; still others are used to address pain or complications arising during labor.

Preterm Labor

The presence of uterine contractions that cause changes in the cervix (effacement or dilation) prior to 37 weeks' gestation is diagnostic of preterm labor. In most circumstances, **tocolytic drugs** are prescribed to stop the labor and allow the pregnancy to continue until the fetus reaches full term, considered to be 38 weeks' gestation, if possible. These drugs work best if given before the cervix dilates to 4 cm and when the bag of waters is intact. One goal of this therapy is to delay the labor long enough for the administration of a corticosteroid (**betamethasone** or **dexamethasone**) to the mother, with the goal of accelerating fetal lung development

and surfactant production prior to birth. Two doses given intramuscularly 12 hours apart significantly reduces the likelihood of **respiratory distress syndrome** in the neonate, if he or she is born prior to the time of full lung maturation (37–38 weeks). These doses can be utilized for at least 2 days. Continuing administration of tocolytics beyond this period has not proven to be effective in preventing preterm labor (Locatelli, Consonni, & Ghidini, 2015).

Tocolytic Medications

Tocolysis is the use of drugs to decrease uterine activity. Tocolytic drugs include beta-sympathomimetic drugs, **magnesium sulfate**, calcium-channel blockers, and prostaglandin inhibitors (King & Brucker, 2011). In general, they are effective for 2 to 7 days.

Beta-mimetic drugs inhibit uterine activity by binding with beta-adrenergic receptors in the uterus. The only drug in this category to be approved for this indication was **ritodrine**. It is no longer prescribed or available in the United States due to its side effects. **Terbutaline** (a β2-receptor agonist), a drug more commonly used for treatment of asthma, is the most frequently prescribed drug in this category, but it is used off-label for preterm labor and it has been used with less frequency following a 2011 FDA black box warning and contraindication for use in preterm labor (Ross, 2017). Most protocols call for subcutaneous administration of 0.25 mg, with a repeat dose in one to six hours if the cardiovascular effects are tolerable. **Terbutaline** is not recommended for continued treatment of preterm labor. The FDA requires that all forms of **terbutaline** (oral, injectable, and subcutaneous pump) carry Black Box warnings and contraindications for use (FDA, 2011) (TABLE 12-3).

Magnesium sulfate is the drug most widely prescribed for preterm labor because its side effects are relatively mild and it effectively stops uterine contractions. The exact mechanism of action is not known. A loading

TABLE 12-3	Drugs Used in Preterm Labor (Tocolytic Agents and Corticosteroid Prophylaxis)		
Drug Name (Drug Class)	Mechanism of Action	Dosage	Side Effects/Nursing Considerations
Terbutaline (beta agonist)	Binds to beta-adrenergic receptors in the uterus, reducing uterine contractions	Subcutaneous injection: 0.25 mg. May repeat every 1–6 hours if maternal heartrate is < 130 beats per minute *Black box warning – see text	Mother: tachycardia, palpitations, cardiac arrhythmias, chest pain, hyperglycemia. Fetus: tachycardia, hyperglycemia during treatment, hypoglycemia after birth
Magnesium sulfate	Smooth muscle relaxant; decreases uterine contractions	4–6 g IV over 20 minutes; 1–4 g/h maintenance dose if uterine contractions persist and depending on urine output	Tachycardia, palpitations, flushing, headaches
Nifedipine (calcium-channel blocker)	Inhibits uterine activity	20 mg orally, repeat, if needed, after 30 minutes 20 mg orally every 3–8 hours for 48–72 hours if contractions persist	Mother: palpitations, flushing, headaches, dizziness, maternal tachycardia, nausea Fetus: decreased amniotic fluid, resolves after treatment
Indomethacin (NSAID)	Inhibits prostaglandin synthesis (not recommended after 32 weeks' gestation due to risk of premature closure of ductus arteriosus in fetus)	Rectal suppository: 100 mg, followed by 50 mg orally every 6 hours for 48 hours	Mother: hyperglycemia
Betamethasone, dexamethasone (corticosteroids)	Accelerates lung maturity in neonate; given antepartum to mother if preterm birth is likely (24–34 weeks' gestation) to accelerate lung maturity in the neonate	Betamethasone: 12 mg intramuscularly; two doses 24 hours apart Dexamethasone: 6 mg intramuscularly every 6 hours for 24 hours (4 doses)	

Data from Ross, M. (2017). Preterm labor. *Medscape*. Retrieved from https://emedicine.medscape.com/article/260998-overview#a6

dose of four to six grams intravenously, followed by a maintenance dose of one to two grams per hour, is the usual protocol.

Indomethacin, an NSAID used for its prostaglandin inhibition properties, has been used effectively to stop preterm labor for a period of 24 to 48 hours. It is not recommended after 32 weeks' gestation due to the possibility of premature closure of the ductus arteriosus in the fetus.

Labor Induction

When medically indicated due to a complication of pregnancy or risk of fetal compromise, labor may be artificially induced. If the cervix is not considered "favorable" based on Bishop's scoring system of cervical characteristics and the descent of the fetus into the pelvis, a two-step process is usually implemented. First, a prostaglandin agent, such as **misoprostol** (a synthetic analog of **PGE1**) or **PGE2** (**dinoprostone**), is inserted vaginally.

The prostaglandin is absorbed locally into the cervix, helping to "ripen" the cervix, making it more likely to dilate in response to **oxytocin** administration. **Oxytocin** binds oxytocin receptors in the myometrium, leading to increased intracellular calcium concentrations, resulting in stimulation of uterine contractions. It will stimulate uterine contractions but will usually not be effective if the cervix is not ripened (**TABLE 12-4**).

PGE2 is inserted as a vaginal gel or insert (suppository), usually 12 hours before **oxytocin** is started. Prostaglandins can stimulate uterine contractions via binding to E-prostanoid receptors (EP), which are G-coupled receptors that mediate the actions of calcium and adenylyl cyclase, ultimately controlling contractility (Blesson & Sahlin, 2014). The patient must be monitored in a labor setting. The drug must be removed 30 minutes prior to labor induction to avoid hyperstimulation of the uterus.

TABLE 12-4	Use of Oxytocin for Labor Induction

Action	**Nursing Considerations**
Stimulate uterine muscles to contract by increasing the excitability of the muscle cells.	Follow ordered protocols carefully, including maximum dose.
Dosage	Continuous fetal monitoring is recommended, along with assessment of contraction pattern.
Must always be diluted; 10 units added to 1,000 mL of isotonic solution for intravenous administration results in a solution containing 10 milliunits (mu) per milliliter. Using an electronic infusion pump, begin at 2 mu/min and increase by 1–2 mu/min until a satisfactory contraction pattern is established. Protocols vary among institutions. IV infusion must be piggybacked into the main IV line at the site nearest the patient so that it can quickly be discontinued if necessary.	Begin monitoring before beginning oxytocin. Assess maternal vital signs hourly or as ordered. Monitor intake and output. Discuss management of pain with the patient.
Side Effects	
Uterine hyperstimulation: can lead to rupture of uterus, abruption of placenta, and rapid labor and birth with possible lacerations and tissue trauma in both mother and baby	
Water intoxication: nausea and vomiting, hypotension	

Although not approved by the FDA for this indication, misoprostol, a prostaglandin E_1 analog, is also used to achieve cervical ripeness for labor induction and is sanctioned for that use by the American Congress of Obstetricians and Gynecologists (ACOG). A 100-mcg tablet must be broken into four pieces to obtain the 25-mcg recommended dose, which may be taken orally or inserted into the vagina. Oxytocin must not be started until four hours after the last administration of misoprostol. As with the other prostaglandin cervical-ripening agents, close observation is required in a labor setting. Extreme care should be observed with misoprostol administration for labor induction, as it can cause uterine rupture. In addition, during pregnancy, misoprostol can cause birth defects, abortion, and premature birth.

If the cervix is favorable for induction, the patient may be admitted for intravenous administration of oxytocin. The goal is to effectively mimic a normal labor pattern, with uterine contractions every two to three minutes, of sufficient duration and intensity to cause progressive dilation of the cervix and descent of the fetus into the birth canal. Oxytocin may also be administered when labor is not progressing normally, either because the contractions are too far apart or are not long enough or of sufficient intensity to cause cervical changes. This use of oxytocin is referred to as *labor augmentation*.

Oxytocin is also used after delivery of the infant and the placenta to help contract the uterine muscle and prevent excessive postpartum bleeding.

Analgesia/Anesthesia

Uterine contractions are the main cause of pain during labor. Because there is the fetus to consider, drug choice for pain relief must take into account the needs of both patients. Due to the prolonged gastric emptying time during labor, oral medications are not used. The intravenous route is preferred, because most drug actions will take effect more quickly and in a more predictable manner. Medications also may be administered intramuscularly or subcutaneously, but will take longer to produce their effects.

Butorphanol tartrate and nalbuphine-hydrochloride are narcotic agonist/antagonist drugs commonly used for pain management in early labor, particularly when epidural anesthesia is unavailable or the patient refuses it. They can be given either intramuscularly or intravenously. Both of these drugs cause severe withdrawal symptoms in women who have been using narcotics. A thorough history must be obtained before using either drug.

Epidural anesthesia is commonly used during labor as well as delivery for management of pain. Under local anesthesia, a catheter is inserted into the epidural space. An opioid drug such as fentanyl as well as a local anesthetic (see the *Pharmacology of Anesthetic Drugs* chapter) are then injected into the catheter. Additional drugs can be administered to provide anesthesia during either vaginal or cesarean birth. Patients must be given an adequate amount (usually 1,000 mL) of a volume-expanding fluid (such as lactated Ringer's solution), prior to being given epidural anesthesia, to compensate for the sudden shift of fluid that occurs with the epidural injection. Blood pressure is monitored closely, every 5 minutes for the first 15 minutes after each administration; hypotension and fever may develop in the mother (Leighton & Halpern, 2002). Labor may slow, so maternal uterine and fetal monitoring are continuous. Epidural anesthesia using low concentrations of local anesthetics, combined with lipid-soluble opioids, does not generally affect Apgar scores, but use of parenteral opioids is associated with more frequent incidence of low 1-minute Apgar scores (Leighton & Halpern, 2002; Silva & Halpern, 2010).

Drugs Used During the Postpartum Period

After delivery of the placenta, oxytocin is usually administered either intravenously in a diluted mixture of intravenous fluids or as a 10-unit intramuscular injection to control postpartum bleeding. If oxytocin is not sufficient to control bleeding due to a failure of the uterus to contract (**atony**), methylergonovine maleate, an ergot alkaloid, is usually ordered. Methylergonovine is an agonist for both serotonin and dopamine receptors. In addition, it antagonizes endothelial-derived relaxation factor. These effects increase uterine tone and decrease uterine bleeding. Because this drug affects all smooth muscles, including the blood vessels, it must not be given to a woman with hypertension,

because it may cause a severe elevation in blood pressure. Methylergonovine is given as an intramuscular injection, 0.2 mg, which may be repeated every 2 to 4 hours if necessary, followed by oral administration of a 0.2-mg tablet every 6 hours for 2 days until bleeding subsides. Both oxytocin and methylergonovine can cause severe uterine cramping, and the nurse should encourage the patient to take prescribed analgesics for pain.

Drugs Administered During Lactation

During lactation, most drugs do penetrate the milk supply, but usually in very small amounts, less than 1% (Hale, 2010). Very few drugs are contraindicated during lactation. It is important for the nurse to be well informed about this issue, because women may feel discouraged from breastfeeding if they must take prescribed medication, for fear of effects on the infant—yet in many cases those fears are not justified. National Institutes of Health (NIH) has established the LactMed site (https://toxnet.nlm.nih.gov/newtoxnet/lactmed.htm) as part of its TOXNET system. This site has valuable information pertaining to use of drugs during lactation and breastfeeding.

Those agents that *do* warrant concern in conjunction with breastfeeding include chemotherapy drugs, drugs of abuse such as cocaine and heroin, and radioactive isotopes (Davidson et al., 2012). Most drugs do penetrate breastmilk, so consideration should be given as to the timing and dosage form of the medication. For example, using a drug with a shorter half-life rather than a longer-acting form will decrease the accumulation of the drug in the breastmilk. Feeding the infant prior to taking medication will also reduce the amount of medication that reaches the breastmilk. When alternatives are available, choose a drug that has a lower tendency to pass into the breastmilk. Certain drugs, while not absolutely contraindicated, will

Best Practices

Most drugs penetrate the breastmilk to some extent. Drugs that must be given to lactating and breastfeeding patients should be evaluated regarding the best dosage form, and the ideal timing of dosing, to minimize the amount of the drug(s) that is transferred to the infant.

diminish the milk supply and so should not be used in breastfeeding women; examples include estrogen and **ergotamine** (King & Brucker, 2011). Encourage women to discuss any medication use with their pediatrician, but avoid causing unnecessary fear; as noted earlier, very few medications have the potential to pass through breastmilk to the infant in sufficient quantity to cause harm.

CHAPTER SUMMARY

Drugs are not tested in pregnant or lactating women; therefore, evidence of their effects in these women and their infants is known only after they are taken and sufficient data have been obtained. All fetal organs are formed by the eighth week of pregnancy. Thus, drug effects may be more significant when medications are taken during this time.

Physiological changes in the woman's body during pregnancy make drug effects both in the mother and in the fetus more difficult to predict. Planning for pregnancy makes it more likely a woman has adequate stores of essential vitamins, such as folic acid, which can help her to avoid potentially fetotoxic substances. Management of common conditions of pregnancy must always be inclusive of both the needs of the mother and the needs of the developing fetus.

Hypertension is the most common complication of pregnancy. Treatment is focused on preventing progression to eclampsia. Because of the effects of antihypertensive medications on the fetus, use of most classes of antihypertensive drugs is contraindicated in pregnant women. If efforts to stabilize blood pressure fail, hospitalization may be necessary.

Medications given during labor and delivery are administered for one of three reasons: to halt preterm labor, to promote nonprogressing labor, and to address pain and other complications of labor and delivery. Oxytocin promotes labor progression and is also used in the postpartum period to control hemorrhage. Pain management during labor and delivery includes the use of narcotic agonist/antagonists during early labor as well as regional (epidural) anesthesia.

Critical Thinking Questions

1. At what stage of development is it most important to avoid fetotoxic medications?

2. List three common side effects for magnesium sulfate.

3. A pregnant woman has been prescribed methylergonovine to stop postpartum bleeding. Which of the following assessments would be most important for the nurse to determine before administration of the medication?
   a. Urinary output
   b. Respiratory rate
   c. Blood pressure
   d. Deep tendon reflexes

4. What are the concerns of epidural anesthesia for the mother? For the neonate?

CASE STUDIES

Case Scenario: Nausea/Vomiting of Pregnancy

SW is a 26-year-old Asian-American female who presents as a new obstetric patient to the private OB-GYN clinic where you are working as a nurse. She is approximately 6 weeks' gestation, gravida 2, para 1, no pregnancy losses. She is married and has a 4-year-old son. Her chief complaint today is nausea with vomiting up to three times per day that has been increasing in severity over the past week. She expresses concern that she might be getting dehydrated as this happened with her last pregnancy, requiring hospitalization with IV fluids. She also complains of fatigue, food aversion, heightened sense of smell, and a 2-pound weight loss from her pre-pregnancy weight during the past week. She reports she is drinking water "constantly" in small amounts throughout the day, but is only able to tolerate a few foods such as dry crackers, toast, and pretzels. She denies diarrhea, constipation, acid reflux, dysuria, dry mouth, dizziness, or headache. She takes one prenatal vitamin daily. Relevant past medical history includes one full-term pregnancy complicated by significant

CASE STUDIES (CONTINUED)

nausea and vomiting with dehydration during the first 20 weeks' gestation. She reports taking ondansetron during her last pregnancy, but she has read that this drug is no longer recommended during pregnancy. She had no complications during childbirth or postpartum. Her sister also experienced severe nausea and vomiting of pregnancy. She does not use any tobacco products, nor does she drink alcohol or use recreational drugs. She is currently full-time at home with her son and reports daily physical activity taking him on walks to the park.

Allergies: NKDA

Vital signs: BP: 120/70; P: 74/minute, regular; Respirations: 12/minute, regular; Oral temperature: 98.4°F; Weight: 125 lbs.; Ht: 63"; BMI: 22.14.

The healthcare provider performs a thorough physical exam, appropriate for initial prenatal clinic visit. Bimanual pelvic exam reveals fundus is not yet palpable above the pubis symphysis; breasts are tender bilaterally; skin is intact with mildly decreased turgor. The remainder of the exam is normal.

Transvaginal ultrasound reveals fetal pole and heartbeat.

Relevant lab values from today's visit: Serum electrolytes: All values are within upper limits of normal range. CBC shows mild hemoconcentration. Urine specific gravity elevated; urine glucose/ketones negative.

The provider determines that SW is approximately 6 to 7 weeks pregnant by menstrual dates and has nausea and vomiting of pregnancy without dehydration. Doxylamine/pyridoxine 10mg/10mg is prescribed. The provider asks you to explain to the patient how to take this medication, its expected effects/side effects, and any warnings or precautions associated with this drug. You are also to counsel her regarding dietary changes and trigger avoidance.

Case Questions

1. Write a nursing diagnosis that addresses this patient's risk for dehydration.

2. What is the drug class for each component of doxylamine/pyridoxine? What is the mechanism of action (pharmacodynamics) for each component?

3. SW asks you if taking this medication will present any risk to her unborn baby. How will you answer this question? What have well-controlled studies shown regarding a risk for fetal abnormalities associated with this drug?

4. How will you explain to SW about the initial dosing of this medication? What is the maximum dose she can take in 24 hours?

5. How will you counsel SW about dietary adjustments to help control nausea? What are some specific foods or beverages that should be eliminated or avoided of she feels nauseated? When should she drink fluids in relation to eating solid foods?

6. SW admits that she has tried taking ginger products such as ginger tea and ginger lollipops during this past week to help curb the nausea. She asks you if it is safe to take these ginger products during pregnancy. How will you respond? Refer to current evidence-based data for your answer.

7. Write one short-term goal that can be met today regarding the nursing diagnosis you identified in question #1.

8. What is one intervention that can you implement during the visit to meet your short-term goal in question #7?

REFERENCES

American Nurses Association (ANA). (2011). Position statement: Non-punitive alcohol and drug treatment for pregnant and breast-feeding women and their exposed children. Retrieved from http://www.nursingworld.org/MainMenuCategories/Policy-Advocacy/Positions-and-Resolutions/ANAPosition Statements/Position-Statements-Alphabetically/Non-punitive-Alcohol-and-Drug-Treatment-for-Pregnant-and-Breast-feeding-Women-and-the-Exposed-Childr.pdf

Blattner, C.M., Danesh, M., Safaee, M., & Murase, J.E. (2016). Understanding the new FDA pregnancy and lactation labeling rules. *International Journal of Women's Dermatology, 2*(1), 5–7. doi:10.1016/j.ijwd.2015.12.005

Blesson, C.S., & Sahlin, L. (2014). Prostaglandin E and F receptors in the uterus. *Receptors & Clinical Investigation, 1,* e115. doi:10.14800/rci.115

Dante, G., Bellei, G., Neri, I., & Facchinetti, F. (2014). Herbal therapies in pregnancy: what works? *Current Opinion in Obstetrics and Gynecology, 26*(2), 83–91. doi: 10.1097/GCO.0000000000000052

Davidson, M., London, M., & Ladewig, P. (2012). *Maternal–newborn nursing and women's health* (9th ed.). Saddle River, NJ: Pearson.

Department of Health and Human Services (HHS). (2012). Panel on Treatment of Pregnant Women with HIV Infection and Prevention of Perinatal Transmission. Recommendations for use of antiretroviral drugs in transmission in the United States. Available at http://aidsinfo.nih.gov/contentfiles /lvguidelines/ PerinatalGL.pdf.

Department of Health and Human Services (DHHS). (2017). Recommendations for the use of antiretroviral drugs in pregnant women with HIV infection and interventions to reduce perinatal HIV transmission in the United States. Retrieved from https:// aidsinfo.nih.gov/guidelines/html/3/perinatal/143 /introduction

Einarson, T.R., Piwko, C., & Koren G. (2013). Prevalence of nausea and vomiting of pregnancy in the USA: a meta analysis. *J Popul Ther Clin Pharmacol.* 20(2):e163–e170.

Food and Drug Administration (FDA). (2011). *FDA Drug Safety Communication: New warnings against the use of terbutaline to treat preterm labor.* Retrieved from https://www.fda.gov/Drugs/DrugSafety /ucm243539.htm

Ford, N., Calmy, A., & Mofenson, L. (2011). Safety of efavirenz in the first trimester of pregnancy: An updated systematic review and meta-analysis. *AIDS, 25*(18), 2301–2304.

Gilboa, S.M., Ailes, E.C., Rai, R.P., Anderson, J.A., & Honein, M.A. (2014). Antihistamines and birth defects: A systematic review of the literature. *Expert Opinion on Drug Safety, 13*(12), 1667–1698. http://doi .org/10.1517/14740338.2014.970164

Hale, T.W. (2010). *Medications and mother's milk* (14th ed.). Amarillo, TX: Pharmasoft.

Kennedy, D.A., Lupattelli, A., Koren, G., & Nordeng, H. (2016). Safety classification of herbal medicines used in pregnancy in a multinational study. *BMC Complementary and Alternative Medicine, 16,* 102.

King, T., & Brucker, M. (2011). *Pharmacology for women's health.* Sudbury, MA: Jones & Bartlett.

Leighton, B.L., & Halpern, S.H. (2002). The effects of epidural analgesia on labor, maternal, and neonatal outcomes: A systematic review. *American Journal of Obstetrics and Gynecology, 186*(5 Suppl.), S69–S77.

Locatelli, A., Consonni, S., & Ghidini, A. (2015). Preterm labor: Approach to decreasing complications of prematurity. *Obstetrics and Gynecology Clinics of North America, 42*(2), 255–274. doi: 10.1016/j .ogc.2015.01.004

London, V., Grube, S., Sherer, D.M., & Abulafia, O. (2017). Hyperemesis gravidarum: a review of recent literature. Pharmacology, 100:161-171.

Madjunkova, S., Maltepe, C., & Koren, G. (2014). The delayed-release combination of doxylamine and pyridoxine for the treatment of nausea and vomiting in pregnancy. Paediatr Drugs. 16(3):199-211. doi: 10.1007/s40272-014-0065-5.

Mittendorf, R. (1995). Teratogen update: Carcinogenesis and teratogenesis associated with exposure to diethylstilbestrol (DES) in utero. *Teratology, 51*(6), 435–445.

Moore, L.E. (2018). Pathophysiology of insulin resistance. In L. Moore (Ed.), *Diabetes in pregnancy* (pp 1–6). Cham, Switzerland: Springer.

Mosley, J.F., Smith, L.L., & Dezan, M.D. (2015). An overview of upcoming changes in pregnancy and lactation labeling information. *Pharmacy Practice, 13*(2), 605.

Mustafa, R., Ahmed, S., Gupta, A., & Venuto, R.C. (2012). A comprehensive review of hypertension in pregnancy. *Journal of Pregnancy, 105918.* doi: 10.1155/2012/105918

Nuangchamnong, N. & Niebyl, J. (2014). Doxylamine succinate–pyridoxine hydrochloride (Diclegis) for the management of nausea and vomiting in pregnancy: an overview. *International Journal of Women's Health.* 6:401-409. doi:10.2147/IJWH.S46653.

Pernia, S., & DeMaagd, G. (2016). The new Pregnancy and Lactation Labeling Rule. *Pharmacy and Therapeutics, 41*(11), 713–715.

Ross, M. (2017). Preterm labor. *Medscape.* Retrieved from https://emedicine.medscape.com/article /260998-overview#a6

Sachdeva, P., Patel, B.G., & Patel, B.K. (2009). Drug use in pregnancy: A point to ponder! *Indian Journal of Pharmacy Science, 71*(1), 1–7.

Sanghavi, M., & Rutherford, J.D. (2014). Cardiovascular physiology of pregnancy. *Circulation, 130,* 1003–1008.

Sax, P. (2014). *HIV essentials.* Burlington, MA: Jones & Bartlett.

Silva, M., & Halpern, S.H. (2010). Epidural analgesia for labor: Current techniques. *Local and Regional Anesthesia, 3,* 143–153.

Trottier, M., Erebara, A., & Bozzo, P. (2012). Treating constipation during pregnancy. *Canadian Family Physician, 58*(8), 836–838.

Vest, A.R., & Cho, L.S. (2012). Hypertension in pregnancy. *Cardiology Clinics, 30*(3), 407–423.

CHAPTER 13

Pharmacology in Dermatologic Conditions

Diana Webber

KEY TERMS

Acne
Atopic dermatitis
Atrophy
Comedogenic
Cream
Dermatopharmacology

Dermatophytosis
Eczema
Emollient
Enteral
Gel
Hyperkeratotic

Integumentary system
Intralesional injection
Keratolytic
Lotion
Microcomedone
Ointment

Parenteral
Pruritic
Systemic administration
Vehicle

CHAPTER OBJECTIVES

At the end of the chapter, the student will be able to:

1. Discuss the basic concepts of drug delivery in dermatologic conditions.

2. Compare the advantages and disadvantages of three methods for drug delivery in dermatologic conditions: topical, intralesional injection, and systemic administration.

3. Describe the use of three common types of topical agents: antimicrobials, steroids, and antifungals.

4. Describe the pharmacology for the drugs discussed in this section: class, therapeutic indication, mechanism of action, interactions, side effects, and toxicity.

5. Identify relevant patient information concepts for medications used for dermatologic conditions.

Introduction

The skin serves as a barrier that protects the body from injury, disease, and environmental conditions. It also functions in temperature regulation, fluid balance, sensory perception, and immunobiology. The three layers of the skin (FIGURE 13-1), the associated glandular structures, plus the mucous membranes, hair, and nails make up the human body's largest organ system: the **integumentary system**. It is no wonder that this system is one of the primary avenues for introduction of pharmacologic agents into the body.

Dermatopharmacology is a term that refers to pharmacology as it applies to dermatologic conditions. Medications for skin disorders may be applied topically, injected intralesionally, or administered systemically. The methods for introducing medication into the body are called routes of drug administration.

The majority of skin conditions are treated with topical medications. To be effective, a topical medication must be able to cross the barrier of the outer layer of the skin. Topical administration in this section refers to the application of a substance to the skin. Otic and ophthalmic preparations are also considered "topical medications," but these are discussed elsewhere in this text (Chapter 10). In only a few instances can a drug be applied directly to the target tissue and exert its effect, as is the case with topically administered drugs. Topical pharmacologic agents may be incorporated into various **vehicles** that will transport the medication across the outer skin barrier to reach the affected site. Common topical drug formulations include **lotions**, **creams**, **gels**, and **ointments** (TABLE 13-1). Topical drug products have many uses, including the following: inflammatory or **pruritic** skin conditions; infectious processes such as bacterial (cellulitis, folliculitis, impetigo), viral (shingles), and fungal conditions; **hyperkeratotic** conditions such as warts and corns; and prevention of skin conditions such as burns from ultraviolet light exposure.

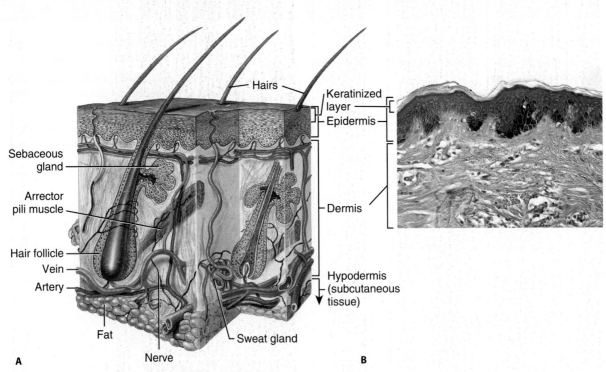

Sebaceous gland
Arrector pili muscle
Hair follicle
Vein
Artery
Fat
Nerve
Sweat gland
Hairs
Keratinized layer
Epidermis
Dermis
Hypodermis (subcutaneous tissue)

A

B

FIGURE 13-1 The layers of the skin.

© Donna Beer Stolz, PhD, Center for Biologic Imaging, University of Pittsburgh Medical School.

TABLE 13-1	Topical Formulations		
	Formulation	Description	Uses
Semi-solids (most common)	Ointment	Oil-based; non-soluble	Hydrating; most absorbent
	Cream	Emulsion of oil in water	Lubricating; absorbs well
	Lotion	A suspension of powder in water (or water and oil)	Cooling; evaporates
	Gel	A gelling agent dispersed in water or alcohol-based medium	Easy to apply; not as well absorbed.
	Foam	Small bubbles suspended in liquid	Easy to apply; not as well absorbed.
	Powder	A solid or semisolid that has been ground into fine particles	Can be used as antifungals in over-the-counter products

Occasionally, a dermatological condition requires treatment with a drug that is administered systemically, as opposed to the topical ROAs shown in Table 13-1, In other words, to produce their desired therapeutic activity, some drugs must first enter the bloodstream to reach their target sites of action, located *inside* the body. Systemic routes of drug administration used to treat skin disorders include **parenteral** (ROA requires a needle, e.g., intravenous, subcutaneous, intramuscular) and **transdermal**. Medications administered by these ROA elicit systemic effects; meaning, the drug enters the bloodstream and is distributed throughout the entire body (Chapter 3).

In contrast, **intralesional injections** provide direct delivery of medication to the site of a lesion without eliciting systemic effects. Steroids are an example of a medication commonly administered via intralesional injection.

Topical Administration

Some common skin conditions treated with topical medications include infections (bacterial, viral, fungal), inflammation, pruritus, hyperkeratosis, and others. Four major factors determine the pharmacologic action or response to topically applied preparations: (1) the type and thickness of skin upon which the preparation is applied, (2) the concentration of the drug being applied, (3) the frequency of drug application, and (4) the vehicle into which the drug is incorporated to facilitate penetration through the skin barrier (Katzung, Masters, & Trevor, 2012).

General principles involving absorption of topical medications include the following:

- More drug is absorbed when the medication is applied to a larger area of skin.
- The more a vehicle moisturizes the skin, the greater the absorption of the drug.
- Absorption is increased by occlusive properties of the agent.
- The more a vehicle is rubbed into the skin, the greater the absorption.
- The longer the vehicle remains in contact with the skin, the greater the absorption.

The goal of topical delivery of medication is to avoid the adverse effects associated with systemic routes of drug administration (such as nausea, dizziness and headache). In general, topical medications have few adverse effects or complications. Topical medications are also convenient, cost-effective, and easy to apply, which collectively increases the likelihood the patient will use them as directed.

There are, of course, some disadvantages to the topical route of administration. Skin irritation or allergic reaction may occur at the application site. Also, due to the size

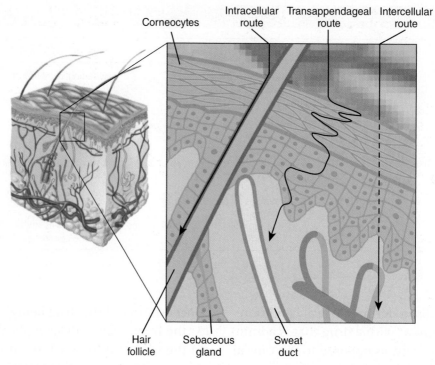

Corneocytes   Intracellular route   Transappendageal route   Intercellular route

Hair follicle   Sebaceous gland   Sweat duct

FIGURE 13-2 Schematic diagram of percutaneous absorption.

and composition of the drug molecule, not all drugs are suitable for absorption through the skin (**FIGURE 13-2**).

Systemic Administration

Although the usual approach to treating cutaneous disorders in immunocompetent persons is with topical pharmacologic agents, sometimes systemic therapy is indicated, such as in widespread infections or **dermatophytosis** (meaning, superficial fungal infections of the skin, hair or nails), or when topical treatments are ineffective. Examples of skin conditions that may require a systemic medication include extensive allergic contact dermatitis, nail and hair infections, widespread dermatophytosis, and chronic nonresponsive yeast infections. When oral therapy is being contemplated, it is imperative to confirm the causative agent and type of skin infection, either by microscopy or by culture.

When a disease condition affects a large area of the skin, **systemic administration** of a pharmacologic agent is advantageous, as widespread infectious or inflammatory conditions may be difficult to treat with a topical preparation. Additionally, adherence to

medication regimens may be enhanced with systemic versus topical medications, particularly in conditions where topical treatment would be prolonged.

A disadvantage of the **enteral** (specifically, oral dosage forms that pass through the GI tract) route for drugs that are highly metabolized by the liver is the first-pass effect (Chapter 2); that is, reduction of the drug's concentration each time if passes through the liver. Cost is also a consideration, as some systemic medications, such as systemic antifungal agents, are quite expensive. Disadvantages of parenterally delivered medications include the pain associated with drug administration, added risk of potentially serious adverse reactions (without recourse of withdrawing the administered dose), and the skill level required for accessing this route.

Intralesional Administration

Common skin conditions treated with intralesional injection include cystic **acne**, psoriasis, keloid scars, hemangiomas, lichen simplex chronicus, and **eczema** that is poorly responsive to topical therapy. Scarring from these conditions is cosmetically unacceptable to patients of both sexes, and often intralesional steroid injection is the only way to reduce the inflammation and skin remodeling that occurs.

Intralesional injection is advantageous in that it places the drug in direct contact with the pathologic tissue.

Although less of the drug administered by intralesional injection is absorbed into the rest of the body (systemic absorption), if large doses are injected, there *may* be a systemic effect. Other disadvantages are localized skin **atrophy** at injection sites and pain associated with injection. Additionally, the medication cannot be self-administered, and the treatment regimen often requires more time and/or repeated visits for maximum effectiveness. Intralesional injection of corticosteroids is not recommended in persons with diabetes due to possible systemic absorption resulting in increased blood glucose.

Physiological Factors Affecting Transdermal Medication Administration

Skin is not uniform over the entire body, nor does it maintain the same qualities throughout the life span. Infants, for example, have skin that is highly sensitive to external stimuli, which is part of the bonding mechanism between a newborn and his or her mother. An infant's skin is soft and fine-grained, but it is generally not thin, and most often there is a relatively thick layer of protective fat beneath it. In an older adult, loss of moisture and elasticity and, in many cases, years of sun damage have toughened the outer surface, but reduced subcutaneous fat and thinning of the epidermal layers (FIGURE 13-3) make skin in older adults more susceptible to damage. This reduction in epidermis and subdermal fat affects how medications cross the skin when applied topically (Story, 2012).

Acne Medications: An Example of Delivery Systems

Acne vulgaris is one of the most common skin conditions affecting adolescents and young adults. One form of acne, termed *rosacea*, develops during adulthood and responds to similar treatment modalities as acne vulgaris. Briefly, the pathogenesis of acne involves the interaction of four factors: sebaceous gland hyperplasia triggered by increased androgen levels, changes in the growth and differentiation of cells lining the hair follicles, bacterial invasion of the follicle by *Propionibacterium acnes*, and subsequent inflammation of the follicle epithelium (FIGURE 13-4).

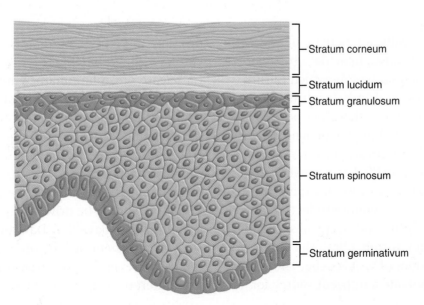

- Stratum corneum
- Stratum lucidum
- Stratum granulosum
- Stratum spinosum
- Stratum germinativum

FIGURE 13-3 The layers of the epidermis.

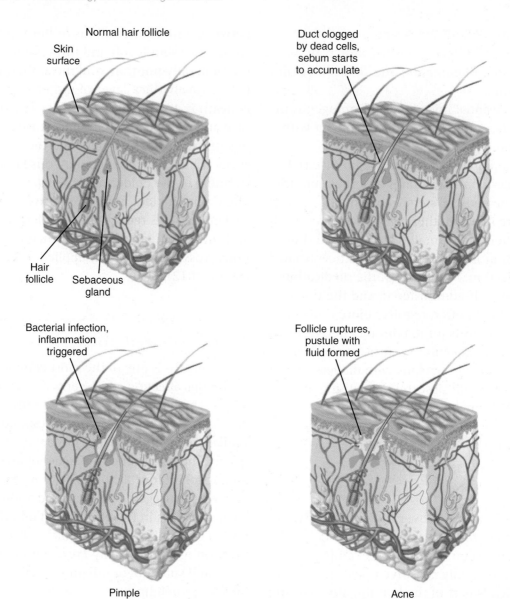

FIGURE 13-4 Pathology of acne.

More specifically, an increase in androgen production first causes follicular obstruction, via epithelial desquamation, which in turn creates **microcomedones** (precursor acne lesions). (Any substance that clogs pores or fosters the formation of precursor acne lesions is known as **comedogenic**; conversely, a topical formulation classified as *noncomedogenic* claims not to directly cause or exacerbate acne vulgaris.) Increased sebum production due to excess circulating androgens fills these obstructed follicles, forming both the open and closed comedones of visible acne. The sebum-rich follicles provide a nutrient source for, and

promote the growth of, *P. acnes* (Kaur, Sehgal, Gupta, & Singh, 2015). The *P. acnes* bacteria release pro-inflammatory mediators that spread to the surrounding dermis when comedones rupture, causing inflammatory papules, pustules, nodules, and cysts to develop. To successfully manage a patient's acne, clinicians must understand these components that contribute to its pathophysiology. Moreover, treatment should be driven by predominant lesion type (Dellavalle & Dawson, 2013).

The treatment of acne often involves the use of several medications that target either different types of acne lesions, different factors involved in the pathogenesis of acne, or different degrees of acne severity. Because acne medications are administered via three different modalities (topical, systemic, and intralesional), acne pharmacologic treatment serves as a model to illustrate dermatologic medication delivery systems.

Pharmacology of Topical Acne Medication

Benzoyl Peroxide

Benzoyl peroxide is a topical antimicrobial agent. Because this medication is lipophilic (i.e., lipid-loving), it is able to penetrate the lipid-lined sebaceous duct. The antimicrobial activity of **benzoyl peroxide** against *P. acnes* is likely due to the release of active or free-radical oxygen into the follicle, which then oxidizes bacterial proteins, causing bacterial death. **Benzoyl peroxide** exerts mild **keratolytic** and comedolytic effects by removing excess sebum and causing mild desquamation (Dutil, 2010; Zaenglein et al., 2016).

Pharmacokinetics

Less than 5% of the applied dose is absorbed through the skin. **Benzoyl peroxide** therapy is limited by concentration-dependent skin irritation associated with the amount of time the drug is in contact with the skin.

Nursing Considerations

Common adverse effects of **benzoyl peroxide** are related to its mechanism of action: oxidation of skin cell proteins causes them to become dry, possibly causing skin irritation and peeling at the site of application. In more pronounced cases, this can lead to pruritus and contact sensitization reactions (topical hypersensitivity reactions). Also, **benzoyl peroxide** is a potent bleaching agent; therefore, patients should be warned that fabrics that come in contact with **benzoyl peroxide**, including towels, bed sheets, and clothing, may be bleached. When evaluating the effectiveness of this medication, the nurse should consider that drug-induced photosensitivity to ultraviolet light may affect an underlying skin condition, causing erythema and irritation (Kraft & Freiman, 2011; Zaenglein et al., 2016).

Salicylic Acid

Salicylic acid is a keratolytic drug that facilitates desquamation by breaking apart intracellular bonds in the stratum corneum. This loosens the keratin and aids in the penetration of other medications through this outermost layer of the epidermis.

Pharmacokinetics

Salicylic acid penetrates only three to four millimeters below the site of application, and it remains biologically active for about two hours.

Nursing Considerations

The nurse should assess the patient's understanding of the drug's potent drying effect on skin and caution the patient to avoid its use on inflamed eczematous skin, as it may induce an eczema flare.

Tretinoin

Tretinoin is a retinoic acid derivative that is available as a topical 0.1% cream or a 0.025% gel. This drug is a naturally occurring derivative of vitamin A that binds to intracellular retinoic acid receptors and regulates epithelial cell reproduction, proliferation, and differentiation. It moderates abnormal keratinization and inflammation by inhibiting the expression of transglutaminases, enzymes that create cross-links between keratin proteins. **Tretinoin** promotes detachment and shedding of keratinized cells from the hair follicle so that the contents of comedones are extruded; this effect reduces the precursor lesions of acne vulgaris (Millikan, 2003).

Pharmacokinetics

Tretinoin demonstrates very little systemic absorption when administered as either a cream or a gel. Its half-life is about 18 hours, and it is excreted through the urine and feces.

Nursing Considerations

To evaluate the full effectiveness of **tretinoin**, the nurse should advise the patient to allow 8 to 12 weeks for optimal clinical improvement. Although the amount of drug absorbed from the skin when using topical retinoid formulations is very low, the risk of systemic absorption still exists. Women should be discouraged from using **tretinoin** during pregnancy and discontinue its use if they do become pregnant (Bozzo, Chua-Gocheco, & Einarson, 2011).

Pharmacology of Systemic Acne Medications

Tetracyclines

Tetracyclines, including **doxycycline**, **tetracycline**, and **minocycline**, are broad-spectrum antibiotics that effectively eradicate *P. acnes*. The drugs bind reversibly to the *P. acnes* bacterial ribosome subunit and block incoming transfer RNA (t-RNA) from binding to their receptor sites. This may result in leakage of intracellular material from bacterial cells, with resultant cell death.

Pharmacokinetics

Only 60% to 70% of **tetracycline** is absorbed after an oral dose, compared to 90% to 100% absorption of **minocycline** and **doxycycline**. The half-life of **tetracycline** is 6 to 8 hours; by comparison, the half-life of **minocycline** and **doxycycline** is 16 to 18 hours, allowing for once-daily dosing of these drugs. All **tetracycline** drugs are primarily excreted in the urine and bile.

Nursing Considerations

The nurse must assess for concurrent use of hormonal contraception in any female patient of childbearing age. **Tetracycline** may decrease oral contraceptive effectiveness by interfering with normal gut flora, thereby decreasing the bioavailability of hormone preparations. Additionally, the use of tetracyclines is not recommended during pregnancy. After long-term use of at least 100 mg/day, **minocycline** may cause a blue-gray skin discoloration, which may take months to years to resolve or may never resolve after the drug is discontinued. The cause of this hyperpigmentation may be related to the fact that **minocycline** turns black when oxidized (Niser et al., 2013). The nurse should advise the patient of this potential adverse effect,

encourage the patient to use a sunscreen with a high SPF rating, and monitor the patient for any skin discoloration, as photosensitivity reactions involving UV light can be a concern with tetracyclines, especially **doxycycline**.

Isotretinoin

Isotretinoin is an oral retinoic acid derivative. Similar to **tretinoin**, **isotretinoin** is a derivative of vitamin A that attaches to skin androgen receptors and alters DNA transcription, resulting in reduced sebaceous gland size, decreased sebum secretion, and inhibited keratin formation. It also has a dermal anti-inflammatory effect. **Isotretinoin** is used primarily for severe nodular acne in patients for whom other treatments fail; it is restricted to this narrow indication because of its safety profile, which includes association with serious mental health disturbances and a well-known, significant teratogenic effect in pregnancy. However, *systemic* **isotretinoin** is the only drug that acts on all etiopathogenic mechanisms of acne (Çinar et al., 2016).

Pharmacokinetics

Isotretinoin is only about 25% bioavailable following an oral dose. The half-life is 10 to 20 hours, and it is excreted via the urine and feces.

Nursing Considerations

Administration of **isotretinoin** requires signed patient consent and regular pregnancy testing for females of childbearing age. Animal or human studies have demonstrated severe fetal abnormalities or fetal risk associated with the use of this drug. The outcomes associated with use of **isotretinoin** while pregnant include high likelihood of pregnancy loss and significant, life-altering malformations to the fetus's central nervous system, face, head, and heart (Zaenglein et al., 2016). So significant is this risk that patients are required to register with a program called iPledge that is intended to ensure that no pregnancies occur in females taking the drug (iPledge, n.d.). Female patients are required to document use of two forms of contraceptive, starting a month prior to use of the drug, or a complete inability to become pregnant (e.g., hysterectomy or menopause) for the drug to be dispensed. Male patients are required to register as well, out of concern that the drug may be present in semen (although no documented cases of birth defects from male use of the drug exist).

In addition, **isotretinoin** has been associated with the development of significant mental health effects in some patients, including depression, psychosis, and suicidal ideation/suicide (Bremner, Shearer, & McCaffery, 2012). It is recommended that all patients be closely monitored at each visit during treatment, and assessed for symptoms of depression, mood disturbance, psychosis, or aggression to determine if further evaluation may be necessary (iPledge, n.d.). The nurse is advised that the patient or a family member may also contact them if the patient develops depression, mood disturbance, psychosis, or aggression, without waiting until the next visit with the prescriber. The recommendation is that the drug should be discontinued if symptoms consistent with depression or psychosis arise.

Hormonal Medications

Oral contraceptives may also be employed for the treatment of acne. For female patients, oral contraceptive pills (OCPs) are effective in reducing both inflammatory and non-inflammatory acne lesions. Although any OCP containing estrogen will improve acne, newer OCPs containing **drospirenone**, **desogestrel**, or **norgestimate** are less androgenic and, as a result, may be more beneficial, as testosterone and other androgens stimulate sebum production.

Drospirenone decreases the levels of ovarian androgens and free testosterone in the blood by counteracting the estrogen-induced stimulation of the renin–angiotensin–aldosterone system and by blocking testosterone from binding to androgen receptors. **Desogestrel** and **norgestimate** combine high progestational activity with minimum androgen effects. They do not counteract the estrogen-induced increase in sex hormone–binding globulin, so a greater amount of circulating testosterone is bound and, therefore, unavailable to the tissues. This results in lower serum levels of free testosterone.

Nursing Considerations

Both smoking and use of OCPs cause increased blood coagulability, with associated increased risk for blood clots. For this reason, the nurse should regularly assess for smoking status and strongly recommend smoking cessation in persons using OCPs.

Myth Buster

A common misconception is that dirty skin, stress, chocolate, and greasy foods cause acne. Hormones, oral contraceptives, pregnancy, heredity, milk, and some medications seem to trigger acne. However, the basic pathology is fourfold: (1) increased sebum production due to androgenic (specifically testosterone) stimulation; (2) excessive keratinization of the cells lining the hair follicles; (3) bacterial invasion of the follicle by *P. acnes*; and (4) inflammation of the follicle epithelium. The interaction of these processes causes swelling, occlusion, and bacterial proliferation in the micro openings (i.e., pores) of the hair follicles and sebaceous glands (Lei & Mercurio, 2009). Treatment focuses on keeping skin pores open and on controlling the bacteria that causes infection of the hair follicle. Topical preparations such as benzoyl peroxide have antibacterial and keratolytic effects, serving to dry the stratum corneum and loosen the keratin so that it is mobilized by the sebum out of the hair follicle duct to the surface of the skin. This helps open the pores so that the antibacterial agent can penetrate the stratum corneum. The presence of bacteria triggers and maintains inflammation; therefore, it is vital that the *P. acnes* bacteria be controlled. The desired outcome is to heal pustules, keep new pustules from forming, prevent scarring, and help reduce the embarrassment from having acne (McKoy, 2008).

Pharmacology of Intralesional Injection Acne Treatment
Intralesional Steroid Injection

Triamcinolone acetonide is a corticosteroid. Corticosteroids decrease inflammation and swelling through suppression of polymorphonuclear leukocytes and reversal of increased capillary permeability. They may also exert vasoconstrictive and antimitotic activity, which may decrease pain. Corticosteroids may reduce scar formation by interfering with oxygen and nutrient delivery to the scar, which inhibits the proliferation of keratinocytes and fibroblasts. Scarring may also be reduced by corticosteroid blockade of alpha-2-microglobulin, a collagenase inhibitor, thereby stimulating digestion of collagen (Fabbrochini et al., 2010).

A 30-gauge needle is used to inject approximately 0.1 mL of a dilute solution of **triamcinolone acetonide** directly into the cavity of the acne lesion. One injection is made into each acne cyst. The injections can be repeated after three weeks (**FIGURE 13-5**).

Nursing Considerations

Injections should not be placed into a site of active skin infection or near a herpes simplex lesion. Corticosteroids may cause a burning sensation for three to five minutes after injection, so the nurse should prepare the patient for this possible discomfort. The nurse should assess for steroid-induced skin changes (e.g., atrophy, telangiectasia, and hypopigmentation) at follow-up visits.

Atopic Dermatitis

Atopic dermatitis (AD; **FIGURE 13-6**) is a common immune-mediated inflammatory skin disorder affecting 8% to 18% of U.S. children younger than 17 years of age (Shaw, Currie, Koudelka, & Simpson, 2011). It is characterized by a pruritic, scaling rash that flares and subsides at intervals. AD is sometimes called "the itch that rashes," as its primary feature is intense pruritus. This condition typically starts in the first year of life, with involvement on the cheeks, chin, and extremities. After the first year, the rash typically transitions to classic involvement of the flexural creases of the arms and legs. AD often improves or resolves as the patient grows older. Because AD is part of an atopic triad that includes asthma and allergic rhinitis, it is important to ask patients and parents whether there is a history of any of these conditions in the patient or family. If there is such a history, AD is more likely.

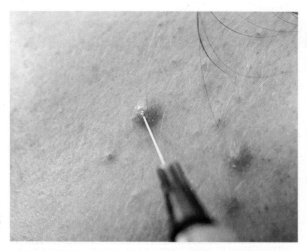

FIGURE 13-5 Intralesional injection.
© Ocskay Bence/Shutterstock, Inc.

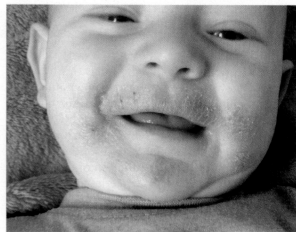

FIGURE 13-6 Infant with atopic dermatitis.
© PHANIE/Science Source.

Typically, treatment begins with a low-potency (Class VI) topical corticosteroid cream twice daily (e.g., **desonide** 0.05%) for the limbs and torso, and an over-the-counter **emollient** ointment for use on the face. If the rash does not improve with the low-potency steroid cream, a medium-potency (Class V) cream or ointment (e.g., **triamcinolone acetonide** 0.1%) will be prescribed for use only on extremities.

Pharmacology of Topical Preparations for AD

Topical corticosteroids are only minimally absorbed when applied to intact, healthy skin. Absorption is increased when the skin is inflamed, such as in AD. Penetration can be increased by increasing the drug concentration, by incorporating the drug into a vehicle that increases its absorption, by occluding the area of application, and by applying the preparation more frequently. Corticosteroids applied to the face, scalp, or genitalia are from 4 to 42 times more potent than when applied to the forearm (Katzung et al., 2012). All of these considerations should be discussed with the patient before use.

Triamcinolone Acetonide

Triamcinolone acetonide is a Class V corticosteroid. Topical corticosteroids are available both as over-the-counter products and as prescription medications. Most are available in generic forms, so often the cost is minimal.

Topical corticosteroids are effective for inflammatory and pruritic conditions. The exact mechanism of anti-inflammatory activity is not clear; however, corticosteroids, in general, may induce phospholipase A_2 inhibitory proteins. These inhibitory proteins target arachidonic acid, the common precursor for inflammatory mediators such as prostaglandins and leukotrienes, thereby controlling mediator biosynthesis. Low-potency steroids are the safest agents for long-term use in the following settings: on large surface areas, on the face or areas of the body with thinner skin, and in children (Rathi & D'Souza, 2012).

Pharmacokinetics

The extent of absorption of **triamcinolone acetonide** is determined by several factors, including concentration, the vehicle, and the integrity of the skin itself. Absorption ranges from approximately 1% in areas of thick stratum corneum (palms, soles, elbows, knees) to 36% in areas with the thinnest skin (genitalia, eyelids, face).

Nursing Considerations

Assess for steroid-related skin changes (e.g., hypopigmentation, atrophy) in areas of chronic AD inflammation. Remind patients to use **triamcinolone acetonide** sparingly for the shortest possible length of time.

Emollient Ointment

Emollients are the first-line topical agents in maintenance treatment for AD. These medications are recommended for restoration of

Myth Buster

Numerous studies have evaluated a variety of dietary, environmental, and alternative approaches to the prevention of AD flare-ups, such as delaying starting solid foods, prolonging breastfeeding, massage therapy, oil of primrose, vitamins, and herbal remedies. Unfortunately, many of these approaches have been shown to be ineffective. Expert opinion supports the use of comfortable fabrics for clothing and bedding, avoidance of known environmental or dietary factors that worsen the rash or itching, avoidance of perfumed soaps and lotions, and avoidance of irritants that worsen skin dryness (Anderson & Dinulos, 2009).

skin barrier function. Emollient vehicles include lotions, creams, and ointments. The exact mechanism for improved barrier function with emollients is not known (Proksch, Brandner, & Jensen, 2008); however, these agents act as moisturizing agents and provide an artificial barrier to transepidermal water loss. No known systemic absorption occurs, but there is substantial penetration into the stratum corneum.

Nursing Considerations

The nurse should evaluate for regular use of emollients after bath and one to two times daily to prevent skin dryness/irritation.

Bacterial Skin Infections

Bacterial skin infections occur when normal flora that reside on the epidermis are able to enter below the surface through breaks in the skin. Such breaks may occur from skin conditions characterized by intense pruritus (such as atopic dermatitis). The vigorous scratching that accompanies such conditions may cause the skin to break (i.e., bleed), allowing the flora (most commonly *Staphylococcus aureus* and various strains of *Streptococcus*), to enter and colonize the affected area. Thus, a former self-limiting skin condition can potentially become much more severe, the most serious of which is the development of bacteremia. In the United States, the most common pathogen to cause skin infections is *methicillin-resistant Staphylococcus aureus* (Dhar, 2018). Bacterial skin infections are treated with oral or topical antibiotics depending on the strain of bacteria causing the infection and the severity of the infection (Chapter 16). Four common bacterial skin infections, *cellulitis, impetigo, boils,* and *folliculitis,* are illustrated in FIGURE 13-7.

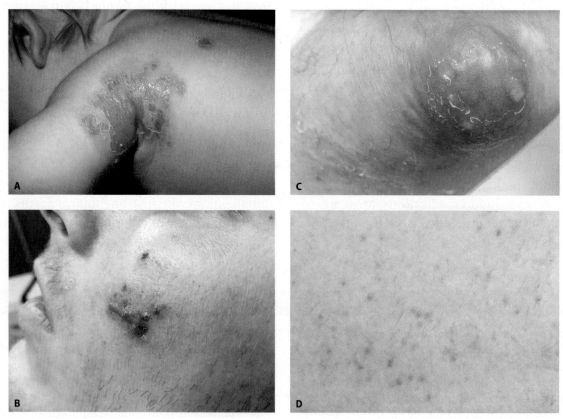

FIGURE 13-7 Bacterial skin rashes.

(A)Courtesy of Allen W. Mathies, MD; (B) © TisforThan/Shutterstock; (C) © andriano.cz/Shutterstock; (D) © Ocskay Mark/Shutterstock

Detailed discussion of bacterial skin infections is beyond the scope of this text; the reader is referred to a more comprehensive dermatology text or resource for further study.

Antifungal Preparations

Superficial fungal infections of the hair, skin, and nails are common human conditions. Essentially, no living tissue is invaded by the fungal organisms; however, a variety of pathological changes may occur in the host because of the presence of the fungus or its metabolic products. The principal fungal organisms include dermatophytes (tinea), a lipophilic yeast (*Malassezia furfur*), and various *Candida* organisms.

Antifungal agents include topical and oral (systemic) preparations. Dermatophytes are fungi that infect hair, skin, and nails, and feed on keratinized nail tissue. Most dermatophytic infections are responsive to topical medications if treatment is started early in the course of the infection; however, once the hair or nails are involved, systemic preparations are required. *Malassezia furfur* and *Candida* infections typically respond well to topical medications; however, if there is treatment failure or if extensive areas are affected, systemic preparations are indicated.

Pharmacology of Common Antifungal Medications
Ketoconazole 2% Cream

Ketoconazole is a drug in the azole class; specifically, it is a synthetic **imidazole**. **Ketoconazole** interferes with fungal biosynthesis of ergosterol via competitive inhibition of fungal cytochrome (CYP) P450 enzyme (**FIGURE 13-8**). A reduction of fungal ergosterol leads to impairment in the integrity of the fungal cell membrane, resulting in increased permeability with loss of essential cell

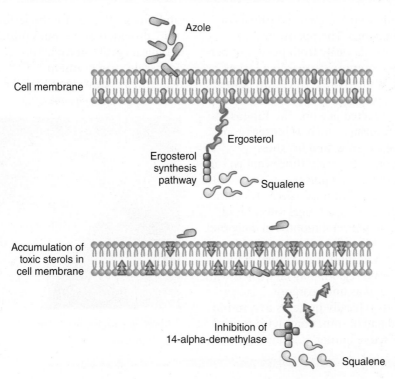

FIGURE 13-8 Diagram of azole antifungal inhibition of ergosterol biosynthesis.

contents. **Ketoconazole** has a strong affinity for keratin in the skin, and it is active against dermatophytes as well as yeast.

Pharmacokinetics

Ketoconazole shows no systemic absorption following topical application unless the affected region is extensive, the skin is broken, or the skin is occluded after application; however, it is well absorbed orally under acid conditions. For this reason, the oral form is not well absorbed in the presence of acid-blocker medications.

Nursing Considerations

The nurse should assess for the location of tinea, as the treatment choice depends on the location of the infection. If the genital region is affected (tinea cruris), instruct the patient not to apply **ketoconazole** near the anus or near other mucous membranes to avoid systemic absorption.

When imidazole derivatives are given orally, they can interfere with the metabolism of other drugs by influencing the cytochrome P450 system (e.g., some statins, **warfarin**, antiepileptic drugs). Use of oral **ketoconazole** with many medications, including inhaled **fluticasone/salmeterol**, will increase plasma concentrations of the substance and, therefore, increase the risk for adverse effects. This interaction typically does not occur with topical **ketoconazole** but should be monitored.

Terbinafine

Terbinafine is both keratophilic (i.e., it targets keratinized tissues such as skin, hair, and nails) and fungicidal. **Terbinafine** interferes with fungal biosynthesis of ergosterol and inhibits the fungal enzyme squalene epoxidase so that squalene, a substance toxic to the fungal organism, is able to accumulate. Similar to **ketoconazole**, **terbinafine** also reduces the ergosterol concentration in the organism, which prevents the synthesis of the fungal cell membrane.

Myth Buster

People often think that "ringworm" (tinea corporis) is not contagious. The opposite is true. Tinea corporis spreads easily from person to person, especially in communal areas like locker rooms and community pools. Tinea can be transmitted even without having skin-to-skin contact with an infected person. The fungus can survive on damp surfaces such as locker room floors, shoes, hats, combs, and brushes.

Tinea infection of the scalp (tinea capitis) can be very difficult to treat, requiring **ketoconazole** shampoo and an oral antifungal agent. Tinea unguium or onychomycosis, a fungal infection of the toenails, requires several months of daily oral antifungal medication rather than a topical formulation for its eradication. Tinea cruris, a fungal infection of the groin region, may be treated with the same medication as tinea corporis.

Tinea corporis typically presents as a round, sharply outlined patch, sometimes with central clearing and an active border of inflammation and pustules. Because the lesions are often pruritic, providers sometimes mistakenly prescribe a topical corticosteroid. This may mask the itching, scale, and erythema; however, the infection will worsen considerably and continue to spread to other people (**FIGURE 13-9**).

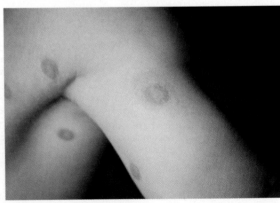

FIGURE 13-9 Ringworm infection.
© Alejandro Rivera/ iStock/ Getty Images

Pharmacokinetics

Terbinafine medication is well absorbed orally and is 40% bioavailable after the first-pass effect. Its half-life is approximately 36 hours at steady state, and it is very slowly eliminated via the skin and adipose tissue.

Nursing Considerations

Assess for preexisting liver disease, as **terbinafine** is hepatotoxic.

CHAPTER SUMMARY

- Dermatologic medications may be delivered through various routes: topical, systemic, and intralesional injection.
- The majority of skin conditions are treated with topical medications; the choice of carrier or vehicle for a topical preparation significantly impacts efficacy.
- When determining route for administration of dermatologic agents, general principles regarding absorption must be considered.
- Superficial fungal infections are a common human malady, which can easily be mistaken for a steroid-responsive or inflammatory condition. When treated with topical steroids, the infection will worsen and become more difficult to identify and treat.

Critical Thinking Questions

1. What problems might a patient encounter with the administration of a topical medication?

2. How does a gel differ from a cream? Under which circumstances might it be better to deliver a drug with one vehicle versus the other?

3. Which changes in skin morphology affect drug absorption in an elderly person? In a person with an inflammatory skin condition?

4. Can you think of a common skin condition for which systemic administration would be superior to topical administration? Why?

5. Intralesional injection is very useful in chronic inflammatory skin conditions such as psoriasis. What might be some barriers for a patient when this form of drug administration is recommended?

6. Which factors might contribute to increased absorption of topical corticosteroids? Why might this be useful or detrimental?

7. Which factors would significantly contraindicate use of isotretinoin in a patient with nodular acne?

CASE STUDIES

Case Scenario 1

A 17-year-old white female, AB, comes to the adolescent clinic very upset and embarrassed about the "zits" on her face. On further questioning, she tells the nurse that she has had this problem for three to four years and has tried many different over-the-counter soaps, creams, and medications, but has seen little improvement. She is currently using either an over-the-counter topical salicylic acid preparation (SalAc) or a benzyl peroxide face wash once daily. The "zits" are now affecting her social life, as AB is afraid to go to social events due to being self-conscious. She currently is not sexually active and is not using any hormone medications such as estrogen/progesterone. She has stopped eating fatty or fried foods and chocolate, as her mother and friends have told her that these items may be causing the problem with her skin. AB is otherwise well. She is allergic to sulfa drugs. She takes no daily medications, vitamins, or supplements.

AB has multiple small open comedones (*blackheads*) and closed comedones (*whiteheads*), and some larger pustules on both cheeks and across her forehead. She has some cysts and scarring. The healthcare provider has graded her acne as moderately severe inflammatory acne. If there were no scarring, the acne would be graded as moderate. Severe acne occurs when nodules, cysts, and scarring are present.

(continues)

CASE STUDIES (CONTINUED)

The provider decides to prescribe both topical and systemic medications for AB. Topical treatment choices include topical retinoids, keratolytics, and antibiotics. Oral choices include antibiotics or isotretinoin. A topical retinoid, tretinoin topical 0.1% once daily at bedtime, was selected. The provider also selected an oral antibiotic, tetracycline 500 mg twice a day for two months, followed by 500 mg once daily for two months. The provider has also discussed intralesional injection of diluted triamcinolone acetonide solution for the acne cysts and scars.

Case Questions

1. What should the nurse tell AB about continuing to use the over-the-counter benzoyl peroxide and salicylic acid preparations?
2. How should AB apply the newly prescribed tretinoin topical 0.1% cream?
3. If the provider prescribed tretinoin 0.025% gel, how would the nurse explain the difference between the cream and gel preparations?
4. Which precautionary information should be provided for AB regarding this medication? What would be the expected results?
5. What are the different tetracycline class medications that could have been prescribed for AB? What are the advantages and disadvantages of selecting any one of these agents?
6. Which precautions should be explained to AB about the use of tetracycline class medications? Are there any interactions that would require AB to take tetracycline separate from food or beverages? Are there any interactions between AB's current medications and tetracycline?
7. If AB were to begin to use any contraceptives, would it be important for her to contact her healthcare provider? Why or why not? If AB suspected she were pregnant, which information should she know about her new medications?
8. At what age could a pediatric patient begin using the topical retinoids or oral tetracycline antibiotics? Why is age important?

CASE STUDIES

Case Scenario 2

CT, a 23-year-old male college student, presents with superficial lesions on his trunk. He recently returned from a summer volunteer experience in a developing country at a sports camp for underprivileged children. Most of the campers come from relatively poor families who do not practice good personal hygiene. As a result, many of them have minor skin and scalp problems. CT's duties at the camp included supervision of swimming classes and other outdoor activities. He also served as the counselor in one of the dormitories in which the children slept and showered.

On examination, CT's vital signs are normal. He has seven distinctive, roughly circular skin lesions on his body. The lesions range from two to eight cm in diameter and have well-demarcated edges. The edges of the lesions are highly inflamed, where there is little or no inflammation in the center of the larger lesions. The borders of the lesions are scaly, slightly raised, and noticeably reddened. The centers of some lesions are hypopigmented. CT states that the lesions first developed about three weeks earlier and have been enlarging steadily since that time. They are quite itchy, but not overtly painful, and only

CASE STUDIES (CONTINUED)

the superficial layer of the skin is involved. The healthcare provider diagnoses CT's skin lesions as tinea corporis, commonly called ringworm due to the raised border of the lesions that appear as if a worm were burrowing under the skin. CT likely contracted the fungal infection from the children at summer camp. CT has a history of persistent asthma for which he takes inhaled fluticasone/salmeterol, two puffs twice a day.

The provider decides to prescribe topical ketoconazole 2% cream applied twice a day for two weeks. After three weeks, CT returns to the provider with no significant improvement in the lesions. Systemic therapy is initiated with terbinafine 250 mg daily for four weeks, which results in complete resolution of the lesions.

Case Questions

1. What is the pharmacologic basis for using the prescribed agents?
2. What should the nurse tell CT about interactions between fluticasone/salmeterol and ketoconazole?
3. For how long after starting the ketoconazole will CT be contagious?
4. CT wants to know if he should continue to use the topical cream even after starting the oral terbinafine. What should the nurse tell him?

CASE STUDIES

Case Scenario 3

KW, a five-month-old girl, presents to the pediatric clinic for her routine well-child exam. KW's mother is concerned about intermittent rashes that seem to be bothersome to her child. She states that the rashes started a few weeks ago, were initially present on her cheeks and around her mouth, and have now appeared on her elbows and knees. There is no rash in her diaper area. Although KW is not able to scratch the affected areas, when the rashes are worse, KW is more irritable. KW's mother has applied various "baby" lotions and does not believe they are helping. She denies other family members being affected by any itchy rashes, and KW does not attend a daycare program. Other than having a rash, KW is healthy and meeting developmental milestones. Her father has a history of seasonal allergies, and her mother had "childhood asthma."

KW is attentive and smiling as her vital signs are checked and found to be within normal limits. Skin assessment reveals symmetric, brightly erythematous, scaling, pink patches on her cheeks and similar, although milder, patches on her knees and elbows. KW's healthcare provider diagnoses this patient with AD, commonly known as eczema, and prescribes hydrocortisone 0.5% ointment (in white petrolatum and mineral oil), to be applied twice daily. A follow-up visit to assess KW's response to the topical corticosteroid is scheduled for four weeks.

Case Questions

1. What is the pharmacologic basis for using the prescribed agents in the particular vehicle?
2. What should the nurse tell KW's mother about the reason why she should not use the steroid cream on KW's face?

(continues)

CASE STUDIES (CONTINUED)

3. KW's mother asks if generic "baby lotion" is one of the emollient creams that are recommended for use on her baby's face. How should the nurse respond?

4. How often and on which occasions should KW's parents apply the emollient cream?

5. What are some signs that would indicate that the parent should stop applying the steroid cream and return to the clinic?

6. KW's mother has been exclusively breastfeeding up to this point, but she planned to introduce solid foods this month. Now she wonders if solid foods will make KW's rash worse. How should the nurse respond to this question?

REFERENCES

Anderson, P.C., & Dinulos, J.G. (2009). Atopic dermatitis and alternative management strategies. *Current Opinion in Pediatrics*, *21*(1), 131–138.

Bozzo, P., Chua-Gocheco A., & Einarson, A. (2011). Safety of skin care products during pregnancy. *Canadian Family Physician*, *57*(6), 665–667.

Bremner, J.D., Shearer, K., & McCaffery, P. (2012). Retinoic acid and affective disorders: The evidence for an association. *Journal of Clinical Psychiatry*, *73*(1), 37–50.

Çinar, L., Kartal, D., Ergin, C., Aksoy, H., Karadag, M.A., Aydin, T., . . . Borlu, M. (2016). The effect of systemic isotretinoin on male fertility. *Cutaneous and Ocular Toxicology*, *35*(4), 296–299. doi: 10.3109/15569527.2015.1119839

Dellavalle, R.P., & Dawson, A.L. (2013). Acne vulgaris. *BMJ*, *346*, f2634 doi: 10.1136/bmj.f2634

Dhar, A.D. (2018). Overview of bacterial skin infections. *Merck manual, professional version*. Kenilworth, NJ: Merck & Co., Inc. Retrieved from https://www.merckmanuals.com/professional /dermatologic-disorders/bacterial-skin-infections /overview-of-bacterial-skin-infections

Dutil, M. (2010). Benzoyl peroxide: Enhancing antibiotic efficacy in acne management. *Skin Therapy Letter*, *15*(10), 5–7. Retrieved from http://www.skintherapy letter.com/2010/15.10/2.html

Fabbrochini, G., Annunziata, M.C., DeArco, V., DeVita, V., Lodi, G., Mauriello, M.C., . . . Monfrecola, G. (2010). Acne scars: Pathogenesis, classification and treatment. *Dermatology Research and Practice*, 893080. doi: 10.1155/2010/893080

iPledge. (n.d.). Home page. Retrieved from https:// www.ipledgeprogram.com/iPledgeUI/home.u

Katzung, B.G., Masters, S.B., & Trevor, A.J. (2012). *Basic and clinical pharmacology* (12th ed.). New York, NY: McGraw-Hill/Lange.

Kaur, J., Sehgal, V.K., Gupta, A.K., & Singh, S.P. (2015). A comparative study to evaluate the efficacy and safety of combination topical preparations in acne vulgaris. *International Journal of Applied and Basic Medical Research*, *5*(2), 106–110. http://doi.org /10.4103/2229-516X.157155

Kraft, J., & Freiman, A. (2011). Management of acne. *CMAJ*, *183*(7), E430–E435. doi: 10.1503 /cmaj.090374

Lei, K.W., & Mercurio, M.G. (2009). Update on the treatment of acne vulgaris. *Journal of Clinical Outcomes Management*, *16*(3), 115–126. Retrieved from http://www.turnerwhite.com/pdf/jcom _mar09_acne.pdf

McKoy, K. (2008). Acne vulgaris. *Merck manual, professional version*. Retrieved from http://www.merck manuals.com/professional/dermatologic_disorders /acne_and_related_disorders/acne_vulgaris.html

Mehta, R. (2004). Topical and transdermal drug delivery: What a pharmacist needs to know. Retrieved from http://www.transderma.com/wp-content/ uploads/2017/07/146-000-01-008-H01.pdf

Millikan, L.E. (2003). The rationale for using a topical retinoid for inflammatory acne. *American Journal of Clinical Dermatology*, *4*(2), 75.

Niser, M.S., Iyer, K., Brodell, R.T., Lloyd, J.R., Shin, T.M., & Ahmad, A. (2013). Minocycline-induced hyperpigmentation: Comparison of 3 Q-switched lasers to reverse its effects. *Clinical, Cosmetic and Investigational Dermatology*, *6*, 159–162.

Proksch, E., Brandner, J.M., & Jensen, J.M. (2008). The skin: An indispensable barrier. *Experimental Dermatology*, *17*(12), 1063–1072. doi: 10.1111/j.1600-0625.2008.00786.x

Rathi, S.K., & D'Souza, P. (2012). Rational and ethical use of topical corticosteroids based on safety and efficacy. *Indian Journal of Dermatology*, *57*(4), 251–259.

Shaw, T.E., Currie, G.P., Koudelka, C.W., & Simpson, E.L. (2011). Eczema prevalence in the United States: Data from the 2003 National Survey of Children's Health. *Journal of Investigative Dermatology*, *131*(1), 67–73.

Story, L. (2012). *Pathophysiology: A practical approach*. Sudbury, MA: Jones & Bartlett.

Zaenglein, A.L., Pathy, A.L., Schlosser, B.J., Alikhan, A., Baldwin, H.E., Berson, D.S., . . . Bhushan, R. (2016). Guidelines of care for the management of acne vulgaris. *Journal of the American Academy of Dermatology*, *74*(5), 945–973.

CHAPTER 14

Pharmacology of Psychotropic Medications

Christopher Footit

KEY TERMS

Acute dystonia
Agranulocytosis
Akathisia
Antihypertensive
Antipsychotics
Anxiety
Ataxia
Atypical antipsychotics
Auditory hallucinations
Barbiturates
Benzodiazepines
Bipolar disorder
Bradykinesia
Cognitive symptoms
Comorbid
Delusional disorders
Delusions
Dependence
Depression

Diaphoresis
Distorted thinking
Dyssomnias
Extrapyramidal symptoms
 (EPS)
Generalized anxiety disorder
Huntington's chorea
Hypertensive crisis
Hyponatremia
Involuntary movements
Mania
Mesolimbic
Metabolic syndrome
Monoamine oxidase inhibitor
 (MAOI)
Mood stabilizers
Motor tics
Negative symptoms

Neuroleptic malignant
 syndrome
Neuropathic pain
Neurotransmission
Obsessive-compulsive
 disorder
Orthostatic hypotension
Palsy
Panic disorder
Paranoia
Parasomnias
Parkinsonian symptoms
Phobic disorders
Positive symptoms
Post-traumatic stress disorder
Prolactin
Psychosis
Psychotropic drugs
Relapse

Remission
Schizophrenia
Selective serotonin reuptake
 inhibitor (SSRI)
Serotonin/norepinephrine
 reuptake inhibitor (SNRI)
Serotonin reuptake pump
Serotonin syndrome
Synaptic space
Tardive dyskinesia (TD)
Tolerance
Tourette syndrome
Treatment-resistant
Tricyclic antidepressant (TCA)
Typical antipsychotics
Tyramine
Visual hallucinations
Withdrawal

CHAPTER OBJECTIVES

At the end of the chapter, the student will be able to:

1. Distinguish between first- and second-generation antipsychotics.

2. Identify key side effects of first- and second-generation antipsychotics.

3. Differentiate the five principal classes of antidepressants and anxiolytics.

Introduction

Psychiatry and the eventual use of psychotropic medication have a long history in Europe and the United States. In 1841 a study of 13 asylums in Europe was conducted to ascertain statistics on the causes, duration, termination, and moral treatment of insanity in Europe and the United States. In 1847 another study involved the construction of government lunatic asylums in hospitals for the insane in London. During the 19th century, asylum doctors and general practitioners wrote texts and papers on "madness," a term that increasingly evolved into *psychiatric*. They began to differentiate the "mind" from the body and to initiate the task of classifying psychiatric illnesses and distinguishing one from another.

In the modern era, the American Psychiatric Association (APA) recognizes more than 400 distinct disorders, as described in the *Diagnostic and Statistical Manual of Mental Disorders, Fifth Edition* (*DSM-5*). This manual undergoes periodic revisions as research develops a more advanced understanding of these conditions.

Psychotropic drugs gained an important role in psychiatry during the mid-20th century. Scientific research into neurology and pharmacology led the way for the development of generations of psychotropic medications. The development and use of psychotropic medications came about as a result of teamwork among the pharmaceutical industry, federal and state governments, and clinical practice and theory. Eventually shifts in social and ethical issues, medical education, and popular culture began to alter the perception of the treatment of mental illness.

Some basic classes of mental illness include the following:

- Organic disorders, in which physical damage to the brain leads to a suite of symptoms such as dementia, motor dysfunction, and hallucinations (e.g., Alzheimer disease, Creutzfeldt-Jakob disease)
- **Delusional disorders**, such as schizophrenia and other psychoses
- Mood (affective) disorders, such as bipolar disorder or depression
- Anxiety disorders, including panic disorders, post-traumatic stress disorder, and phobias
- Behavioral syndromes with physiological disturbances, including eating disorders, some forms of sexual dysfunction, and postpartum depression
- Personality disorders, including obsessive–compulsive personality disorder, pathological gambling, and narcissistic disorder
- Behavioral disorders with childhood onset, including attention-deficit/hyperactivity disorder (ADHD), tic disorders, and conduct disorders
- Developmental disorders, including dyslexia, autism, and learning disabilities

Many of these conditions arise from imbalances in brain chemistry, most specifically from excessive or inadequate levels of specific neurotransmitters, such as dopamine, serotonin, and norepinephrine, among others. Such imbalances are typically treated with medication. Other mental illnesses may arise from disorders of nerve signaling. Although this chapter cannot look comprehensively at the medications used for all disorders, it will examine the pharmacology of key classes of medications for major forms of psychiatric illness.

Delusional Disorders (Psychoses): Schizophrenia and Antipsychotic Medications

According to the World Health Organization (WHO, n.d.), **schizophrenia** affects approximately 24 million people worldwide. Schizophrenia is a treatable disorder, although treatment may be more effective in its early stages. It strikes mostly individuals between the ages of 15 and 35. More than half of affected persons do not receive appropriate care even though the cost of treatment can be as little as $2 per month. The earlier the treatment is initiated, the more effective it will be.

The symptoms of schizophrenia can be divided into three distinct categories: positive symptoms, negative symptoms, and cognitive symptoms:

- **Positive symptoms** include **distorted thinking. Paranoia**, **auditory hallucinations**, **visual hallucinations**, and **delusions** may be present.
- **Negative symptoms** include poor insight and judgment, lack of self-care, emotional and social withdrawal, apathy, agitation, blunted affect, and poverty of speech.
- **Cognitive symptoms** include difficulties with the ability to pay attention and to focus, as well as the presence of significant learning and memory problems and disordered thinking.

Antipsychotic Medications

Antipsychotic medications were introduced in the 1950s, essentially revolutionizing the management of psychoses, ending an era of institutional care, and beginning the treatment of schizophrenic persons in the community setting. The **antipsychotic** medications are grouped as a class of drugs used to treat a broad range of disorders including schizophrenia, psychoses, delusional disorders, bipolar disorder, and depression. In addition, antipsychotics are used to treat emesis, **Tourette syndrome**, and **Huntington's chorea**. Antipsychotic medications are classified as either first-generation antipsychotics (FGAs), sometimes called **typical antipsychotics**, or second-generation antipsychotics (SGAs), otherwise known as **atypical antipsychotics**.

Antipsychotic medications do not cure schizophrenia or other psychotic disorders, but rather offer partial or complete relief of symptoms. The length of treatment depends on whether the patient is experiencing his or her first psychotic episode or a subsequent episode. The first episode should be treated for at least one year. Subsequent episodes may require lifelong maintenance.

First-Generation Antipsychotics (FGAs)

FGAs were initially developed for controlling the symptoms of nausea and vomiting associated with cancer chemotherapy and gastroenteritis. **Chloroperazine** and **perphenazine** are still in use today for this purpose.

FGAs work primarily by blocking dopamine-2 (D_2) receptors in the **mesolimbic** area of the brain (TABLE 14-1). They also block the acetylcholine, histamine (H_1), and norepinephrine receptors thereby reducing the positive symptoms of **psychosis** as well as reducing agitation and hyperactive behavior. Additional actions include blockade of some muscarinic and alpha-1 adrenergic receptors in the brain.

The FGAs' action reduces the positive symptoms associated with acute psychosis, such as auditory and visual hallucinations and delusions. These medications are less effective for treating the negative symptoms such as emotional and social withdrawal and blunted affect. Psychotic symptoms can improve as soon as one week after FGA administration is begun and may continue to improve over the succeeding four to six weeks.

TABLE 14-1	First-Generation Antipsychotic Medications (FGAs)	
Generic Name	Drug Class	Notes
Chlorpromazine	Phenothiazine	
Haloperidol	Antiemetic/ antipsychotic	
Perphenazine	Phenothiazine	Brand-name products are currently sold only as combinations of perphenazine and amitriptyline. Perphenazine without amitriptyline is available only as a generic.
Trifluoperazine	Phenothiazine	

Data from Youdim, Moussa & Edmondson, Dale & F Tipton, Keith. (2006). The therapeutic potential of monoamine oxidase inhibitors. Nature reviews. Neuroscience. 7. 295-309. 10.1038/nrn1883. Retrieved from https://www.researchgate.net/figure/7227442_fig1 _Figure-5-The-mechanism-of-potentiation-of-cardiovascular-effects-of-tyramine-the.

FGAs can also be used to treat episodes of acute bipolar mania (discussed later in this chapter), but only until control of the symptoms is gained. After control is attained, a mood stabilizer or atypical antipsychotic (second-generation antipsychotic, SGA) should be employed for ongoing treatment. FGAs are also indicated for use with Tourette syndrome, a disease not associated with schizophrenia or bipolar disorder. They can be effective for control of **motor tics**, uncontrolled use of obscene language, and other symptoms related to this disorder.

Nursing Considerations

First-generation antipsychotics are indicated for use with Tourette syndrome. FGAs can help control motor tics, uncontrolled use of obscene language, and other Tourette symptoms.

Adverse Reactions

The blocking of D_2, acetylcholine, H_1, norepinephrine, muscarinic, and alpha$_1$-adrenergic receptors in multiple areas of the brain leads to the medications' benefits. Unfortunately, it can also lead to common, potentially troubling, and dangerous side effects.

Extrapyramidal symptoms (EPS) include **acute dystonia**, a syndrome of abnormal muscle contractions that produces repetitive involuntary twisting movements and abnormal posturing of the neck, trunk, face, and extremities; **Parkinsonian symptoms**, which are dopamine-mediated, characterized by rhythmic muscular tremors, rigidity of movement, and droopy posture; and mask-like facies, characterized by an immobile, expressionless face with staring eyes and slightly open mouth. Other types of EPS include shaking **palsy**; trembling palsy; **akathisia**, which is characterized by unpleasant sensations of "inner" restlessness that manifest as an inability to sit still or remain motionless; and **tardive dyskinesia (TD)**, the involuntary movement of the facial muscles and tongue. The shaking palsy, akathisia,

and TD can progress to the limbs, hands, feet, and trunk.

Acute dystonia can have an onset within a few hours of the initial drug administration. Its features include spasms of the muscles of the tongue, face, neck, throat, and back. This is a crisis that requires the addition of anticholinergic agents such as **benztropine**, which works by blocking acetylcholine, to counter dopamine blockade effects, to relieve the crisis.

Parkinsonian symptoms can begin 5 to 30 days after drug therapy is started. Their features include **bradykinesia**, which presents as slow movement and muscle rigidity. In addition, mask-like facies, tremors, rigidity, shuffling gait, drooling, and stooped posture may be present. Again, the use of anticholinergic agents is the treatment of choice.

Onset of akathisia can occur between 5 and 60 days after FGAs are started. Its features include restless movement and symptoms of anxiety and agitation. Drugs used to treat symptoms of akathisia include benzodiazepines, beta blockers, and anticholinergics.

TD can have an onset of months to years and is related to drug dose and duration of treatment. TD is often persistent and can develop as a late complication of antipsychotic therapy; thus it is more likely to be seen with long-term use of typical antipsychotic agents. In many cases, this condition is irreversible. Symptoms include **involuntary movements** of the tongue, mouth, and face. There is no reliable treatment for TD, but the use of benzodiazepines and reduction of dosage of the FGAs can be beneficial.

Other dangerous dopaminergic-mediated adverse effects that can occur with the use of FGAs include **neuroleptic malignant syndrome**, which is characterized by high fever, stiffness of the muscles, altered mental status (paranoid behavior), wide swings of blood pressure, excessive sweating, and excessive secretion of saliva. Blockade of the hypothalamic D_2 receptors by FGAs creates an elevated temperature set point and impairs cutaneous vasodilation, sweating, and other mechanisms for dissipating heat. Other, less severe adverse effects related to FGA use include anticholinergic effects, **orthostatic hypotension**, sedation, and cardiac arrhythmias. The cardiac arrhythmias can manifest as prolongation of the QT interval as measured by an electrocardiogram.

Drug-Drug Interactions

Because of the inherent central nervous system (CNS) depression associated with FGAs, care should be taken when combining FGAs with alcohol due to the potential for excessive CNS depression. Caution should also be used when combining these agents with medications that affect the FGAs' anticholinergic actions, with other CNS depressants, and with medications that activate dopamine receptors (such as **levodopa**) because these medications would directly oppose the actions of the FGAs. Other medications that can interact with antipsychotics include the **selective serotonin reuptake inhibitors (SSRIs) paroxetine**, **fluoxetine, carbamazepine**, and **fluvoxamine**. These drugs can cause an increase in serotonin levels and increase the risk of serotonin syndrome because both FGAs and SSRIs inhibit the reuptake of serotonin; thus, using them together can lead to a synergistic effect on serotonin levels.

The combination of FGAs with **carbamazepine** can cause an increased risk of CNS depression, cardiac arrhythmias, and **hyponatremia**. When FGAs are combined with **antihypertensive** agents, there is an increased risk of hypotension and changes in cardiac rhythms due to blockade of alpha$_1$-adrenergic receptors.

Prescribing Considerations

FGAs are considerably less expensive than SGAs. Patients with an inadequate response to SGAs may respond to FGAs. Weight gain, which may or may not be desirable, occurs more frequently with SGAs and tends to be minimal with FGAs. FGAs and SGAs are available in injectable depot formulations, which offer the benefits of long duration of effect (Llorca et al., 2013). No adequate or well-controlled human studies have been done regarding teratogenic effects of FGAs; however, potential benefits may outweigh potential risks. Pregnant women should be counseled per the Pregnancy and Lactation Labeling Rule (PLLR).

Second-Generation Antipsychotics

SGAs (TABLE 14-2) are commonly referred to as "atypicals" because they generally do not cause the same degree of kinesthetic side effects observed with the "typical" (FGA) antipsychotic medications. Most work by blocking dopamine-D$_2$ receptors as well as strongly blocking multiple serotonin receptors. In addition, norepinephrine, acetylcholine, alpha$_1$-adrenergic and, to a lesser extent, histamine and muscarinic receptors in the brain are blocked by SGAs. Although much is understood about how the various neurotransmitters are affected by the SGAs, little is known about why these changes in brain chemistry have a positive outcome in terms of controlling the symptoms of schizophrenia.

The SGAs have been more commonly used than the FGAs since the 1990s. Whereas the FGAs help control the auditory and visual hallucinations and delusions as well as reduce the emotional and social withdrawal, the SGAs reduce both positive and negative symptoms associated with schizophrenia. Efficacy of the medication cannot be accurately determined for at least 4 to 6 weeks, and negative symptoms may require 16 to 20 weeks to show a beneficial response (Lehne, 2015). Duration of treatment is similar to that with FGAs. SGAs can also be used to treat acute mania and bipolar depression, for maintenance of bipolar disorder, and to treat behavioral disorders and disorders associated with impulse control and agitation.

Adverse Reactions

The blockade of D$_2$ receptors and alpha$_1$-adrenergic receptors, and to a lesser extent

TABLE 14-2	Second-Generation Antipsychotic Medications	
Generic Name	Drug Class	Notes
Aripiprazole	Partial dopamine agonist (atypical antipsychotic) with 5-HT$_{2A}$ antagonism	Also used in treating bipolar disorder, depression, and autism-related irritability
Asenapine	Atypical antipsychotic, Dopamine antagonist with 5-HT$_{2A}$ antagonism	Also used in treating bipolar disorder
Clozapine	Benzodiazepine (atypical antipsychotic)	Carries "black box" warnings for agranulocytosis, seizures, myocarditis, unspecified respiratory/cardiovascular effects, and increased mortality in elderly patients with dementia
Iloperidone	Dopamine antagonist	Only used for treatment of schizophrenia
Lurasidone	Dopamine antagonist	Also used for treatment of bipolar disorder
Olanzapine	Thienobenzodiazepine, Dopamine and 5-HT$_2$ antagonist (atypical antipsychotic)	Principal side effects are weight gain and metabolic effects (e.g., hyperglycemia or diabetes)
Paliperidone	Dopamine antagonist (atypical antipsychotic)	Also used in treating bipolar disorder and schizoaffective disorder
Quetiapine	Atypical antipsychotic	Also used in treating bipolar disorder, psychosis related to Parkinson disease, and, in concert with other medications, major depressive disorder
Risperidone	Dopamine antagonist (atypical antipsychotic)	Also used in treating bipolar disorder, schizoaffective disorder, and autism-related irritability
Ziprasidone	Dopamine/serotonin antagonist with 5-HT$_{2A}$ antagonism (atypical antipsychotic)	Also used in treating bipolar disorder

H$_1$ and muscarinic receptors, can cause significant side effects. Common side effects of atypical antipsychotics include dizziness, sedation, and hypotension, all of which can be associated with blockade of alpha$_1$-adrenergic receptors. More serious side effects include an increased risk of **metabolic syndrome**. Features of this syndrome include weight gain for which the mechanism is unknown. As a result of the weight gain, there is a concomitant increase in incidence of diabetes and dyslipidemia. SGAs are also associated with an increased risk of dangerous arrhythmias and elevated **prolactin** levels due to their blocking of D$_2$ receptors in the pituitary. **Clozapine** has been associated with an increased risk of **agranulocytosis** and is considered a drug of last resort for this reason; however, it also has been shown to reduce suicidality in schizophrenia and may be used with caution to help reduce this risk. When compared to FGAs, SGAs have a significantly lower risk for EPS and TD.

What's in a Name? FGAs Versus SGAs

Going by the classification alone, it is tempting to think of "first-generation" antipsychotics as being older, and possibly less effective, formulations. While it may be true that some of these drugs preceded the development of second-generation antipsychotics, the presumed difference in efficacy does not exist. In fact, second-generation antipsychotic drugs are not derived from the first-generation medications at all. They are a completely different set of medications with completely different mechanisms of action, and whether they are more or less effective for a patient's condition depends on the patient. A 2009 meta-analysis of first- versus second-generation antipsychotics noted that selection should depend on efficacy, side effects, and cost (Leucht et al., 2009). The results of this review are similar in some respects to another recent systematic review of SGAs versus FGAs, although the 2009 Leucht et al. review is broader in scope in terms of medications included, patient populations, and outcomes.

Drug-Drug Interactions

In general, caution should be used when combining SGAs with medications that increase the risk of CNS depression, such as antihistamines and over-the-counter sleep aids. CNS depressants such as alcohol and benzodiazepines should be used with caution or avoided altogether for the same reason. **Levodopa** may adversely affect SGAs through D_2-receptor agonism, a mechanism that opposes the desired D_2 blockade.

The combination of **clozapine** with an SSRI can also increase the risk of serotonin syndrome. Neuroleptic malignant syndrome is another possible serious adverse reaction when combining SGAs or using them in combination with SSRIs or a similar class of medications, the **serotonin/norepinephrine reuptake inhibitors (SNRIs)**.

Prescribing Considerations

All antipsychotic agents should be prescribed at the lowest possible effective dose to reduce the possibility of side effects. Injectable depot formulations offer the benefits of long-acting efficacy, and in some situations may be preferable to orally administered versions (Llorca et al., 2013). These formulations should be considered if a patient has memory problems and forgets to take the medication, or if the patient is considered to be at a great risk of doing harm to self or others if nonadherent with taking the medication by mouth.

Choice of SGAs can be made according to side effects. Some patients may benefit from the sedating effect of SGAs, whereas others may benefit from the activating effects. In some cases, weight gain may be beneficial for those patients who have a low body mass index. Patients receiving SGAs should always be closely monitored for signs and symptoms of metabolic syndrome.

Depression and Anxiety

The *DSM-5* describes major depressive disorder as a common mental disorder that presents with a depressed mood, loss of interest in daily activities, lack of pleasure, feelings of guilt or low self-worth, disturbed sleep or appetite, low energy and poor concentration, and possibly, suicidal thoughts. **Depression** can lead to substantial impairments in an individual's ability to take care of his or her everyday responsibilities. WHO estimates depression affects more than 300 million people worldwide and is among the leading causes of disability (WHO, 2017).

It is hypothesized that depression is caused by deficiencies in the monoamine neurotransmitters, norepinephrine, dopamine, and serotonin, at CNS receptors. Therefore, the focus of pharmacologic treatment is to increase the concentrations/levels of these neurotransmitters. In general, all antidepressants boost the synaptic action of one or more of these neurotransmitters, in most cases by blocking the presynaptic transporters, which normally act to decrease, or recycle, the neurotransmitter (FIGURE 14-1).

The National Institute of Mental Health (2012) describes **anxiety** as a normal reaction to stress that in some situations can be beneficial. However, in approximately 18% of adults in the United States, anxiety can become excessive—and in nearly one-fourth of these persons, anxiety can become so severe that it negatively affects day-to-day living. This condition is characterized by worry, fear, muscle tension, irritability, sleep changes, arousal, fatigue, breathing changes, and concentration difficulties.

Anxiety triggers the endocrine system connected to the amygdala and the hypothalamus to increase the levels of the adrenal hormone cortisol. The autonomic nervous system is also triggered, which causes the fight-or-flight response. Chronic increases in cortisol can lead to coronary disease, type 2 diabetes, and stroke.

Anxiety disorders can be divided into six major classes: **generalized anxiety disorder**, **panic disorder**, **obsessive–compulsive disorder**, **phobic disorders**, **post-traumatic stress disorder**, and **acute stress disorder**.

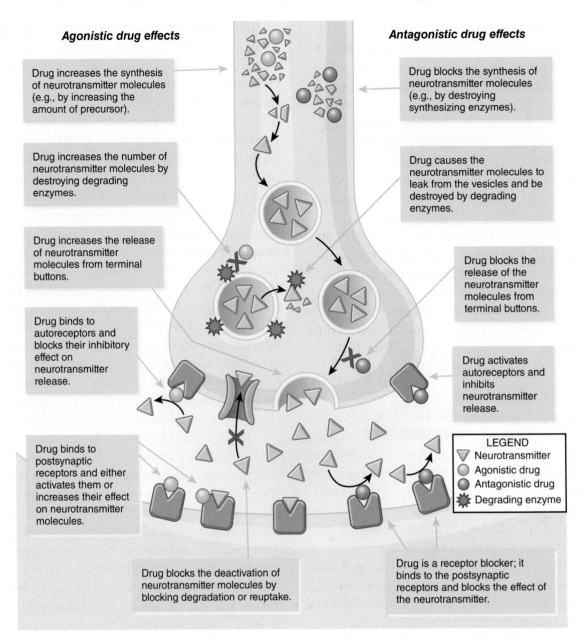

Agonistic drug effects

Drug increases the synthesis of neurotransmitter molecules (e.g., by increasing the amount of precursor).

Drug increases the number of neurotransmitter molecules by destroying degrading enzymes.

Drug increases the release of neurotransmitter molecules from terminal buttons.

Drug binds to autoreceptors and blocks their inhibitory effect on neurotransmitter release.

Drug binds to postsynaptic receptors and either activates them or increases their effect on neurotransmitter molecules.

Antagonistic drug effects

Drug blocks the synthesis of neurotransmitter molecules (e.g., by destroying synthesizing enzymes).

Drug causes the neurotransmitter molecules to leak from the vesicles and be destroyed by degrading enzymes.

Drug blocks the release of the neurotransmitter molecules from terminal buttons.

Drug activates autoreceptors and inhibits neurotransmitter release.

LEGEND
▽ Neurotransmitter
○ Agonistic drug
● Antagonistic drug
✳ Degrading enzyme

Drug blocks the deactivation of neurotransmitter molecules by blocking degradation or reuptake.

Drug is a receptor blocker; it binds to the postsynaptic receptors and blocks the effect of the neurotransmitter.

FIGURE 14-1 Neuronal junction, with receptors and reuptake for various neurotransmitters, and sites for drug actions.

Use of medications is one of the modalities for treatment of depression and anxiety. The four major types of antidepressant medications are **tricyclic antidepressants (TCAs)**, SSRIs, SNRIs, and **monoamine oxidase inhibitors (MAOIs)**. In general, anxiety responds well to **benzodiazepines** and/or SSRIs or SNRIs.

Depression and anxiety are often **comorbid** conditions. They share many symptoms in common, making it difficult to separate the diagnoses in many cases. The psychopharmacologic treatments for both depression and anxiety are often similar as well. The antidepressant medications will be addressed first, followed by anxiolytic (antianxiety) medications. The section on SSRIs/SNRIs considers both antidepressant and anxiolytic indications. At the end of the section, the discussion turns to the benzodiazepines and **buspirone**, which are used to treat anxiety disorders.

Psychotherapy should always be considered before initiating antidepressant and anxiolytic medications. As noted when discussing the adverse reactions for each drug class, whenever antidepressant medications are prescribed for and used by a patient, that individual should routinely be evaluated for the emergence of suicidal thoughts, particularly if the patient is a young adult (younger than 25 years) or an adolescent (Gibbons et al., 2015; Hawthorne, 2017; Hussain, Dubicka, & Wilkinson, 2017).

Nursing Considerations

Adolescents and young adults using antidepressant medications should be routinely evaluated for the emergence of suicidal thoughts.

Serotonin Syndrome

Of special note is the drug reaction called **serotonin syndrome**, a disorder that can develop with the use of any medication that prevents the reuptake of serotonin. It develops when suppression of serotonin reuptake causes an excess concentration of serotonin in the brain stem and spinal cord. Symptoms include alterations in mental status and coordination, **diaphoresis** (excessive sweating), tremor, rapid heartbeat, muscle spasms, blood pressure fluctuations, and fever. The condition can be fatal owing to a potentially lethal combination of side effects, including hyperthermia, seizures, coma, and brain damage. Yet it is a condition that is easily overlooked, as initial symptoms (e.g., agitation) sometimes mimic the signs associated with activity of SSRIs and other antidepressants.

Clinicians using any of the medications described in this section, as well as any other medications that increase serotonin levels (many of which are not considered psychoactive drugs), should be aware of the signs of serotonin syndrome and educate their patients to respond proactively should they occur; that is, in the context of a high fever, the patient should go to a hospital or physician for treatment rather than attempt to self-treat, even if the patient believes that the fever may be related to an infection. Notably, in a study of physician overrides of drug–drug interaction alerts, slightly more than one in five of the overrides deemed inappropriate by the reviewers involved an interaction between an antidepressant and another drug that put the patient at risk of serotonin syndrome (Slight et al., 2013); it is likely that the clinicians were unaware of the pharmacology behind the warning, because physician awareness of serotonin syndrome is low (Arora & Kannikeswaran, 2010; Spies, Pot, Willems, Box, & Kramers, 2016).

Serotonin syndrome can occur because of drug–drug interactions and, in some instances, drug–food interactions. The risk of this syndrome developing due to consumption of foods rich in **tyramine**, such as aged cheeses, is one reason that MAOIs—otherwise highly effective medications—are now considered drugs of last resort.

Care must also be taken when switching patients from one class of antidepressant medication to another, as many of these medications have long half-lives and can produce residual effects that could potentially lead to serotonin syndrome, even in patients who have not taken the medication for several weeks.

Medications with Potential to Cause Serotonin Syndrome*

Drug Classification	Specific Agent Reported
Analgesics	Tramadol, meperidine, fentanyl; opioids
Anti-Parkinson agents	Selegiline, L-dopa
Antibiotics	Linezolid
Anticonvulsants	Carbamazepine
Antidepressant/ antianxiety	All agents in the SSRI, SNRI, TCA, and MAOI classes; buspirone, St. John's wort
Antiemetic	Ondansetron, metoclopramide
Antihistamine	Chlorpheniramine
Antimigraine agents (triptans)	All agents have potential for interaction; specific case examples are limited and disputed
Antipsychotics	Mirtazapine, olanzapine, risperidone, phenelzine, quetiapine
Cough suppressant	Dextromethorphan (found in many OTC medications)
Muscle relaxant	Cyclobenzaprine

*List is not comprehensive.

Monoamine Oxidase Inhibitors

As the name indicates, monoamine oxidase inhibitors (MAOIs) block the action of monoamine oxidase (MAO), which is the enzyme that degrades the neurotransmitters norepinephrine, serotonin, dopamine, epinephrine, and tyramine and makes these neurotransmitters less available in the brain (**FIGURE 14-2**). It is theorized that by blocking MAO, MAOIs increase the availability of norepinephrine, serotonin, and dopamine (D_2) **neurotransmission** in the brain, which in turn provides a powerful antidepressant effect (**TABLE 14-3**). Conversely, withdrawing MAOIs decreases availability of norepinephrine, serotonin, and dopamine and so may cause "depressive" symptoms (Kosinski & Rothschild, 2012).

MAOIs are indicated for depression, treatment-resistant depression, treatment-resistant panic disorder, and treatment-resistant social anxiety disorder (Flockhart, 2012). **Treatment-resistant** refers to those disorders that do not respond to, or only partially respond to, multiple trials of medications, and continue to be problematic. The onset of action of MAOIs often is delayed by two to four weeks, and a dosage increase may be required if the medication is not helpful by six to eight weeks. The goal of treatment is symptom **remission** as well as **relapse** prevention. Symptoms of depression may recur after the medication is stopped.

Adverse Reactions

Side effects of MAOIs include symptoms of **CNS stimulation**, such as anxiety, insomnia,

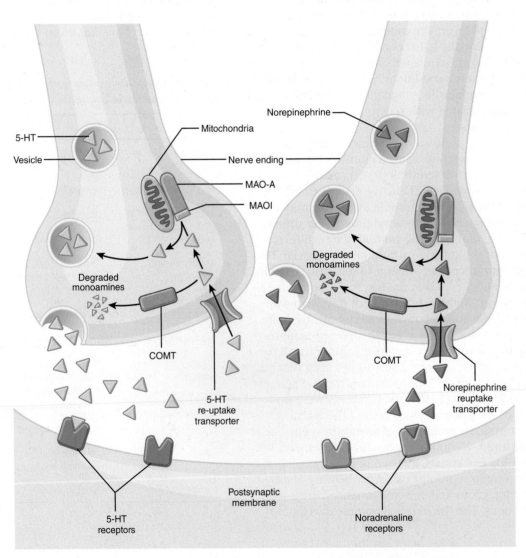

FIGURE 14-2 Metabolism of monoamines by catechol-o-methyl transferase (COMT) and monoamine oxidase (MAO).

TABLE 14-3	Monoamine Oxidase Inhibitors for Depression
Generic Name	**Notes**
Phenelzine	Phenelzine has been linked to vitamin B$_6$ deficiency.
Selegiline	Low-dose selegiline is often used to treat Parkinson disease. It is the only member of its class that is also available as a transdermal patch.
Tranylcypromine	Contraindicated in patients with low body weight or eating disorders, particularly anorexia.

agitation, and elevated mood, in addition to the more troubling side effects such as reduced sleep, constipation, dry mouth, nausea, diarrhea, weight gain, changes in appetite, orthostatic hypotension, and sexual dysfunction. A life-threatening side effect of the MAOIs can be **hypertensive crisis** caused by eating certain foods and beverages that contain tyramine (Flockhart, 2012). This occurs because the neurotransmitter MAO-A, which normally would prevent excessively high levels of norepinephrine in the gut (thus controlling blood pressure), is less available in people who take MAOIs. High levels of tyramine, which can occur when a patient eats foods such as certain aged cheeses, yeast products, aged fish or meat, chocolate, some vegetables, some alcoholic beverages, and some fruits, cause a significant increase in the neurotransmitter norepinephrine in the gut, leading to a dangerous hypertensive crisis (FIGURE 14-3). The patient prescribed oral MAOIs must be carefully educated and provided with materials that identify which foods must be avoided. A transdermal form of one MAOI, **selegiline**, is available and is thought to reduce the impairment of MAO-A in the gut by allowing a larger portion of the dose to reach the CNS and avoid first-pass metabolism (Finbert & Rabey, 2016).

In addition to the tyramine-related issues, other life-threatening side effects that can occur with MAOI use include seizures and liver toxicity.

Drug–Drug Interactions

Starting an MAOI when a patient is taking an SSRI or SNRI can cause a life-threatening serotonin surge by inhibiting the breakdown and reuptake of serotonin, leading to an excessive amount of serotonin in the neuronal synapse. Therefore, a "washout" period of at least five weeks should be observed before either starting or stopping an MAOI if the patient has been taking or is to be switched to an SSRI or SNRI. Other medications to use with caution or avoid altogether in patients taking MAOIs include antihypertensives, TCAs, **meperidine**, decongestants that contain **phenylephrine**, and stimulants such as amphetamines or methylphenidates, as these are metabolized by the same pathway. Street drugs should, of course, be avoided at all times, but drugs that hyperstimulate the CNS, such as cocaine, are particularly dangerous in combination with MAOIs due to the risk of hypertensive crisis. The herb St. John's wort, long used as a natural remedy for depression, increases serotonin levels and could potentially interact with MAOIs to produce a serotonin surge (Klemow et al., 2011). The adverse events occur when MAOIs are combined with the previously mentioned medications. This causes excessive alpha$_1$ and noradrenergic stimulation and can result in elevated blood pressure or hypertensive crisis.

Prescribing Considerations

In general, MAOIs are reserved for use as second-line antidepressants. They can sometimes be beneficial in patients with whom SSRIs and SNRIs have failed. A patient should consult with a healthcare professional before taking other prescriptions or over-the-counter medications or supplements. MAOIs can be of benefit for the treatment-resistant client and should be carefully considered as an option for treatment (Stahl, 2005). Pregnant women (or those attempting to achieve pregnancy) should be counseled about potential teratogenic effects.

Best Practices

As with all antidepressants, clinicians should monitor patients for suicidal ideation, particularly in younger individuals (younger than 25 years).

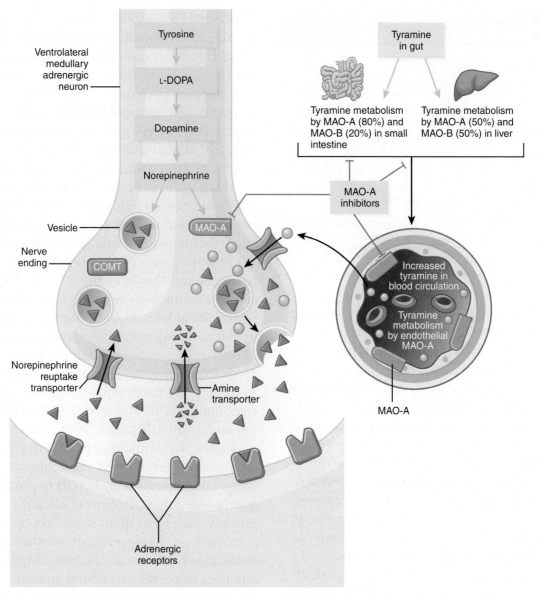

FIGURE 14-3 Tyramine chemistry and its relation to MAOI hypertensive crises induction.

Tricyclic Antidepressants (TCAs)

TCAs were introduced as first-line antidepressants in the 1950s. They work by blocking the norepinephrine reuptake pump and the **serotonin reuptake pump** in the **synaptic space**, thereby boosting the availability of the neurotransmitters serotonin, norepinephrine, histamine, muscarine, acetylcholine, and dopamine in the brain.

TCAs (**TABLE 14-4**) are indicated for depression, bipolar disorder, **neuropathic pain**, panic disorder, and obsessive–compulsive disorder. Improvement of symptoms can often be delayed up to two to four weeks and may require a dosage increase of the particular TCA if improvement is not seen by six to eight weeks. The goals of treatment are remission of depressive symptoms as well as prevention of relapse. Symptoms of depression may recur after the medication is stopped.

Acting on the same neurotransmitters, TCAs are also beneficial for anxiety and chronic pain; patients may require long-term treatment of months to years or as long as the anxiety and chronic pain persist. Chronic pain includes fibromyalgia, a condition that occurs when descending norepinephrine is deficient in the dorsal region of the brain.

TABLE 14-4	Tricyclic and Tetracyclic Antidepressants
Generic Name	**Notes**
Amitriptyline	Single-ingredient amitriptyline is available only as a generic. Brand-name formulations of combined amitriptyline and perphenazine are also available.
Amoxapine	Also used to treat anxiety and agitation. Amoxapine has been studied as a resistance-modifying agent for MRSA.
Desipramine	Off-label use includes treatment for anxiety, ADHD, bulimia, and panic attacks.
Doxepin	Medication is also sold in cream form for use in treating eczema.
Imipramine	Sometimes used in children to treat bedwetting.
Maprotiline	Maprotiline is a tetracyclic antidepressant; it is also used for treating bipolar disorder and anxiety disorders.
Nortriptyline	Sometimes used to treat panic disorders and postherpetic neuralgia, and as an antismoking agent.
Protriptyline	A tricyclic antidepressant that is FDA-approved to treat attention deficit-hyperactivity disorder, narcolepsy, and headaches.
Trimipramine	Trimipramine has more antihistaminic and sedative properties than imipramine.

Adverse Reactions

Side effects of the TCAs, many related to anticholinergic actions of the drugs, include orthostatic hypotension and anticholinergic effects such as dry mouth, constipation, blurred vision, and sedation. In addition, weight gain, dizziness, sexual dysfunction, nausea, and vomiting are common. Life-threatening side effects include seizures, arrhythmias, hepatic failure, and EPS. EPS may include acute dystonia, a syndrome of abnormal muscle contraction that produces repetitive involuntary twisting movements and abnormal posturing of the neck, trunk, face, and extremities. In addition, Parkinsonian symptoms characterized by rhythmic muscular tremors, rigidity of movement, and droopy posture may occur. Other potential side effects include mask-like facies, shaking palsy, and trembling palsy. Weight gain and sedation are common. As with all antidepressants, clinicians should monitor patients for suicidal ideation, particularly in younger individuals (younger than 25 years).

Drug–Drug Interactions

TCAs should not be used in combination with MAOIs, anticholinergic agents, or CNS depressants. Caution should be used when these agents are given in combination with some SSRIs, such as fluvoxamine, which is metabolized through the CYP enzyme pathway, and with antihypertensive agents and methylphenidate, which compete for the same enzymes. There have been reports of serious cardiac effects with concomitant TCA and CYP-inhibiting SSRI use (English, Dortch, Ereshefsky, & Jhee, 2012).

Prescribing Considerations

TCAs can be beneficial for chronic pain related to increased norepinephrine reuptake inhibition and sleep disorders related to an increase in histamine receptors' availability. They continue to be useful for treatment-resistant depression. These medications are considered second-line options for treatment of depression compared to the SSRIs and SNRIs (the first-line options) because of their significant side-effect profile. More importantly, TCAs have a narrow therapeutic index; for this reason, overdoses are associated with a greater risk of fatality than the newer classes of antidepressant medications. Therefore, patient history of suicidality should be considered when initiating TCA pharmacotherapeutic treatment of depression. TCA overdose can cause QT prolongation, cardiac toxicity, cardiac contractility, and hypotension. Treatment includes activated charcoal up to two hours post-ingestion, benzodiazepines for seizures, and sodium bicarbonate for hemodynamically unstable patients. Pregnant women should be counseled about potential teratogenic effects.

SSRIs and SNRIs

The SSRIs were introduced in the mid-1980s and are now the first-line antidepressant and anxiolytic medications. They work by blocking the serotonin reuptake pump in the synaptic space, thereby increasing the concentration of the neurotransmitter serotonin in the brain (FIGURE 14-4); recently, they have also been identified as having significant anti-inflammatory properties that are being explored in the context of their effects on depression and anxiety (Walker, 2013).

SNRIs are also considered a first-line choice for antidepressant and antianxiety medications. Introduced in the mid-1990s, they block both the serotonin and norepinephrine pumps in the synaptic space (Figure 14-4), thereby boosting the availability of the neurotransmitters serotonin and norepinephrine in the brain. Increased levels of serotonin and norepinephrine in the synaptic space have been shown to cause a decrease in depression and anxiety symptoms in patients (Stahl, 2008).

SSRIs and SNRIs (TABLE 14-5) are indicated for depression and numerous anxiety disorders, including panic disorder, general anxiety disorder, post-traumatic stress disorder, and obsessive–compulsive disorder. Members of these drug classes are effective in these disorders because increasing serotonin and norepinephrine has been shown to decrease anxiety symptoms in patients, which in turn improves the symptoms of the anxiety disorders. Drug response can often be delayed by two to four weeks, and patients may require an increase in dose if the medication is not helpful in six to eight weeks. The goal of treatment is the remission of symptoms of depression and anxiety as well as prevention of relapse. Symptoms of depression and anxiety may recur after the medication is stopped. Use of SSRIs or SNRIs to treat anxiety disorders may require long-term treatment of months to years.

Adverse Reactions

In general, SSRIs and SNRIs are the safest and best-tolerated antidepressant and anxiolytic medications (compared to TCAs and MAOIs). The most commonly reported side effects with these drugs are sexual dysfunction, defined as reduced libido, erectile dysfunction, or ejaculatory difficulties, caused by stimulation of serotonin receptors in the spinal cord. Nausea, another common side effect, is caused by the stimulation of serotonin receptors in the hypothalamus or brain stem. Headaches and nervousness also can occur, caused by the action of serotonin in the prefrontal cortex. Insomnia is caused by stimulation of serotonin receptors in the brain stem's sleep centers, which disrupts slow-wave or stage III and IV sleep; this can contribute to a lack of restorative sleep and cause daytime fatigue. Life-threatening side effects are rare, although patients should routinely be evaluated for suicidal thoughts.

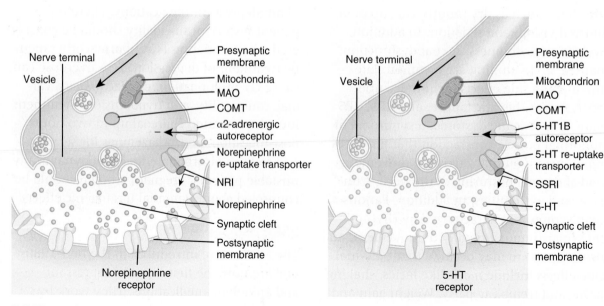

FIGURE 14-4 Serotonin and norepinephrine reuptake pathways.

| TABLE 14-5 | Selective Serotonin and Selective Norepinephrine Reuptake Inhibitors Used for Depression and Anxiety* |

Generic Name	Class	Notes
Citalopram	SSRI	
Desvenlafaxine	SNRI	
Duloxetine	SNRI	Also used for generalized anxiety disorder, diabetic neuropathy, fibromyalgia, and bone/muscle pain.
Escitalopram	SSRI	Also used for generalized anxiety disorder.
Fluoxetine	SSRI	Also used to treat OCD, bulimia, and panic disorder.
Fluvoxamine	SSRI	Primarily used in the treatment of OCD, but may also be used for depression.
Levomilnacipran	SNRI	
Paroxetine	SSRI	Also used to treat panic disorder, OCD, social anxiety disorder, generalized anxiety disorder, and PTSD.
Sertraline	SSRI	Also used to treat panic disorder, OCD, PTSD, social anxiety disorder, and premenstrual dysphoric disorder.
Venlafaxine	SNRI	Also used for generalized anxiety disorder, social anxiety disorder, and panic disorder.
Vilazodone	SSRI	
Vortioxetine	SNRI	

*Other drugs in these classes (e.g., tramadol) are not used for treating anxiety or depression. However, any drug in this class should not be used in conjunction with antidepressants in the SSRI/SNRI class due to the risk of serotonin syndrome.

Studies have shown a small (approximately 4%; Bridge et al., 2007) but significant risk for suicidal ideation and behavior, with use of antidepressants in children and adolescents (Termorshuizen, Smeets, Boks, & Heerdink, 2016). Clinicians prescribing antidepressants to children and adolescents should monitor them closely for both response and adverse reactions. Studies show that the benefit-to-risk ratio is favorable and that the use of antidepressants in children and adolescents should be a personal decision made through collaboration among clinicians, family, and patient. The reason for the increased suicidal risk is unclear, but may be related to the short half-life of some antidepressants. It is also theorized that suicidal risk could be related to the activating/drive-enhancing effects or side effects of the medication such as akathisia. Personality disturbances such as borderline personality should also be considered (Moller, 2006).

Weight gain may occur with SSRIs and SNRIs. Sedation is not often reported. Most side effects occur early in treatment and often resolve within a week, as a patient's neurologic system accommodates the medication. Lowering the dosage can reduce the side effects.

Drug–Drug Interactions

The number of potential SSRI and SNRI drug–drug interactions is extremely extensive. Therefore, a general list of medications that may interact with SSRIs and/or SNRIs is provided here. More broadly, caution should be used when combining SSRIs and SNRIs with **tramadol**, **codeine**, **thioridazine**, **warfarin**, **sumatriptan**, **simvastatin**, **lovastatin**, and **atorvastatin**. These interactions arise related to the liver's cytochrome P450 enzyme, which is involved in the metabolism of most drugs and can lead to excessive or reduced blood levels of these medications.

Extreme caution must be used when exchanging SSRIs or SNRIs with MAOIs; clinicians should never combine the medications and should wait at least 14 days until the MAOI has "washed out" of the patient's system before initiating an SSRI or SNRI or switching from an SSRI or SNRI back to an MAOI. Concomitant use of SSRIs or SNRIs with MAOIs could cause serotonin syndrome, a potentially fatal side effect (described earlier in this chapter).

Prescribing Considerations

To avoid withdrawal effects such as rebound depression, anxiety, dizziness, nausea, or sweating, SSRI and SNRI dosages should be slowly tapered when these medications are being decreased or discontinued. Withdrawal effects can occur as a result of reducing the neurotransmitter concentrations in the brain that were artificially boosted by the medications.

Buspirone

Buspirone is a medication used for the treatment of anxiety and treatment-resistant anxiety disorders. Its exact mechanism of action is unknown; however, it binds to serotonin and dopamine (D_2) receptors.

Adverse Reactions

Side effects of buspirone are often benign but can include dizziness, drowsiness, and nausea. Buspirone does not appear to cause **dependence** or **withdrawal** symptoms. It is best used as an adjunct agent for other antianxiety medications but can also be effective when used alone.

Drug–Drug Interactions

As mentioned earlier, buspirone is a serotonergic medication, so it should not be used with other medications that affect serotonin levels in the brain. Buspirone is metabolized via the cytochrome P450 3A4 (CYP3A4) pathway, which means it is likely to interact with a great many other medications processed via this mechanism. Medications such as azole antifungal drugs (e.g., itraconazole), carbamepazine, and rifampin are metabolized via this pathway as well and may increase or decrease the plasma levels of buspirone. Grapefruit juice is a known inhibitor of CYP3A4 metabolism and can significantly increase plasma levels of buspirone. Use of the herb St. John's wort, which increases serotonin levels, while taking buspirone has been reported as a possible cause of serotonin syndrome

(Borrelli & Izzo, 2009; Dannawi, 2002). Concomitant use with MAOIs is contraindicated due to the possibility of hypertensive crisis. Linezolid, an antimicrobial, has also been reported to produce serotonin syndrome in concert with buspirone and other serotonergic agents (Morrison & Rowe, 2012).

Benzodiazepines

Benzodiazepine drugs (BZD) are one of the most widely prescribed pharmacologic categories in the United States. They are prescribed for numerous indications, including anxiety, insomnia, muscle relaxation, relief from spasticity caused by central nervous system pathology, and epilepsy. They are also used intraoperatively because of their amnesic and anxiolytic properties. Benzodiazepines act primarily on the CNS and are often the first-line treatment for anxiety. This is due to BZDs' mechanism of action. Benzodiazepines act on the gamma-aminobutyric acid (GABA)-A receptor, a ligand-gated chloride-selective ion channel. GABA is the most common neurotransmitter in the central nervous system, found in high concentrations in the cortex and limbic system. GABA is an inhibitory neurotransmitter in nature and thus reduces the excitability of neurons, producing a calming effect on the brain (FIGURE 14-5).

There is no evidence that any one benzodiazepine is more effective for alleviating anxiety than another (TABLE 14-6).

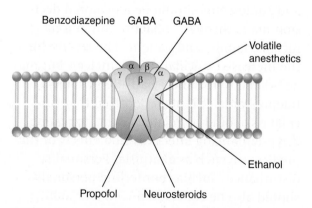

FIGURE 14-5 Benzodiazepine receptor and flow chart.

The GABA chloride channel has multiple receptor sites, including those for benzodiazepines. When GABA receptors are bound, chloride ions enter the neuron cell body, moving the cell away from firing, causing a dampening effect on the neuron cell.

TABLE 14-6	Benzodiazepines Commonly Used for Anxiety*
Generic Name
Alprazolam
Chlordiazepoxide
Clonazepam
Clorazepate
Clotiazepam
Diazepam
Lorazepam
Oxazepam

*This class of medications has a wide range of additional examples used for anxiety as well as for sedation and anticonvulsant indications. This list includes only a subset of the class.

It is their rapid onset of action that makes some benzodiazepines a good choice for short-term relief of anxiety, although this is not necessarily true for the entire class. A specific benzodiazepine is chosen based upon its pharmacodynamic and pharmacokinetic properties, including the half-life, onset time, and duration of action. Certain conditions may require quick onset, whereas other conditions may require a longer duration of action (Bostwick, Casher, & Yasugi, 2012). BZDs are classified in terms of their elimination half-life. Short-acting BZDs have a median elimination half-life of 1 to 12 hours, intermediate-acting BZDs have an average elimination half-life of 12 to 40 hours, and long-acting BZDs have an average elimination half-life of 40 to 250 hours.

Benzodiazepines can also be used to augment the anxiolytic effects of SSRIs and SNRIs, as they do not affect serotonin or norepinephrine levels and, therefore, incur no risk of serotonin syndrome. They are also helpful for alleviating insomnia, due to their sedative properties (Griffin, Kaye, Bueno, & Kaye, 2013). Further, benzodiazepines can be used to prevent common seizures and alcohol withdrawal due to their inhibiting actions in the cerebral cortex, mediated through GABA receptors.

Adverse Reactions

Overall, benzodiazepines are well tolerated and safe. Long-term use of these medications may lead to dependence or **tolerance** and cause withdrawal symptoms when the dosage is reduced or the drug is discontinued. Therefore, slow tapering of benzodiazepines is often required in these instances. There is the potential for abuse, particularly if treatment periods are longer than 12 weeks in length. Patients with a history of substance abuse should be carefully evaluated to determine whether benzodiazepines are an appropriate choice. Use of benzodiazepines should be closely monitored for signs of abuse and inappropriate or illegal use. Sedation, fatigue, dizziness, **ataxia**, and confusion are common side effects, and memory loss can occur with long-term use of benzodiazepines. A change in body weight is not often seen with benzodiazepines.

Drug–Drug Interactions

Increased CNS depression is possible when benzodiazepines are combined with other CNS depressants, such as additional benzodiazepines, alcohol, and opioids. Coma and death are possible with overdosing of a combination of these CNS depressants. **Cimetidine**, **valproic acid**, **fluvoxamine**, and grapefruit juice can reduce the liver's ability to clear benzodiazepines from the body, thereby increasing benzodiazepine plasma levels and effects.

Prescribing Considerations

As previously mentioned, decreasing benzodiazepine dose or discontinuing a benzodiazepine should be accomplished through tapering of the dose rather than abrupt reductions in dose. However, tapering patients off benzodiazepines can be performed rapidly if the patient has not been taking a benzodiazepine for longer than seven days. Long-term use of benzodiazepines requires a much slower taper because the risk of rebound anxiety, hypertension, muscle twitches, and seizures. Caution should be used with benzodiazepine dosing in elderly patients because of the increased risk of unsteadiness, oversedation, and injuries related to falls. Use of benzodiazepines should be avoided in pregnancy.

Bipolar Disorder

According to the National Institute of Mental Health (2017), 2.8% of U.S. adults and as many as 3% of adolescents have been diagnosed with **bipolar disorder**, also known as manic–depressive disorder. The onset of bipolar disorder often occurs between the ages of 15 and 25 years but can occur in children or later in life. The prevalence of child-onset bipolar disorder is not well established, but 82.9% of adult bipolar disorder is classified as severe, characterized by severe mood swings between depression and mania. Only 48.8% of those diagnosed with bipolar disorder are receiving treatment, and many are receiving only minimally adequate treatment.

Bipolar disorder is often unrecognized or misdiagnosed and therefore, is not treated or medicated properly. It can often take years before the patient receives the correct diagnosis. Early diagnosis of bipolar disorder is preferred and should include input from family members, to give important historical insight (U.S. National Library of Medicine, 2011). This can help differentiate between unipolar symptoms, defined as typical depression without the mood swings, and bipolar symptoms. Patients often fail to report symptoms of mania because they do not see them as debilitating, but family members are much more likely to observe early behavioral symptoms of mania and report them as a problem. All too often patients are misdiagnosed with unipolar disorder, which presents as signs and symptoms similar to depression, and then treated with antidepressants. Patients can then go on to exhibit symptoms of bipolar disorder and will require a change in medications.

Symptoms of bipolar disorder include unusual shifts in mood between depression and **mania**. Energy, activity levels, and ability to carry out daily activities can be significantly increased or decreased according to the mood.

Manic episodes may last from hours to days to months. Symptoms include being easily distracted, reduced need for sleep, poor judgment, loss of temper, reckless behavior, poor impulse control, hyperactivity, excessive energy, grandiose thoughts, racing thoughts, excessive talking, and agitation or irritability. Psychotic symptoms, such as auditory and visual hallucinations and delusional thoughts, may also be present.

Hypomania is defined as a mild form of mania. Its symptoms are similar to mania but not as severe. The patient's mood tends to be elevated, and irritability and agitation are often prominent.

Major depressive episodes include sadness, fatigue, appetite changes, sleep changes (evidenced by either excessive or inadequate sleep), isolation, thoughts of death or suicide, and feelings of hopelessness and worthlessness.

Mixed episodes include mood swings between manic and depression. Symptoms include agitation and irritability as well as feelings of depression and/or mania.

The drugs of choice for treatment of bipolar disorder generally are classified in one of two categories: mood stabilizers and antipsychotics.

Mood Stabilizers
First-Line Medications: Lithium, Valproic Acid, and Carbamazepine

Mood stabilizers are often the first choice of medications to treat bipolar disorder. The goal of treatment is to stabilize the patient's mood and eliminate mood swings, or make them less frequent and less severe. Three medications are indicated to treat the symptoms of bipolar disorder: **lithium**, **valproic acid**, and **carbamazepine**.

The exact mechanism of action of **lithium** is unknown and complex, although it is believed to alter the distribution of calcium, sodium, and magnesium ions as well as alter the synthesis and release of norepinephrine, serotonin, and dopamine in the brain. **Valproic acid** and **carbamazepine** are antiseizure agents that have been approved to reduce symptoms during manic and depressive episodes. Valproic acid is believed to work by altering the brain's sodium channels and the concentration of GABA. Carbamazepine works by inhibiting the brain's sodium channels so as to increase the release of glutamate, an agonist at several important CNS stimulatory receptors.

Mood stabilizers, used with or without antipsychotic medications, are effective in relieving acute mania and depressive episodes and can help with maintaining mood stability by preventing reoccurrence of both mania and depression. The onset of action of the mood stabilizers is fairly rapid and should be seen within a few days; however, it may take weeks to months for optimal effects on mood stabilization to be seen.

Adverse Reactions

Common side effects that may occur with lithium, valproic acid, and carbamazepine include sedation, dizziness, tremors, nausea, vomiting, diarrhea, unsteadiness, headache, weight gain, and hematological changes. It is good practice to monitor the patient's blood levels for all three agents, so as to titrate any necessary dose adjustments, determine efficacy, and check for possibly life-threatening toxicity, which can occur if the blood levels of these drugs are too high. Also, complete blood counts, including electrolytes and platelets, should be closely monitored, as well as lipids and liver, thyroid, and renal function tests. Because weight gain is one of the potential adverse effects of the mood-stabilizing drugs, the patient's weight, body mass index, and blood pressure should also be monitored on a regular basis.

Serious side effects of lithium can include renal impairment, arrhythmias, and hypothyroidism. Serious side effects of valproic acid can include thrombocytopenia, pancreatitis, and liver failure. Serious side effects of carbamazepine include leukopenia, anemia, and thrombocytopenia.

Drug-Drug Interactions

Caution is advised when combining lithium, valproic acid, and carbamazepine with the medications listed here. Interactions can alter the blood levels of the mood stabilizers or alter the metabolism of the other medications listed, thereby causing side effects or increasing plasma levels of these drugs.

- Lithium: Caution should be used when combining lithium with nonsteroidal anti-inflammatory drugs, diuretics, calcium-channel blockers, angiotensin-converting enzyme inhibitors, and metronidazole.
- Valproic acid: Caution should be used when combining valproic acid with lamotrigine, carbamazepine, aspirin, phenytoin, and phenobarbital.
- Carbamazepine: Caution should be used when combining carbamazepine with phenobarbital, phenytoin, fluoxetine, fluvoxamine, and hormonal contraceptives.

Lamotrigine

A fourth medication, the anticonvulsant lamotrigine, has been approved for long-term maintenance treatment of bipolar disorder and is regarded as a first-line agent in adults (but not children) by the APA (2002). It acts by inhibiting the voltage-dependent sodium channels within the cell, which decreases presynaptic glutamate and aspartate (which, again, are normally stimulatory neurotransmitters) release. Studies show that this drug is most effective at stabilizing depressive phases but is not particularly useful in acute manic phases; however, it can be paired with other medications to stabilize mood acutely and transition the patient into preventive therapy (El-Mallakh, Elmaadawi, Gao, Lohano, & Roberts, 2011).

Adverse Effects

The key adverse effect of lamotrigine is a serious rash that can develop, particularly when the drug is paired with valproic acid or the anticonvulsant divalproex, which is sometimes used to manage manic-phase symptoms. This rash can take one of several forms severe enough to require hospitalization (e.g., Stevens-Johnson syndrome, DRESS syndrome, and toxic epidermal necrolysis) and should be treated proactively. Skin reactions of this sort are most likely to occur in the first two to eight weeks of treatment but may appear at any time. Because these reactions are more common in children, the drug should not be used in patients younger than 16 years of age. In 2010, the Food and Drug Administration (FDA) also issued a warning (which is still current) stating that lamotrigine can cause aseptic meningitis.

Drug-Drug Interactions

The use of lamotrigine in patients taking valproic acid affects serum levels of both drugs, with lamotrigine increasing in the serum as valproic acid decreases. The risk of skin reaction is also increased with this combination. Concomitant use with carbamazepine leads to increases in side effects such as blurred vision and dizziness, although the mechanism is unknown. Drugs such as phenytoin, phenobarbital, rifampin, and oral contraceptives containing estrogen increase liver metabolism of lamotrigine significantly, resulting in a reduction of 40% to 50% in the drug's serum concentration.

Antipsychotic Drugs in Bipolar Disorder

FGA and SGA medications, which were described in terms of their pharmacology in an earlier section, are indicated to treat acute manic episodes, stabilize mood beyond the acute episode, and continue to manage symptoms of acute manic episodes over longer periods of time (known as the maintenance phase). They are particularly valuable in managing the psychotic symptoms that may occur during acute manic episodes, including delusions, hallucinations, thought disorders, and other symptoms that are similar to those seen with schizophrenia. The difference between psychotic symptoms in bipolar disease and schizophrenia is that in the latter disease, psychotic symptoms are present on an ongoing,

persistent basis and are firmly embedded in the patient's belief system, whereas with bipolar disorder, psychotic symptoms are present only during acute manic episodes and abate when the patient's mood has normalized. Manic symptoms are generally absent in schizophrenia. Agitation and irritability are often associated with bipolar disorder and can be managed effectively with antipsychotics.

For descriptions of the mechanisms of action and adverse reactions associated with antipsychotics, refer to the section describing these drugs earlier in the chapter.

Prescribing Considerations for Drugs Used To Treat Bipolar Disorder

As noted earlier, bipolar disorder is often misdiagnosed as major depression and anxiety and may take years to be correctly diagnosed and treated with the appropriate medications. Patients who take mood stabilizers or antipsychotics should always be closely monitored for worsening symptoms of depression or emerging signs of suicidal risk. The increased potential for impulsive action associated with bipolar disorder can increase the risk of suicide. Lithium can be helpful to reduce suicidal thoughts. Lithium and valproic acid may be helpful as adjuncts to boost the efficacy of SGAs.

Attention-Deficit Disorder and Attention-Deficit/Hyperactivity Disorder

Both attention-deficit disorder (ADD) and ADHD are often characterized by symptoms that include hyperactivity, lack of attention, lack of focus and concentration, distractibility, and difficulty organizing and completing tasks. For diagnostic purposes, these symptoms must have been present since childhood, although they may or may not have been recognized. In fact, ADD or ADHD is often not diagnosed until the patient is an adult. In addition, the symptoms must interfere with school, employment, or social functioning. Criteria for the diagnosis of ADHD are laid out in the *Diagnostic and Statistical Manual of Mental Disorders* and were revised for the fifth edition. Changes to the criteria include shifting the age of onset requirement from the presence of symptoms and impairment by age 7 years to the presence of some symptoms by age 12 years; reducing the number of symptoms required for a diagnosis for individuals 17 years of age and older; and providing clinical examples of symptoms that are more age appropriate for older adolescents and adults (APA, 2013).

The *DSM-5* reports the prevalence of ADHD to be approximately 5% of school-age children, and around 2.5% of adults in the general population (APA, 2013). Other estimates, however, place the prevalence higher, at about 9% of children aged 6 to 11 years, and almost 12% for those aged 12 to 17 (Pastor, Reuben, Duran, & Hawkins, 2015). Boys are twice as likely to be diagnosed with ADHD as girls (Pastor et al., 2015). As of 2017, parents of 2.7 million youth aged 4 to 17 years reported use of medications to treat ADHD. Children with a history of ADHD are almost 3 times more likely to encounter peer group problems and 10 times as likely to have difficulties that interfere with friendships. They are also at greater risk for injury. Young adults and adults are a greater risk for involvement in motor vehicle accidents, drinking and driving, and traffic violations (Centers for Disease Control and Prevention [CDC], 2017).

Stimulant Medications

The most commonly used class of medications used to treat ADD/ADHD is stimulants (**TABLE 14-7**) (Albert, Rui, & Ashman, 2017). These controlled substances work by blocking reuptake and facilitating release of norepinephrine and dopamine (D_2) in areas of the brain that control impulsivity, including the dorsolateral prefrontal cortex, basal ganglia, and medial prefrontal cortex (**FIGURE 14-6**). Frontal cortex neuronal transmission is too slow in patients with ADD/ADHD, allowing for more "impulsive" behavior (e.g., speech, motor). Stimulant medications are categorized as either *amphetamines* or *methylphenidates*; both are Schedule II controlled substances

TABLE 14-7	Stimulant Medications Used for Treating ADD/ADHD	
Generic Name	Class	Notes
Amphetamine/ dextroamphetamine mixed salts	Amphetamine	Comes in IR and ER formulations
Dextroamphetamine	Amphetamine	Comes in IR and ER formulations
Lisdexamfetamine dimesylate	Amphetamine	A prodrug formulation that is metabolized to dextroamphetamine; is preferred in adolescents and children due to lower risk of abuse and better side-effect profile
Methylphenidate HCl	Methylphenadine	Comes in IR, SR, and ER formulations

All medications listed are Schedule II controlled substances. Use of IR formulations can be problematic in children for this reason.

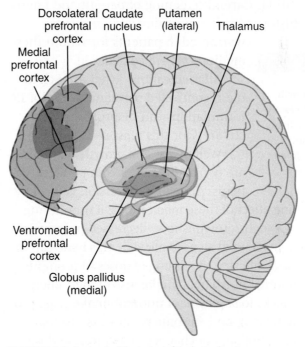

FIGURE 14-6 Anatomical illustration of the brain showing dorsolateral prefrontal cortex, basal ganglia and medial prefrontal cortex.

(Goodman, 2010). Neither category is superior to the other, although patients sometimes will respond better to one than the other, and determining the most efficacious agent in a particular patient often is a matter of trial and error.

Two types of drug release systems are used for these medications: instant release (IR), which has a duration of action of approximately 4 hours, and extended release (ER) or sustained release (SR) formulations, which have durations of actions of 6 to 12 hours.

Adverse Effects

Reports for all of the stimulant drugs associate medication use with increases in heart rate of one to two beats per minute on average (although some considerably higher rates have been noted) as well as elevation of blood pressure by as much as 10 mm Hg. These changes were noted in both adult and pediatric populations. The increases, on average, are relatively small, but in patients already predisposed to cardiac issues or hypertension, they could create potential harm in a long-term use scenario (Graham et al., 2011). Careful screening of patient and family history to rule out cardiovascular disease is, warranted in patients for whom these medications are considered.

All medications listed are Schedule II controlled substances. Use of IR formulations can be problematic in children for this reason.

Weight loss and growth retardation are two additional risks in pediatric patients. Appetite suppression is one key side effect of these medications; if monitoring of weight/growth shows decreased progression, management steps to alleviate this issue can include altering the timing of doses to promote optimal nutritional intake, use of high-energy snacks to supplement nutrient intake (e.g., protein bars), and, in some patients, occasional drug holidays or changes in medication dose or type (Graham et al., 2011), which has been shown to produce a rebound growth effect.

Sleep disturbance may occur in some patients, with a variety of causative factors. Patients with a history of sleep disturbance *preceding* medication use probably should be prescribed atomoxetine, which is a *non-stimulant* ADHD/antidepressant drug (acting in part by inhibiting norepinephrine reuptake), instead of stimulants, as there is a lower incidence of insomnia side effects associated with

Best Practices

Weight and growth rate should be closely monitored in patients taking stimulants, particularly children.

atomoxetine use. Sleep hygiene and behavioral modification therapies may work best for patients whose sleep disturbance predates their medication for ADHD (Graham et al., 2011).

Long-term use of stimulants can result in physical dependence. When discontinuing the stimulant, the patient may experience excessive fatigue, depression, and craving for the stimulant. Slow titration is the best method for discontinuing the medication. Patients should always be monitored closely for signs of abuse. Abuse of stimulants should be approached with a treatment plan that focuses on addressing the substance abuse.

Drug–Drug Interactions

Amphetamines taken in concert with fluoxetine, duloxetine, escitalopram, or a variety of other antidepressant/antipsychotic drugs can cause serotonin syndrome because of redundancy of transporter reuptake blockade. A number of medications taken concurrently with amphetamines increase the risk of seizures, including acetaminophen, bupropion, and tramadol. Using amphetamines with linezolid, procarbazine, or isocarboxazid can produce a hypertensive crisis.

Nonstimulant Medications

A variety of nonstimulant medications are also used to treat ADD/ADHD. They are most often prescribed for patients who cannot tolerate stimulants or who have a history of stimulant abuse, although these agents are generally less effective at improving attention span and concentration. Most fall into one of two classes (TABLE 14-8): antidepressant medications (atomoxetine, bupropion, nortriptyline) or centrally acting α_2-adrenergic agonists (guanfacine, clonidine).

Atomoxetine is a nonstimulant medication in the SNRI class that works by increasing the concentrations of the neurotransmitters norepinephrine at the norepinephrine receptors and dopamine at the D_2 receptors in the frontal cortex in the brain. It is not a controlled substance and is more

TABLE 14-8	Nonstimulant Medications Used for Treating ADD/ADHD		
Generic Name	Class	Notes	
Atomoxetine	Selective norepinephrine uptake inhibitor		
Bupropion	Antidepressant		
Clonidine	Antihypertensive/ central α₂ adrenergic agonist	Affects cardiac conduction and should be used with caution in patients with a personal or family history of arrhythmia	
Guanfacine	Antihypertensive/ central α₂ adrenergic agonist		
Nortriptyline	Tricyclic antidepressant	Used off-label as a second-line therapy in ADHD	

closely related to antidepressant medications described earlier. Because it affects the norepinephrine in the brain, **atomoxetine** can also have a calming effect.

Atomoxetine has several advantages. First and foremost, it is not a controlled substance because it lacks the addictive potential of stimulants, and there are no legal repercussions or controls on its distribution, which makes it attractive for use in children and adolescents as well as adults with a history of substance abuse, who might otherwise be difficult to treat with stimulants. This drug is cost-effective to use and does not differ greatly in efficacy from IR stimulants, although it has significantly lower efficacy than the ER/SR methylphenidates (Garnock-Jones & Keating, 2009). **Atomoxetine** is generally well tolerated and adherence to the prescribed regimen is usually good, even in adolescents (Barner, Khoza, & Oladapo, 2011).

Nortriptyline is a TCA that was mentioned in the earlier section detailing use of those medications for depression, and acts in the same fashion as **amitriptyline**.

The α₂-adrenergic agonists **guanfacine** and **clonidine** are not approved in IR form

for use in ADHD but have a long history of off-label use for this indication (Barner et al., 2011); ER formulations of both drugs have been approved for the ADHD indication. Response to these agents is not as robust as with stimulants or **atomoxetine**, but they do help with comorbid tics and lack the appetite suppressive effects observed with stimulants. Like **atomoxetine**, **guanfacine** and **clonidine** carry a lower risk of abuse and are good candidates for patients with a history of addiction to stimulant-type drugs. Because they are antihypertensive agents, these drugs can cause orthostatic hypotension and may cause reactive hypertension if withdrawn suddenly. In combination with **methylphenidate**, **clonidine** was associated with sudden death in children, although no causative factor could be established. Nevertheless, patients should be screened for cardiac anomalies and monitored if placed on this regimen (Barner et al., 2011).

Bupropion is an atypical antidepressant, most often used to help with smoking cessation due to its activity as a nicotinic acetylcholine receptor antagonist. Its mechanism of action in depression is not well understood, but it appears to act (weakly) as both a norepinephrine and a dopamine reuptake inhibitor (Reimherr, Hedges, Strong, Marchant, & Williams, 2005). **Bupropion** is slow to take effect, with patients showing a response at approximately four weeks (Reimherr et al., 2005), which makes it somewhat less attractive than the faster-acting stimulant medications or **atomoxetine**. It is not currently considered a first-line agent for ADD/ADHD but may be useful in patients for whom stimulants or **atomoxetine** are contraindicated or ineffective.

Adverse Reactions

For all nonstimulants, increases in norepinephrine and D₂ in the extraneuronal space in the brain and increases in the nontherapeutic acetylcholine receptors in the body and the brain can cause autonomic side effects. These effects include tremors, tachycardia, hypertension, cardiac arrhythmias, insomnia, agitation, irritability, and psychosis. The medications can also aggravate motor tics and Tourette syndrome. Other reports cite the occurrence of seizures, headaches, nervousness, nausea, dry mouth, anorexia, and weight loss. Children may experience temporary slowing of growth, particularly with atomoxetine, although long-term growth does not seem to be affected (Poulton, Bui, Melzer, & Evans, 2016; Reed et al., 2016). Bupropion, in particular, bears the caveat that dose-dependent incidence of seizures is notably higher than with most other antidepressant or ADHD therapies (Alper, Schwartz, Kolts, & Khan, 2007).

Drug–Drug Interactions

Patients who are being treated for hypertension should be evaluated for elevations in blood pressure related to the use of ADD/ADHD medications. Other medications that block the reuptake of norepinephrine, such as SNRIs or antipsychotics, may increase the CNS and cardiovascular effects of the stimulants. Great care should be used when combining stimulants with mood stabilizers and antipsychotics. A condition such as bipolar disorder or psychosis that requires treatment with mood stabilizers or antipsychotics may be aggravated by the use of stimulants, resulting in aggravated mood instability and psychosis. The use of stimulants and atomoxetine should be avoided in patients who have a history of heart disease, stroke, or neurovascular disorders because of the increased risk of cardiac arrhythmias and increased blood pressure. These drugs should not be administered with an MAOI agent.

Prescribing Considerations for Drugs Used for ADD/ADHD

Both stimulants and atomoxetine can improve attention, focus, concentration, organizational skills, and the ability to initiate and complete tasks. They can also increase wakefulness and reduce hyperactivity by increasing the concentrations of norepinephrine and D_2 at their respective receptors. In addition, these medications may improve the symptoms of depression and fatigue, have a calming effect, and reduce sleepiness. Results may include increased productivity at home, school, and work; improved self-esteem and self-image; and, therefore, reduced anxiety and depression.

The effects of the stimulants may be observed as early as the first day of their use, but often dose adjustments are necessary to achieve the optimal benefits. When atomoxetine (and other antidepressant drugs) are prescribed, it can take weeks before benefits are noted, and these medications often require dose adjustments to realize the optimal therapeutic benefit. Treatment can be continued indefinitely, as long as benefits are present. Acceptable use of stimulants can span from childhood to adulthood. Stimulant doses should be slowly tapered when these drugs are discontinued.

Stimulant drugs can be helpful as adjunct therapies in the treatment of depression and treatment-refractory depression because of their enhancement of dopamine and norepinephrine release and binding in the medial prefrontal cortex and hypothalamus. Overall, the potential for developing drug abuse in children and adults may be diminished or prevented when medications are used for the treatment of ADD/ADHD.

There is another, unrelated use for the stimulant drugs. They can be used effectively to reduce sedation and fatigue caused by opioid analgesic use because of their ability to increase alertness and wakefulness by increasing the concentration of dopamine and norepinephrine in the hypothalamus and the medial prefrontal cortex. Dosing of stimulants should be timed to avoid interference with sleep. It is good practice to monitor the patient's weight. Pregnant women (or those attempting to achieve pregnancy) should be counseled about potential teratogenic effects.

Sleep Disorders

The *DSM-5* identifies 10 sleep-wake disorders, all of which include patient dissatisfaction with the quality and amount of sleep as a major complaint. Previously, the primary sleep disorders were categorized as either *dyssomnias* or *parasomnias*. **Dyssomnias** include primary insomnia, which is defined as the inability to sleep well and pertains to the improper amount, quality, or timing of sleep. **Parasomnias** are defined as abnormal behavioral or physiological events that occur while sleeping. The CDC (2012) has made it one of the agency's missions to raise awareness about the problem of sleep insufficiency and sleep disorders, and to emphasize the importance of sleep.

The CDC (2012) estimates that 70 million Americans suffer from chronic sleep problems. Difficulty with falling asleep or daytime sleepiness affects approximately 35% to 40% of U.S. adults and approximately one-third of adults report not getting the recommended amount of sleep (National Center for Chronic Disease Prevention and Health Promotion, 2017). The high prevalence of complications related to sleep insufficiency in sleep disorders, concomitant illnesses, and untreated symptoms has immense cost implications (Hafner, Stepanek, Taylor, Troxel, & van Stolk, 2016). Sleep deprivation is associated with injuries from accidents, chronic disease (e.g., coronary heart disease), and metabolic and endocrine complications. Also associated with sleep deprivation are mental illnesses such as depression, poor quality of life, and feelings and perceptions of diminished well-being, such as marital and social problems. Lack of sleep can be correlated with increased healthcare costs and loss of work productivity as well.

Sleep problems tend to be under-addressed. There are three categories of dyssomnias:

- Difficulty initiating sleep
- Difficulty maintaining sleep
- Early awakening

Parasomnias include the following conditions:

- *Nightmare disorder:* Defined as nightmares that repeatedly awaken the affected individual.
- *Sleep terror disorder:* Defined as recurrent episodes of abrupt awakening from sleep with intense fear and autonomic arousal such as tachycardia, rapid breathing, and sweating. During the episode, the individual is difficult to awaken or comfort. No dream is recalled, and the patient often does not remember the event the following day.
- *Sleepwalking disorder:* Characterized as repeated episodes of motor activity during sleep, including getting out of bed and walking around.

Primary sleep disorders can be further classified as *acute* or *chronic* insomnias. Acute insomnia lasts for no more than a few weeks and ends without treatment. Chronic insomnia occurs at least three nights per week and lasts longer than three months; it often requires treatment. Acute or chronic insomnia can be caused by a medical problem, such as respiratory disease, acute or chronic pain, hypothyroidism, sleep apnea, or restless legs syndrome. Acute or chronic insomnia can also be caused by life changes such as chronic stress, depression, and emotional difficulties (Sateia, Buysse, Krystal, Neubauer, & Heald, 2017).

Medications used as sleep aids are summarized in TABLE 14-9.

Sleep Hypnotic Drugs

The sleep hypnotic drugs work by suppressing the CNS. Benzodiazepines, which are used as anxiolytic agents at lower doses, promote sleep at higher doses via their inhibitory actions in the sleep centers. The benzodiazepine-like drugs such as zolpidem, zaleplon, and eszopiclone work in a fashion similar to the benzodiazepines and are the preferred agents for treating sleep disorders because they are generally well tolerated, are eliminated rapidly by the liver, and have

TABLE 14-9	Commonly Used Sleep Aids (Nonbarbiturate)		
Generic Name	Class	Notes	
Clonazepam	Benzodiazepine	By prescription only	
Diazepam	Benzodiazepine	By prescription only	
Diphenhydramine	Antihistamine	Sold OTC as an allergy medication; commonly found in OTC "PM" analgesic formulations	
Doxylamine (+ diphenhydramine)	Antihistamine	Sold OTC as a sleep aid	
Eszopiclone	Nonbenzodiazepine sedative	By prescription only	
Lorazepam	Benzodiazepine	By prescription only	
Melatonin	Endogenous biochemical	Sold as OTC supplement	
Promethazine	Antihistamine	By prescription only	
Triazolam	Benzodiazepine	By prescription only	
Zaleplon	Nonbenzodiazepine sedative	By prescription only	
Zolpidem	Nonbenzodiazepine sedative	By prescription only	

a low abuse potential. Historically, **barbiturates** were used in the treatment of anxiety, epilepsy, as anesthetics, and to induce sleep. Barbiturates also bind GABA receptors, but they have a high abuse potential and can be fatal with overdosage, so they are not normally considered drugs of choice for sleep disorders and are rarely prescribed for these indications. However, barbiturates may be cautiously considered if other treatments have failed. For example, phenobarbital, a long-acting barbiturate, is indicated for use as a sedative and anticonvulsant. Its onset of action occurs within 30 minutes, and the duration of action ranges from 5 to 6 hours.

The sleep hypnotics help induce *and* improve the quality of sleep in patients with dyssomnias and parasomnias. The total hours of sleep may be increased and the number of nighttime awakenings may be decreased, thereby affording patients improved sleep quality. These drugs also can be effective for managing anxiety, especially when the anxiety adversely affects the sleep cycle.

Adverse Reactions

All of the sleep hypnotics cause CNS depression. Their side effects include daytime drowsiness, dizziness, problems with motor coordination, and possibly cognitive changes, including memory deficits, with long-term use. Amnesia and forgetfulness can occur. Behaviors such as sleep-driving and preparing and eating foods in an amnesic state have been reported.

Benzodiazepines and benzodiazepine-like medications are generally well tolerated. Barbiturates, in contrast, can produce tolerance and dependence, and have a high abuse potential. Rebound anxiety and rebound insomnia have been reported with benzodiazepine *and* barbiturate withdrawal, but the incidence is lower with benzodiazepine-like medications. Tolerance can occur with benzodiazepine-like medications but the incidence is very low. Tolerance and medication dependence can occur with the benzodiazepines, especially at the higher doses, but again, the incidence is fairly low.

The benzodiazepines are designed for short-term use or as-needed use. Long-term use, for periods greater than 30 days, and higher doses can lead to more serious withdrawal symptoms. Abrupt cessation of benzodiazepines and barbiturates use should be avoided. Instead, tapering of dosages is recommended, normally over a period of weeks or months.

Withdrawal symptoms include rebound anxiety and rebound insomnia, lack of restfulness, orthostatic hypotension, confusion, and disorientation. In serious cases, hypertension, paranoia, seizures, cardiovascular collapse, and death are possible from withdrawal. Pregnant women should not be prescribed benzodiazepines.

Drug–Drug Interactions

Caution should be used when combining benzodiazepines, benzodiazepine-like drugs, or barbiturates with medications or other substances that may increase the depressive effects of the CNS system, including alcohol and opioids. Such a combination can cause respiratory depression, coma, and even death. Oral contraceptives may increase the clearance of (and so lower the plasma concentration of) lorazepam. Valproic acid may reduce the clearance and increase the plasma levels of lorazepam. Sertraline may reduce the clearance and increase the plasma levels of zolpidem. Sleep hypnotics should be used with caution with patients who have respiratory problems or obstructive sleep apnea because they can further depress the respiratory system.

Other Sleep Aids

Trazodone and mirtazapine are atypical antidepressants because they react differently to neurotransmitters than do SSRIs or SNRIs. They are often used as sleep medications on an off-label basis because they have a sedating side effect and can be very effective in initiating and maintaining sleep. Trazodone's sedative effects are related to H_1 properties and blockade of serotonin 2A receptors. Mirtazapine's sedative effects seem to be related to H_1 receptor antagonism.

Other over-the-counter medications such as melatonin and diphenhydramine (an antihistamine) can also be considered as options for sleep. Patients should be warned against combining these readily available options with prescription CNS depressants, and to avoid concomitant use of any "PM" formulations of analgesics, as these products almost always contain diphenhydramine to promote sleep.

Prescribing Considerations for Sleep Aids

All sleep medications can lead to troubling adverse reactions, and their use should be limited to avoid dependency and abuse. Benzodiazepines and benzodiazepine-like medications are the most popular sleep agents and the most frequently used. They tend to have a short half-life because they are metabolized quickly in the liver. These drugs also have fewer side effects than other sleep agents. Pregnancy risk must be evaluated carefully, and women counseled as to the benefits and potential risks. In general, the barbiturates should be avoided and relegated to "last resort" status for treating individuals with severely disturbed sleep and no contraindicating health issues.

Sleep hygiene, behavioral changes, and treatment of other underlying medical problems should always be addressed before medications are prescribed for sleep problems. All sleep hypnotic medications are indicated for short-term use only—that is, two to three nights in a row—and caution should be used if they are prescribed for longer periods of time or for chronic insomnia because tolerance may develop. Rebound insomnia can occur with the discontinuation of a hypnotic medication (Roth & Culpepper, 2008). The sleep hypnotic eszopiclone, however, has been approved for long-term use and does not appear to lead to tolerance.

CHAPTER SUMMARY

Mental health issues encompass a wide range of biochemical imbalances and dysfunctions. Depression, anxiety, psychosis, bipolar disorder, ADHD, and sleep disturbances are among the most common—and, unfortunately, the most likely to be undertreated or misdiagnosed—psychiatric conditions seen. Identifying the appropriate medical therapies is important, but awareness of the potential for severe side effects related to enhanced neurotransmitter levels, particularly with respect to serotonin, is of key importance to safe and effective treatment. A number of psychiatric medications, including antidepressants, stimulants, and sedatives, are prone to abuse, and patients taking these agents should be monitored.

Critical Thinking Questions

1. Which three neurotransmitters are affected by most antidepressant drugs?

2. What causes serotonin syndrome?

3. Which antipsychotic drugs are indicated for bipolar disorder?

4. Which key drug interactions must be identified and avoided when treating a patient with concomitant anxiety and insomnia?

5. Why are MAOIs subject to significant dietary restrictions?

6. Which considerations might make atomoxetine a better choice than a stimulant drug for treating a 16-year-old male with history of mild episodic depression who has been recently diagnosed with ADHD?

CASE SCENARIO 1

M.T. is a 22-year-old male who has been transported to the emergency department via the police department from a local coffee shop. Police were notified after M.T. was found to be agitated, with a disheveled appearance and loudly speaking to another person despite the fact that he was alone at the table and there was no one else in the coffee shop other than the employee. He was upset and shouting curse words and appeared to feel threatened, stating, "I'll get you before you get me."

Upon examination in the emergency department, M.T. exhibited similar behavior. His lab work and vital signs were normal. He stated that he takes medications for voices and paranoia but stopped the medications 10 days prior because "They make me tired and fat."

M.T. reluctantly agreed to take a combined intramuscular injection of the antipsychotic haloperidol and the antianxiety medication lorazepam to control the auditory hallucinations, agitation, and paranoia. He became much calmer and less psychotic over the following two hours. M.T. was released and referred to his psychiatric prescriber and support services for a follow-up appointment.

Case Questions

1. What evidence supports that this patient may be psychotic?

2. What evidence of positive and negative symptoms is present?

3. What evidence of adverse reactions to use of antipsychotic medications is present?

4. Which medications were used to treat the acute psychotic symptoms and agitation, and which other treatment recommendations were made?

CASE SCENARIO 2

Mrs. A. is a 45-year-old woman who presents at her primary care physician's office with complaints of fatigue, sadness, lack of interest, lack of pleasure of normally pleasurable life events, excessive sleep, frequent crying, and difficulty with focusing and paying attention. These symptoms have been present for the past three months, after she lost her job and her only child moved to another state to attend college. Mrs. A. also states she has been increasingly anxious, avoids social gatherings and crowds, and is increasingly uncomfortable leaving the house. The lab work and physical exam are normal. Mrs. A. states she has a family history of depression.

Case Questions

1. What evidence supports that this patient may have a depressive or an anxiety disorder?
2. Which category of medication is the first-line choice for treatment of depression and anxiety?
3. What would be some of the signs of positive response to treatment, and in what time period would you expect to see benefits from the medication?

CASE SCENARIO 3

S.T. is a 22-year-old man who informed his therapist that he has experienced significant mood swings recently. He reports episodes of feeling sad and depressed, crying, lack of motivation and energy, excessive time in bed, and vague thoughts of suicide. These episodes can last for up to 7 to 10 days. S.T. then experiences a rapid mood change to episodes of feeling elated and very happy with excessive energy and lack of need for sleep. During the last episode he was involved with risky behavior such as drug use and unsafe sex on multiple occasions, and impulsive behavior such as unwise spending of his money. This episode also lasted 7 to 10 days. S.T. was arrested for driving under the influence of alcohol at excessive speed. He tells his therapist, "My mood is all over the place. I lost my job because I got into an argument with my boss. I just want to feel normal again." Referral to a psychiatric prescriber resulted in a trial of lithium in an effort to stabilize S.T.'s mood and reduce or eliminate the episodes of mania and depression.

Case Questions

1. What evidence is present to indicate a diagnosis of depression? Of mania?
2. Which medication was prescribed, and what was the rationale for prescribing the medication?

CASE SCENARIO 4

Mr. F. has been struggling with an inability to complete his work and to stay productive both in the office and at home. His boss and his wife state that he has difficulty paying attention, focusing, concentrating, and staying on task. He often starts a task and then is easily distracted, going on to another task before completing the original task. His boss has placed him on probation because of inconsistencies in his work.

Mr. F's eight-year-old son was recently diagnosed with ADHD and has been prescribed an amphetamine. Mr. F. recognizes similar problems with his own behavior. His general practitioner has considered a trial with amphetamine, methylphenidate, or atomoxetine. He decided to initiate an amphetamine because Mr. F's son has responded well to the medication and is now slowly titrating the dosage according to the response. Mr. F. reports that he is better able to pay attention, focus, concentrate, and stay on task. He reports he is less distracted and thus able to complete tasks and increase his productivity.

Case Questions

1. Which symptoms are present that indicate a diagnosis of ADD/ADHD?
2. Which medications are used to treat the disorder?
3. Which benefits from the medication did Mr. F. report?

CASE SCENARIO 5

Mrs. B. has recently experienced an increase in stress due to relationship problems at home as well as financial stressors. She has had an increase in symptoms of anxiety and notes "sleep changes." She has difficulty falling asleep and wakes every two to three hours throughout the night. Often the worries and concerns of the day are present in her thoughts when lying awake in bed. Mrs. B. feels sleepy during the day and has noted that she is less productive at home and at work.

Her nurse practitioner reviewed Mrs. B's sleep hygiene and then recommended a two-week trial with clonazepam at bedtime, as well as a referral to a psychotherapist for talk therapy to address her problems and concerns. Mrs. B. reported feeling more relaxed after taking the medication before bedtime and was able to fall asleep and remain sleeping for six to eight hours. Feeling more rested during the day helped her to function better at home and at work. She also made an appointment with a therapist to address her problems and concerns and learn a nonpharmacologic approach for insomnia, including cognitive-behavioral therapy.

Case Questions

1. Which symptoms are present that indicate a sleep disorder?
2. Which interventions are used to treat the sleep disorder?
3. What are the benefits of the sleep medication?
4. Which adverse events might be monitored in a patient taking this medication?

REFERENCES

Albert, M., Rui, P., & Ashman, J.J. (2017). *Physician office visits for attention-deficit/hyperactivity disorder in children and adolescents aged 4–17 years: United States, 2012–2013*. NCHS Data Brief No. 269. Hyattsville, MD: National Center for Health Statistics. Retrieved from https://stacks.cdc.gov/view/cdc/49009

Alper, K., Schwartz, K.A., Kolts, R.L., & Khan, A. (2007). Seizure incidence in psychopharmacological clinical trials: An analysis of Food and Drug Administration (FDA) summary basis of approval reports. *Biology and Psychiatry, 62*(4), 345–354.

American Psychiatric Association (APA). (2002). Practice guideline for the treatment of patients with bipolar disorder (revision). *American Journal of Psychiatry, 159*(Suppl.), 1–50.

American Psychiatric Association (APA). (2013). *Diagnostic and statistical manual of mental disorders* (5th ed.). Washington, DC: Author.

Arora, B., & Kannikeswaran, N. (2010). The serotonin syndrome—the need for physician's awareness. *International Journal of Emergency Medicine, 3*(4), 373–377. doi: 10.1007/s12245-010-0195-7

Barner, J., Khoza, S., & Oladapo, A. (2011). ADHD medication use, adherence, persistence and cost among Texas Medicaid children. *Current Medical Research and Opinion, 27*(Suppl. 2), 13–22.

Borrelli, F., & Izzo, A.A. (2009). Herb–drug interactions with St John's wort (*Hypericum perforatum*): An update on clinical observations. *The AAPS Journal, 11*(4), 710. doi: 10.1208/s12248-009-9146-8

Bostwick, J., Casher, M., & Yasugi, S. (2012). Benzodiazepines: A versatile clinical tool. *Current Psychiatry, 11*(4), 55–62.

Bridge, J.A., Iyengar, S., Salary, C.B., Barbe, R.P., Birmaher, B., Pincus, H.A., . . . Brent, D.A. (2007). Clinical response and risk for reported suicidal ideation and suicide attempts in pediatric antidepressant treatment: A meta-analysis of randomized controlled trials. *JAMA, 297*, 1683–1696.

Centers for Disease Control and Prevention (CDC). (2012). Retrieved from https://www.cdc.gov/sleep/index.html

Centers for Disease Control and Prevention (CDC). (2017). Attention-deficit/hyperactivity disorder (ADHD): Facts about ADHD. Retrieved from http://www.cdc.gov/ncbddd/adhd/facts.html

Dannawi, M. (2002). Possible serotonin syndrome after combination of buspirone and St John's wort. *Journal of Psychopharmacology, 16*(4), 401.

El-Mallakh, R.S., Elmaadawi, A.Z., Gao, Y., Lohano, K., & Roberts, R.J. (2011). Current and emerging therapies for the management of bipolar disorders. *Journal of Central Nervous System Disease, 7*(3), 189–197.

English, B.A., Dortch, M., Ereshefsky, L., & Jhee, S. (2012). Clinically significant psychotropic drug-drug interactions in the primary care setting. *Current Psychiatry Reports, 14*(4), 376–390. doi: 10.1007/s11920-012-0284-9

Finbert, J.P.M., & Rabey, J.M. (2016). Inhibitors of MAO-A and MAO-B in psychiatry and neurology. *Frontiers in Pharmacology, 18*. doi: 10.3389/fphar.2016.00340

Flockhart, D.A. (2012). Dietary restrictions and drug interactions with monoamine oxidase inhibitors: An update. *Journal of Clinical Psychiatry, 73*(Suppl. 1), 17–24.

Food and Drug Administration (FDA). (2010). *FDA drug safety communication: Aseptic meningitis associated with use of Lamictal (lamotrigine)*. Retrieved from http://www.fda.gov/drugs/drugsafety/postmarketdrugsafetyinformationforpatientsandproviders/ucm221847.htm

Garnock-Jones, K.P., & Keating, G.M. (2009). Atomoxetine: A review of its use in attention-deficit hyperactivity disorder in children and adolescents. *Paediatric Drugs, 11*(3), 203–226.

Gibbons, R.D., Coca-Perraillon, M., Hur, K., Conti, R.M., Valuck, R.J., & Brent D.A. (2015). Antidepressant treatment and suicide attempts and self-inflicted injury in children and adolescents. *Pharmacoepidemiology Drug Safety, 24*, 208–214, doi: 10.1002/pds.3713

Goodman, D.W. (2010). Lisdexamfetamine dimesylate (Vyvanse), a prodrug stimulant for attention-deficit/hyperactivity disorder. *Pharmacy and Therapeutics, 35*(5), 273–276, 282–287.

Graham, J., Banaschewski, T., Buitelaar, J., Coghill, D., Danckaerts, M., Dittmann, R.W., . . . Taylor, E. (2011). European guidelines on managing adverse effects of medication for ADHD. *European Child and Adolescent Psychiatry, 20*(1), 17–37.

Griffin, C.E. III, Kaye, A.M., Bueno, F.R., & Kaye, A.D. (2013). Benzodiazepine pharmacology and central nervous system–mediated effects. *Ochsner Journal, 13*(2), 214–223.

Hafner, M., Stepanek, M., Taylor, J., Troxel, W.M., & van Stolk, C. (2016). *Why sleep matters – The economic costs of insufficient sleep: A cross-country comparative analysis*. Cambridge, United Kingdom: Rand Corporation.

Hawthorne, M. (2017). Patients unaware of the risks of antidepressants – TGA. *Australian Medicine, 29*(1), 9.

Hussain, H., Dubicka, B., & Wilkinson, P. (2017). Newer generation antidepressants for young people: Real-life evidence needed. Commentary on . . . Cochrane Corner. *British Journal of Psychiatry, 23*(2), 75–80. doi: 10.1192/apt.bp.116.016717

Klemow, K.M., Bartlow, A., Crawford, J., Kocher, N., Shah, J., & Ritsick, M. (2011). Medical attributes of St. John's wort (*Hypericum perforatum*). In I.F.F. Benzie & S. Wachtel-Galor (Eds.), *Herbal medicine: Biomolecular and clinical aspects* (2nd ed.). Boca Raton, FL: CRC Press.

Kosinski, E., & Rothschild, A. (2012). Monoamine oxidase inhibitors: Forgotten treatment for depression. *Current Psychiatry, 11*(12), 20–26.

Lehne, R. (2015). *Pharmacology for nursing care* (9th ed.). St. Louis, MO: Saunders.

Leucht, S., Corves, C., Arbter, D., Engel, R.R., Li, C., & Davis, J.M. (2009). Second-generation versus first-generation antipsychotic drugs for schizophrenia: A meta-analysis. *Lancet, 373*(9657), 31–41.

Llorca, P.M., Abbar, M., Courtet, P., Guillaume, S., Lancrenon, S., & Samalin, L. (2013). Guidelines for the use and management of long-acting injectable antipsychotics in serious mental illness. *BMC Psychiatry, 13*(1), 340.

Moller, H. (2006). Is there evidence for negative effects of antidepressants on suicidality in depressive patients? *European Archives of Psychiatry and Clinical Neuroscience, 256,* 476–496.

Morrison, E.K., & Rowe, A.S. (2012). Probable drug–drug interaction leading to serotonin syndrome in a patient treated with concomitant buspirone and linezolid in the setting of therapeutic hypothermia. *Journal of Clinical Pharmacy and Therapeutics, 37*(5), 610–613.

National Center for Chronic Disease Prevention and Health Promotion, Division of Population Health. (2017). Sleep and sleep disorders. Retrieved from https://www.cdc.gov/sleep/index.html

National Institute of Mental Health. (2012). *Any anxiety disorder among adults.* Retrieved from https://www.nimh.nih.gov/health/statistics/any-anxiety-disorder.shtml

National Institute of Mental Health. (2017). *Bipolar disorder.* Retrieved from https://www.nimh.nih.gov/health/statistics/bipolar-disorder.shtml

Pastor, P.N., Reuben, C.A., Duran, C.R., & Hawkins, L.D. (2015). *Association between diagnosed ADHD and selected characteristics among children aged 4–17 years: United States, 2011–2013.* NCHS Data Brief No. 201. Hyattsville, MD: National Center for Health Statistics.

Poulton, A.S., Bui, Q., Melzer, E., & Evans, R. (2016). Stimulant medication effects on growth and bone age in children with attention-deficit/hyperactivity disorder: A prospective cohort study. *International Clinical Psychopharmacology, 31*(2), 93–99. doi: 10.1097/YIC.0000000000000109

Reed, V.A., Buitelaar, J.K., Anand, E., Day, K.A., Treuer, T., Upadhyaya, H.P., . . . Savill, N.C. (2016). The safety of atomoxetine for the treatment of children and adolescents with attention-deficit/hyperactivity disorder: A comprehensive review over a decade of research. *CNS Drugs, 30*(7), 603–628.

Reimherr, F.W., Hedges, D.W., Strong, R.E., Marchant, B.K., & Williams, E.D. (2005). Bupropion SR in adults with ADHD: A short-term, placebo-controlled trial. *Neuropsychiatry Disease and Treatment, 1*(3), 245–251.

Roth, T., & Culpepper, L. (2008). Insomnia management in primary care. *Clinical Symposia, 58*(1), 18–19.

Sateia, M.J., Buysse, D.J., Krystal, A.D., Neubauer, D.N., & Heald, J.L. (2017). Clinical practice guideline for the pharmacologic treatment of chronic insomnia in adults: An American Academy of Sleep Medicine clinical practice guideline. *Journal of Clinical Sleep Medicine, 13*(2), 307–349.

Slight, S.P., Seger, D.L., Nanji, K.C., Cho, I., Maniam, N., & Dykes, P.C. (2013). Are we heeding the warning signs? Examining providers' overrides of computerized drug–drug interaction alerts in primary care. *PLoS One, 8*(12), e85071.

Spies, P.E., Pot, J.L.W., Willems, R.P.J., Box, J.M., & Kramers, C. (2016). Interaction between tramadol and selective serotonin reuptake inhibitors: Are doctors aware of the potential risks in their prescription practice? *European Journal of Hospital Pharmacy.* doi: 10.1136/ejhpharm-2015-000838

Stahl, S. (2005). *The prescriber's guide.* New York, NY: Cambridge University Press.

Stahl, S. (2008). *Stahl's essential psychopharmacology.* New York, NY: Cambridge University Press.

Termorshuizen, F., Smeets, H.M., Boks, M.P.M., & Heerdink, E.R. (2016). Comparing episodes of antidepressants use with intermittent episodes of no use: A higher relative risk of suicide attempts but not of suicide at young age. *Journal of Psychopharmacology, 30*(10), 1000–1007.

U.S. National Library of Medicine. (2011). Bipolar disorder. Retrieved from http://www.ncbi.nlm.nih.gov/pubmedhealth/PMH0001924/

Walker, F.R. (2013). A critical review of the mechanism of action for the selective serotonin reuptake inhibitors: Do these drugs possess anti-inflammatory properties and how relevant is this in the treatment of depression? *Neuropharmacology, 67,* 304–317.

World Health Organization (WHO). (n.d.). *Mental health: Schizophrenia.* Retrieved from http://www.who.int/mental_health/management/schizophrenia/en/

World Health Organization (WHO). (2017). *Depression.* Retrieved from http://www.who.int/mediacentre/factsheets/fs369/en/

CHAPTER 15

Pharmacology of Anesthetic Drugs

Dwayne Accardo

Amide (anesthetic)
Anesthetic adjunct
Chemoreceptor trigger
 zone (CTZ)
Conduction blockade
Depolarizing
Epidural

Ester (anesthetic)
Hypnotics
Induction anesthesia
Infiltrative anesthesia
Inhalational anesthetic
Laryngospasm
Local anesthetic

Maintenance anesthesia
Minimum alveolar
 concentration (MAC)
Nondepolarizing
Offset
Onset
Opioid receptors

Postoperative nausea
 and vomiting (PONV)
Pruritus
Sedation
Topical anesthetic

CHAPTER OBJECTIVES

At the end of the chapter, the reader will be able to:

1. Discuss the various types of anesthetic drugs and various forms of anesthesia.

2. Explain how each type of anesthesia is administered, and under which circumstances it is used.

3. Describe the potential benefits and drawbacks of inhalational versus intravenous general anesthesia.

4. Identify specific anesthetics that offer unique benefits for specific patient populations.

5. Describe various anesthetic adjuncts and explain why they are used.

Introduction

Anesthetic drugs are medications intended to reduce or eliminate sensation. In addition, several drugs also affect the patient's awareness of surroundings or reduce consciousness. Anesthetics are used in patients who are (or may be) experiencing pain or other unpleasant sensations (e.g., **pruritus**) and are of particular importance for patients who are undergoing surgical procedures or other forms of therapy that can be painful or difficult to tolerate.

Anesthetics produce their effects via a variety of mechanisms, including those that are central nervous system (CNS) depressants that act on gamma-aminobutyric acid (GABA) and *N*-methyl-D-aspartate (NMDA) receptors in the brain and spinal column. Important mechanisms will be discussed here.

Types of Anesthesia

There are a number of disparate drugs considered anesthetics, and they are not all administered via the same route. **Topical anesthetics** are medications provided in creams, ointments, gels, or other vehicles for use on superficial skin conditions that cause pain or itching. These pass through the skin to soothe pain or inflammation in muscles or joints. **Local anesthetics** are used to block pain or other sensations in a specific area of the body when complete or partial sedation is not desired or is contraindicated. These medications are primarily drugs with the suffix "caine," of which the best-known example is **procaine**, commonly used in oral or dental surgery to create **conduction blockade** in the nerves of the mouth. Other types of nerve blockade are applied through **epidural** and spinal injection, which offer regional anesthesia by means of application of local anesthetic to a particular set of nerves feeding the region in which sensory, motor, or autonomic nerve blockade is desired (most often this involves injecting the agent into the spine). **Inhalational anesthetics** are inhaled drugs, for which *general anesthesia* (complete unconsciousness) or *partial anesthesia* (semi-consciousness), are the most common applications. These drugs are used for patients undergoing surgery or other invasive, stressful, or complex procedures that require the patient to remain still for long stretches of time. Inhalational agents come either as gases (e.g., **nitrous oxide**) or volatile liquids (e.g., **sevoflurane**). Alternatively, intravenous agents may be used to accomplish the same goals without inhalational medications, or in addition to them. These include barbiturates, opioids, benzodiazepines, and nonbarbiturate **hypnotics**, which are used most often to provide general anesthesia or modified sedation as well as, in some cases, pain relief. Inhalational and intravenous agents are often used simultaneously or in succession so that their complementary effects may work to the patient's advantage.

In general anesthesia, subcategories of therapies exist, including induction anesthesia, maintenance anesthesia, and anesthetic adjuncts. **Induction anesthesia** is the process of creating a state of unconsciousness or semi-consciousness (**sedation**) prior to a painful or unpleasant procedure. Diverse drugs administered by various means may be considered based on patient characteristics, goals of the anesthesia, and other factors—for instance, a patient with a fear of needles might do better with an inhalational agent, whereas a patient prone to respiratory illnesses might have a superior response to an intravenous medication. **Maintenance anesthesia** is the use of agents to prolong the unconscious or sedated state for procedures that require a time frame longer than the induction agent usually lasts; often, the maintenance agent used differs from the induction agent, and it may even be administered via a different method. Often, **anesthetic adjuncts** (usually administered intravenously) are used to limit the patient's pain and enhance the sedating effects of the maintenance anesthetic. A few of these adjuncts may also address other factors of concern during surgery, including nausea or vomiting (which may be directly caused by some anesthetics, particularly volatile agents), and the unwelcome possibility that the patient may move or twitch during delicate procedures. Nonanesthetic adjuncts such as muscle relaxants and antiemetic drugs support patient well-being during and immediately after procedures by reducing these complicating factors.

Not all anesthesia requires patients to become unconscious or semi-conscious. Anesthetic drugs may be used simply to deaden sensation in a particular area so that a procedure may be undertaken without the patient feeling discomfort. This practice is common in dentistry, dermatology, and obstetrics. It is also used in certain types of neurosurgery where the patient's ability to produce a voluntary movement or report sensations is helpful to the surgeon. The medications used for this purpose may include a topical anesthetic drug, used to "deaden" skin sensation for superficial procedures (often simply as a precursor to injecting another medication or setting an intravenous line), or a local anesthetic injected to block nerve impulses in a specific region of the body for the duration of a short, relatively superficial procedure. Most of the agents used in topical and local anesthesia are the same, but they are delivered by diverse means and are intended to have varying levels of effect upon the nerves.

Topical and local anesthetics are used far more commonly than are those for systemic anesthesia. For example, topical anesthetics that contain **benzocaine** are sold over-the-counter for temporary pain relief caused from sunburn pain, for soothing painful gums, and to relieve severe itching. Topical anesthetics are also included in lozenges intended for temporary relief of sore throat pain. Topical and local anesthetics will be addressed first in this chapter, as they are more likely to be encountered and are used frequently in general nursing practice. Other forms of anesthetic/analgesic drugs are usually encountered in the context of surgery or postsurgical recovery or critical care nursing.

Local and Topical Anesthesia

Local anesthetics are commonly used in anesthetic practice, especially for regional anesthesia and peripheral nerve blocks. Local anesthetics are classified as either **amides** or **esters**; the majority fall in the amide class of drugs, largely because those in the ester class are more likely to induce allergic responses. TABLE 15-1 lists agents commonly used for local and topical anesthesia.

TABLE 15-1	Local Anesthetic Drugs		
Drug	Class	Uses	Cautions
Benzocaine	Ester	Used primarily for treatment of pain in the oral cavity, in dentistry, and treatment of ear pain. Many over-the-counter products for sore throat or teething pain (lozenges, sprays, gels) include this medication.	Limited risks when used as directed. Persons with hypersensitivity to other ester-class anesthetics should not use this product.
Bupivacaine	Amide	Used in local infiltrative anesthesia, regional (epidural and spinal), and transdermally for postherpetic neuralgia.	Contraindicated for use in obstetrics or in children younger than age 12. Must not be used in combination with epinephrine on distal surfaces (e.g., ear, nose, toes). In epidural and spinal anesthesia, preparations containing preservatives should be avoided. Concomitant use with chloroprocaine is toxic and contraindicated. Do not use in patients with personal or familial history of malignant hyperthermia.

(continues)

TABLE 15-1   Local Anesthetic Drugs *(continued)*

Drug	Class	Uses	Cautions
Chloroprocaine	Amide	Used for epidural, infiltrative, and peripheral nerve blockade in adults only, as safety in children has not been established.	In epidural anesthesia, preparations containing preservatives should be avoided. Must not be used in combination with epinephrine on distal surfaces (e.g., ear, nose, toes). Concomitant use with bupivacaine is toxic and contraindicated. Do not use in patients with personal or familial history of malignant hyperthermia.
Cocaine	Ester	Applied to mucous membranes of the mouth, nose, or larynx for local anesthesia in a 1% to 10% solution. Not widely used due to safety concerns.	Serious toxicity (seizures, cardiac arrest) is a key concern in elderly and pediatric patients, particularly when used topically admixed with epinephrine. Do not use in patients with personal or familial history of malignant hyperthermia.
Etidocaine	Amide	Primarily used as an infiltrative anesthetic in dentistry. May be used in epidural regional blockade but is not recommended for obstetric use due to inadequate safety data.	In epidural anesthesia, preparations containing preservatives should be avoided. Should not be used in patients with heart block. Safety in children has not been established. Do not use in patients with personal or familial history of malignant hyperthermia.
Lidocaine (xylocaine)	Amide	Used in topical liquid, ointment (5%), cream, or gel formulations for sunburn or superficial pruritus; oral gels for pain associated with teething or gum soreness; as a transdermal patch for mild, superficial muscle pain; or injected as a local infiltrative anesthetic (often in combination with epinephrine) to reduce bleeding. May be used in epidural or spinal anesthesia if no cardiac contraindications are present. In topical or transdermal uses, it is sometimes combined with prilocaine, bupivacaine, or tetracaine. A lidocaine/prilocaine combination (EMLA) is commonly used prior to needle puncture for blood collection or other purposes.	Lidocaine is a Class IB antiarrhythmic; thus, it should not be used in patients with certain cardiac conditions (e.g., those who require a pacemaker or who are being concurrently treated with other Class I antiarrhythmic agents). It can be toxic to the CNS in excessive doses (plasma levels >6–10 mcg/mL), with early signs of toxicity manifesting as seizures and later signs manifesting as respiratory depression or arrest. Combinations with epinephrine or epinephrine/tetracaine should not be used on broken skin or on distal surfaces (e.g., nose, ear, toes). Do not use in patients with personal or familial history of malignant hyperthermia.
Mepivacaine	Amide	Used in infiltration anesthesia, spinal/epidural anesthesia.	In epidural or spinal anesthesia, preparations containing preservatives should be avoided. Do not use in patients with personal or familial history of malignant hyperthermia. Concomitant use with bupivacaine is toxic and contraindicated.
Prilocaine	Amide	Infiltrative anesthesia, usually in dentistry. Combined in topical formulations with lidocaine (e.g., EMLA cream, EMLA patch, and generic variants of both).	In high doses (more than 600 mg), may cause methemoglobinemia. Combinations with epinephrine should not be used on broken skin or on distal surfaces (e.g., nose, ear, toes). Do not use in patients with personal or familial history of malignant hyperthermia.
Procaine	Ester	Used primarily for infiltrative local anesthesia, to reduce pain of penicillin G injections, and in dentistry. Not selected for other uses due to the availability of more effective and less allergenic alternatives such as lidocaine.	Risk of CNS depression and hypersensitivity response, cardiac arrest.
Ropivacaine	Amide	Used in epidural and spinal anesthesia (including obstetrics).	Do not use in children younger than age 12. Do not use in patients with personal or familial history of malignant hyperthermia. Combinations with epinephrine should not be used on broken skin or on distal surfaces (e.g., nose, ear, toes).
Tetracaine	Ester	Used in spinal anesthesia, ophthalmic anesthesia, and in spray form for the larynx. A topical combination containing epinephrine and cocaine (TAC) for surgical repair of skin lesions has fallen into disuse in favor of a safer formulation of lidocaine, epinephrine, and tetracaine (LET).	In spinal anesthesia, preparations containing preservatives should be avoided. Combinations with epinephrine or epinephrine/lidocaine should not be used on broken skin or on distal surfaces (e.g., nose, ear, toes). Do not use in patients with personal or familial history of malignant hyperthermia. TAC should not be used on intact skin.

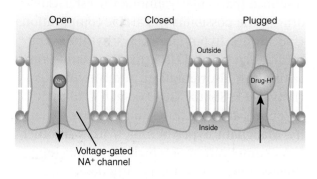

Open   Closed   Plugged

Outside

Na⁺   Drug-H⁺

Inside

Voltage-gated
NA⁺ channel

FIGURE 15-1 Voltage-gated sodium channels.

Most local anesthetics work by interfering with nerve signaling, thereby reducing permeability of voltage-gated sodium channels (**FIGURE 15-1**). When sodium cannot pass through these channels, the ability of the channels to conduct signals is reduced, effectively interrupting the transmission of the nerve's "message" of pain to the brain. Local anesthetics bind to sodium channels most efficiently when the channels are in an activated state, meaning that the drugs take effect more rapidly in neurons that are excited than in those that are quiescent. As a consequence of this state-dependent blockade, a topical medication—for instance, EMLA cream composed of 2.5% lidocaine and 2.5% prilocaine—will work faster in a patient whose skin has a rash or a sunburn than it will in a patient whose skin is undamaged and whose dermal nerves are not in a state of excitement.

Administration of the drugs is performed via a variety of means. Topical administration, in which the drug is added to a vehicle (e.g., an oil-based cream or ointment, a gel, or a liquid solution that can be sprayed or wiped onto the surface to be treated), is an extremely common route of delivery. Many topical preparations containing anesthetic drugs are sold as over-the-counter products for home treatment of burns, rashes, sore throat, or minor wounds. Some popular products for treating sunburn, for example,

contain a combination of lidocaine, which blocks the pain signals, and aloe, which promotes healing and protects the damaged skin from further drying and abrasion. In recent years, transdermal patches have gained in popularity as a means of administering topical anesthetics for relief of discomfort either on the skin itself or immediately subdermally (e.g., muscle pain).

Infiltrative anesthesia is delivered via direct injection to the nerves that require blockade. There are several purposes for which this technique is used:

- *Infiltrative nerve blockade* is a conduction block used to eliminate sensation in a specific location that is to undergo an invasive procedure. It is preferred for any form of relatively minor surgery in which it is undesirable for the patient to move or feel the procedure but he or she need not be unconscious for the surgery to be performed. Local conduction blocks, such as a brachial plexus block, numb the arm and shoulder; this type of nerve blockade might be used prior to repair of torn ligaments or rotator cuff, for example.
- *Intra-articular injections* are used to manage postsurgical pain or arthritis pain in joints such as the knee or the hip.
- *Epidural anesthesia* is a form of conduction blockade in which the local anesthetic is injected into the epidural space surrounding the spinal cord's dura mater. It is commonly used in obstetrics because it is somewhat safer than spinal anesthesia.
- *Spinal anesthesia* is a form of infiltrative nerve blockade similar to epidural anesthesia in that it targets the spinal cord, but in which the local anesthetic is injected *through* the dura mater into the subarachnoid space to produce paralysis and lack of sensation in the lower body. The needle is introduced between the lumbar vertebrae (usually L4 and L5). In some instances, the anesthetic may disperse to the upper thoracic region, so that the patient

may require support in the form of mechanical ventilation (Smeltzer, Bare, Hinkle, & Cheever, 2008); such risks, along with the obvious risk of direct damage to the spinal nerves and/or introduction of infection into the cerebrospinal fluid, are the main reason why epidural anesthesia is preferred if possible in most patients.

- *Subcutaneous infiltration* is used to deaden multiple layers of skin quickly and thoroughly for invasive procedures such as intravenous line placement, skin biopsies, or wound repair using sutures or staples. It is superior to simple topical application of anesthetic because the anesthetic agent is absorbed much more rapidly and more thoroughly.

- *Submucosal infiltration* is used in dental procedures and for repair of mucosal lacerations. Injection is preferred to topical application in these circumstances because complete coverage of the nerves needing blockade is guaranteed; the main drawback is that infiltration lasts longer and produces effects that generally outlast the need (as anyone who has left the dentist with numbed lips and tongues will know).

- *Wound infiltration* is used to manage postoperative pain at the site of a surgical incision or a laceration that has been repaired.

While local anesthesia via infiltrative techniques may be administered by clinicians in most cases, spinal and epidural anesthesia are always administered by a specialist due to the need for significant training and expertise in penetrating the correct spinal structure without damaging the spinal cord. Because such cases are always in the care of an anesthesia provider, the discussion of the local anesthetic drugs provided here will, for the most part, assume that they have been used for less invasive procedures.

Adverse Effects

Among the key effects of concern with local anesthetics are the potential for allergic response (particularly among the ester-class drugs), the possibility of cardiac complications (specifically, hypotension, dysrhythmia, and cardiac arrest), and CNS toxicity, manifesting as tinnitus, disorientation, and convulsions (Dewaele & Santos, 2013). Such CNS toxicity occurs at lower doses than cardiac toxicity. Malignant hyperthermia (MH) is another, rarer complication of which clinicians nonetheless must be aware, as early detection, cessation of anesthesia, and treatment with **dantrolene sodium** and sodium bicarbonate are essential to prevent mortality (Schneiderbanger, Johannsen, Roewer, & Schuster, 2014). MH is a type of severe reaction in susceptible individuals triggered by either volatile (inhaled) anesthetics or **succinylcholine**, a depolarizing muscle relaxant.

Inhalational Anesthesia

Inhalational anesthetics are used for the maintenance of general anesthesia and induce anesthesia by acting on the brain and spinal cord. They are effective by virtue of their access to the pulmonary circulation, which allows rapid uptake and distribution to the brain. Several theories have been proposed to explain how they work, but their overall mechanism of action remains unknown. The depth of anesthesia is reflected by the degree of suppression of consciousness and autonomic and motor reflexes.

To better understand the importance and the role of inhalational agents in anesthesia, it will help to cover a few basics regarding how they work in the body. Unlike ingested or injected agents, inhaled agents become distributed in the body along pressure gradients, rather than via absorption into serum and circulation. Equilibration occurs when the partial pressures of the inspired gas and the gas distributed into alveoli, blood, and tissues are the same (Becker & Rosenberg, 2008).

Solubility refers to how the body's tissues become saturated with the agent, with solubility of the agent in blood and in adipose tissue being the key reference points. The higher-solubility agents take longer to saturate the body and will be retained longer in the body after the agent is discontinued. Highly soluble agents also take longer to reach the brain to achieve their desired effect (**onset**) and dissipate from tissues more slowly (**offset**). Thus, the solubility and the rapidity of onset/recovery of an agent are important considerations affecting selection. In some circumstances, rapid onset and recovery are desirable; in others, they are not.

Another important factor in choosing an agent is *pungency*. A pungent agent is one with a very strong, ethereal odor that can make a patient breath-hold or cough with an inhalational induction. Pungency can be problematic for patients with strong gag reflexes, or for children.

Dosing is guided by the agent's **minimum alveolar concentration (MAC)**, which represents the alveolar concentration that prevents patient movement in 50% of patients in response to surgical stimulation. The MAC values are designed for patients aged 30 to 55 years, and the values for MACs are expressed as a percentage of 1 atmosphere at sea level (760 mm Hg). Obviously, if the patient is outside the rather narrow age range, the MAC for the agent must be adjusted to compensate. Similar adjustments must be made to account for factors that can alter concentration or solubility of the gas, such as the ambient temperature, the patient's alcohol consumption, electrolyte imbalances, pregnancy, coadministration with other drugs, and any preexisting disease processes in the patient.

Drugs Used for Inhalational Anesthesia

Currently available modern inhalational anesthetics include **nitrous oxide**, **isoflurane**, **desflurane**, and **sevoflurane**. Two other similar anesthetics, **halothane** and **enflurane**, are no longer used due to their dangerous side effects; both are linked to acute liver injury (National Institutes of Health [NIH], 2018a, 2018b). Although the chemical structures of **isoflurane**, **desflurane**, and **sevoflurane** are all very

similar, their respective mechanisms of action remain unknown. **Nitrous oxide** is a gas; the other three inhalational anesthetics are volatile liquids, meaning that the active ingredient is obtained by breathing in the fumes of the agent rather than taking in the agent itself (Smeltzer et al., 2008). All of these medications are combined with oxygen when administered, although the proportion of inhalant to oxygen varies depending on the agent, the goal of the anesthesia protocol (e.g., general anesthesia versus partial anesthesia), and the factors influencing the MAC. TABLE 15-2 provides MAC values for the four commonly used inhalational anesthetics.

Nitrous Oxide

Nitrous oxide (N_2O) is an odorless, colorless gas that has been in use as an anesthetic for more than 170 years. Its MAC is 104%, considerably higher than the MACs of other agents; **nitrous oxide**, therefore, cannot be used alone to produce general anesthesia due to the fact that the patient would

TABLE 15-2	MAC Values of Commonly Used Inhalational Anesthetics	
Agent	Patient Age	MAC
Nitrous oxide	~40 years	104*
	~80 years	81
Isoflurane + 100% oxygen	26 ± 4 years	1.28
	44 ± 7 years	1.15
	64 ± 5 years	1.05
Isoflurane + 70% nitrous oxide	26 ± 4 years	0.56
	44 ± 7 years	0.50
	64 ± 5 years	0.37
Desflurane + 100% oxygen	~40 years	6.6
	~80 years	5.1
Sevoflurane + 100% oxygen	~1 year	2.3
	~40 years	1.8
	~80 years	1.4

*As a single agent. Values of nitrous oxide combined with other agents are given separately where available.
Data from Nickalls, R.W.D., & Mapleson, W.W. (2003). Age-related iso-MAC charts for isoflurane, sevoflurane, and desflurane in man. British Journal of Anesthesia, 91(2), 170–174. Table 1. For full discussion of how age-related MACs are calculated, view this article at http://bja.oxfordjournals.org /content/91/2/170.full

become hypoxic long before the concentration reached the minimum level. However, doses considerably below the MAC, generally in the range of 0.1 to 0.5, provide acceptable levels of sedation to conduct most routine dental procedures (Becker & Rosenberg, 2008). **Nitrous oxide** may be combined with other inhaled agents or with intravenous agents (Becker & Rosenberg, 2008) for general anesthesia. It has an impressive safety profile when used alone, but when combined with other agents, the possibility of synergistic depression of respiratory and cardiac function must be considered (Becker & Rosenberg, 2008).

Adverse Effects

Concerns around **nitrous oxide** relate to its significantly greater blood:gas partition coefficient (0.46) compared to that of nitrogen (0.014). Substituting a mixture of oxygen and **nitrous oxide** for the room air produces a situation in which the **nitrous oxide** enters gas-filled spaces 30 times faster than nitrogen leaves it, causing an increase in volume or pressure of such spaces (Becker & Rosenberg, 2008). For this reason, the use of nitrous oxide may be very dangerous in the following conditions: air embolism, pneumothorax, bowel obstructions, intracranial air, pulmonary air cysts, and intraocular bubbles. Chest pain, hypertension, and indications of stroke are warning signs of potential pressure-related complications.

Nursing Considerations

Nitrous oxide alone does not produce the ventilation or cardiovascular depression characteristic of other agents, but when it is used in combination with sedatives or opioids, the patient's vital signs should be closely monitored. Hypoxia is the most significant concern, aside from the risk of pressure-related adverse events as noted previously; officially termed "diffusion hypoxia," **nitrous oxide** is eliminated from the lungs so rapidly it will significantly decrease the partial pressure of oxygen leading to hypoxia. At the end of the procedure, best practice is to shut off the nitrous oxide and deliver pure oxygen for a few minutes prior to removing the patient's mask (Becker & Rosenberg, 2008). Chronic exposure to **nitrous oxide** can produce toxic effects including vitamin B_{12} deficiency, which is a consideration not only for patients undergoing repeated procedures using this agent, but also for nurses or clinical staff who administer it on a regular basis.

Isoflurane

Isoflurane is the oldest of the three currently used modern inhalational anesthetic agents. It is a pungent agent, making it unsuitable for inhalational induction of general anesthesia; however, it may be combined with **nitrous oxide** for induction. **Isoflurane** does not significantly alter the heart rate or cardiac output, making it a cardiac-stable agent. Its main disadvantage is its high solubility, which means that the desired effects are realized slowly compared to the other two flurane agents and the process of patient recovery is relatively slow.

Adverse Effects

Isoflurane has neurologic effects that are incompletely understood, including the potential for neurodegeneration and possibly cognitive effects, particularly in young children and older adults (Schifilliti, Grasso, Conti, & Fodale, 2010). These concerns are still under investigation, but in patients younger than 10 years, older than 65 years, or with existing cognitive impairment, use of alternative agents should be considered. **Isoflurane** produces significant respiratory depression, more so than other agents. All of the flurane inhalants have been associated with malignant hyperthermia, although this adverse effect occurs only rarely.

Nursing Considerations

Due to **isoflurane's** respiratory depressant effects, careful monitoring of patients' oxygen intake and blood oxygen levels is necessary. It is important to note that this respiratory depression may not be observable, as the effects are seen in tidal volume and not in respiration rate. Supportive oxygen supplementation must be available at all times. Isoflurane can also potentiate muscle relaxant drugs used simultaneously, so caution should be exercised when determining the doses of such medications during or immediately after use of isoflurane anesthesia.

Desflurane

Desflurane is the least soluble of the modern inhalational agents, making its onset and offset very rapid. Its main drawback is its pungency, which makes it unsuitable as a single agent for inhalational induction (causes coughing, salivation, breath holding, and laryngospasm), although desflurane can be mixed with nitrous oxide for that purpose. Its rapid onset and offset make desflurane a preferred agent for outpatient procedures. However, it sometimes causes respiratory irritation, which makes it less attractive for use in pediatric patients.

Nursing Considerations

Desflurane has been associated with tachycardia, hypertension, or rarely, myocardial ischemia when used in high concentrations or when the inspired concentration is rapidly increased.

Adverse Effects

Malignant hyperthermia and tachycardia are the principal concerns with desflurane. Patients should be monitored for signs of these complications.

Sevoflurane

Sevoflurane is the only modern agent that is not pungent, making it ideal for inhalational induction of general anesthesia. It is the primary inhalational anesthetic used for pediatric patients for this reason. It is more soluble in the blood than desflurane, but less soluble than isoflurane, putting its onset and offset somewhere between those of these other two inhalational agents. Sevoflurane may cause agitation, coughing, or gagging during administration or emergence delirium after administration in pediatric patients, but aside from that, its side-effect profile is relatively mild. Unlike desflurane and isoflurane, sevoflurane is not metabolized to trifluoroacetate (a metabolite that is connected to liver toxicity) and has not been associated with liver injury (Eger, 2004).

Adverse Effects

Malignant hyperthermia is the principal concern with sevoflurane. Patients should be monitored for signs of increased body temperature.

Nursing Considerations

Sevoflurane can form carbon monoxide during exposure to dry CO_2 absorbents; postoperative serum carboxyhemoglobin (HbCO) levels may be ordered.

Sevoflurane has the least effect on blood pressure and heart rate (will see tachycardia with MAC >1.5).

Intravenous Anesthetics

Intravenous administration of anesthetics offers an attractive adjunct or alternative to inhalational agents. There is a much greater variety of intravenous agents available that may be used alone or in conjunction with other agents; these drugs can be used for either general anesthesia (complete lack of consciousness) or partial anesthesia (mild to moderate sedation). As a rule, most of these agents are relatively pleasant at onset (unlike some inhalational agents, which have an overpowering, unpleasant odor that may induce discomfort) and produce few aftereffects once the patient awakens. They are, however, somewhat more expensive to use than inhalational anesthetics and are less attractive to use in needle-phobic adults or in children. Moreover, some drugs have side effects that may complicate procedures or produce unwanted after-effects during recovery, including significant alterations of respiration, heart rate, and blood pressure. In many cases, these side effects may be reduced by coadministration of adjunct medications. TABLE 15-3 lists the main types of drugs used for intravenous anesthesia.

TABLE 15-3	Types of Drugs Used in Intravenous Anesthesia		
Agent Class	Common Use	Examples	Notes
Anesthetics/Analgesics			
Induction + maintenance anesthetics	Induction and maintenance; sedation with regional anesthesia	Propofol	Propofol is the most commonly used anesthetic due to its dual capacity as an induction and maintenance agent.
Induction anesthetics	Induction of general or regional anesthesia	Ketamine, etomidate, and barbiturates (e.g., thiopental, sodium methohexital)	Their rapid onset makes these drugs useful for induction. Often paired with a secondary agent for maintenance.
Adjuncts			
Opioid analgesics	Surgical analgesia	Morphine, fentanyl	Sedating effect is secondary to pain relief; not used for induction and usually used in conjunction with another agent.
Neuromuscular blocking agents (depolarizing)	Muscle relaxation for intubation, short-duration procedures	Succinylcholine	Its rapid onset and short duration make this agent useful only for very short-term treatment.
Neuromuscular blocking agents (nondepolarizing)	Muscle relaxation for intubation, maintenance of relaxation for moderate- to long-duration procedures	Atracurium, rocuronium, metocurine	Several agents produce histamine release.
Hypnotics/anxiolytics	Used as adjuncts to induction anesthetics	Benzodiazepines (e.g., diazepam, midazolam)	May be given as preprocedure medication to reduce patient anxiety. Most often used for local/regional anesthesia.

Induction Anesthetics

Propofol

Propofol is an alkyl phenol hypnotic/amnestic agent that has become the most commonly used intravenous induction/sedation medication in anesthesia. It has a very rapid onset as well as a rapid offset due to its rapid redistribution (Hemmings, 2010); an intravenous injection of propofol induces anesthesia within 40 seconds, which is roughly the amount of time it takes blood from the arm to circulate to the brain (propofol injectable emulsion USP, package insert). Its rapid metabolism leads to a more alert patient when the propofol has cleared from the body. In addition, the drug has an antiemetic characteristic of unknown origin, although some researchers have speculated that it is related to the fact that—unlike other drugs (e.g., thiopental)—propofol produces uniform CNS depression that includes the subcortical centers such as the **chemoreceptor trigger zone (CTZ)** that antiemetic drugs typically affect (Golembiewski, Chernin, & Chopra, 2005). Propofol is also considered a bronchodilator and anticonvulsant though it offers no analgesia.

Nursing Considerations

The lack of lasting effects and its overall safety profile along with antiemetic properties makes propofol an ideal choice for the majority of procedures and patient populations, as it does not alter the heart rate or decrease blood pressure, respirations, cerebral blood flow, and intracranial pressure. Propofol can burn on administration, cause hypotension, cause apnea with larger doses, and is contraindicated in shock states and in patients with an ejection fraction <30%.

Ketamine

Ketamine is a phenocyclidine (PCP) derivative that can be used for the induction of general anesthesia. Of all of the intravenous induction agents, it is the only one

Best Practices

Currently, Propofol is considered the first-line agent for intravenous general anesthesia induction due to its rapid onset and good safety profile.

with analgesic properties, which may be a product of its noncompetitive blockade of NMDA-receptor calcium-channel pores (Pai & Heining, 2007). This drug's anticholinergic effects also reduce its potential for creating respiratory depression; in fact, ketamine is a potent bronchodilator, which can be beneficial in the patient with asthma. It is considered a dissociative anesthetic due to the fact that it can cause hallucinations and out-of-body experiences, but it is not a drug that promotes seizures; indeed, it appears to have anticonvulsive and neuroprotective properties (Pai & Heining, 2007). Some of these effects may be related to ketamine's agonist actions on mu and kappa opioid receptors as well as its antagonism of a variety of adrenergic receptors (Pai & Heining, 2007). At high doses, ketamine produces a local anesthetic response as well, which can be useful in some surgical procedures.

Ketamine is commonly used in hemodynamically compromised patients because it is a sympathetic nervous system stimulant due to its induction of increased sympathetic nervous system outflow from the CNS; through that mechanism, it can increase heart rate, cardiac output, and blood pressure. This characteristic does, however, mean use of ketamine is contraindicated in patients with head trauma, because intracranial pressure can be increased by this mechanism, leading to brain herniation. In patients in whom such cardiovascular effects pose a risk, it is possible to reduce the side effects by administering ketamine via continuous infusion and giving a benzodiazepine (Pai & Heining, 2007). Ketamine should be used with caution in patients with known psychiatric disease, as it has significant psychotic effects in as many as 30% of patients, and has been shown to activate psychosis in patients with schizophrenia. As with the cardiac side effects, concomitant use of other sedative-hypnotic drugs (e.g., benzodiazepines) has been shown to attenuate this problem (Pai & Heining, 2007).

Nursing Considerations

Close vital sign monitoring is necessary with sympathetic nervous system activation with ketamine use. Hypersalivation is a common effect; patients should be able to handle their own secretions effectively. Ketamine administration is especially useful with uncooperative patients and helps to preserve airway reflexes due to its minimally depressing cardiorespiratory effects. It can cause dysphoria and hallucinations; therefore, coadministration with a benzodiazepine (with its amnestic effect) is useful to prevent awareness or memory of these effects.

Etomidate

Etomidate is a short-acting, nonbarbiturate anesthetic drug that produces hypnosis, amnesia, and inhibition of sensory responses via agonist actions at GABA-A receptors (Forman, 2011). It also inhibits adrenal hormone (aldosterone, cortisol) synthesis and reduces pain on injection (Forman, 2011). Its inhibitory effects on corticosteroid synthesis mean that etomidate does not increase heart rate and decreases blood pressure, respirations, cerebral blood flow, and intracranial pressure. These effects make it a good choice for patients with poor cardiac health; the drug's overall effects on patients' hemodynamic profiles are mild and may benefit those patients experiencing circulatory stress. At the same time, in patients who are critically ill and who would potentially benefit from a higher metabolic rate, there have been concerns that etomidate might have an adverse effect on survival (Forman, 2011). A variety of studies comparing etomidate to other agents, such as ketamine or opioids, offer little guidance as to when its use is appropriate in critically ill patients who require intubation (Forman, 2011).

Due to the decreased demand on the heart, at-risk cardiac patients are less likely to have an induced myocardial infarction from anesthesia induction when etomidate is compared to other agents that tend to increase heart rate and cardiac output, placing undue stress on this patient population. This effect may far outlast the sedative effects of the drug, however, so resumption of medical treatment for hypertension or similar

> **Best Practices**
>
> Ketamine is a good choice in hemodynamically compromised patients but should not be used in patients with head trauma because it increases blood and intracranial pressure.

conditions should be undertaken with caution in patients who discontinued such therapies prior to surgery (Forman, 2011).

Nursing Considerations

Post anesthetic nausea and vomiting (PONV) is a frequent problem and antiemetic prophylaxis should be given before emergence. Pain on IV injection is possible. **Etomidate** should not be administered to patients at risk for seizures as **etomidate** can lower the seizure threshold and accelerate seizure foci.

Barbiturates

Barbiturates is a class of CNS depressant medications that produce sleepiness and relaxation via GABA-A agonism. They were the primary intravenous induction agents used in anesthesia before the introduction of **propofol**, which has since become the drug of choice for intravenous induction. Nevertheless, there are good reasons why barbiturates might still be used for anesthesia. For one thing, they can be more useful than **propofol** or other induction agents under specific circumstances. For another thing, occasional manufacturers' shortages of preferred drugs such as **propofol** mean that availability dictates the use of barbiturates in lieu of **propofol**; such shortages occurred in 2009 and 2010, leading to selection of drugs based as much on availability as on pharmacologic properties (Hemmings, 2010).

Barbiturates do have some significant detrimental effects that mean they must be used cautiously. In general, all barbiturates increase heart rate and lower blood pressure, respirations, and cerebral blood flow, via mechanisms that are still unclear. They also decrease intracranial pressure, potentially increasing the risk of seizure, which can be a significant complication for patients undergoing surgery. Because safer intravenous alternatives are now available, barbiturate drugs are now rarely used for general anesthesia unless other induction agents are contraindicated.

The two barbiturates that were most commonly used in anesthesia are **thiopental** and **methohexital**. A third agent, **thiamylal**, is sometimes used as well, although it has been shown to promote clotting, which may be problematic in a surgical setting. Due to shortages of **thiopental** that have occurred in recent years, in general **methohexital** is the only such drug still being used in the United States (Hemmings, 2010). Its principal use is for the induction of anesthesia for electroconvulsive therapy (ECT), in which the lower seizure threshold of barbiturates works to the advantage, rather than the disadvantage, of the therapeutic intervention. For this indication, **methohexital** is preferred over **thiopental** or **thiamylal** because it is considerably more potent than either of the latter agents (Hemmings, 2010); the induction dose needed is about half that of **thiopental**, making **methohexital** less likely to create dose-dependent adverse effects. Moreover, **methohexital** does not induce the kind of electrocardiographic anomalies that are seen with other similar drugs (Pitts, Desmarais, Stewart, & Schaberg, 1965).

Barbiturates, in oral form, are sometimes used as anxiolytics (albeit infrequently), headache pain relievers, and anticonvulsants (as noted in the *Pharmacology of Psychotropic Medications* chapter). Patients who take oral barbiturate medications should be managed with great care when they are undergoing any form of anesthesia, but particularly if they are being sedated with a barbiturate, due to concerns of excessive CNS depression and seizures. Although all medications and patient health history should be reviewed before anesthesia as a matter of good practice, patients who report a history of seizure, recurrent or "cluster" headaches, or anxiety should prompt closer review.

Nursing Considerations

Use barbiturates with caution in elderly patients due to post administration sedation and confusion. Give IV doses via the largest bore peripheral IV as possible, as barbiturate use leads to soft tissue damage with extravasation of drug outside the blood vessel into surrounding tissues.

Barbiturates may be used as an anesthetic, an anticonvulsant, and for brain protection as they decrease the cerebral metabolic rate and intracranial pressure. Barbiturate use carries a risk of a histamine reaction, cardiopulmonary depression (negative inotrope), and laryngospasm or bronchospasm.

Anesthetic Adjuncts

Benzodiazepines

Benzodiazepines are anxiolytic drugs commonly used in anesthesia as adjunct medications, acting as GABA-A receptor agonists; they are often given prior to anesthesia to help patients relax. Numerous benzodiazepines are available, but the primary one used is midazolam, which is currently the shortest-acting benzodiazepine available, making it an ideal choice in the anesthesia setting. The agent for reversal specifically for benzodiazepines is flumazenil, a benzodiazepine receptor antagonist; it is used in case of a suspected benzodiazepine overdose or in an elderly patient who is showing new onset confusion or deep sedation postoperatively.

Nursing Considerations

Use decreased doses in patients with liver or kidney disease. Elderly patients have increased sensitivity to benzodiazepines with possible CNS effects (sedation, disorientation) and risk of falls, thus they are often not given to patients older than 70 years of age. Benzodiazepines can be used for antegrade amnesia, anxiolysis, and as an anticonvulsant but they offer no analgesia and can depress ventilation and blood pressure.

Opioids

Opioids are medications that agonize opioid receptors in the brain and nervous system (see Chapter 4). There are three major opioid receptors: delta (δ) opioid receptors (DOP), kappa (κ) opioid receptors (KOP), and mu (μ) opioid receptors (MOP), as well as a fourth receptor designated as a nociceptive, opioid-like receptor (NOP). Activation of these different receptors has a variety of effects that can be useful, but also sometimes harmful, in patients who require sedation or pain relief. For example, stimulation of the MOP receptors produces analgesia and sedation, but can also trigger respiratory and cardiac depression as well as nausea and vomiting—all of which are unwanted effects in a patient undergoing surgery (Pathan & Williams, 2012). MOP receptor stimulation is also implicated in opiate addiction (Goodman, Le Bourdonnec, & Dolle, 2007). Thus, when selecting an opioid drug, it is important to understand which receptors it affects, how it affects them (i.e., stimulation versus blockade), and which response that effect produces in the body. TABLE 15-4 lists the various receptors and effects of stimulation; TABLE 15-5 lists opioid drugs by class and effects.

In the setting of general or partial anesthesia, opioid drugs offer two basic benefits. First, using them alongside another anesthetic—an inhaled anesthetic such as sevoflurane or an intravenous induction anesthetic such as propofol—can reduce the

TABLE 15-4	Opioid Receptors and Their Effects
Receptor	Effects of Stimulation
DOP (δ)	Spinal and supraspinal analgesia, reduced gastric motility, euphoria, physical dependence
KOP (κ)	Spinal analgesia, diuresis, dysphoria, inhibition of vasopressin release
MOP (μ)	Analgesia, sedation, respiratory depression, bradycardia, nausea and vomiting, reduction in gastric motility, physical dependence
NOP	Analgesia/hyperalgesia,* allodynia; antagonism of these receptors may reduce opioid tolerance

*Dose dependent

Data from Fine, P. G., & Portenoy, R.K. (2004). The endogenous opioid system. In A clinical guide to opioid analgesia (pp. 9–15). New York, NY: McGraw-Hill; McDonald, J., & Lambert, D.G. (2005). Opioid receptors. Continuing Education in Anaesthesia, Critical Care, and Pain , 5 (1), 22–25.; Pathan, H., & Williams, J. (2012). Basic opioid pharmacology: An update. British Journal of Pain , 6 (1), 11–16.

TABLE 15-5	Opioid Medications Used in Anesthesia		
Drug	Opioid Subclass	Effects	Uses
Alfentanil	Opioid agonist	Increases pain threshold and alters pain perceptions. Immediate onset; duration: 30 to 60 minutes; half-life: approximately 90 minutes in adults. Produces increased intracranial pressure and respiratory depression.	Used as an analgesic adjunct to anesthesia with barbiturate/nitrous oxide/oxygen for short-duration (less than 1 hour) surgical procedures, by continuous infusion as a maintenance analgesic, or as the analgesic component for monitored anesthesia care.
Buprenorphine	Mixed opioid agonist	Strong affinity for MOP receptors that provide analgesia at relatively low concentrations; exerts agonistic effects at MOP and DOP receptors but antagonistic effects at KOP receptors. Produces dose-dependent respiratory depression. Onset: 15 minutes IM; duration: 4 to 10 hours; half-life: approximately 2 hours.	Generally not used in anesthesia, but may be used for postoperative pain. May induce withdrawal symptoms in opioid-dependent patients.
Butorphanol	Mixed opioid agonist	Agonist for KOP and partial agonist of MOP receptors. Inhibition of ascending pain pathways causes altered pain response; also produces analgesia, respiratory depression, and sedation. Onset: less than 10 minutes; half-life: 4 to 6 hours; duration: 3 to 4 hours.	Used as an anesthetic adjunct during induction; also given as a preinduction medication.
Fentanyl	Opioid agonist	Reduces MAC by approximately 50% when given 30 minutes before procedure. Similar reduction is seen in propofol induction. Excellent hemodynamic stability but the patient may maintain some awareness (this is good in cases where partial anesthesia is preferred). IV onset is immediate; duration: 30 to 60 minutes: half-life: 2 to 4 hours.	Most commonly used opioid for surgical or postsurgical analgesia. Has 10 times the potency of morphine, but is short acting. May be used as the sole agent in small (<100 kg) patients.
Hydromorphone	Opioid agonist	MOP agonist with lesser effects at other receptors. Inhibition of ascending pain pathways alters pain response; respiratory depression, sedation, and cough suppression are additional effects. Onset: 10 to 15 minutes IV; duration: 3 to 4 hours; half-life: 2 to 3 hours.	Principal use is analgesic rather than anesthetic or sedative. Is best used in opiate-naïve patients.
Meperidine	Opioid agonist	Second-line analgesic with anesthetic and vagolytic effects. May produce histamine release, bronchospasm, and hypotension. Onset is rapid; duration: 2 to 4 hours; half-life: 2.5 to 4 hours.	Due to side effects and drug interactions, this drug is not recommended for analgesia unless other options are unavailable. Avoid in patients taking MAOI inhibitors. May cause seizure.
Morphine sulfate	Opioid agonist	Generalized opioid receptor agonist; inhibits ascending pain pathways and produces analgesia, respiratory depression, and sedation; suppresses cough by acting centrally in medulla. When used with an inhalational induction anesthetic, reduces MAC by as much as 65% in a dose-dependent manner. Even in significant respiratory depression, patients may still be readily aroused. May produce histamine release at higher doses. Onset: less than 5 minutes IV; duration: up to 7 hours; half-life: 1.5 to 4 hours.	Often administered via the intrathecal or epidural route for postoperative pain. Elimination half-life: 3 hours.
Nalbuphine	Mixed opioid agonist	Agonist for KOP and partial antagonist of MOP receptors. Inhibition of ascending pain pathways causes altered pain response; also produces analgesia, respiratory depression, and sedation. Onset: 2 to 3 minutes IV, 15 minutes IM; duration: 3 to 6 hours; half-life: 5 hours.	May produce withdrawal signs in opiate-dependent patients due to MOP antagonism effects.

TABLE 15-5	Opioid Medications Used in Anesthesia (*continued*)

Drug	Opioid Subclass	Effects	Uses
Naloxone	Opioid antagonist	Rapid-acting antagonist that reverses effects of opioid drugs; is especially active at MOP receptors. Used to counteract effects of opioids administered during surgery. Onset: 1 to 2 minutes IV, 2 to 5 minutes IM; duration: 1 to 4 hours, depending on route of administration; half-life: 30 to 90 minutes.	Preferred agent used in case of excessive respiratory depression. With careful titration, respiratory depression may be reversed without sacrificing analgesia.
Pentazocine	Mixed opioid agonist	Produces dose-dependent respiratory depression, but to a lesser extent than a pure opioid agonist. This drug has highest incidence of psychotomimetic effects of all drugs in this class and should be avoided in concert with ketamine. Onset: two to three minutes; duration: one hour IV, two hours IM; half-life: two to three hours.	Used preoperatively for pain or for analgesia/sedation before general anesthesia. Also used as an adjunct during surgery. May produce withdrawal in opioid-dependent patients.
Remifentanil	Opioid agonist	Ultra-short-acting analgesic that must be given via continuous infusion to have lasting effects, but is extremely potent so that small doses are needed to obtain effects. Inhibits ascending pain pathways and alters the patient's response to pain (increased pain threshold); produces analgesia, respiratory depression, and sedation. Onset: one to three minutes IV; half-life, three to ten minutes.	Rapid metabolism allows for prolonged continuous infusion without tissue accumulation. Used as an adjunct to volatile anesthetics to lower MAC during induction. Often used in surgical cases where the patient must be awakened quickly at the end of surgery for assessment (e.g., can they move their toes, grip their hands, stick their tongue out). Patients must receive longer-acting narcotics once remifentanil is stopped for analgesia.

MAC or dose needed to obtain the desired level of sedation, while simultaneously producing pain relief. Opioids are often given prior to induction as a way of minimizing the discomfort associated with some induction medications (**propofol** and **etomidate** are both known to cause pain upon injection). Second, opioids block the stress response, inhibiting release of catecholamines, vasopressin, and cortisol, better than volatile anesthetics, which in theory could produce a better outcome for the patient.

There are three basic variants of opioid drugs:

- Opioid **agonists**, which stimulate a maximal response from opioid receptors
- Opioid **antagonists**, which bind to the receptor but stimulate no response and block other opiates, whether produced by the body or administered as a drug, from binding to the receptor ("blockade")

- Partial opioid agonists, which bind to the receptor but produce only a partial response from the receptor no matter what dose of drug is administered (Pathan & Williams, 2012)

Opioid Agonists

There are numerous opioid agonist drugs available for use concomitantly with an anesthetic (see Table 15-5). Of these, **fentanyl**, **sufentanil**, and **hydromorphone** are the most commonly used intravenous opioids due to their favorable onset and duration of action (but, as noted earlier, these medications also carry a significant risk of respiratory depression).

Nursing Considerations

There is great variability in the dosing of opioids needed to produce pain relief, even among patients having identical surgical procedures. Opioid agonist medications carry a significant risk of respiratory depression and other negative side effects and risks including opioid dependence, and severe nausea and vomiting.

Mixed-Agonists

Some opioid drugs selectively stimulate specific opioid receptors while not affecting others. The mixed-agonists (also called opioid agonist-antagonists) encompass a group of drugs that are structurally similar to **morphine**; unlike **morphine** and other drugs in the morphine family, however, mixed-agonist drugs stimulate select opioid receptors, and, they may simultaneously *antagonize* other opioid receptors. For example, the mixed-agonist drug **pentazocine** partially agonizes DOP and KOP receptors but antagonizes MOP receptors (Kimura, Ohi, & Haji, 2016; Mori et al., 2015). As the MOP receptors are the principal source of some of the negative effects of opioids, this characteristic reduces the unwanted side effects to a certain extent. Moreover, when given as pain medications, these drugs have lower risk of promoting drug-seeking or addictive behaviors due to the lower stimulation of opioid receptors (Pathan & Williams, 2012). The main advantage of this class of drugs is that the agents produce analgesia without the same significant risk of depression of ventilation; although they produce lower maximal analgesic effects than the opioids, they have limited toxic effects as well. Two commonly seen medications in this subclass are **nalbuphine** and **butorphanol**.

Nursing Considerations

An important factor to keep in mind is that partial agonists can reduce the responsiveness of full agonists. For example, if a patient is sedated with an inhalant plus a partial agonist opioid (given to maintain analgesia and/or sedation) and then switched to a full agonist opioid while the partial agonist remains in effect, the partial agonist will block the effects of the full agonist, potentially reducing the patient's level of sedation or pain relief at an inopportune

time unless a larger dose of the full agonist is given—which itself has risks, as the higher dose could then produce overdose once the partial agonist drug is eliminated from the patient's body unless correctly titrated down.

Opioid Antagonists

The pure opioid antagonists are drugs that competitively antagonize all opioid receptors. This action makes them "antidotes" to opioid drugs—an important consideration given the potential for overdose or adverse effects with the opioids.

The opioid antagonist class includes a variety of medications, but the most commonly used agent in anesthetic practice is **naloxone**. This drug is used in overdose or the presence of excessive opioid effects, such as sedation and respiratory depression, following surgery. It is favored to the exclusion of other drugs in this class specifically because of the speed with which it works: **Naloxone**, given intravenously, can usually reverse opioid-induced respiratory depression within 1 to 2 minutes, whereas **naltrexone** (another drug in this class that is primarily used for treating opiate addiction) has an onset of 15 to 30 minutes when given intramuscularly (it is not administered intravenously). In a patient who is at risk due to respiratory depression, the time difference in the opioid antagonist's onset may be the determinant of whether the outcome is good or bad; thus, **naloxone** is indicated as a "rescue" medication whenever opioid drugs are used in anesthesia. It has similar effects in counteracting benzodiazepines (Solhi, Mostafazdeh, Vishteh, Ghezavati, & Shooshtarizadeh, 2011), making it an important agent in managing overdose of either opioid or benzodiazepine adjuncts.

Nursing Considerations

The duration of action of some opioids may exceed that of **naloxone**; the patient must be kept under continuous surveillance for the life of the given opioid. Repeat doses of **naloxone** may be needed depending upon the amount, type and route of administration of the opioid being antagonized.

Nonanesthetic Adjuncts

As noted earlier, a variety of drugs that offer neither anesthesia nor analgesia are used as adjuncts to anesthesia. They offer benefits for the patient on several fronts. Some act on the patient's muscles to prevent them from moving during the procedure; this is more important than it might seem, because even a slight, involuntary twitch could prove catastrophic in, for example, a patient undergoing eye or heart surgery. Other adjunct medications suppress nausea and vomiting. TABLE 15-6 describes many of the medications used as nonanesthetic adjuncts to surgery.

TABLE 15-6	Additional (Nonanesthetic) Adjuncts	
Drug	Class	Notes
Aprepitant	Neurokinin-1 (NK1) receptor antagonist (antiemetic)	Hypersensitivity reaction (rare) is usually immediate; symptoms include flushing, erythema, and dyspnea during infusion. Discontinue if symptoms occur.
Atracurium	Nondepolarizing muscle relaxant	May cause transient hypotension and release of histamine; its metabolite laudanosine is toxic and may show greater accumulation in patients with renal failure. Onset: approximately 2 minutes; duration: 30 minutes.
Atropine	Anticholinergic	Inhibits acetylcholine activity in smooth muscle, CNS, and secretory glands. Increases cardiac output and dries secretions. Onset: approximately 1 hour; duration: 4 hours.
Cisatracurium	Nondepolarizing muscle relaxant	Generally does not cause histamine release. Onset: approximately 2.5 minutes; duration: 60 minutes.
Dimenhydrinate	Histamine-receptor antagonist (antiemetic)	CNS depressant, anticholinergic, antiemetic, antihistamine (H_1), and local anesthetic effects. Immediate onset if given IV; onset is 20 to 30 minutes if given IM.
Diphenhydramine	Histamine-receptor antagonist (antiemetic)	Antihistamine (H_1) with moderate to high anticholinergic and antiemetic properties. Onset: 15 to 30 minutes; duration: 4 to 6 hours.
Dolasetron	Serotonin-receptor antagonist (antiemetic)	Binds to 5-HT3 receptors in GI tract to block vagal signaling to CTZ.
Droperidol	Dopamine-receptor antagonist (antiemetic)	Reduces motor activity and anxiety, and causes sedation; also possesses adrenergic-blocking, antifibrillatory, antihistaminic, and anticonvulsive properties. Antiemetic effects stem from dopamine receptor blockade in brain. Onset: 3 to 10 minutes; duration: 2 to 4 hours typically but may last up to 12 hours.
Edrophonium	Acetylcholinesterase inhibitor	Increases presence of acetylcholine to offset actions of nondepolarizing muscle relaxants. Onset: within 1 minute; duration: 5 to 10 minutes.
Glycopyrrolate	Anticholinergic	Inhibits action of acetylcholine competitively to reduce salivation and tracheobronchial secretions; also increases heart rate and blood pressure. Onset: within 1 minute; duration: 2 to 3 hours.
Granisetron	Serotonin-receptor antagonist (antiemetic)	Binds to 5-HT3 receptors in peripheral and central nervous system; effects are strongest in GI tract. May be given IV preoperatively or transdermally for procedures such as radiotherapy.
Haloperidol	Dopamine-receptor antagonist (antiemetic)	An antipsychotic; blocks dopamine D_1 and D_2 receptors in brain. Onset: 30 to 60 minutes; duration: variable depending on formulation (long-acting formula lasts up to 3 weeks). Contraindicated in patients with glaucoma and dementia-related psychosis (black box warning).
Metoclopramide	Dopamine-receptor antagonist (antiemetic)	Antagonizes dopamine receptors in CTZ; sensitizes tissues to acetylcholine; increases upper GI motility but not secretions. May cause irreversible tardive dyskinesia and should not be used with other drugs that cause extrapyramidal symptoms (black box warning).
Neostigmine	Acetylcholinesterase inhibitor	Increases presence of acetylcholine to offset actions of nondepolarizing muscle relaxants. Onset: 1 to 20 minutes; duration: 1 to 2 hours.

(continues)

TABLE 15-6	Additional (Nonanesthetic) Adjuncts (*continued*)	
Drug	Class	Notes
Ondansetron	Serotonin-receptor antagonist (antiemetic)	Binds to 5-HT3 receptors both in periphery and in CNS, with primary effects in GI tract. Onset: 30 minutes.
Palonosetron	Serotonin-receptor antagonist (antiemetic)	Binds to 5-HT3 receptors both in periphery and in CNS, with primary effects in GI tract. Onset: 30 minutes.
Pancuronium	Nondepolarizing muscle relaxant	May produce slight elevation in heart rate and blood pressure. Onset: 90 minutes; duration: up to 3 hours.
Physostigmine	Acetylcholinesterase inhibitor	Increases presence of acetylcholine to offset actions of nondepolarizing muscle relaxants.
Promethazine	Histamine-receptor antagonist (antiemetic)	Antihistamine (H_1) that blocks mesolimbic dopamine receptors and α-adrenergic receptors in the brain. Onset: 3 to 5 minutes; duration: 4 to 6 hours.
Rocuronium	Nondepolarizing muscle relaxant	May increase heart rate via vagolytic effects. Onset: 75 minutes; duration: 45 to 60 minutes.
Scopolamine	Anticholinergic	Blocks transmission of cholinergic signaling to CTZ. Onset: 10 minutes; duration: 2 hours.
Succinylcholine	Depolarizing muscle relaxant	Drug of choice for muscle relaxation in emergency situations due to its rapid onset and short duration of action. Onset: within 1 minute; duration: 2 to 10 minutes.
Vecuronium	Nondepolarizing muscle relaxant	Generally does not cause histamine release or cardiovascular effects. Onset: 60 minutes; duration: 30 minutes.

Muscle Relaxants

Neuromuscular blocking drugs, more often referred to as muscle relaxants or paralytics, are commonly used as intravenous adjunct medications with anesthesia agents to induce muscle paralysis. They are used for intubation of the trachea as well as to induce muscle relaxation for surgical procedures. Two subclasses of neuromuscular blocking drugs are distinguished, based on their respective mechanisms of action: **nondepolarizing** and **depolarizing**. Both classes work by blocking the function of acetylcholine receptors on skeletal muscle, but the mechanisms by which they act differs significantly.

The majority of neuromuscular blocking drugs used today belong to the nondepolarizing class, which blocks the acetylcholine receptors on skeletal muscle without activating them—behaving much like a key that fits in a lock, but does not turn the tumblers. The blockade of acetylcholine receptors causes flaccid paralysis of skeletal muscles to allow relaxation, prevent movement during surgery, and aid in surgical exposure. Although a variety of nondepolarizing agents is available, the choice of drug used is based highly on duration of action and provider preference.

Succinylcholine is the only depolarizing neuromuscular blocking drug. It similarly blocks acetylcholine stimulation in muscles, but by a different means: Instead of binding to the receptors without stimulating them, it depolarizes the plasma membrane of the skeletal muscle fiber, which makes the muscle fiber resistant to stimulation by acetylcholine. In contrast to the nondepolarizing agents, this drug's action is like a key that fits a lock and turns the tumblers, but does not complete the turn to open the door—yet it stops another key from doing so while it remains in place. **Succinylcholine** also leads to flaccid paralysis of skeletal muscle, but only after the muscles have contracted or fasciculated. The fasciculations induced by **succinylcholine** explain why a patient's muscles may twitch following its administration.

Nursing Considerations

Obviously, muscle relaxants are not given unless the patient is sedated and intubated on ventilatory support.

Succinylcholine administration can lead to an increase in serum potassium levels and should be avoided in hyperkalemic patients (e.g., patients in end-stage renal disease on hemodialysis, severe burns, paralysis). Other adverse side effects such as cardiac dysrhythmias, and bradycardia and/or asystole (especially in children or in a repeat dose in adults) can occur.

Acetylcholinesterase Inhibitors

Acetylcholinesterase inhibitors are intravenous medications used as reversal agents of motor blockade for nondepolarizing muscle relaxants. These medications prevent the enzyme acetylcholinesterase, which breaks down acetylcholine, from functioning, leading to an increased concentration of acetylcholine in the neuromuscular junction. The presence of acetylcholine is required to compete with nondepolarizing muscle relaxants on skeletal muscle. When acetylcholinesterase is blocked, more acetylcholine is made available in the neuromuscular junction, thus countering the effects of nondepolarizing neuromuscular blocking agents. Acetylcholinesterase inhibitors do not reverse the actions of a depolarizing block and can actually cause the block to last longer.

Nursing Considerations

Acetylcholinesterase inhibitors will NOT reverse the effects of succinylcholine and can actually make the paralytic effect last longer.

Because the anticholinesterase drugs used to reverse nondepolarizing muscle relaxants also act on nerve endings in areas other than the neuromuscular junction, they must be administered with an anticholinergic drug. Acetylcholinesterase inhibitor side effects include bradycardia, asystole, bladder and bowel incontinence, and increased bronchial and salivary secretions.

Anticholinergic Drugs

Anticholinergic drugs are used to oppose the acetylcholine actions of the parasympathetic nervous system, via muscarinic and nicotinic blockade. Some of the effects they have are to increase cardiac output—which can be valuable in counteracting the hypotensive effects of some anesthetics—and to reduce secretion of saliva and (to a lesser extent) mucus. The antisialagogue (saliva-suppressive) effect is an important mechanism to lessen secretions in the airway that can lead to laryngospasm, a spasm of the vocal cords that can occlude the airway, making ventilation impossible.

Three anticholinergic medications are commonly used in anesthesia: atropine, scopolamine, and glycopyrrolate. Atropine is primarily used to raise the heart rate during episodes of bradycardia. Scopolamine causes some sedation and prevents motion sickness, which is helpful for patients prone to postoperative nausea and vomiting (PONV). Glycopyrrolate, which does not cross the blood–brain barrier, lacks the sedative effects that can be found with scopolamine but is useful as an antisialagogue (decreases production of saliva) and is the most commonly used anticholinergic administered with acetylcholinesterase inhibitors to offset the undesirable side effects that they produce.

Nursing Considerations

Anticholinergics can be used to treat a variety of conditions (diarrhea, overactive bladder/incontinence, and asthma), to dilate the pupil to prep for an ophthalmic exam, or in the treatment of motion sickness, but in the anesthetic arena, these drugs are given to prevent negative side effects from the use of anticholinesterase drugs in neuromuscular relaxation reversal. They can cause urinary retention, constipation, and dry mouth; closely monitor the patient's vital signs to assess for hypertension and tachycardia.

Antiemetics

Nausea and vomiting can be significant side effects of anesthetic medications. Finding ways to suppress or relieve these symptoms is important not only during induction but also postoperatively, as the involuntary motions associated with vomiting are powerful enough to potentially tear sutures or displace recently repaired anatomic structures. All of the volatile anesthetics can cause postoperative nausea and vomiting, and many adjuncts trigger histamine release and thereby promote PONV indirectly. Managing this effect is one of the main challenges in anesthetic practice. Countless studies have been performed involving antiemetic therapy for PONV, yet the exact mechanism that induces it remains unknown. It is known that such nausea and vomiting can be triggered by a variety of substances. The most common of these stimulate the area in the medulla known as the chemoreceptor trigger zone. Five receptors in this zone, when stimulated by their respective agonists, produce nausea and vomiting: serotonin (5HT-3), histamine, muscarinic, opioid, and dopamine receptors. The majority of drugs that are currently used to prevent and treat PONV are antagonists of these receptors.

Serotonin-receptor antagonists include **ondansetron**, **granisetron**, **dolasetron**, and **palonosetron**. **Ondansetron** was the first agent developed in this class and is one of the most commonly used antiemetics in anesthetic practice for the prevention and treatment of PONV. **Palonosetron** is the newest member of the 5HT-3–specific receptor antagonists, acting at both central and peripheral 5HT-3 receptors. It has a longer half-life and therapeutic effect than the other drugs in this class.

Histamine-receptor antagonists include **dimenhydrinate**, **diphenhydramine**, and **promethazine**. They work by slowing production of histamine and reducing stimulation of the histamine receptors.

Dopamine-receptor antagonists work similarly on dopamine receptors; those used for PONV include **droperidol**, **haloperidol**, and **metoclopramide**. The U.S. Food and Drug Administration has issued black box warnings for all three of these drugs due to their serious side effects at higher doses.

Neurokinin-1 (NK1) receptor antagonists block receptors that are also found in the GI tract, stimulation of which is responsible for the vomiting reflex. **Aprepitant**, one of the newest drugs used in the prevention of PONV, is a NK1-receptor antagonist that appears to be very effective.

Other medications with antiemetic properties include the following:

- *Corticosteroids.* **Dexamethasone** is commonly used in combination with other antiemetics.
- *GABA-receptor agonists.* **Propofol** and benzodiazepines occupy GABA receptors and have been used successfully in the prevention of PONV.
- *Muscarinic-receptor antagonists.* The sole example of this class used for PONV is **scopolamine**, which is administered primarily as a transdermal patch.
- **Alvimopan.** This mu opioid receptor antagonist is used primarily when PONV is thought to be due to opioids.

Nursing Considerations

Side effects from antiemetics are as varied as the classes of drugs used to prevent or treat nausea and vomiting and too numerous to include in this chapter, but can include life-threatening events. Clear knowledge and understanding of the patient's history and disease state is imperative before administering a particular antiemetic.

CHAPTER SUMMARY

Anesthesia is primarily a method of blocking nerve impulses to reduce sensation and, if needed, consciousness, muscle activity, and nausea. Particularly in patients undergoing general or partial sedation, the potential for systemic effects on the heart and respiration is a key consideration. With surgical patients, consideration of postoperative pain and nausea is also of key importance due to the potential for these factors to produce complications and affect recovery. Anesthetics, analgesics, and adjunct medications may be administered in concert to avoid such complications.

1. Which of the following anesthetic inhalational agents would you not use on a patient with a pneumothorax? Why?
   a. Desflurane
   b. Isoflurane
   c. Sevoflurane
   d. Nitrous oxide

2. Which of the following induction agents would be the best option to use in an outpatient setting due to the rapid emergence from anesthesia? Why?
   a. Ketamine
   b. Propofol
   c. Methohexital
   d. Fentanyl

3. Which of the following medications is a depolarizing neuromuscular blocker? Why would you avoid use of an acetylcholinesterase inhibitor with this medication?
   a. Rocuronium
   b. Vecuronium
   c. Succinylcholine
   d. Atracurium

4. Which of the following induction agents would be the best choice to use in a hemodynamically compromised patient? Why?
   a. Ketamine
   b. Propofol
   c. Etomidate
   d. Methohexital

5. Which of the following inhalational agents is used for inhalational induction of anesthesia, especially in pediatric patients? What makes it different from the other agents so that it is preferred for this use? Why would it be preferable to an intravenous induction agent?
   a. Desflurane
   b. Isoflurane
   c. Sevoflurane
   d. Nitrous oxide

6. Anticholinergic drugs are often utilized in anesthesia. Which of the following drugs is generally devoid of the sedating effects that can be seen with the others?
   a. Atropine
   b. Glycopyrrolate
   c. Scopolamine
   d. None

7. Two types of local anesthetics are used in regional and peripheral nerve blocks. Which of the following drugs is *not* a member of the ester class?
   a. Chloroprocaine
   b. Cocaine
   c. Lidocaine
   d. Tetracaine

8. Which of the following is *not* one of the receptors in the brain that, if stimulated, may lead to PONV?
   a. Acetylcholine
   b. Serotonin
   c. Histamine
   d. Opioid
   e. Dopamine

9. Opioid antagonists can be used if there is excessive sedation or respiratory depression following surgery. Which one is generally used and reverses the untoward side effects within one to two minutes?
   a. Nalmefene
   b. Naltrexone
   c. Flumazenil
   d. Naloxone

10. Of the following, which drug is known to be a specific antagonist for benzodiazepines?
    a. Fentanyl
    b. Flumazenil
    c. Naltrexone
    d. Naloxone

CASE SCENARIO 1

An 82-year-old female patient has just been brought to the recovery room after having general anesthesia for a fractured hip repair. She is confused to time, place, and date and very fearful but states she is not in any pain and her vital signs are stable. Her husband states that she had a "sharp mind" and was not confused before surgery. You look at her anesthesia record and see that she received Isoflurane volatile anesthetic, fentanyl 200 mcg IV and a preoperative dose of midazolam 2 mg.

Case Questions

1. What anesthetic drug most likely caused her new onset confusion?
2. What drug would you give to reverse its effects?

Answers: *Midazolam:* Elderly patients have increased sensitivity to benzodiazepines with possible CNS effects (sedation, disorientation) and risk of falls and are often not given to patients older than 70 years of age.

Flumazenil is a benzodiazepine antagonist.

CASE SCENARIO 2

A 38-year-old male patient is admitted onto the neurosurgical stepdown unit after having a craniotomy for aneurysm clipping. You hear the patient yelling about a "horrible headache" as he is coming down the hall. The recovery nurse giving report states she doesn't understand why the patient is so uncomfortable as he "received a continuous dosing of remifentanil in the operating room."

Case Questions:

1. What is the duration of action of remifentanil?
2. What other drug class does this patient need for pain control?

Answers: The half-life of remifentanil is 3–10 minutes. This patient has had his cranium opened surgically and needs a strong opioid agonist for pain control.

REFERENCES

Becker, D.E., & Rosenberg, M. (2008). Nitrous oxide and the inhalation anesthetics. *Anesthesia Progress, 55*(4), 124–131.

Dewaele, S., & Santos, A.C. (2013). Toxicity of local anesthetics. New York School of Regional Anesthesia. Retrieved from https://www.nysora.com/toxicity-of-local-anesthetics

Eger, E.II. (2004). Characteristics of anesthetic agents used for induction and maintenance of general anesthesia. *American Journal of Health-System Pharmacy, 61*(Suppl. 4), S3–S10.

Fine, P.G., & Portenoy, R.K. (2004). The endogenous opioid system. In *A clinical guide to opioid analgesia* (pp 9–15). New York, NY: McGraw-Hill.

Forman, S.A. (2011). Clinical and molecular pharmacology of etomidate. *Anesthesiology, 114*(3), 695–707.

Golembiewski, J., Chernin, E., & Chopra, T. (2005). Prevention and treatment of postoperative nausea and vomiting. *American Journal of Health-System Pharmacy, 62*(12), 1247–1260.

Goodman, A.J., Le Bourdonnec, B., & Dolle, R.E. (2007). Mu opioid receptor antagonists: Recent developments. *ChemMedChem, 2*(11), 1552–1570.

Hemmings, H. (2010). The pharmacology of intravenous anesthetic induction agents: A primer. *Anesthesia News* (Special Edition). Retrieved from http://www.anesthesiologynews.com/download /Induction_ANSE10_WM.pdf

Kimura, S., Ohi, Y., & Haji, A. (2016). Mechanisms of pentazocine-induced ventilatory depression and antinociception in anesthetized rats. *Journal of Pharmacological Sciences, 130*(3), 181–184.

McDonald, J., & Lambert, D.G. (2005). Opioid receptors. *Continuing Education in Anaesthesia, Critical Care, and Pain, 5*(1), 22–25.

Mori, T., Itoh, T., Yoshizawa, K., Ise, Y., Mizuo, K., Saeki, T., . . . Suzuki, T. (2015). Involvement of µ- and δ-opioid receptor function in the rewarding effect of (±)-pentazocine. *Addiction Biology, 20,* 724–732. doi:10.1111/adb.12169

National Institutes of Health (NIH). (2018a). Drug record: Enflurane. *LiverTox: Clinical and Research Information on Drug-Induced Liver Injury.* Retrieved from https://livertox.nlm.nih.gov//Enflurane.htm

National Institutes of Health (NIH). (2018b). Drug record: Halothane. *LiverTox: Clinical and Research Information on Drug-Induced Liver Injury.* Retrieved from https://livertox.nlm.nih.gov//Halothane.htm

Nickalls, R.W.D., & Mapleson, W.W. (2003). Age-related iso-MAC charts for isoflurane, sevoflurane and desflurane in man. *British Journal of Anaesthesia, 91*(2), 170–174.

Pai, A., & Heining, M. (2007). Ketamine. *Continuing Education in Anaesthesia, Critical Care, and Pain, 7*(2), 59–63.

Pathan, H., & Williams, J. (2012). Basic opioid pharmacology: An update. *British Journal of Pain, 6*(1), 11–16.

Pitts, F.N. Jr., Desmarais, G.M., Stewart, W., & Schaberg, K. (1965). Induction of anesthesia with methohexital and thiopental in electroconvulsive therapy: The effect on the electrocardiogram and clinical observations in 500 consecutive treatments with each agent. *New England Journal of Medicine, 273,* 353–336.

Schifilliti, D., Grasso, G., Conti, A., & Fodale, V. (2010). Anaesthetic-related neuroprotection: Intravenous or inhalational agents? *CNS Drugs, 24*(11), 893–907.

Schneiderbanger, D., Johannsen, S., Roewer, N., & Schuster, F. (2014). Management of malignant hyperthermia: Diagnosis and treatment. *Therapeutics and Clinical Risk Management, 10,* 355–362. http://doi .org/10.2147/TCRM.S47632

Smeltzer, S.C., Bare, B.G., Hinkle, J.L., & Cheever, K.H. (2008). *Brunner & Suddarth's textbook of medical-surgical nursing* (11th ed.). Philadelphia, PA: Wolters Kluwer/Lippincott Williams & Wilkins.

Solhi, H., Mostafazdeh, B., Vishteh, H.R., Ghezavati, A.R., & Shooshtarizadeh, A. (2011). Benefit effect of naloxone in benzodiazepines intoxication: Findings of a preliminary study. *Human and Experimental Toxicology, 30,* 535–540.

CHAPTER 16

Pharmacology of Antimicrobial Drugs

Blaine Templar Smith

KEY TERMS

Anthelmintic
Antibacterial
Antibiotic
Antifungal
Anti-infective
Antimicrobial
Antiviral
Bactericidal
Bacteriostatic
Bacterium (bacteria)
Beta-lactamase
Broad spectrum

Combination therapy
Culture
Dihydropterate
    synthetase
Drug resistance
Fungus (fungi)
Gram negative
Gram positive
Helminth
Host factors
Hypersensitivity reaction
Influenza-type viruses

Maximum tolerable
    concentration
Minimum inhibitory
    concentration
Narrow spectrum
Non-retrovirus
Nosocomial
Nucleoside
Nucleoside reverse
    transcriptase inhibitors
    (NRTIs)
Parasite

Peptidoglycan
Protozoan
Resistant
Retrovirus
Sensitivity
Specificity
Superinfection
Susceptible
Virus

CHAPTER OBJECTIVES

At the end of the chapter, the reader will be able to:

1. Describe the classes of antibacterial and antiviral drugs.

2. Distinguish the various mechanisms of action antibacterial and antiviral drugs utilize.

3. Describe the pharmacology of various antimicrobials in humans.

4. Define the difference between bacteriostatic and bactericidal effects.

5. Broadly apply specific drugs to correct bacterial and viral species.

6. Explain the limitations and major side effects or interactions that exist for specific drugs.

Introduction

Antimicrobial therapy is a story of drug discovery and microbial evasion. It is also the story of dual pharmacology: that of the pathologic organisms that drugs are intended to target, and of the human hosts who, though not the therapeutic target, must absorb, distribute, metabolize, and eliminate antimicrobials they are administered or take. As with all organisms, microbes can acquire new capabilities through mutation and acquisition of novel DNA or RNA. For microbes, this enables them to become invulnerable to drugs designed to disable or destroy them. They *select* for strains that have emergent resistance, and they *acquire* abilities to resist new environmental hazards via selection, and from other microbes. Often, this resistance is accelerated by improper or inappropriate use of antimicrobial drugs. Thus, the escalation of resistance, followed by novel drug development, continues. Following proper guidelines for use of antimicrobial drugs will help slow the evolution of resistance, but, by nature, the cycle may well never stop. In addition, it is important to consider the effects these drugs have on the host. Unless designed specifically to alter or enhance a natural immune response, *all* antimicrobial actions on humans are considered "side effects."

This chapter emphasizes antibacterial and antiviral drugs, as these are the most commonly encountered anti-infectives in practice. Because many pathogens are living organisms, treatment of microbial diseases involves the pharmacology of both the host and the pathogen. Antimicrobial drugs are designed to act preferentially upon pathogens; part of the discussion will focus on the mechanisms by which pathogens are inhibited or killed by antimicrobials. Drugs target specific, essential microbial biochemical and physiological pathways, but also often affect the host. Therefore, **minimum inhibitory concentration** and **patient maximum tolerable concentrations** in-vivo are important considerations for both drug efficacy and patient safety. There is a saying: The dose makes the poison. Antimicrobial therapy is a balance between toxicities: While we "poison" the microbe, we must spare the host, as much as possible.

Terminology of Antimicrobial Drugs

Although terms like *antibiotic*, *antimicrobial*, and *anti-infective* are used interchangeably in practice, there are essential distinctions to be made among them.

An **anti-infective** is a drug that treats an infection caused by an organism; thus, this term encompasses treatments for infections involving not only microbes, but also macrobiotic organisms such as helminths. When speaking of microbial pathogens, **antimicrobial** is a more accurate term. Either of these might be considered interchangeable with *antibiotic*, but there is a distinction: An **antibiotic** refers to a drug that targets *any* organism in the body, including symbiotic (nonpathogenic) microbes as well as micro-and macro-organismal pathogens.

In popular parlance, *antibiotic* is often used to mean drugs used to treat bacterial infections, but a more accurate term would be **antibacterial**, just as drugs that target **viruses** are called **antivirals** and those that target **fungi** are **antifungals**. A further delineation is made with regard to the drug's mechanism of action: Antimicrobials that directly kill (eradicate) the target organism are termed-*cidal* (e.g., **bactericidal**, fungicidal); antimicrobials that only inhibit the growth of the organism, reproduction, or health are termed-*static* (e.g., **bacteriostatic**, fungistatic). "Static" drugs suppress the growth, or weaken the pathogen sufficiently to allow the patient's immune system to complete the recovery process, as opposed to "cidal" drugs that directly eradicate the invading microorganism. A **broad-spectrum** antimicrobial is effective against many strains of microorganisms, whereas a **narrow-spectrum** antimicrobial is effective against only a few strains. Each antimicrobial drug offers a unique profile of pharmacokinetics, specificity, spectrum, and resistance. *Antimicrobial drugs* is the most inclusive term.

Some antimicrobials kill the target organism, and so will be described as *-cidal*, while others inhibit the organism, allowing the patient's immune system to complete the recovery process, and will be described as *-static*. Technically, there will differences in meaning among the terms *antibacterial, antibiotic,* and *anti-infective*. However, in practice these terms are used interchangeably. Each antimicrobial drug offers a unique profile of pharmacokinetics, **specificity**, spectrum, and resistance.

Antibacterials

There are some general targets against which antimicrobial drugs have traditionally been aimed. Those for various **bacteria** are summarized in FIGURE 16-1.

Antibacterials include agents that are bacteriostatic, and those that are bactericidal. The various classes of antibacterials are introduced in roughly their order of discovery and use.

Sulfonamides

Sulfonamides were the first therapeutic antibacterial agents and were discovered in the 1930s (TABLE 16-1). Sulfonamides are derived

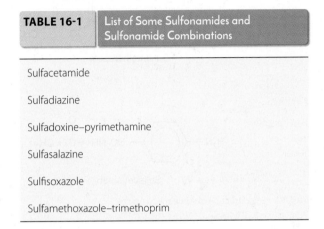

TABLE 16-1	List of Some Sulfonamides and Sulfonamide Combinations
Sulfacetamide	
Sulfadiazine	
Sulfadoxine–pyrimethamine	
Sulfasalazine	
Sulfisoxazole	
Sulfamethoxazole–trimethoprim	

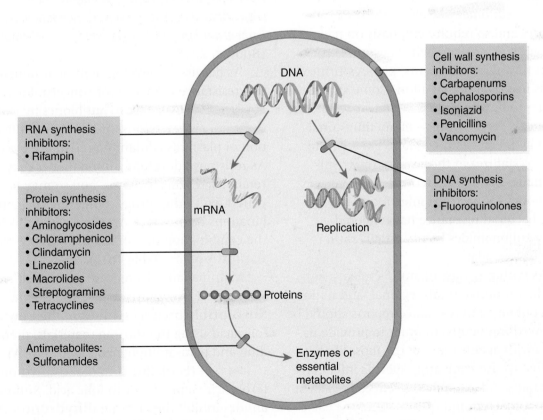

FIGURE 16-1 Mechanisms of action of some antibiotics.

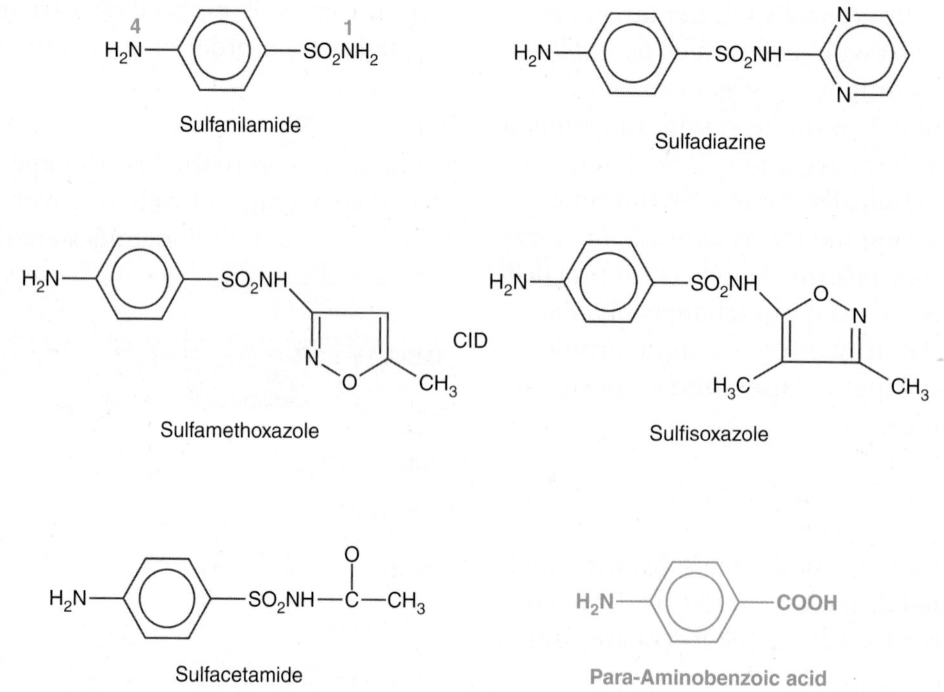

FIGURE 16-2 Structure of some sulfonamides.

from para-aminobenzenesulfonamide, or sulfanilamide (see **FIGURE 16-2**).

Most sulfonamides are fairly water insoluble, and so require emphasis on patient hydration in order to better eliminate these drugs through the patients' kidneys/urine. It is this insolubility that allows some sulfonamides to be effective agents for urinary tract infections, as the drugs—many times unaltered by metabolism—tend to concentrate (and crystallize) in the urinary tract. Sulfonamides are considered broad-spectrum antibiotics for bacterial infections. However, bacterial resistance has rendered many sulfonamides bacteriostatic, rather than bactericidal.

As with any class of antimicrobials, current institutional, local, regional, and national susceptibility and resistance reports should be reviewed frequently, in order to provide patients with agents that are the most likely to be effective for combating specific infections. Generally, sulfonamides are effective against **Gram-positive** and **Gram-negative** bacteria. The most common microorganisms that *may* be treatable with sulfonamides include:

Streptococcus pyogenes, Streptococcus pneumoniae, Haemophilus influenzae, Haemophilus ducreyi, Nocardia, Actinomyces, Calymmatobacterium granulomatis, and *Chlamydia trachomatis* (Boothe, 2018).

As discussed, development of antimicrobial resistance is a constant concern. Bacteria can become **resistant** to antibiotics by random genetic mutations, or through acquisition of plasmids containing resistance genes. As resistance develops, sulfonamides may retain bacterio*static* effects, and so may be paired with other drugs, rendering the combinations bacteri*cidal*. An example of this is the combination of **sulfamethoxazole** with **trimethoprim** (Table 16-1).

Mammalian cells require preformed folic acid and cannot synthesize their own. **Susceptible** bacteria synthesize their own folic acid using the starting materials, pteridine and para-aminobenzoic acid (PABA) (**FIGURE 16-3**) (Petri, 2011) to make dihydropteroic acid, a precursor to folic acid. Sulfonamides inhibit the enzyme **dihydropterate synthetase**, which is required for this first step. Sulfonamides have structures similar

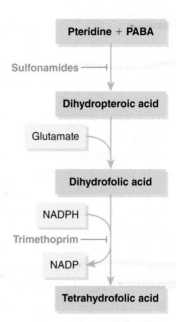

FIGURE 16-3 Folic acid synthesis in bacteria.

TABLE 16-2	Classification of Sulfonamides
Classification	Sulfonamide
Orally absorbed and rapidly excreted (renally)	Sulfadiazine
	Sulfadimidine
	Sulfamethoxazole
	Sulfamethizole
	Sulfadiazone
	Sulfisoxazole
Orally absorbed poorly	Sulfasalazine
Long-acting (half-life of ≥35 hour)	Sulfadimethoxine
	Sulfalene
	Sulfametomidine
	Sulfametoxydiazine
	Sulfaperin
	Sulfamerazine
	Sulfaphenazole
	Sulfamazone
Topical	Silver sulfadiazine
	Sulfanilamide (in vaginal suppositories)
	Ophthalmic sulfacetamide

to that of PABA and are mistakenly used by susceptible bacteria in this reaction, resulting in inhibition of folic acid synthesis. Because mammalian (patient) cells do not use this reaction, their folic acid supply is unaffected by the presence of sulfonamides. Trimethoprim, which is not a sulfonamide, often is paired with a sulfonamide, to augment sulfonamide action and circumvent bacterial adaptations that counter sulfonamide action in the first step of folic acid synthesis (Figure 16-3). Trimethoprim inhibits microbial dihydrofolate reductase, the enzyme that converts dihydrofolate to tetrahydrofolate, thereby adding a second obstacle to bacterial folic acid synthesis.

Sulfonamides can be classified by their oral absorption and excretion characteristics: (1) orally absorbed and excreted (renally) rapidly, (2) orally absorbed poorly, (3) topical, (4) orally long-lasting (absorbed rapidly, but also excreted slowly). Sulfonamides that are in these categories are shown in TABLE 16-2 (Petri, 2011). Sulfonamides and some of their notable characteristics and applications appear in TABLE 16-3.

Sulfonamides with rapid oral absorption and excretion are used for treatment of systemic infections as well as urinary tract

TABLE 16-3	Sulfonamides	
Drug	Characteristics	Uses
Sulfisoxazole	Rapid absorption/ excretion	UTIs, STDs, otitis media, eye infections, and CNS infections (meningococcal)
Sulfamethoxazole	Rapid absorption/ excretion	Wide range of infections, particularly in combination with trimethoprim, including UTIs, otitis media, bronchitis, pneumocystic pneumonia, traveler's diarrhea, and shigellosis
Sulfadiazine	Rapid absorption/ excretion	UTIs; combined with pyrimethamine, used for toxoplasmosis and malaria
Sulfasalazine	Poor absorption	Infections of the bowel
Sulfacetamide	Topical	Bacterial infections of eye, ear, and skin
Silver sulfadiazine	Topical	Prevention of wound infections
Sulfadoxine	Rapid absorption/ slow excretion	Primarily used in combination with pyrimethamine for prevention and treatment of malaria

infections (notably, the combination of sulfamethoxazole and trimethoprim). Poorly absorbed sulfonamides can be useful for treating infections of the gastrointestinal tract. Topical uses of sulfonamides include prevention and treatment of ophthalmic and skin infections from compromised skin, such as burns. Sulfadoxine, a long-acting sulfonamide, combined with pyrimethamine, is occasionally used for prevention and treatment of malaria (*Plasmodium falciparum*, a protozoan parasite). Sulfonamides are renally excreted, and if a patient is insufficiently hydrated, can cause *crystaluria*, in which drug crystals form in the urine, causing pain and irritation.

The most important adverse reactions associated with sulfonamides include hypersensitivity reactions (e.g., toxic epidermal necrolysis and Stevens-Johnson syndrome), crystalluria, and some anemias. Toxic epidermal necrolysis and Stevens-Johnson syndrome are thought to be caused by a T-cell-mediated cytotoxicity in keratinocytes (Gonzalez, 2018), though more immediate skin reactions suggest type-I hypersensitivity mechanisms may also be involved. Crystalluria is generally not a concern, except for with the N-4 acetylated sulfonamides, which have deceased water solubility, and thus occasionally present an issue, especially in poorly hydrated patients. Sulfonamides have been implicated in occasional photosensitivity reactions, probably caused by UV-induced free-radical production from the drugs (Moore, 2002). Therefore, general guidelines include ensuring patients have adequate-to-increased hydration for the duration of treatment, increased awareness, observation for signs of hypersensitivity and blood reactions, and adequate protection from sun exposure for the duration of therapy. Patients should be advised to wear more sunscreen than normal due to the increased possibility of burning while taking sulfonamides.

Drug Interactions and Contraindications

Sulfonamides are closely related to the sulfonylurea class of drugs used in the treatment of type 2 diabetes (Loubatières-Mariani, 2007), so sulfonamides may produce a reduction of blood glucose levels that can be significant with concomitant use of oral hypoglycemics (e.g., **tolbutamide**, **glyburide**, **glipizide**). This increases the risk of hypoglycemia in diabetic patients due to the enhancing effect of the antibacterial sulfonamide with the oral hypoglycemic drugs. Patients with allergies to sulfonamide-based diuretics are more likely to elicit hypersensitivity reactions to sulfonamide anti-infective drugs.

A similar enhancing effect is seen with the anticonvulsant phenytoin and the anticoagulant warfarin. Patients using any of these drugs should be carefully monitored for signs of overmedication.

In patients with renal failure, concurrent use of sulfonamides with cyclosporine increases the risk for nephrotoxicity and should be avoided; these drugs should be used with caution (generally as a last resort) in patients who have any history of kidney disease or kidney stones. Sulfonamides cross-react with sulfonylureas and in theory may also cross-react with loop or thiazide diuretics (Tan, Holmes, Kuo, Raji, & Goodwin, 2015); they should be used cautiously, if at all, in patients taking these drugs. Sulfonamides should be avoided if possible in pregnant or lactating women.

Nursing Considerations

Most sulfonamides are given orally; however, sulfamethoxazole-trimethoprim is also given intravenously. When IV administration is used, it should be slow or via drip. Oral preparations should be taken with 8 ounces of water on an empty stomach, and patients should be advised to maintain a fluid intake of at least 1,200 mL/day (8 to 10 glasses of water per day) because of the characteristics of sulfonamides' concentration in the kidneys.

The most important adverse reactions associated with sulfonamides include hypersensitivity reactions (e.g., Stevens-Johnson syndrome), crystalluria, and some anemias. Thus, one nursing consideration is to monitor the patient's complete blood count and assess for hemolysis so that the drug may be discontinued should a hematologic adverse response (e.g., thrombocytopenia, aplastic anemia, hemolytic anemia, or agranulocytosis) develop. General guidelines for patient teaching include ensuring patients have adequate hydration for the duration of treatment, and an increased awareness and observation for signs of hypersensitivity and blood reactions.

Sulfonamides also have been implicated in occasional photosensitivity reactions. Patients should be advised to avoid sun exposure if possible and wear SPF-15 sunblock and protective clothing if sun exposure is unavoidable, due to the increased possibility of burning while taking sulfonamides.

Tetracyclines

Tetracyclines (FIGURE 16-4) are bacteriostatic agents composed of three natural drugs derived from a common soil mold, *Streptomyces*—that is, tetracycline, demeclocycline, and oxytetracycline—as well as two other drugs derived semi-synthetically—doxycycline and minocycline—and have a broad range of bacteria for which they are useful. In addition to both Gram-negative and Gram-positive bacteria, tetracyclines are effective against infections caused by Rickettsia, *Coxiella burnetii, Mycoplasma pneumoniae,* Chlamydia species, Legionella species, and Ureaplasma. Also, tetracyclines may be useful for treatment of infections caused by some atypical Mycobacteria, and Plasmodium species that are resistant to antimicrobials directed against bacterial cell walls (MacDougall &

Chambers, 2011a). Tetracyclines were first used in the late 1940s. Those drugs included in the tetracycline class include tetracycline, chlortetracycline, oxytetracycline, demeclocycline, methacycline, doxycycline, and minocycline. Doxycycline and minocycline are most commonly used today.

Glycylcyclines are newer, synthetic analogs of tetracyclines, and are useful for overcoming tetracycline resistance. Currently, the only approved glycylcycline is tigecycline. Tetracyclines and glycycyclines act by binding susceptible bacterial 30s ribosomes, blocking tRNA access to its mRNA binding site, thereby inhibiting bacterial protein synthesis (FIGURE 16-5).

Tetracyclines readily chelate metal ions in the stomach and gastrointestinal tract. Binding of ions by tetracyclines inactivates the drugs. So, patients should be counseled to avoid concomitant (within one to two hours) ingestion of dairy products (calcium), vitamins (several ions), and antacids (magnesium and/or calcium ions) with oral tetracyclines. Tetracyclines are contraindicated in patients with a history of severe allergic reaction to them (which is rare) and during pregnancy and lactation. They should not be given to children younger than the age of eight and should be used with caution in clients with kidney or liver dysfunction (Herbert-Ashton & Clarkson, 2008). The reason for

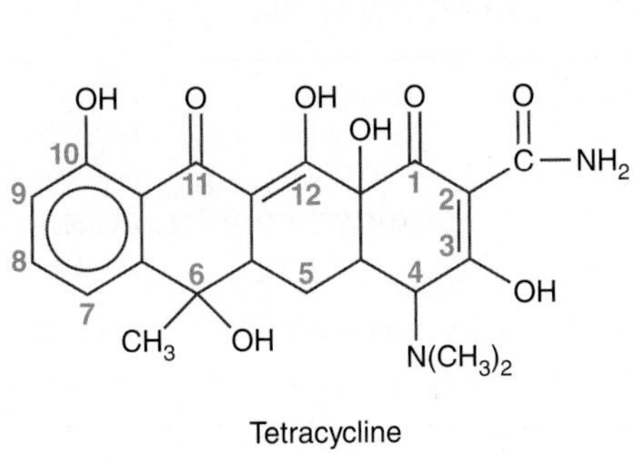

FIGURE 16-4 Structure of tetracycline.

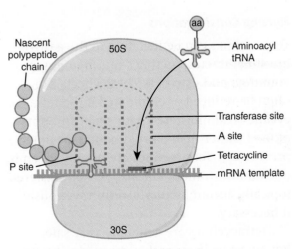

FIGURE 16-5 Mechanism of action for tetracyclines.

avoiding the use in children is because they are still forming teeth, and, as tetracyclines bind to calcium, they can cause permanent staining of preemergent teeth.

Tetracyclines are well distributed to most body fluids and tissues, except for cerebrospinal fluid (CSF), and are excreted by the kidney and liver. Bioavailability of doxycycline and minocycline is 90% to 100% even in the presence of food. With the other agents, bioavailability is lower and can be significantly decreased by food, especially substances containing minerals; for this reason, medications should be taken on an empty stomach if possible.

Although a great deal of microbial resistance has developed against members of this group over the years, and newer medications have been developed that are less toxic and more effective, the tetracyclines remain the drugs of choice for a number of specific infections, including those already listed and *Vibrio cholerae*, *Borrelia burgdorferi*, and gastric infections of *Helicobacter pylori*. Other diseases in which they are used include endocervical, rectal, and urethral infections caused by *Chlamydia*; acne; combination therapy with other anti-infective agents to treat pelvic inflammatory disease and STIs; and traveler's diarrhea caused by *E. coli*. Demeclocycline also has a use unrelated to infectious disease, as a treatment for the syndrome of inappropriate secretion of antidiuretic hormone.

Nursing Considerations

Tetracyclines can be irritating to the gastrointestinal tract, sometimes causing nausea, vomiting, and diarrhea. These effects can often be reduced or eliminated if the tetracycline is administered with small amounts of food (other than dairy products, as noted previously). Tetracyclines are usually given by oral administration, but may be administered topically, intramuscularly, or intravenously if necessary.

Tetracyclines are generally very safe, but adverse effects and interactions of note include the potential for photosensitivity and discoloration of undeveloped teeth. Therefore, patients should be warned that exposure to sunlight may result in burning of the skin more quickly than normal (most notably with demeclocycline and doxycycline). Patients should be advised to wear SPF-15 sunscreen and a hat, and to cover any exposed skin if exposure cannot be avoided. As previously stated, because of the potential for effects on teeth, use of tetracyclines or glycylcyclines should be avoided in pregnant women and children younger than eight years of age.

Review the history of any tetracycline reactions with patients. Each dose should be taken with eight ounces of water on an empty stomach. Doxycycline and minocycline can be taken with food. Review the patient's medications and dietary preferences and advise the patient that the drug must not be taken with, or within two hours of, antacids, iron preparations, or dairy products. Monitor for diarrhea, vaginal itching, or anal itching; report black, "furry" tongue immediately to the prescriber. These may be signs of adventitious infection. Offer small, frequent meals if nausea and vomiting occur.

β-Lactam Antibiotics

β-lactam antibiotics are bacteriostatic antibiotics, and include penicillins, cephalosporins, and other β-lactam structurally related antibiotics (TABLE 16-4). The beta-lactam (β-lactam) class derives its name from the beta-lactam

TABLE 16-4	β-Lactam Classes	
Drug Classification	Prototype Drug	Related Drugs
Natural penicillins	Penicillin G potassium	Penicillin G benzathine Penicillin G procaine Penicillin V
Penicillinase-resistant penicillins	Methicillin	Cloxacillin Dicloxacillin Nafcillin Oxacillin

Drug Classification	Prototype Drug	Related Drugs
Aminopenicillins	Ampicillin	Amoxicillin Bacampicillin Epicillin Hetacillin Metampicillin Pivampicillin Talampicillin
Ureidopenicillins	Mezlocillin	Azlocillin Piperacillin
Penicillin/beta-lactamase inhibitor combinations	Ampicillin/sulbactam	Amoxicillin clavulanate Piperacillin/tazobactam Ticarcillin/clavulanate
Carboxypenicillins	Carbenicillin	Ticarcillin
Extended-spectrum penicillins*	Mecillinam	Sulbenicillin
First-generation cephalosporins	Cephadroxil Cephazolin Cephalexin Cephradine	
Second-generation cephalosporins (includes cabacephams)	Cefaclor Ceforanide Cefotetan Cefoxitin Cefprozil Cefuroxime acetil Cefuroxime Cefmetazole Loracarbef	
Third-generation cephalosporins	Cefdinir Cefditoren pivoxil Cefibuten Cefixime Cefotaxime Cefpodoxime proxetil Cefperazone Ceftizoxime Ceftazidime Ceftriaxone Ceftibuten	
Fourth-generation cephalosporins	Cefepime	

*Aminopenicillins, carboxypenicillins, and ureidopenicillins are all considered extended-spectrum penicillins. However, aminopenicillins lack activity against *Pseudomonas* species.

ring that is the source of their bactericidal activity against numerous Gram-positive and some Gram-negative bacteria. The class includes a wide range of antibacterial drugs, including penicillins, cephalosporins, carbacephems, clavams (oxapenems), monobactams, and carbapenems.

In general, β-lactams are very safe drugs, although injection-related reactions do occasionally occur. β-lactams have a reputation of being "risky" drugs to administer due to the widespread *perception* that they often induce allergic reactions, even though the *incidence* of allergic response to penicillins is actually relatively low (1% to 2% of patients). The difference between the perception and the reality is that to many patients (and even some practitioners), *any* adverse response may be interpreted as allergy, when most of the time the "reaction" actually involves a non-immune effect or even an effect unrelated to the drug's activity. For example, among patients with acute Epstein-Barr virus infection who are given amoxicillin, it is common for a pruritic, macropapular rash to emerge that is often mistaken for an anaphylactoid reaction. These patients may take the same drug under other circumstances and experience no reaction.

Incidence of allergic reaction to cephalosporins is still lower; even in those patients known to have an allergy to penicillins, true allergic reactions to cephalosporin (as opposed to non-immune-mediated sensitivity responses) occur in only a small percentage. The anaphylactic cross-sensitivity between penicillins and first-generation cephalosporins has been estimated to be as high as 40% (i.e., 40% of 1.2%, or 0.4% of patients), whereas cross-sensitivity between penicillins and third- or fourth-generation cephalosporins appears to be negligible (Campagna, Bond, Schabelman, & Hayes, 2012).

Nevertheless, many people *are* allergic to one or more penicillin, *and* lactams in general. Therefore, penicillins (and cephalosporins) should be used with caution in patients whose response (history) is unclear. In those patients with a history of a bona fide allergic response, these agents should be completely avoided.

As with most broad-spectrum antibiotics, prolonged oral use can lead to overpopulation by yeast or fungi in the gastrointestinal tract or mouth (i.e., thrush). Occasionally, use of β-lactams can lead to severe infection by intestinal flora. These effects are due to the destruction of nonpathogenic bacteria along with the targeted organism(s). Use of probiotic preparations to restore gut flora as a means of curtailing or offsetting these effects has been recommended by some sources (Hempel et al., 2012), but approached with caution by others (Hickson, 2011).

Mechanism of Action

Beta-lactam antibiotics act by inhibiting bacterial cell wall synthesis. They do so by entering into the bacterial cell wall and binding to a specific protein within the peptidoglycan layer of the cell wall, which is essential for cell wall integrity (the protein is called, appropriately enough, the penicillin-binding protein). After attaching to this protein, the drug then interrupts normal cell wall synthesis; the bacteria usually die from lysis.

Penicillins

Penicillin was discovered in 1928 but was not formally used in patients until the early 1940s. Though the central portion of the **penicillin** molecule is responsible for most β-lactam effects, the side chain attached to the central portion dictates the unique pharmacology of each drug, and so the antibiotic spectrum each β-lactam derivative exhibits (FIGURE 16-6).

Recall that **peptidoglycan** is an important component of bacterial cell walls, and that Gram-positive bacteria have thicker cell walls than do Gram-negative bacteria. Both penicillins and cephalosporins act by inhibiting the final step of bacterial peptidoglycan synthesis, blocking proper bacterial cell wall formation and lysis. The mechanisms by which these occur are presently being clarified, but understanding of the details is still incomplete. Unless protected by chemically added groups, the basic β-lactam structure is susceptible to the enzymes β-lactamase (also called penicillinase) and amidase, which are produced by bacteria (Figure 16-6). These enzymes destroy the structural integrity of the β-lactams and compromise their effectiveness.

The penicillins are most commonly used to kill Gram-positive bacteria: *Staphylococcus,*

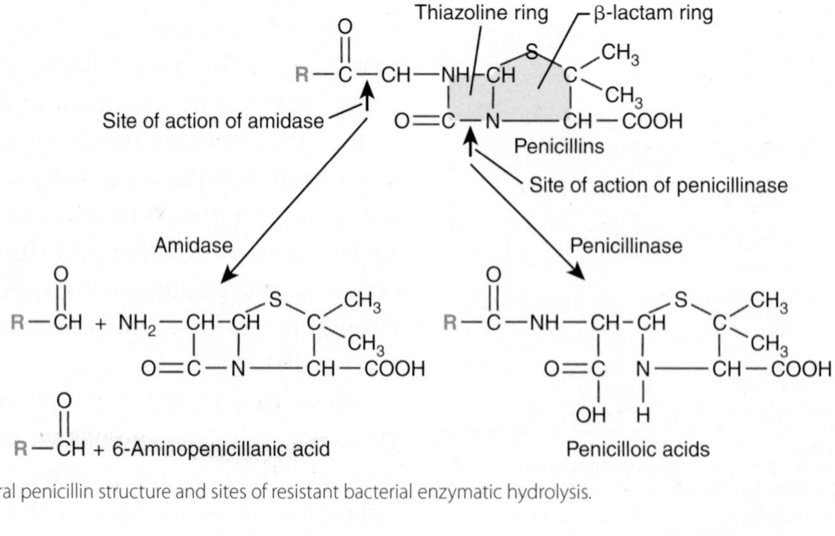

FIGURE 16-6 General penicillin structure and sites of resistant bacterial enzymatic hydrolysis.

Enterococcus, and *Streptococcus*. These drugs have been classified into four groups, based upon chemical structure and the type of bacteria they are able to kill:

- Natural penicillins
- Penicillinase-resistant penicillins
- Aminopenicillins
- Extended-spectrum penicillins, including carboxypenicillins and ureidopenicillins

The extended-spectrum penicillins, including the aminopenicillins, carboxypenicillins, and ureidopenicillins, have activity against Gram-negative bacteria, such as *Pseudomonas*, *Enterobacter*, and *Proteus* species.

Some combination drugs contain both penicillins and beta-lactamase inhibitors (TABLE 16-5). The beta-lactamase inhibitors prevent destruction of the penicillin with which they are paired.

Penicillins in general have few adverse effects and are well tolerated. Whether given orally, intravenously, or intramuscularly, they tend to be well distributed to most body tissues and fluids and are eliminated by the kidneys. However, many bacteria species have developed resistance to these drugs, as mentioned previously (mostly *Staphylococcus* species), via **beta-lactamase**, which breaks down the molecular integrity of beta-lactam antibiotics (the enzyme targets and destroys the beta-lactam ring), rendering the drug inactive, and thereby unable to destroy the bacterial cell wall.

Natural penicillins are the agents of choice for pneumonia and meningitis caused by *Streptococcus pneumoniae*; pharyngitis caused by *Streptococcus pyogenes*; infectious endocarditis caused by *Streptococcus viridans*; meningitis caused by *N. meningitidis*; and syphilis caused by *T. pallidum*. These drugs are also used for anthrax, tetanus, gas gangrene, and prophylactically for rheumatic fever *and* bacterial endocarditis in individuals with mitral valve prolapse, congenital heart disease, and prosthetic heart valves.

Aminopenicillins such as **ampicillin** are useful for the same infections targeted by

TABLE 16-5	Penicillins	
Prototype Drug	Related Drugs	Drug Classification
Penicillin G potassium	Penicillin G benzathine	Natural penicillins
	Penicillin G procaine	
	Penicillin V	
Methicillin	Cloxacillin	Penicillinase-resistant penicillins
	Dicloxacillin	
	Nafcillin	
	Oxacillin	
Ampicillin	Amoxicillin	Aminopenicillins
	Bacampicillin	
	Epicillin	
	Hetacillin	
	Metampicillin	
	Pivampicillin	
	Talampicillin	
Mezlocillin	Azlocillin	Ureidopenicillins
	Piperacillin	
Ampicillin/ sulbactam	Amoxicillin clavulanate	Penicillin/ beta-lactamase inhibitor combinations
	Piperacillin/ tazobactam	
	Ticarcillin/ clavulanate	
Carbenicillin	Ticarcillin	Carboxypenicillins
Mecillinam	Sulbenicillin	Extended-spectrum penicillins*

*Aminopenicillins, carboxypenicillins, and ureidopenicillins are all considered extended-spectrum penicillins. However, aminopenicillins lack activity against *Pseudomonas* species.

natural penicillins but are also active against the following Gram-negative bacteria: *Haemophilus influenzae*, *Escherichia coli*, *Salmonella*, and *Shigella*. These agents are used in bacterial meningitis, otitis media, septicemia, gonorrhea, and sinusitis.

Extended-spectrum penicillins such as **ticarcillin** are mainly used for infections of *Pseudomonas aeruginosa* and are usually given in combination with an aminoglycoside (such as **gentamicin**) antibiotic to help increase the killing of the *Pseudomonas* bacteria.

Penicillin–beta-lactamase inhibitor combinations, such as **ampicillin-sulbactam**, are used in infections that are caused by bacteria resistant to beta-lactam antibiotics.

Penicillins are roughly categorized as discussed here, and summarized in Table 16-5. Again, current susceptibilities and resistances should be periodically reviewed to ensure drug choices that allow the least chance of resistance, and optimum patient risk (Doi & Chambers, 2015).

1. Penicillin G and penicillin V are very susceptible to penicillinase, so they are effective against Gram-positive cocci, but not most *S. aureus* strains.
2. Nafcillin, oxacillin, and dicloxacillin are *penicillinase-resistant*, but less active than penicillin G and penicillin V against susceptible bacteria (i.e., *S. aureus* and *S. epidermidis*).
3. Ampicillin and amoxicillin possess the activity of the above penicillins, *plus* some Gram-negative bacterial coverage, such as *H. influenza*, *E. coli*, and *Proteus mirabilus*, and are known as the *extended (spectrum) amino-penicillins*. Clavulanate or sulbactam can be added to prolong action by inhibiting class A β-lactamases, which degrade many penicillins.
4. The carboxypenicillins and ureidopenicillins class, which includes carbenicillin indanyl with clavulanate, have *extended Gram-negative* activity including *Pseudomonas*, *Enterobacter*, and *Proteus* species.
5. Mezlocillin and azlocillin (both now discontinued in the United States) have a further extended Gram-negative spectrum, with improved activity against *Pseudomonas*, *Klebsiella*, and some other Gram-negative bacteria.

Drug Interactions and Contraindications

Penicillin decreases the effectiveness of oral contraceptives and warfarin. NSAIDs compete with penicillin for protein-binding sites and cause more free penicillin to circulate in the body. Probenecid enhances the effectiveness of penicillin. Food interferes with the absorption of penicillin. Penicillins given intravenously should never be mixed with aminoglycosides in the same intravenous (IV) solution, as penicillins can inactivate aminoglycosides, and so the two drug classes are considered "incompatible" with regard to mixing them in the same container. However, once delivered to the patient, this incompatibility does not exist in-vivo. Bacteriostatic drugs should not be given with a penicillin, as this combination could decrease the effectiveness of the penicillin; instead, the penicillin should be administered first, followed by the bacteriostatic drug a few hours later.

The penicillins are contraindicated in patients with history of severe allergic reaction to them, and/or to cephalosporins. Counsel pregnant women according to benefits and potential risks.

Nursing Implications

When considering prescribing a penicillin, review the history of any penicillin reactions with the patient. Patients prescribed oral penicillin should be instructed to take the full course of medication at evenly spaced intervals around the clock to maintain blood concentration above the minimum effective concentration (MIC). Oral penicillin should be taken with six to eight ounces of water, but without food, in order to avoid acidic stomach fluids, as these degrade the drug. Alert patients to the symptoms of superinfections (e.g., candidiasis), and treat them appropriately if these concomitant infections arise.

For parenteral dosing, monitor the patient for 30 minutes after giving the parenteral dose of any penicillin for signs of allergic reaction. Monitor the patient for decreasing signs of infection and kidney function (especially in patients with decreased kidney function). Dilute intramuscular (IM) doses in the diluent recommended by the drug manufacturer and rotate injection sites. Monitor IV sites closely for irritation. Monitor patients on sodium restriction closely who are receiving high doses of sodium penicillin G, carbenicillin, and ticarcillin for signs of sodium overloading, and follow serum sodium levels and cardiac status. In patients receiving high doses of potassium penicillin G, check serum potassium levels before initiating the medication, and then monitor for hyperkalemia.

Women taking oral contraceptives should be advised to add a second method of protection (e.g., a barrier method) at least for the duration of therapy. This is true for many broad-spectrum antibiotics, due to their effects on the enterohepatic recirculation of oral estrogens, resulting in subtherapeutic estrogen concentrations.

Cephalosporins

Cephalosporins were discovered in the late 1940s and came into clinical use in the 1960s. Chemically, they appear very similar to each other, and to penicillins (FIGURE 16-7). The core

Cephem nucleus

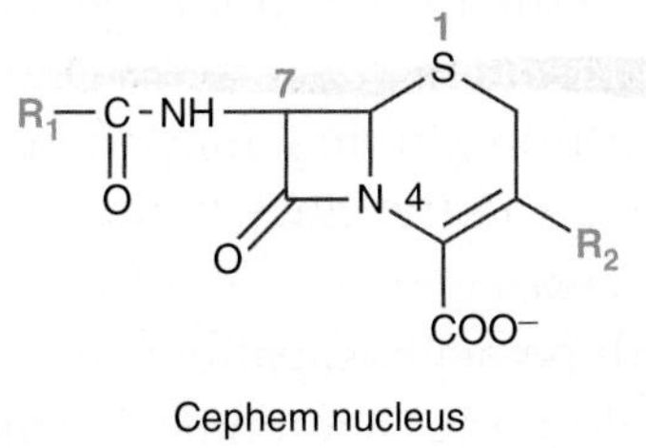

FIGURE 16-7 Basic structure of the cephalosporins.

structure differs slightly among cephalosporins, and slightly—but of significance—between cephalosporins and penicillins. Like the penicillins, the cephalosporins inhibit bacterial cell wall synthesis. The categories of cephalosporins are shown in TABLE 16-6. The most common method of classification is by "generation" (first to fourth), which, more or less, follows their usefulness from Gram-positive to more Gram-negative organisms. The fourth-generation cephalosporins are used in hospitalized patients who have infections with Gram-positive bacteria, Enterobacteriaceae, or *Pseudomonas*.

Though the β-lactams may have earned a reputation of being risky drugs to administer due to the stereotype of induction of allergic reactions, the incidence with penicillins is actually relatively low (about 1% to 2% of patients). The incidence of severe allergic reactions to cephalosporins is lower than that of penicillins (from 1% to 10%, with rare anaphylaxis (<0.02%) (Annè & Reisman, 1995), and, though they share structural similarities, the cross-sensitivity between penicillins and cephalosporins is quite low (0.012%

TABLE 16-6	Cephalosporin Antibacterial Drugs by Generation		
Generation	Generic Names	Organisms Targeted	Resistant Organisms
First	Cefazolin, cephalexin, cefadroxil, cephradine	*Streptococcus* spp., *Staphylococcus aureus*.	*Acinetobacter* spp., *Listeria monocytogenes*, *Legionella* spp., MRSA, penicillin-resistant *Streptococcus* spp., *Xanthomonas maltophilia*.
Second	Cefuroxime, cefuroxime axetil, cefotetan, cefoxitin, cefprozil, cefmetazole, loracarbef	*Escherichia coli*, *Haemophilus influenzae*, *Klebsiella* spp., *Moraxella catarrhalis*, *Proteus* spp., *Streptococcus* spp., *Staphylococcus aureus*. Cefmetazole and loracarbef: All of the above plus *Bacteroides* spp.	*Acinetobacter* spp., *Listeria monocytogenes*, *Legionella* spp., MRSA, *Xanthomonas maltophilia*. Has less activity against Gram-positive species than first-generation agents. Activity of cefmetazole and loracarbef against *S. aureus* is somewhat reduced.
Third	Cefotaxime, ceftriaxone, cefdinir, cefditoren, ceftibuten, cefpodoxime, ceftizoxime, cefoperazone, ceftazidime	Enterobacteriaceae, *Neisseria gonorrhoeae* (ceftriaxone only), *Providencia* spp., *Pseudomonas aeruginosa*, *Serratia*, *Streptococcus pneumoniae*, *Streptococcus pyogenes*, *Staphylococcus aureus*. Some activity against *Bacteroides* spp., but less than second-generation drugs. Cefotaxime has greatest activity against *S. pyogenes* and *Staph. aureus*.	*Acinetobacter* spp., *Listeria monocytogenes*, *Legionella* spp., MRSA, *Xanthomonas maltophilia*. Most strains of *N. gonorrhoeae* have become resistant to all but ceftriaxone.
Fourth	Cefepime	Similar to third-generation spectrum, but with greater resistance to beta-lactamases.	*Acinetobacter* spp., *Listeria monocytogenes*, *Legionella* spp., MRSA, *Xanthomonas maltophilia*.

of patients), meaning, in most cases, patients allergic to penicillins are not also allergic to cephalosporins. However, many people *are* allergic to these classes, and especially the penicillins are notable for induction of type-I anaphylactic reactions, and there is no reliable test to predict or confirm penicillin allergy (Romano, Mondino, Viola, & Montushi, 2003). It has been estimated that only about 1.2% of patients who report "penicillin allergy" are, in fact, allergic, though such allergies are rarely confirmed, and practitioners take a cautious approach when prescribing (Albin & Agarwal, 2014). The cross-sensitivity between penicillins and first-generation cephalosporins has been estimated to be as high as 40% (i.e., 40% of 1.2%, or 0.4% of patients), with cross-sensitivity between penicillins and third-or fourth-generation cephalosporins appearing to be negligible (Campagna, Bond, Schabelman, & Hayes, 2012). Therefore, penicillins (and perhaps cephalosporins) should be used with caution in patients, and if there is a history of bonafide allergy, should be completely avoided. In general, β-lactams are very safe drugs, with mechanical, injection-related reactions occasionally occurring. As with most broad-spectrum antibiotics, prolonged oral use can lead to overpopulation by yeast or fungi in the mouth or gastrointestinal tract (i.e., thrush). Occasionally, use of β-lactams can lead to severe infection by intestinal flora. These effects are due to the destruction of nonpathogenic gut bacteria along with the targeted organism(s).

Drug Interactions and Contraindications

The cephalosporins are contraindicated in patients with a history of severe allergic reaction to them and/or to penicillins. If the patient is known to have had a mild or moderate adverse response to either class in previous usage, clinicians should consider alternative options; if no better antibiotic option is available for treatment, patients known to have had adverse responses in the past should be carefully monitored for similar reactions. Patients should be warned to abstain from alcohol during therapy and for the first 72 hours after completing therapy, as alcohol in combination with some cephalosporins can cause a disulfiram-like reaction.

Counsel pregnant women according to benefits and potential risks of cephalosporins. These agents have been found to enter breastmilk, so they should be used with caution in breastfeeding mothers.

Nursing Implications

Review the history of any penicillin or cephalosporin reactions with the patient; consider alternative therapy in patients with a known beta-lactam allergy. When administering a cephalosporin parenterally, the IM injection should be given deeply into a large muscle mass. IV forms should be well diluted, and the IV site should be monitored for signs of redness, tenderness, and swelling. Check prothrombin time for patients taking **cefazolin**, **cefmetazole**, **cefoperazone**, and **cefotetan**.

As with penicillins, patients prescribed oral cephalosporins should be instructed to take the full course of medication at evenly spaced intervals around the clock to maintain blood levels. Oral cephalosporins should be taken with six to eight ounces of water; avoid taking them with acidic fluids as these will destroy the drug. Prolonged use may lead to superinfection, and clinicians should be alert for *Clostridium difficile*–associated diarrhea in patients who present with persistent diarrhea after use. Alert patients to the symptoms of superinfections and treat them appropriately if these infections arise. Oral forms of cephalosporins should be taken on an empty stomach if possible, but patients may take them with milk or food if gastric problems occur.

Carbapenems

Carbapenems are a class of beta-lactam antibiotics that are distinguished by a fused beta-lactam ring and a five-member ring system. The drugs in this class—**imipenem**, **meropenem**, **ertapenem**, **doripenem**, **panipenem**, and **biapenem**—have a broader spectrum of activity compared to the penicillins and cephalosporins; they are considered potent agents against severe infections. More importantly, the carbapenems are called extended-spectrum beta-lactamases (ESBLs) because they are the only agents available that have activity against organisms capable of resisting not only standard beta-lactam antibiotics but also the combination agents that utilize a beta-lactamase inhibitor to reduce the microbe's ability to hydrolyze the antibiotic (Hawkey, 2012). These properties make carbapenems the agents of choice for mixed aerobic and anaerobic infections resistant to treatment with other antibiotics, especially for cephalosporin-resistant *Enterobacter* infections. Hospitalized patients with serious infections may be treated with carbapenems if the suspected organism is a cephalosporin-resistant or penicillin-resistant bacterium. Note, however, that some strains of *Enterobacter* have begun to develop resistance to carbapenems (Hawkey, 2012).

Imipenem, panipenem, and doripenem are very effective against Gram-positive bacteria (Papp-Wallace, Endimiani, Taracila, & Bonomo, 2011), including streptococci, enterococci, staphylococci, and *Listeria*. For imipenem, the list of susceptible pathogens includes penicillin-resistant strains of *S. pneumoniae* and some strains of MRSA as well as anaerobes. Meropenem, biapenem, ertapenem, and doripenem have slightly greater efficacy against Gram-negative organisms (Papp-Wallace, Endimiani, Taracila, & Bonomo, 2011).

Meropenem and doripenem have an antimicrobial spectrum of activity similar to that of imipenem, with greater activity against Gram-negative aerobes but less activity against Gram-positive aerobes. All three drugs are effective against *Pseudomonas aeruginosa* and *Acinetobacter baumannii*, although resistance to them is spreading in *A. baumannii* (Hawkey, 2012). Doripenem has lower MICs than do imipenem and meropenem versus *P. aeruginosa* and *A. baumannii*, making it attractive as a first choice against these bacteria,

if possible; of all the members of this class, doripenem is least susceptible to hydrolysis by carbapenemases.

Drug Interactions and Contraindications

Drug sensitivity is the most serious concern with the carbapenem drugs, although the frequency of hypersensitivity is estimated at less than 3% (Hawkey, 2012). As stated previously regarding penicillins and cephalosporins, cross-sensitivity among individuals with allergies both to penicillin and carbepenem is low, approximately 1%; in severe infections, the low likelihood of allergic reaction should be weighed against the need for aggressive therapy. Because of issues of resistance, carbapenems should be avoided in patients with known *C. difficile* infection or high likelihood of contracting such an infection (Hawkey, 2012).

For all agents in this class, nephrotoxicity, neurotoxicity (including status epilepticus), and immunomodulation have been reported. Seizures in patients with renal impairment are a specific risk, and patients with renal impairment should have doses adjusted in accordance with the guidelines specific to the agent used. Therefore, renal function should be monitored in these patients. Liver function should be monitored, particularly in those patients with known or likely hepatic impairment.

Nursing Considerations

Review the history of any penicillin or cephalosporin reactions with patients; consider alternative therapy in patients with known beta-lactam allergy. Assess for and adjust doses in the presence of renal or hepatic impairment. Do not mix carbapenems with other medications in the IV. Assess patients for CNS or seizure-related disorders and GI disorders such as colitis, nausea, vomiting, and pseudomembranous colitis, which are known adverse effects associated with this class. Monitor patients for abscess or inflammation at the injection site as well as for phlebitis or rash. Use of carbapenem drugs may lead to superinfection, and clinicians should be alert for persistent diarrhea after use. Alert patients to the symptoms of super-infections and treat the symptoms appropriately if these infections arise.

Monobactams

Monobactams are similar to other beta-lactam antibiotics but contain a monocyclic beta-lactam ring. Aztreonam, the only monobactam available in the United States, is relatively resistant to beta-lactamases. Its spectrum of activity includes Gram-negative rods, but it has no activity against Gram-positive bacteria or anaerobic organisms. It is used primarily in treatment of UTIs, dermal infections, septicemia, intra-abdominal infections, and gynecologic infections involving the following organisms: *Citrobacter, Enterobacter, E. coli, H. pneumoniae, Klebsiella, N. gonorrhoeae, Proteus, Providencia, Pseudomonas, Salmonella,* and *Serratia.*

Drug Interactions and Contraindications

Aztreonam is well tolerated, with few adverse reactions reported. This agent *lacks* cross-sensitivity in patients with documented allergies to penicillin or cephalosporin antibiotics, but should nonetheless be used with caution in patients with significant type-I anaphylactic (immediate)-type beta-lactam hypersensitivity.

Nursing Considerations

For IV injection, after constituting aztreonam with a diluent in accordance with the manufacturer's instructions, the medication should be administered immediately and any excess discarded; do not reserve extra constituted drug for later use.

Beta-Lactamase Inhibitors

The drugs in the beta-lactamase inhibitor class (clavulanate, sulbactam, and tazobactam) are similar in structure to beta-lactam molecules but have only limited direct effects on bacteria. Their value lies, as their name suggests, in their ability to deactivate the

beta-lactamase enzymes produced by resistant organisms, thereby preventing these enzymes from halting the actions of beta-lactam antibiotics. The result is prolongation of beta-lactam MIC concentrations, without necessitating drug doses that would potentially be toxic to the patient. As adjunct medications, they are beneficial in terms of their ability to boost the potency (duration/sustained concentration) of antibacterial agents that otherwise might not be effective against particular organisms or specific resistant strains due to intolerably high MICs. When combined with beta-lactamases, beta-lactams can be used at serum concentrations that are lower than would be required without the beta-lactamases, allowing tolerable drug concentrations in patients. However, increased use has led to the emergence of organisms that are resistant even to the combination drugs—in particular, strains of *E. coli* and *K. pneumoniae* that show resistance to sulbactam and clavulanate (Drawz & Bonomo, 2010).

Each beta-lactamase inhibitor agent has slightly different pharmacology, stability, and potency, but the efficacy of the combination against the organism at issue is determined by the antibiotic with which the beta-lactamase inhibitor is paired, coupled with the (weak) intrinsic activity of each component of the combination therapy. Therefore, sensitivity and susceptibility of pathogens should be known. It should be clear that, *alone*, beta-lactamase inhibitors are not useful. They are only considered *adjuncts* to specified beta-lactams.

Drug Interactions and Contraindications

Beta-lactamase inhibitors as a class have limited toxicity, and most adverse effects seen in patients are due to the coadministered antibacterial drug (Lehne, 2012). Allergy to clavulanic acid has been observed, however (Tortajada Girbés et al., 2008).

Aminoglycosides

Aminoglycosides (the prototype streptomycin is shown in FIGURE 16-8) were discovered in 1943 (Rogers, 2009), are of primary

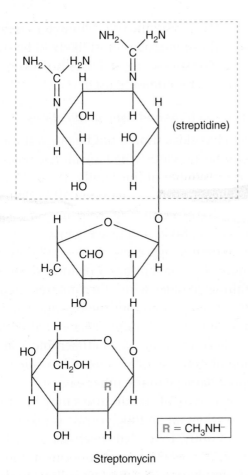

use against aerobic Gram-negative bacteria, and are bactericidal. They act by first traversing bacterial porin protein channels into bacterial periplasmic space, then being transported across the inner membrane, eventually binding RNA polysomes (30s, with effects on 50s). Binding of polysomes causes misreading of the mRNA, causing premature termination of mRNA translation, and leading to incomplete and incorrect protein synthesis by the susceptible bacteria (FIGURE 16-9). It is thought these aberrant proteins are inserted into the bacterial cytoplasmic membrane, causing leakage, and eventually disruption of the bacterial cell envelope.

The aminoglycosides include amikacin, gentamicin, kanamycin, neomycin, netilmicin, paromomycin, streptomycin, and tobramycin. Most aminoglycosides are administered via IM injection. Neomycin and paromomycin are administered orally.

The aminoglycosides tend to be more toxic (or have more narrow *therapeutic indices*) than other antibiotics, with nephro- and ototoxicities being the most notable. Their major

FIGURE 16-8 Structure of streptomycin, the prototype aminoglycoside.

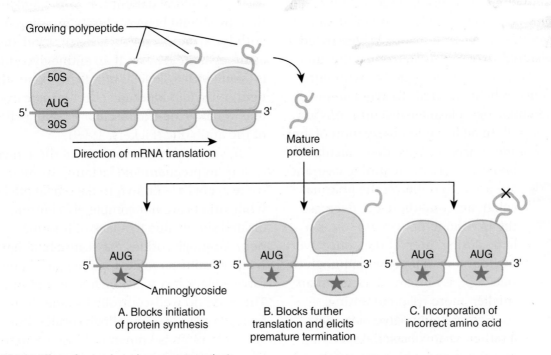

FIGURE 16-9 Effects of aminoglycosides on protein synthesis.

use is for systemic Gram-negative infections, including those resulting from *E. coli*, *Serratia*, *Proteus*, *Klebsiella*, and *Pseudomonas* (MacDougall and Chambers, 2011b). They can sometimes be effective against methicillin-resistant *Staph. aureus* (MRSA). In some circumstances, aminoglycosides are used in combination with other antibiotics to improve spectral coverage or avoid bacterial resistance. Bacterial killing is concentration dependent, so a challenge often is to maintain the highest possible aminoglycoside concentration in the patient, without surpassing the concentration where the likelihood of nephrotoxicity or ototoxicity becomes too great.

Toxicities caused by aminoglycosides can occur when administered by any of the available dosage routes (oral, injectable, rectal, and even topical). Ototoxicity occurs from toxic effects on hair cells and neurons in the cochlea, and, eventually the auditory nerve. Nephrotoxicity is caused by actions of aminoglycosides in the proximal tubules. This can lead to decreased glomerular filtration rate (GFR) and increased serum creatinine concentrations (Rougier et al., 2003). Once it occurs, ototoxicity is often irreversible, whereas nephrotoxicity is usually reversible, because proximal tubules can regenerate. These problems are more often encountered when aminoglycosides are administered systemically than topically, unless a large surface area, such as with burn patients, is being treated. To avoid aminoglycoside toxicities, plasma concentrations are monitored. In addition to observation of aminoglycoside concentrations, dose calculations based on patient creatinine clearance are used. To optimize the pharmacokinetics (and therefore decrease the likelihood of toxicity), often a large dosing interval (i.e., once every 24 hours) with a higher aminoglycoside dose, is employed, rather than smaller, more frequent dosing.

Because aminoglycosides have a rather narrow bacterial spectrum of activity, and a high potential for

toxicity, their systemic use is limited to treatment of those microbes most likely to be susceptible. For smaller topical uses however, they are very commonly used.

Drug Interactions and Contraindications

Aminoglycosides should not be taken if the patient has previously had an allergic reaction to a member of this family. They must be used cautiously in patients with Parkinson disease, dehydration, liver or kidney disease, myasthenia gravis, and hearing loss due to the potential to aggravate these conditions or promote additional injury. Coadministration of aminoglycosides with other innately nephrotoxic drugs compounds the existing risk for kidney damage and should be avoided. Similarly, the concurrent use of ethacrynic acid (a loop diuretic) with an aminoglycoside can promote damage to the inner ear.

The activity of certain drugs may be enhanced when an aminoglycoside is taken concomitantly. Extended-spectrum penicillins (e.g., **ticarcillin**) inactivate the aminoglycosides; however, other penicillins produce a synergistic effect when combined with these drugs. Aminoglycosides increase anticoagulant activity when taken with an anticoagulant. Therefore, patients on anticoagulant therapy should be very closely monitored, both for aminoglycoside concentration and anticoagulant activity. If an aminoglycoside is taken with a skeletal muscle relaxant, the neuromuscular blockade effect is increased due to native neuromuscular blocking effects of the antibiotic (Fiekers, 1999).

It is advisable to avoid use of these medications in pregnant and lactating women, as some agents are known to have fetal effects while others are not completely contraindicated simply due to a lack of information. Aminoglycosides may cause fetal harm when administered during pregnancy and carry a black box warning for this reason. There are no well-controlled studies in pregnant women for all aminoglycosides, but **streptomycin** is known to cause harm to the fetus in-utero. Others have not been shown to cause fetal harm. However, all aminogly-cosides should be used cautiously in pregnant patients, and these patients should be properly apprised of potential risks versus benefits from use of these drugs. Likewise, generally only small amounts of aminoglycoside doses partition into breastmilk. Because the potential for harm exists, breastfeeding patients should be apprised of the risks and benefits prior to their use during nursing.

Nursing Considerations

Review the history of any aminoglycoside reactions with patients. Aminoglycosides may be administered via the oral, topical, IM, and IV routes. Oral forms should be taken on an empty stomach, and the patient advised to take the full course of medication. IV doses should be administered slowly, over 30 minutes or more; peak and trough levels must be monitored. Peak levels greater than 12 mcg/mL and trough levels greater than 2 mcg/mL are associated with toxicity. If the patient is also receiving an extended-spectrum penicillin, administer the aminoglycoside and penicillin at least 2 hours apart.

Nurses should monitor for adverse effects of aminoglycoside drugs, which may include any of the following conditions: weakness, depression, confusion, numbness, tingling, and neuromuscular blockade; hypertension, hypotension, and palpitations; ototoxicity; nausea, vomiting, diarrhea, stomatitis, and weight loss; nephrotoxicity; bone marrow depression; joint pain; superinfection; and apnea. The patient's BUN, creatinine clearance, and input and output (I & O), as well as hearing, in particular, should be monitored, especially if administering other ototoxic or nephrotoxic drugs in tandem with aminoglycosides. IV calcium gluconate can reverse the neuromuscular blockade caused by aminoglycosides (Herbert-Ashton & Clarkson, 2008).

Macrolides

Macrolide antibiotics were introduced in the 1950s. This class of antimicrobials includes erythromycin (FIGURE 16-10), clarithromycin, and azithromycin. A variety of newer macrolides has been developed, including azithromycin, clarithromycin, dirithromycin, roxithromycin, and the ketolide variant telithromycin. Macrolides bind bacterial 50s ribosomes and block actions of tRNA. The results include inhibition of bacterial protein synthesis (FIGURE 16-11). Macrolides are usually bacteriostatic, though they can be bactericidal at higher concentrations. They are most useful for treatment of infections caused by aerobic Gram-positive cocci and bacilli, including *Staphylococci* and

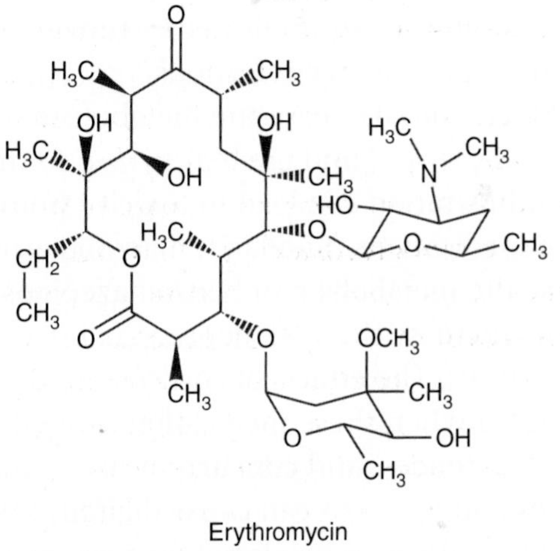

Erythromycin

FIGURE 16-10 Structure of erythromycin.

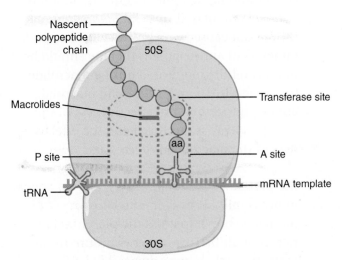

FIGURE 16-11 Mechanism of macrolide antibiotics: Bacterial protein synthesis.

Streptococci. The macrolides can also be useful for the treatment of *H. pylori*–related stomach ulcers. The most important adverse effects of the macrolides include gastric distress, when taken orally. Therefore, oral macrolides should be taken with food if gastric distress, nausea, vomiting, or diarrhea prove to be problematic.

Drug Interactions and Contraindications

The macrolides are contraindicated in patients who are allergic to them. They should be used cautiously in patients with liver disease, gastrointestinal disease, impaired hearing, and cardiac arrhythmias. The ophthalmic preparation is contraindicated in fungal, viral, and mycbacterial eye infections.

Macrolides decrease the metabolism of **carbamazepine** and **cyclosporine**, so their coadministration can lead to toxicity from these medications. Similarly, macrolides decrease the metabolism of benzodiazepines and so increase the CNS depression effects of these drugs. The effects of corticosteroids are increased when these medications are taken with macrolides, and concurrent use of macrolides and **digoxin** can cause digitalis toxicity. If patients *must* be placed on a regimen of a macrolide, extra care should be taken to assess **digoxin** plasma levels, especially for longer-duration macrolide therapy. In addition, combination of oral anticoagulants and macrolides can cause increased bleeding, so parameters of anticoagulant therapy should be more carefully monitored during macrolide treatment. If **theophylline** and macrolides are taken together, the effectiveness of the **theophylline** is increased and the effectiveness of the macrolide is decreased.

Erythromycin and azithromycin cross the placenta in small amounts, and do appear in breastmilk. However, **clarithromycin** has been shown to cross the placental barrier, though first-trimester exposure in humans has not shown adverse fetal effects in humans. In animals, there has been

harm shown. Spontaneous abortion is statistically higher for pregnant patients taking **clarithromycin** in the first trimester. Small amounts of **clarithromycin** appear in breastmilk, but do not appear to be unduly deleterious to the infant (AbbVie, 2017). Therefore, **erythro mycin** and **azithromycin** appear to have less evidence of fetal or infant harm than does **clarithromycin**. Pregnant and nursing patients should be apprised of the relative risks and benefits before use of these drugs.

Nursing Considerations

Macrolides can be administered orally or parenterally. **Erythromycin** solutions must be used within 8 hours if stored at room temperature; solutions stored in the refrigerator must be used within 24 hours.

When these drugs are taken orally, the most significant adverse effects include gastric distress. For this reason, oral macrolides should be taken with food if gastric distress, nausea, vomiting, or diarrhea proves to be problematic. However, food will decrease absorption of non-enteric-coated erythromycin tablets; thus, if the patient has been prescribed this formulation, he or she should be switched to an enteric-coated formulation, if one exists, when gastric adverse effects warrant dosing of **erythromycin** with food.

Each dose should be taken with eight ounces of water. Instruct the patient about whether the specific prescription may be taken with food. Monitor for diarrhea, vomiting, abdominal pain, jaundice, dark-colored urine, light-colored stools, and lethargy, as these are signs of liver damage. Also report the following signs of ototoxicity: nausea, tinnitus, dizziness, and vertigo.

Quinolones and Fluoroquinolones

Quinolones and fluoroquinolones were first discovered in the early 1960s (Takahashi, Hayakawa, & Akimoto, 2003), specifically, **nalidixic acid.** The introduction of *fluoro*quinolones (6-fluorinated quinolones) improved the spectrum over the quinolones, so they are now more predominantly used than quinolones. Quinolones include **nalidixic acid** and **cinoxacin**. The fluoroquinolones include **ciprofloxacin**, **ofloxacin**, **moxifloxacin**, **levofloxacin**, and others. The general structure of this class appears in FIGURE 16-12.

The fluoroquinolones are bactericidal via their action of interfering with DNA gyrase, which is an enzyme needed to synthesize bacterial DNA. The inability to synthesize DNA kills the bacterial cell. The quinolones/fluoroquinolones have a very broad spectrum of antibacterial activity. They act on bacterial DNA gyrase and/or topoisomerase IV (Strahilevitz & Hooper, 2005). DNA gyrase is the major target in Gram-positive bacteria (e.g., *S. aureus*), while topoisomerase IV is the major target in most Gram-negative bacteria (Cozzarelli, 1980) (FIGURE 16-13).

Bacterial DNA gyrase normally binds and twists two segments of DNA, creating a DNA superhelix. Further DNA gyrase action induces a supercoil in the DNA. Quinolones and fluoroquinolones inhibit these activities of DNA gyrase. At higher concentrations, they also block topoisomerase IV actions. Inhibiting DNA gyrase and/or topoisomerase IV inhibits bacterial growth.

The fluoroquinolones are very dominant in their range of activity and are bactericidal while generating few adverse reactions. They are useful for the treatment of UTIs, STDs, and gastrointestinal, abdominal, respiratory, bone and joint, and soft-tissue infections. Fluoroquinolones are generally safe, with the major problems pertaining to mild nausea, vomiting, and gastrointestinal cramps. Some patients report mild headaches or dizziness.

The fluoroquinolones are active against most aerobic Gram-negative bacteria and a few Gram-positive strains. Notably, they are effective against *Campylobacter jejuni*, *E. coli*, *Klebsiella*, *Pseudomonas aeruginosa*, *Haemophilus influenzae*, *Salmonella*, *Shigella*, meningococci, and numerous streptococci. They are also useful in the treatment of multidrug-resistant TB, gonorrhea, *Mycobacterium avium* complex (MAC) infections in patients with acquired immune deficiency syndrome (AIDS), and fever in patients with cancer who have neutropenia (Tanne, 2008; Sendzik, Shakibaei, Schäfer-Korting, & Stahlmann, 2005).

Even though this group of medications is new, a great deal of microbial resistance has already developed due to misuse of the drugs. In particular, *Clostridium difficile* has often been found to be resistant (Spigaglia,

Best Practices

Patients should be advised that common minerals found in antacids, antidiarrheals, and supplements, as well as caffeine, will interact with fluoroquinolones.

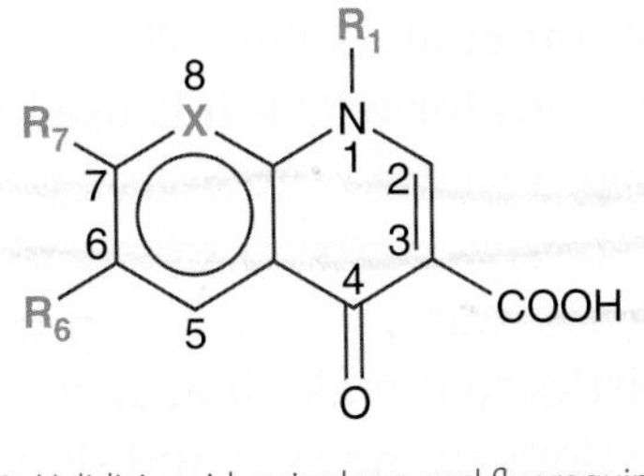

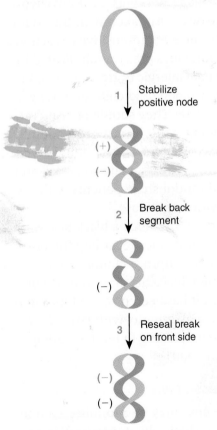

FIGURE 16-12 Nalidixic acid, quinolone, and fluoroquinolone structures.

FIGURE 16-13 Mechanism of action of quinolones and fluoroqinolones.

Barbanti, Dionisi, & Mastrantonio, 2010), and fluoroquinolones generally have little effect against anaerobes.

The fluoroquinolones can be given orally, parenterally, and topically, although many are given only in the oral form because they have excellent absorption. They are absorbed by the gastrointestinal tract and well distributed in the body. The principal organ for excretion is the kidneys.

Drug Interactions and Contraindications

Concurrent administration of a fluoroquinolone with any of the following medications *decreases* absorption of the fluoroquinolones: sucralfate; antacids; didanosine; salts of aluminum, magnesium, calcium, zinc, and iron; and food.

Theophyllines taken with fluoroquinolones can cause theophylline toxicity. Fluoroquinolones can decrease blood levels of the hydantoins and increase the incidence of seizures. These drugs interfere with liver metabolism of caffeine and decrease the effectiveness of birth control pills. St. John's wort (*Hypericum perforatum*), taken with fluoroquinolones, can cause photosensitivity reactions.

Fluoroquinolones are contraindicated in patients who are allergic to them, pregnant and lactating women, and children younger than the age of 18. They should be used cautiously in patients with liver disease, kidney disease, gastrointestinal disease, and dehydration. Ciprofloxacin stimulates the CNS and must be used cautiously in patients with CNS and cerebrovascular disease.

In 2008 the FDA added a black box warning for fluoroquinolones regarding the potential for tendon rupture (Tanne, 2008). The mechanism by which this rare event occurs is unclear, but it has been proposed that fluoroquinolones may interact with tenocyte regulatory proteins, leading to tendon damage (Sendzik et al., 2005).

Nursing Considerations

Fluoroquinolones may be administered orally, parenterally, or topically. IV preparations should be given over one hour via a large vein. Any sudden joint pain should be reported, particularly in the area of the Achilles tendon, as tendon rupture has been associated with these agents (Kim, 2010).

Antacids should not be given within four hours of an oral fluoroquinolone, and urine pH should be monitored and alkalized to decrease the risk of crystalluria. Increase fluid intake to two to three L/day. Offer small frequent meals to patients with gastrointestinal upset.

Lincosamides

The lincosamide class originated with **lincomycin**, a derivative of the soil bacterium *Streptomyces lincolnensis*. **Lincomycin** has since been replaced by a second-generation drug, **clindamycin**, which shows more extensive activity against both bacterial and protozoan pathogens (e.g., *Toxoplasmosis*, *Plasmodium*). **Clindamycin** is currently the only lincosamide antibiotic available for human use, although others are in development due to concerns about the spread of bacterial resistance (Morar, Bhullar, Hughes, Junop, & Wright, 2009). The mechanism of action for **clindamycin** is via interference with protein synthesis by binding to 50S ribosomal subunits in bacterial cells.

When delivered orally or via IM/IV injection, **clindamycin** becomes distributed via a one-compartment model to nearly all areas of the body, including the bones; however, it does not distribute well to the CSF and should not be used for treatment of meningitis.

Systemically, **clindamycin** is administered orally or parenterally to treat infections with streptococci, staphylococci, *Bacteriodes*, and other anaerobic bacteria, including MRSA (Morar et al., 2009). The types of serious infections for which it is used include lower respiratory tract, bone and joint, gynecologic, and skin structure infections as well as septicemia. **Clindamycin** has certain characteristics that make it attractive for serious infections of the skin and skin structure such as necrotizing fasciitis: It reduces the toxicity of the virulent *S. aureus* and *S. pyogenes* microbes that cause these infections and has a small anti-inflammatory effect. However, resistance has been noted, particularly among staphylococci (Mahesh, Ramakant, & Jagadeesh, 2013); due to similarities in the drug's mechanisms of action, it can be generally stated that any microbe resistant to a macrolide will likely also resist clindamycin.

Clindamycin is also used topically to treat vaginosis (Eriksson, Larsson, Nilsson, & Forsum, 2011) and epidermal infections, including acne. For those patients with a penicillin allergy, clindamycin is an excellent second choice, especially for prevention and treatment of oral/gum infection, due to its ability to partition into tissues including the gums and bone.

Drug Interactions and Contraindications

Hypersensitivity to clindamycin is rare; when it does occur, it tends to emerge as severe skin-related eruptions (Thong, 2010). For this reason, the drug should be used cautiously in patients with a history of atopic dermatitis (eczema) or other forms of atopy (e.g., asthma). Clindamycin has a long-established association with pseudomembranous colitis (Tedesco, 1977), so its systemic use is contraindicated in patients with a history of regional enteritis, ulcerative colitis, or antibiotic-associated colitis. Topical preparations have minimal systemic absorption and, therefore, may be used cautiously in such patients, but should be immediately discontinued if gastrointestinal symptoms arise. Caution should be used in patients with hepatic and renal dysfunction and in infants, as the drug is associated with gasping syndrome. *C. difficile* resistance to clindamycin has been noted, and clindamycin should be discontinued and treatment versus *C. difficile* initiated should the patient present with persistent, severe diarrhea suggestive of *C. difficile* superinfection. Coadministration with rifampicin may reduce serum levels of clindamycin (Bouazza et al., 2012). There is increased

neuromuscular blockade with neuromuscular blocking agents and decreased gastrointestinal absorption with agents containing kaolin or aluminum salts (e.g., antidiarrheal agents, antacids).

Clindamycin does transfer into breast-milk, so it should not be used in lactating women due to the potential for gastric disturbance in the infant.

Nursing Considerations

Review of the patient's history for hypersensitivity, atopy, and gastrointestinal symptoms should be undertaken before clindamycin is administered. Researchers have noted that patient body weight seems to affect clearance of this drug (Bouazza et al., 2012), so that higher doses may be needed to achieve MIC in patients weighing more than approximately 75 kg.

IV infusion should be done slowly, as there is a risk of cardiac arrest when the drug is rapidly infused. Monitor for sterile abscess with IM administration and for thrombophlebitis with IV administration.

For oral preparations, patients should be instructed to take clindamycin with a full glass of water or with food and to complete the full prescribed course of the drug unless instructed to cease taking it by a healthcare provider.

For all systemically administered regimens, monitor patients for adverse effects such as nausea and vomiting; patients may eat frequent, small meals if this occurs. Monitor for superinfections in the mouth or vagina and instruct patients to use frequent hygiene measures (provide treatment if these infections are severe). Report severe or watery diarrhea, abdominal pain, inflamed mouth or vagina, and skin rash or lesions to the physician.

For topical dermatologic administration (acne), instruct patients to apply a thin film of solution to the affected area twice daily, taking care to avoid the eyes, mucous membranes, and broken or inflamed skin. Any medication that contacts non-intact skin should be rinsed away thoroughly with cool water. Patients should be advised to report any symptoms of abdominal pain or diarrhea while using the medication.

For vaginal preparations, the medication should be used for three or seven consecutive days (as prescribed), preferably at bedtime. The patient should not use vaginal douches, deodorants, or vaginally inserted contraceptive products, and should likewise refrain from sexual intercourse during treatment with this product. Patients should be advised to report lack of improvement (e.g., ongoing vaginal irritation or itching) as well as diarrhea that develops during treatment.

Vancomycin

The vancomycins currently have only one member of the group, which is the prototype for which the class is named. This drug is a naturally occurring bactericidal antibiotic used in the treatment of severe infections. Because it produces very severe toxic effects, however, its use is limited, and reserved for use against specific bacteria and in narrowly defined disease conditions. Initially, vancomycin had very widespread use in the treatment of *Staphylococcus aureus* and *Enterobacter* infections, but the CDC has recommended decreased use of vancomycin to limit the spread of vancomycin-resistant organisms (National Institute of Allergy and Infectious Diseases [NIAID], 2011). Vancomycin prevents cell wall synthesis in bacteria by attaching to pentapeptides of bacterial peptidoglycan monomers in the bacterial cell wall that are necessary for peptidoglycan synthesis; the drug also alters bacterial membrane permeability and RNA synthesis. This, in turn, leads to death of the bacteria.

Vancomycin is usually given intravenously for serious infections not responsive to other anti-infective medications. The oral route is used only when treatment of susceptible GI bacteria is necessary, as the absorption from the gastrointestinal tract for systemic uses is unsatisfactory, rendering oral vancomycin useful for gastrointestinal infections but little else. Parenterally, it is the drug of choice for infection with MRSA or *Staphylococcus epidermides*; via oral route, it is the drug of choice for pseudomembranous colitis caused by *C. difficile*.

When delivered parenterally, vancomycin becomes distributed into almost all body fluids and tissues and has a serum half-life of 4 to 6 hours in patients with normal kidney function. In those with impaired kidney function and in elderly patients, the half-life can last as long as 146 hours. The IV form of the drug is excreted mainly through the kidney, while the oral form is excreted in the feces.

Drug Interactions and Contraindications

As mentioned earlier, the list of toxicities and contraindications for vancomycin is long (TABLE 16-7). This drug should not be used in patients who are allergic or who have suspected or past vancomycin-resistant *Enterobacter* (VRE) or *S. aureus* (VRSA) infections.

Vancomycin is contraindicated in pregnancy. Lactating women need to have breast-fed neonates and infants monitored for toxic levels of drug, with dose and dosing interval adjustments made, as necessary (Herbert-Ashton & Clarkson, 2008).

Nursing Considerations

Patients should take vancomycin according to the prescriber's directions. They must take the entire prescription and take doses at evenly spaced intervals around the clock to keep blood levels even.

Patients should report hearing abnormalities to the physician immediately; they should also advise the physician of any skin rash, fever, or sore throat. The report for ordered blood work should include a complete blood count (CBC), as well as peak and trough drug levels. Healthcare providers should develop awareness of patients' I & O when taking this drug. They should also assess patients' liver and kidney function. Concentrations of 60 to 80 mcg/mL may cause ototoxicity.

TABLE 16-7	Toxicities and Contraindications Associated with Vancomycin	
Systemic Toxicities	**Adverse Effect**	**Comments**
Central nervous system	Vertigo, ataxia	
Eyes, ears, nose, and throat	Ototoxicity causing tinnitus, hearing loss (considered the most serious effect)	Ototoxicity is significant with this drug. Do not use in hearing-impaired patients if an alternative is available. Do not use concomitantly with other ototoxic agents. Monitor hearing, especially in older or very young patients.
Gastrointestinal	Nausea	
Genitourinary	Nephrotoxicity, uremia	
Hematologic	Thrombocytopenia, eosinophilia, leukopenia	
Immunologic	Hypersensitivity; "red neck" or "red man" syndrome	Associated with rapid IV infusion and caused by histamine release. Symptoms include redness of face, neck, and upper body; hypotension; fever; chills; tachycardia; pruritus; and paresthesias.
Other	Thrombophlebitis at IV injection site	
Drug Interactions		
Cholestyramine and colestipol	Concurrent use interferes with absorption of oral vancomycin	
Known ototoxic drugs (e.g., aminoglycosides, ethacrynic acid, furosemide, salicylates)	Increased risk of ototoxicity with concurrent use	Especially with IM administration.
Known nephrotoxic drugs (e.g., aminoglycosides, amphotericin B, cisplatin, cyclosporine, polymixin B)	Increased risk of nephrotoxicity with concurrent use; renal disease requires cautious use	
Metformin	Concurrent use may cause lactic acidosis	
Nondepolarizing muscle relaxants (e.g., atracurium, metocurine)	Concurrent use may cause an increase in neuromuscular blockade	
Special Populations		
Patients with inflammatory bowel disease	Cautious use of oral preparation due to increased drug absorption and possibility of drug toxicity	
Pregnancy	Contraindicated due to safety concerns	
Older adults	Use with caution and monitor for toxicity	

The IV preparation of **vancomycin** should be infused over 60 minutes or longer; *never* infuse it quickly. Assess the IV site frequently for extravasation, as serious skin complications (necrosis, tissue sloughing) may occur. In some patients, it may be necessary to administer an antihistamine before IV dosing of **vancomycin** is performed. Assess blood pressure and pulse during IV administration.

Newer Anti-Infective Drugs for Resistant Infections

The newest anti-infective agents are drugs that developed specifically for use against resistant strains of bacteria. The first class of novel agents comprises the streptogramins, which were introduced in 1999 (Karch, 2008). There are two drugs in this group (used together), **quinupristin** and

dalfopristin. They have a synergistic effect, by binding to different sites on the 50S ribosomal units of susceptible bacteria, inhibiting bacterial protein synthesis. They also used for other serious infections caused by methicillin-resistant and vancomycin-resistant bacteria as well as *S. aureus* and *S. epidermides*. This therapy must be used very judiciously to prevent the development of **drug resistance** to these agents; they should *only* be used in patients who have known resistant infection.

The oxazolidinones were introduced in 2000, when the first and (as yet) only member of the group, **linezolid**, was approved for use in the United States (Herbert-Ashton & Clarkson, 2008). **Linezolid** is a synthetic drug that, like the streptogramins, was developed to treat serious infections caused by methicillin-resistant and vancomycin-resistant bacteria. **Linezolid** acts by binding to bacterial 23S rRNA (part of the 50S subunit), preventing bacterial protein translation. It also possesses monoamine oxidase (MAO) inhibition, an enzyme necessary for monoamine metabolism. It is bactericidal when used against anaerobic, Gram-positive, and Gram-negative bacteria. It is primarily used against **nosocomial** or community-acquired pneumonia caused by *Streptococcus pneumoniae* or MRSA, as well as complicated skin infections caused by MRSA and bacteremia caused by VREF (Food and Drug Administration [FDA], 2011). Again, this drug must be used cautiously, and numerous healthcare facilities require their Infectious Disease Committee to approve its use (Aschenbrenner, Cleveland, & Venable, 2006).

Both classes of newer antibiotic agents (strepto-gramins and oxazolidinones) act by inhibiting protein synthesis in bacterial cells, but via slightly different mechanisms, as just briefly described. **Quinupristin/dalfopristin** is given intravenously. It is well distributed to the skin and soft tissues and excreted through bile via feces. **Linezolid**

> **Best Practices**
>
> Never infuse IV vancomycin quickly; instead, infuse it over one hour or longer.

can be given orally and intravenously. It is distributed all over the body after quick absorption from the gastrointestinal tract and is excreted via the urine (Herbert-Ashton & Clarkson, 2008).

Drug Interactions and Contraindications Quinupristin/Dalfopristin

Quinupristin/dalfopristin increases serum concentrations of **alprazolam**, **cyclosporine**, **diazepam**, **erythromycin**, **lidocaine**, **nifedipine**, **verapamil**, and vinca alkaloids. Therefore, it should be used with caution in patients taking any of these medications or compounds with a similar structure. It may be used cautiously in pregnant women, but in lactating women, breastfeeding should be halted for the duration of therapy. **Quinupristin/dalfopristin** is not approved for use in children. Monitor patients with decreased liver function.

Linezolid

The FDA issued a warning in 2011 of serious CNS reactions, specifically serotonin syndrome, in patients taking drugs that promote increased serotonin availability such as selective serotonin reuptake inhibitors (SSRIs; see the *Pharmacology of Psychotropic Medications* chapter). Concurrent use of **linezolid** with SSRIs, monoamine oxidase inhibitors, sympathomimetics, or **levodopa** can cause serotonin syndrome or hypertensive crisis. Foods that contain tyramine can likewise increase blood pressure in patients who are taking **linezolid**. Herbal remedies such as ephedra, ginseng, and ma-huang can cause nervousness, headache, and/or increased blood pressure. The oral suspension of **linezolid** should be used cautiously when given to patients with phenylketonuria, as it contains aspartame, and when given to patients with blood dyscrasias, as it may cause bone marrow suppression. Pregnant women should be counseled regarding the potential teratogenic effects of this drug.

Nursing Considerations
Quinupristin/Dalfopristin

Quinupristin/dalfopristin is administered intravenously. Monitor patients' liver function tests, IV site, and superinfection risk when they are taking quinupristin/dalfopristin. Superinfection with *C. difficile* may lead to prolonged diarrhea and indicates a need for secondary treatment. Watch for candidiasis.

Linezolid

Linezolid may be given either via IV or orally. The oral form should not be shaken, and it can be taken with or without food. Patients should be counseled about which foods contain tyramine and that avoidance or restriction of tyramine intake is essential to prevent a drug reaction. Patients should not breastfeed and should avoid caffeine and alcohol. They must be informed of the need to consult with the prescriber or pharmacist before taking any over-the-counter drug, as there are many interactions between linezolid and over-the-counter medications.

Antitubercular Drugs

Tuberculosis (TB) is an ancient disease that continues to be found worldwide. It is estimated that 8 million new cases of TB occur each year, most of which arise in developing countries (World Health Organization [WHO], 2012). Reasons for the continuing presence of TB include the development of multidrug-resistant mycobacteria and AIDS (Nunn, 2012). Drugs used to treat tuberculosis differ in their pharmacology, and so a summary is provided in TABLE 16-8.

TABLE 16-8	Antitubercular Drugs		
Drug	Mechanism of Action	Cautions	Use
Isoniazid (INH)	Prevents synthesis of mycolic acid, which is an integral part of the mycobacteria's cell wall. Also, interferes with DNA, lipid, carbohydrate, and nicotinamide adenine dinucleotide (NAD) biochemistry.	Do not drink alcohol. Do not breastfeed. Stop use of the drug if symptoms occur: jaundice, dark urine, clay-colored stools, chills, fever, or skin rash. Report numbness or tingling in the hands and feet to the physician.	Given alone for prophylaxis; given in combination with other antitubercular agents for treatment.
Ethambutol	Prevents RNA synthesis, by inhibiting arabinosyl transferases, enzymes involved in the synthesis of mycobacteria cell wall, thus stopping growth.	Do not breastfeed. Report any eye problems.	Used in combination with other antitubercular agents to treat pulmonary TB.
Ethionamide	Inhibits mycolic acid synthesis.	Do not drink alcohol. Do not breastfeed. Change position slowly to avoid postural hypotension.	Given to treat active TB after primary drugs have not worked; must be given in combination with other antituberculosis drugs.
Pyrazinamide (PZA)	Prodrug of pyrazinoic acid, but the mechanism of action of the active drug is unclear.	Do not breastfeed. Tell the physician about any urination problems. Increase fluids.	Given to treat TB after primary drugs have not worked. Appears to work best in the early stages of treatment.
Rifampin	Hinders DNA-dependent RNA polymerase, which stops RNA synthesis and, ultimately, protein synthesis.	Do not breastfeed. Do not stop and restart use of the drug, as a flu-like syndrome may occur. Body secretions will be red-orange colored. Contact lenses may be permanently stained red-orange. Additional birth control is necessary if taking oral contraceptives.	Drug of choice for pulmonary TB; used in combination with other antitubercular agents.
Streptomycin	See mechanism of action for aminoglycosides.	See the discussion of aminoglycosides.	Used for TB that is resistant to other medications.

Reproduced from Herbert-Ashton, M., & Clarkson, N. (2008). Quick look nursing:Pharmacology (2nd ed.). Sudbury, MA: Jones & Bartlett.

Isoniazid (INH) is the prototype drug for TB: It is included in all treatment regimens except one—that for **INH**-resistant TB. The drugs used for treatment of TB are used in combination, a strategy that allows the drugs to act on the bacterium at different phases of its life cycle as well as to reduce development of resistant strains (Lehne, 2012).

Compliance tends to be a problem, as treatment for TB is a long-duration affair; patient education is very important for compliance. Baseline tests of sputum **culture** and sensitivity and chest X-ray are generally ordered so that the combination of drugs that is most likely to work without promoting resistance may be selected. Table 16-8 lists antitubercular drugs and their mechanisms of action.

Drug Interactions and Contraindications
Isoniazid (INH)

Drinking alcohol or taking the drug concomitantly with **rifampin** or **pyrazinamide (PZA)** increases the chance of liver damage. Concurrent use with **phenytoin** causes **phenytoin** toxicity. Food interferes with absorption. Contraindications include acute liver disease and known hypersensitivity; use cautiously in lactating women, patients with chronic alcoholism, individuals older than 35 years of age, patients with chronic liver disease, and patients with seizure disorder.

Ethambutol

Antacids containing aluminum interfere with absorption. Contraindications include hypersensitivity, lactation, age younger than 13 years, and optic neuritis.

Ethionamide

Concurrent use with **INH** or **cycloserine** increases patients' risk for nerve damage. Contraindications include hypersensitivity. Use this medication cautiously in patients with liver disease and diabetes mellitus, particularly in those patients with neuropathy.

Pyrazinamide (PZA)

Concurrent use with **INH** or **rifampin** increases patients' risk for liver damage. The

presence of liver disease and known hypersensitivity are the only contraindications.

Rifampin

Drinking alcohol or taking this drug with **INH** or **PZA** increases patients' risk for liver damage. **Rifampin** decreases the effectiveness of numerous drugs; the medications for which this possibility is the most significant concern include corticosteroids, oral contraceptives, thyroid hormones, oral sulfonylureas, **warfarin**, **phenytoin**, and **digoxin**. Contraindications (aside from medication interactions) include hypersensitivity, lactation, and recent history or presence of diseases caused by meningococci. Use **rifampin** cautiously in patients with a history of alcoholism and in patients with liver disease.

Streptomycin

See the earlier discussion of this drug's interactions and contraindications in the aminoglycosides section.

Nursing Considerations

The agents used against TB are markedly powerful and, therefore, produce a spectrum of adverse effects. These adverse effects contribute to patient difficulty in complying with and maintaining the months-long regimen. This issue has contributed to development of multidrug-resistant (MDR) and extensively drug-resistant (XDR) TB strains (Cox et al., 2007; Tabarsi et al., 2011).

One strategy to promote greater compliance is to use directly observed therapy (DOT). Although a Cochrane review of randomized, controlled trials of the use of DOT for TB treatment showed no significant benefit to patient outcomes (Karumbi & Garner, 2015), WHO still suggests DOT as a consideration (WHO, 2017).

Isoniazid

INH causes a variety of adverse effects for which the nurse should assess, including peripheral neuropathy; paresthesias; dyspnea; visual disturbances and optic neuritis; elevated liver enzymes and frank hepatitis; urinary retention in males; hematologic effects such as aplastic or hemolytic anemia; fluid and electrolyte disturbances, including hyperkalemia, hypocalcemia, and hypophosphatemia; and decreased pyridoxine (vitamin B$_6$).

This medication is administered orally and via IM injection. Assess the patient's blood pressure during initial therapy as orthostatic hypotension may occur; also assess eye function. Monitor liver function tests and ensure the patient is taking supplemental pyridoxine (vitamin B$_6$).

Ethambutol

Adverse effects of ethambutol include dizziness, hallucinations, confusion, and paresthesias; retrobulbar optic neuritis, loss of red-green color spectrum, photophobia, and eye pain; abdominal pain; and loss of appetite. Assess the patient's eyes using an ophthalmoscope to obtain baseline data; reassess the patient's eyes monthly. Monitor I & O.

Ethionamide

Adverse effects of ethionamide use include peripheral neuritis, restlessness, hallucinations, and convulsions; postural hypotension; hypothyroidism; menorrhagia; nausea, vomiting, anorexia, diarrhea, and metallic taste; hepatitis; and erectile dysfunction. Ethionamide is administered orally. The patient should take supplemental pyridoxine (vitamin B$_6$). Monitor the following tests: complete blood count, urinalysis, and kidney and liver function.

Pyrazinamide

PZA adverse effects include headache; urticaria; liver toxicity; urination problems, elevated uric acid, and gout; hemolytic anemia; photosensitivity; and arthralgia. This medication is administered orally. Assess the patient for liver toxicity and bleeding tendencies, and monitor uric acid levels; stop use of the drug if gout or liver reactions occur.

Rifampin

Rifampin produces adverse effects including fatigue, drowsiness, confusion, dizziness, and extremity pain; visual impairments; nausea, vomiting, abdominal cramps, and diarrhea; liver injury and hepatitis; hematuria and renal failure; anemia and thrombocytopenia; a red-orange discoloration of body secretions; and flu-like syndrome. This drug is administered orally or intravenously. Assess liver function tests and obtain a daily prothrombin time if the patient is receiving an anticoagulant.

Streptomycin

Streptomycin adverse effects and nursing considerations were discussed in the aminoglycoside section.

Antifungal Agents

Antifungal drugs are divided into three groups: (1) systemic antifungals, (2) azole antifungals (which also treat systemic fungal infections but are a newer class of drugs), and (3) topical medications that treat fungal infections of the mucous membranes and skin. As topical medications are better addressed in the context of medications for dermatologic conditions (see Chapter 13, *Pharmacology in Dermatologic Conditions*) and gynecologic conditions (see the *Pharmacology of the Genitourinary System* chapter), this discussion will focus on systemic uses.

The principal classes of systemic antifungals include the polyene macrolides, such as amphotericin B; the azoles, which are in turn grouped into the subclasses of imidazoles (ketoconazole is the only one with systemic use; all others are used topically) and triazoles (e.g., itraconazole and fluconazole); echinocandins such as caspofungin and micafungin; and the allylamines, such as terbinafine. A variety of unclassified systemic antifungal agents, including griseofulvin and flucytosine, are also used (TABLE 16-9).

Antifungal medications, as a class, act by binding to sterols, especially ergosterol, increasing the permeability of the fungal cell wall, causing leakage of cellular components, death of the cell and failure of the cell to

TABLE 16-9	Systemic Antifungal Agents	
Drug Name	Drug Class	Use
Amphotericin B	Polyene antimycotic	Oral or IV treatment of candidiasis, cryptococcal meningitis, leishmaniasis, *Coccidiodes immitis, Fusarium oxysporum*
Anidulafungin	Echinocandin	Aspergillosis, candidemia/invasive candidiasis; often used for strains resistant to azoles
Caspofungin	Echinocandin	Aspergillosis, candidemia/invasive candidiasis
Fluconazole	Triazole antifungal	Candidemia/invasive candidiasis, cryptococcal meningitis
Flucytosine	Unclassified systemic antifungal	Candidiasis, aspergillosis, chromoblastomycosis, cryptococcal meningitis
Griseofulvin	Unclassified systemic antifungal	Oral therapy for fungal infections of the skin, nails, and scalp
Itraconazole	Triazole antifungal	Wide range of fungal and yeast infections, including aspergillosis, histoplasmosis, blastomycosis, sporotrichosis, cryptococcosis, candidiasis, coccidioidomycosis, paracoccidioidomycosis, leishmaniasis, zygomycosis
Ketoconazole	Imidazole antifungal	Aspergillosis, histoplasmosis, blastomycosis, sporotrichosis, cryptococcosis, candidiasis, coccidioidomycosis, paracoccidioidomycosis, leishmaniasis
Micafungin	Echinocandin	Aspergillosis, candidemia/invasive candidiasis
Nystatin	Polyene antimycotic	Candidiasis
Posaconazole	Triazole antifungal	Aspergillosis, candidiasis
Terbinafine	Allylamine	Oral therapy for fungal infections of the nails, scalp, or skin
Voriconazole	Triazole antifungal	Aspergillosis

reproduce. Azoles, in particular, exert a fungistatic effect by targeting CYP-dependent 14α-demethylase, required for the synthesis of ergosterol, part of the cell membrane. All these drugs do not use the same mechanism to perform this action, however. For example, **amphotericin B** attaches to ergosterol and opens pores in the cell wall, whereas the azoles inhibit a specific enzyme in the fungal cell, lanosterol 14-alpha-demethylase, that is needed to synthesize ergosterol (Zonios & Bennett, 2008). In each instance, the antifungal agent affects the functioning of the fungal cell membrane and thereby suppresses or kills the fungus.

As with other antimicrobial drugs, resistance has developed to a number of antifungal agents (Vandeputte, Ferrari, & Coste, 2012), and many serious fungal infections are now treated with combination therapies. Triazole antifungals have emerged as being among the best broad-spectrum agents (Lass-Flörl, 2011), but resistance to them is expanding. This trend poses a significant threat given that the microbes targeted by these drugs tend to be present in immunocompromised persons and may prove lethal in that setting.

Some fungal infections respond better to drugs outside the realm of typical antifungal medications. For example, *Pneumocystis jiroveci*, a fungus that causes pneumocystic pneumonia, which is particularly dangerous in AIDS patients, is treated not with an antifungal medication but rather with either a combination of **sulfamethoxazole** and **trimethoprim** or, in case of resistance, **clindamycin** combined with the antimalarial drug **primaquine** (Bennett, Gilroy, & Rose, 2013). The clinician should keep in mind the instances in which a drug outside the antifungal class may be indicated for treating infection by a mold or yeast.

Drug Interactions and Contraindications

A wide range of drug interactions is noted with all classes of antifungal medications. Drug interactions with amphotericin B cause nephrotoxicity, hypokalemia, and blood dyscrasias (Albengres, Le Louët, & Tillement, 1998; Depont et al., 2007). Amphotericin B increases toxicity of flucytosine but may facilitate its antifungal activity. This agent also has hematologic and renal adverse effects that are exacerbated when it is used in conjunction with nephrotoxic drugs administered concurrently; furosemide, cyclosporine, and corticosteroids were associated with significant amphotericin B drug interactions in one study (Depont et al., 2007). This risk is especially noteworthy when amphotericin B is used for treatment of fungal infections in patients with HIV, as the antiviral agents frequently used in HIV therapy may compound renal toxicity. An increased risk of hypokalemia is present with concurrent corticosteroid use. Synergism is likely to occur when QT interval–modifying drugs (terfenadine) and drugs that induce hypokalemia (amphotericin B) are coadministered (Depont et al., 2007).

Azole antifungals affect the cytochrome P450 pathway and significantly decrease the serum levels and activity of numerous drugs, including histamine H_1-receptor antagonists, warfarin, cyclosporine, tacrolimus, felodipine, lovastatin, midazolam, triazolam, methylprednisolone, rifabutin, protease inhibitors, and nortriptyline. Similarly, concomitant use with other CYP450-metabolized medications such as carbamazepine, phenobarbital, and rifampicin can cause unusually rapid metabolism of azole antifungals (Albengres et al., 1998). Ketoconazole and itraconazole bioavailabilities are is also reduced by H_2-receptor antagonists and proton pump inhibitors. In contrast, concurrent use of the azoles with some drugs—namely, warfarin, phenytoin, oral hypoglycemics, digoxin, and cyclosporine—results in elevated blood levels of these drugs.

Life-threatening cardiovascular episodes may occur if azoles are taken concurrently with midazolam, lovastatin, triazolam, or simvastatin (Herbert-Ashton & Clarkson, 2008).

Griseofulvin is an enzymatic inducer of coumarin-like drugs and estrogens, whereas terbinafine seems to have a low potential for drug interactions.

Flucytosine produces significant nephrotoxicity when it is given in combination with amphotericin B and other nephrotoxic drugs (Vermes, Guchelaar, & Dankert, 2000).

Contraindications to all antifungal agents include hypersensitivity, lactation, and liver or kidney disease. All systemic antifungals should be used with caution in pregnant women, who should be counseled per Pregnancy and Lactation Labeling Rule (PLLR) guidelines. Amphotericin B may be the least risky systemic antifungal for use in pregnant women.

Nursing Considerations

In the context of systemic fungal infection, particularly in patients who are immunocompromised, treatment may last for an extended time. Due to the likelihood of emerging resistance and drug interactions, patients should be instructed to take all of the medication and to take over-the-counter preparations only after checking with their prescriber or pharmacist. Patients should be advised to report fever, chills, vomiting, abdominal pain, and skin rash.

Lactating women who are taking antifungal drugs should not breastfeed their infants. All oral forms of antifungals except ketoconazole can be taken with food if gastrointestinal upset occurs.

Healthcare providers should assess patients who are taking these medications for adverse effects, including headache, visual problems, peripheral neuritis, dizziness, seizures, and insomnia; arrhythmias, tachycardia, and hypertension; rash, urticaria, photosensitivity, and hives; endocrine dysfunction (e.g., hypothyroidism, hypoadrenalism); transient hearing loss; nausea, vomiting, diarrhea, anorexia, cramps, and liver toxicity; erectile dysfunction, or vaginal burning and itching; renal dysfunction; anemia, bone marrow suppression, thrombocytopenia, and leukopenia; and fever, chills, malaise, and arthralgias. Monitor for hypokalemia and hyponatremia as well.

In intravenously administered antifungal therapy, infuse IV medication slowly (over two to four hours) and assess the IV site for phlebitis. With oral and IV formulations, monitor the patient's liver and kidney lab studies and I & O. Monitor nutrition and offer frequent small meals if gastrointestinal symptoms are present; oral medications may be taken with food if gastrointestinal symptoms are present except for **ketoconazole**, which must be taken on empty stomach. Administer analgesics and antipyretics to assist in controlling fever, headache, and chills.

Antiparasitic Agents

Human beings are susceptible to infection by a variety of **parasites**—some microbial, and some "macro" organisms such as **helminthes**.

Protozoal Infections

Protozoa cause numerous serious infections, such as malaria, toxoplasmosis, leishmaniasis, giardiasis, trichomoniasis, trypanosomiasis, and amebiasis. These infections affect billions of individuals worldwide, but fortunately are uncommon in the United States among otherwise healthy persons. However, it is not uncommon for tropical protozoal infections to appear in individuals who have traveled outside the United States, especially to tropical climates. For example, a visit to the Caribbean can expose travelers to malaria, or a trip to Egypt may expose tourists to *Cryptosporidium* (Putignani & Menichella, 2010). Further, an individual may develop a zoonotic disease via direct contact with infected animals' feces, contact with water that has been contaminated by animal feces, or—an

increasingly common vector—by eating fruits and vegetables grown in contaminated water (Feng & Zhao, 2011). Two protozoal infections common in the United States, *Toxoplasma gondii* and *Giardia duodenalis* (also known as *G. lamblia*) are zoonotic diseases.

The average person is fairly resistant to protozoal infections; however, individuals with suppressed immune systems, such as pregnant women and patients with HIV or AIDS, are highly susceptible to such infections (Herbert-Ashton & Clarkson, 2008), as are infants infected in utero by the onset of infection in the mother. For most persons infected with toxoplasmosis, the vector is a household pet that may have acquired the parasite by eating wild rodents or birds that carried it.

Antiprotozoal Medications

A variety of medications are used to treat protozoal infections (TABLE 16-10). Some were developed specifically to be effective against *Plasmodium*, the organism that causes malaria and, therefore, are classified as "antimalarials" (although they often treat other protozoan infections and even some nonprotozoan organisms as well, particularly the fungus *Pneumocystis jiroveci*). Antimalarial drugs may be used to prevent infection, to treat established infection, or for both purposes. Other antiprotozoal medications are used for a variety of organisms, but generally are not effective against *Plasmodium*.

Drug Interactions and Contraindications

All antimalarials should be used with caution in pregnant women, except **quinine**, which should not be used. Other antiprotozoal drugs should be used with caution and pregnant women should be counseled about the benefits and potential risks of using these drugs, taking into account the drug and the number of weeks' gestation of the fetus.

Antiprotozoal agents have a wide spectrum of interactions and cross-reactivity with other agents and with specific disease states. While these adverse events are too numerous

TABLE 16-10	Agents Used for Prevention or Treatment of Protozoal Infections			
Drug Class	Drug Generic Name	Organism	Mechanism of Action	Uses
Antimalarials	Chloroquine	*Plasmodium* spp. (protozoan) *Entamoeba histolytica* (protozoan)	Inhibits biocrystallization of heme in red blood cells, possibly by changing vesicle pH.	Prophylaxis and treatment of malaria; treatment of *E. histolytica*–related liver abscess (may be combined with other medications to expand efficacy)
	Artemether/ lumefantrine	*Plasmodium* spp. (protozoan)	Artemether inhibits calcium ATPase, inhibiting nucleic acid and protein synthesis. Lumefantrine's mechanism is unclear, but it may complex hemin, inhibiting β-hematin formation.	Treatment of uncomplicated malaria
	Hydroxychloroquine	*Plasmodium* spp. (protozoan)	Changes vesicle pH, inhibiting heme polymerization; inhibits DNA-enzyme interactions.	Prophylaxis and treatment of malaria
	Mefloquine	*Plasmodium* spp. (protozoan)	Interacts with phospholipids, but mechanism(s) unclear.	Prophylaxis and treatment of malaria; considered second-line therapy for treating chloroquine-resistant strains
	Primaquine	*Plasmodium* spp. (protozoan) *Pneumocystis jiroveci* (also known as *P. carinii*) (fungus)	Inflicts oxidative damage to target cells, though the complete mechanism is unclear.	Treatment of malaria and Pneumocystis jiroveci pneumonia (PCP); may be used for malarial prophylaxis if other agents are unsuitable
	Pyrimethamine	*Plasmodium* spp. (protozoan) *Toxoplasma gondii* (protozoan)	Inhibits target cell dihydrofolate reductase, and so inhibits tetrahydrofolic acid synthesis.	Treatment of malaria and toxoplasmosis; combined with sulfadiazine for the latter
	Quinine	*Plasmodium* spp. (protozoan)	Binds hemozoin, and inhibits synthesis of nucleic acids, proteins, and inhibits glycolysis, all through mechanisms that remain unclear.	Prophylaxis/treatment of last resort for malaria due to availability of newer, more effective agents
Antiprotozoal agents	Atovaquone, atovaquone-proguanil	*Toxoplasma gondii* (protozoan) *Babesia microti* (protozoan) *Pneumocystis jiroveci (P. carinii)* (fungus) *Plasmodium* spp. (protozoan)	Block two separate pyrimidine/ nucleic acid synthesis pathways: Atovaquone blocks parasite mitochondrial electron transport. Proguanil is a prodrug of cycloguanil, which inhibits dihydrofolate reductase, and so deoxythymidylate synthesis.	In *Babesia* infection ("Texas fever"), used in conjunction with azithromycin For PCP, used only for mild cases for which usual treatments are not tolerable For malaria, may be prophylaxis or treatment and is combined with proguanil
	Benznidazole	*Trypanosoma cruzi*	Interferes with RNA and DNA polymerases and templates, blocking protein synthesis, though complete mechanism(s) unclear.	Treatment of Chagas disease

(continues)

TABLE 16-10 Agents Used for Prevention or Treatment of Protozoal Infections (*continued*)

Drug Class	Drug Generic Name	Organism	Mechanism of Action	Uses
	Metronidazole	*Entamoeba histolytica* (protozoan) *Giardia lamblia* (protozoan) *Trichomonas vaginalis* (protozoan)	Inhibits DNA synthesis, though the mechanism is unclear.	Treatment of amoebiasis, giardiasis, and trichomoniasis as well as a variety of bacterial diseases
	Nifurtimox	*Trypanosoma brucei* *Trypanosoma cruzi*	Breakage of parasitic DNA via a nitro-anion radical metabolite of the drug; production of superoxide (toxic to parasitic cell); complete mechanism(s) unclear.	Treatment of trypanosomiasis and Chagas disease
	Nitazoxanide	*Cryptosporidium parvum* (protozoan) *Giardia lamblia* (protozoan)	Prodrug of tizoxanide, which may interfere with the pyruvate:ferredoxin oxidoreductase (PFOR) enzyme-dependent electron transfer reaction, a reaction that is essential to anaerobic metabolism.	Treatment of giardiasis and cryptosporidiosis
	Pentamidine	*Pneumocystis jiroveci* (aka *P. carinii*) (fungus) *Leishmania* spp. *Trypanosoma brucei*	Mechanism unclear but may be via inhibition of nucleotide incorporation into RNA and DNA, interfering with RNA, DNA, protein and phospholipid production.	Prophylaxis/treatment of PCP; use against leishmaniasis and trypanosomiasis is off-label
	Tinidazole	*Entamoeba histolytica* (protozoan) *Giardia lamblia* (protozoan) *Trichomonas vaginalis* (protozoan)	Mechanism unclear, but may interfere with the pyruvate:ferredoxin oxidoreductase (PFOR) enzyme-dependent electron transfer reaction, a reaction that is essential to anaerobic metabolism.	Similar to metronidazole in activity

to describe in detail for all drugs, healthcare practitioners should be aware that the interactivity of the class as a whole means that the potential for adverse effects and adverse events—some of them potentially serious or even fatal—is high. Consequently, a thorough pharmacologic cross-check should be performed before initiating therapy.

Chloroquine cross-reacts with antacids and laxatives containing aluminum and magnesium, which decrease absorption of chloroquine. Concurrent administration of chloroquine with valproic acid decreases serum levels of valproic acid and increases risk of seizures. Chloroquine is contraindicated in patients with chloroquine hypersensitivity,

kidney disease, lactation, porphyria, and retinal disease; it should be used cautiously in patients with liver disease, neurologic disease, and alcoholism. Taking chloroquine concurrently with vaccination against rabies can disrupt the vaccine response.

Mefloquine carries a risk of cardiac arrhythmia, and it also interacts with several categories of drugs. First, use of this drug should generally be avoided in persons with history of seizure, as it lowers plasma levels of anticonvulsants such as valproic acid, carbamazepine, phenobarbital, and phenytoin. Second, use concomitantly with other antimalarial agents should be avoided, particularly concurrent use with artemether/lumefantrine, as fatal cardiac rhythm effects may occur (Youngster & Barnett, 2013). Coadministration of mefloquine and other drugs that may affect cardiac conduction is not currently considered to be contraindicated, but it should be undertaken with caution or avoided in patients taking antiarrhythmic or beta-blocking agents, calcium-channel blockers, antihistamines, H_1-blocking agents, tricyclic antidepressants, or phenothiazines. Finally, mefloquine can lead to increased levels of calcineurin inhibitors and mTOR inhibitors, while the serum level of mefloquine itself may be increased by concomitant use with potent CYP3A4 inhibitors. CYP3A4 inducers may reduce plasma concentrations of mefloquine, so their concurrent use should be avoided.

Atovaquone and atovaquone-proguanil should not be used concurrently with tetracycline, rifampin, and rifabutin due to these drugs' capacity to reduce plasma levels of atovaquone. Bioavailability of atovaquone is reduced in the presence of the antiemetic metoclopramide; thus, if vomiting occurs while using atovaquone, an alternative antiemetic should be sought. Patients on anticoagulants may need a dose reduction or closer monitoring of prothrombin time while taking atovaquone-proguanil (Youngster & Barnett, 2013).

Metronidazole may increase serum lithium levels if taken concurrently with that antipsychotic drug; in contrast, elevated metronidazole metabolism is seen if taken with phenobarbital. Metronidazole should not be taken with disulfiram or (because of a disulfiram-like reaction) with alcohol; with IV administration of nitroglycerin, sulfamethoxazole, or trimethoprim; or with oral solutions of lopinavir/ritonavir, citalopram, or ritonavir. Transient neutropenia can occur when metronidazole is administered concurrently with azathioprine and/or fluorouracil, and hypoprothrombinemia may arise with concurrent use of oral anticoagulants.

Nursing Considerations

Key considerations for this class of agents focus on avoiding adverse drug–drug interactions, ensuring that the correct organism is paired with an appropriate agent, and supporting patient compliance with completing the regimen.

Anthelmintic Agents

Worm or helminthic infections are a problem found all over the world. It is estimated that 1 billion individuals have worms somewhere in their bodies. The worms that are commonly found in human infections include tapeworms, flukes, and roundworms. As anthelmintic drugs destroy specific worms (TABLE 16-11), it is very important to correctly identify the worm causing the infection so

TABLE 16-11	Anthelmintic and Antiparasitic Agents	
Drug	Mechanism of Action	Uses
Mebendazole	Inhibits the formation of the worm microtubules and causes worm glucose depletion.	Pinworms (*Enterobius* spp.), roundworms (*Ascaris lubricoides*), tapeworms (*Cestoidea*), hookworms (*Necator americanus*), whipworms (Trichuris trichiura)
Albendazole	Causes degeneration of cytoplasmic microtubules in intestinal and tegmental cells of intestinal helminths and larvae, glycogen depletion, impairment of glucose uptake and cholinesterase secretion are impaired. These result in intracellular accumulation of desecratory substances, and decreased ATP production, which then results in energy depletion, immobilization, and worm death.	Broad spectrum; not approved for use in humans in the United States but used off-label for a variety of nematode and flatworm infections

(continues)

TABLE 16-10	Agents Used for Prevention or Treatment of Protozoal Infections *(continued)*	
Drug	Mechanism of Action	Uses
Ivermectin	Binds to glutamate-gated chloride ion channels in target organism muscle and nerve cells of the microfilaria, causing increased permeability of the cell membrane to chloride ions, causing hyperpolarization of the cell, leading to paralysis and death of the parasite. May also act as a gamma-aminobutyric acid (GABA) agonist, disrupting GABA-mediated central nervous system (CNS) neurosynaptic transmission. May also impair normal intrauterine development of *O. volvulus microfilariae* and may inhibit their release from the uteri of gravid female worms.	Used against arthropods (e.g., scabies mites), lice, bed bugs, and a variety of worms (e.g., strongylids, ascarids, trichurids)
Oxamniquine	May inhibit target organism nucleic acid metabolism, but mechanism is unclear.	Used for schistosomiasis
Praziquantel	Causes increased schistosome cell permeability to calcium, inducing strong contractions and paralysis of worm musculature, leading to detachment of suckers from the blood vessel walls and then to dislodgment.	Used for flatworm infections, schistosomiasis, and flukes
Thiabendazole	Inhibits helminth-specific enzyme fumarate reductase. Also, suppresses egg or larval production, and may inhibit subsequent development of eggs or larvae in the stool of the patient.	Used for roundworm and hookworm infections

that the appropriate drug can be prescribed. (A few medications, such as **ivermectin**, also work on arthropods such as mites and lice.)

The action of each anthelmintic agent differs, because each works on particular metabolic processes in the specific worm. The prototype drug, **mebendazole**, prevents the uptake of glucose and other nutrients, which in turn prevents worm reproduction and eventually causes helminth death.

Drug Interactions and Contraindications

All anthelmintic agents should be used with caution in pregnant women except **albendazole**, which is a known teratogen and contraindicated in pregnancy. **Praziquantel** has shown less risk than other anthelmintic agents. Concurrent use with **phenytoin** or **carbamazepine** increases the metabolism of **mebendazole** and reduces the bioavailability of **praziquantel**. **Praziquantel** bioavailability may increase if it is taken concurrently with **cimetidine**. Use of **praziquantel** concurrently with **dexamethasone** is contraindicated due to a potentially lethal reduction in plasma concentration. **Albendazole** induces liver enzymes of the cytochrome P450

system; thus it may interact with **theophylline**, anticonvulsants, oral contraceptives, and oral hypoglycemic. A similar risk exists with **thiabendazole**. Use of alcohol while taking **ivermectin** can exacerbate adverse effects or increase serum ivermectin levels; use of antiviral medications (e.g., **efavirenz**) may reduce serum **ivermectin** levels.

Nursing Considerations

Patients should be advised to wash their hands after touching contaminated articles; shower frequently; change towels, bedding, and underwear often; and sleep alone during the treatment period. All medication must be taken. If one person in a family is infected, all persons should be treated. If the infection is still present three weeks post initiation of treatment, a second round of medications is indicated.

Antivirals

Antivirals are relatively new, with most being discovered and used since the 1990s. Viruses are obligate intracellular parasites, relying completely on the host for their own building materials. They are classified using either the Baltimore System, or the system created by the International Committee on Taxonomy of Viruses (ICTV). This text will use the Baltimore System, which separates viruses according to nucleic acid type (DNA- or RNA-based), method of replication (positive- or negative-sense), and the number of strands (single or double). Viruses consist of either single- or double-stranded DNA (ssDNA or dsDNA) or RNA, surrounded by a protein coat. Examples for each class of the Baltimore System are shown in TABLE 16-12.

Herpesviridae include herpes simplex viruses (HSV) I and II, varicella-zoster virus (VZV), cytomegalovirus (CMV), Epstein-Barr virus (EBV), and herpesvirus-6. HSV-1 can cause infections of the eye, mouth, lips, and genitalia, though it is less frequently associated with genital infections than is HSV-II, which causes genital warts. HSV (I and II) can remain latent in ganglial cells for many years before becoming activated (or reactivated), as can VZV. VZV causes chicken pox (where it is referred to as varicella), and, sometimes later in life, shingles (where it is referred to as zoster). Though it is the same virus, zoster (shingles) occurs because of reactivation of the latent VZV in nervous ganglia. EBV is the causative agent of mononucleosis, though a very large majority of people carry EBV without any associated disease. EBV is also associated with Burkitt lymphoma, a B-cell malignancy, that can be induced via viral mutations of B-cell MYC genes.

Besides classification by system (Baltimore, ICTV), viruses can also be divided into two major types—**non-retrovirus** and **retrovirus**. Within the non-retroviruses there are three subdivisions: herpes-type viruses, **influenza-type viruses**, hepatitis-type viruses, and other viruses. Retroviruses include, among others, HIV. Accordingly, antiviral drugs can be classified as follows:

A. Non-retroviral antiviral agents
1. Anti-herpesvirus agents
2. Anti-influenza agents
3. Anti-hepatitis agents

B. Antiretroviral Agents
1. Nucleoside reverse transcriptase inhibitors (NRTIs)
2. Non-nucleoside reverse transcriptase inhibitors (NNRTIs)
3. Protease inhibitors (PI)
4. Entry inhibitors
5. Integrase strand transfer inhibitors

Antiviral agents have a more restricted spectrum compared to antibacterial agents. Most of the current agents inhibit viral replication, but the host immune system must participate to eradicate the virus, and affect a cure, and current drugs do not target non-replicating or latent viruses. Many antiviral agents must be activated by viral or host cell enzymes before exerting their effects, and, like bacteria, viruses often mutate. Sometimes a mutation of a single viral nucleotide is sufficient to render a medication useless. Non-retrovirus agents will be discussed first.

TABLE 16-12	Baltimore Classification	
Class	**Descriptor**	**Examples**
I: dsDNA viruses	Double-stranded DNA viruses	Adenoviruses, Poxviruses, Herpesviruses
II: ssDNA viruses	Single-stranded positive-sense DNA viruses	Parvoviruses
III: dsRNA viruses	Double-stranded RNA viruses	Reoviruses
IV: (+)ssRNA viruses	Single-stranded positive-sense RNA viruses	Picornaviruses (poliovirus, rhinovirus), Togaviruses
V: (-)ssRNA viruses	Single-stranded negative-sense RNA viruses	Orthomyxoviruses, Rhabdoviruses
VI: ssRNA-RT virusus	Single-stranded positive-sense reverse transcriptase RNA viruses	Retroviruses
VII: dsDNA-RT viruses	Double-stranded reverse transcriptase DNA viruses	Hepadnaviruses

Non-retroviral viruses and non-retroviral antivirals appear in TABLE 16-13. The table illustrates the three major subdivisions (along with a fourth, "miscellaneous" category) of drugs used for non-retroviruses.

Anti-Herpesvirus Agents

The herpesvirus (a DNA virus) replication cycle is illustrated in FIGURE 16-14. The anti-herpes (herpes simplex virus, HSV) agents are mostly nucleoside analogs (Table 16-6, Figure 16-14), of which **acyclovir** is a prototype. They act first by being taken up by infected host cells as a prodrug, being phosphorylated as "faux" nucleosides, and interfering with correct DNA synthesis by target viruses, by virtue of their similarity in chemical structure to regular DNA nucleosides. Most of these drugs are converted by viral and cellular enzymes to their active **nucleoside** triphosphate forms, such as *acyclovir triphosphate*. The triphosphate forms compete with endogenous viral nucleoside triphosphates and inhibit *viral* (not host) DNA polymerase. Some drugs are incorporated into viral DNA (Figure 16-14). Because nucleoside analogs lack a 3′ hydroxyl group, chain termination occurs at the point where the analog is incorporated. Additionally, some antivirals known as **nucleoside reverse transcriptase inhibitors (NRTIs)** get incorporated into nascent DNA leading to chain termination. **Ganciclovir** and **penciclovir** do have a 3′ hydroxyl group, so do not cause chain termination (Figure 16-14). Acyclovir (and its relative, **valacyclovir**) is excreted in the urine, and adverse effects are often related to compromised renal function. CNS side effects, such as confusion, hallucinations, headache, and nausea, are seen with buildup of **acyclovir**. These may be related to induction of crystalline nephropathy by the drug.

Other viruses that **acyclovir** and **valacyclovir** may be used to treat include varicella-zoster virus. **Cidofovir** is useful for treating herpes, papilloma, polyoma, pox, and adenoviruses.

TABLE 16-13	Agents for Treatment of Non-Retroviral Viruses	
Class	Anti-Non-Retroviral Drugs	Subclass
Anti-herpesvirus Agents	Acyclovir	Nucleoside analog
	Cidofovir	Nucleoside analog
	Famcyclovir	Nucleoside analog
	Foscarnet	Other (triphosphate cleavage inhibitor)
	Fomivirsena	Antisense RNA
	Gancicyclovir	Nucleoside analog
	Idoxuridine	Nucleoside analog
	Penciclovir	Nucleoside analog
	Trifluridine	Nucleoside analog
	Valacyclovir	Nucleoside analog
	Valgancyclovir	Nucleoside analog (prodrug to Gancyclovir)
Anti-influenza agents	Amantidine	Tricyclic amine
	Oseltamivir	Sialic acid TSA*; neuraminidase inhibitor
	Rimantadine	Tricyclic amine (a-methyl derivative of Amantidine)
	Zanamivir	Sialic acid TSA; neuraminidase inhibitor
Anti-hepatitis agents	Adefovir dipivoxil	Hepatitis B; Phosphonate nucleotide analog
	Entecavir	Hepatitis B; nucleoside analog
	Interferon alfa-N1	Hepatitis C
	Interferon alfa-N3	Hepatitis C
	Interferon alfacon-1	Hepatitis C
	Interferon alfa-2B	Hepatitis C
	Interferon alfa-2A	Hepatitis C
	Lamivudine	Hepatitis B; nucleoside analog
	Peginterferon alfa-2A	Hepatitis C
	Peginterferon alfa-2B	Hepatitis C; nucleoside analog
	Ribavirin	
	Telbivudine	Hepatitis B; nucleoside analog
	Tenofovir	Hepatitis B; nucleotide analog
Other antiviral agents	Imiquimod	Cytokine inducer

*TSA: transition state analog

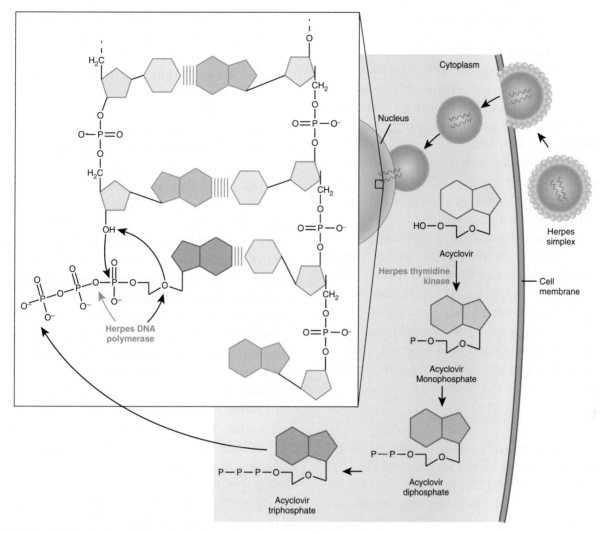

FIGURE 16-14 Mechanism of action of acyclovir (a nucleoside analog) in HSV-infected cells.

Foscarnet, useful against cytomegalovirus (CMV), acts at the site where viral DNA polymerase binds pyrophosphate, preventing removal of pyrophosphate from nucleoside triphosphates. This halts any further attachment of nucleoside precursors that would be used for viral primer template extension of the DNA chain.

Fomivirsen, an antisense antiviral, is effective against CMV. **Fomivirsen** is a complementary strand to viral mRNA coding for the major immediate-early transcription region of the virus. The effect on the virus is to inhibit its binding to target cells.

Idoxuridine is an iodinated thymidine analog. By virtue of the attached iodine, its incorporation into viral DNA inhibits replication.

The anti-herpesvirideae agents are generally safe. Occasionally patients may complain of nausea, diarrhea, rash, or headache. **Valacyclovir** is a prodrug (a drug that is converted in-vivo to the active drug) of **acyclovir**. The important adverse effects/side effects of the nucleoside analogs include occasional headache and neurotoxicity (confusion, hallucinations). The occurrence of hallucinations is often due to renal toxicity of the drugs, or preexisting reduced renal function in the patient. **Cidifovir** and **foscarnet** are sometimes associated with nephrotoxicity.

Anti-Influenza Agents

Anti-influenza agents include amantadine, rimantadine, oseltamivir, and zanamivir (Table 16-13). Amantidine and rimantidine act by inhibiting an early step, thought to be the uncoating step, by blocking the M2 channel in viral replication. Oseltimivir and zanamivir (FIGURE 16-15) are transition state analogs (TSA) of sialic acid, which inhibits neuraminidases in influenza viruses. Side effects associated with amantadine and rimantidine include nervousness, light-headedness, and nausea, but are usually minor. The most notable side effect of oseltamavir is nausea, so it should be administered with food.

The replication cycles for herpesviruses and influenza viruses, and where drugs are thought to act against them are shown in FIGURE 16-16.

Anti-Hepatitis Agents

Infectious hepatitis can be caused by bacteria (hepatitis A) or viruses (hepatitis B, C). The hepatitis viral lifecycles are illustrated in FIGURE 16-17. Anti-hepatitis virus agents include adefovir, entecavir, lamivudine, telbivudine, tenofovir, and clevudine (for hepatitis B); interferons and ribavirin (for hepatitis C), although interferons are less recommended now.

Interferons (IFNs) are natural cytokines, possessing potent antiviral, immunomodulatory, and antiproliferative effects on viruses, notably for this section, hepatitis B and C viruses. Normally, these proteins are produced by host cells in response to various stimuli, including viruses. Interferons cause cellular biochemical responses that lead to states of viral resistance. After binding, INFs activate JAK-STAT signaling, leading ultimately to multiple proteins that contribute to a cell's viral resistance (FIGURE 16-18). Of the three major classes of interferons (α, β, and γ), the INFas are currently most useful as anti-hepatitis drugs. As these are immunomodulators, the major adverse effects of their use, as expected, may include myelosuppression, granulocytopenia, and thrombocytopenia. Non-immune-related adverse effects include behavioral changes, and rarely, seizures. Pegylated interferons are modified by attaching a polyethylene glycol (PEG) molecule to interferons. This has no direct antiviral activity, but the chemical modification prolongs duration of each interferon dose, decreasing dosing frequency.

Recently, there has been a proliferation of very effective antiviral agents for treatment of hepatitis C. These mainly fall in three categories: NS3/4A polymerase inhibitors, NS5A inhibitors, and NS5B polymerase inhibitors. The reader is encouraged to refer to a virology

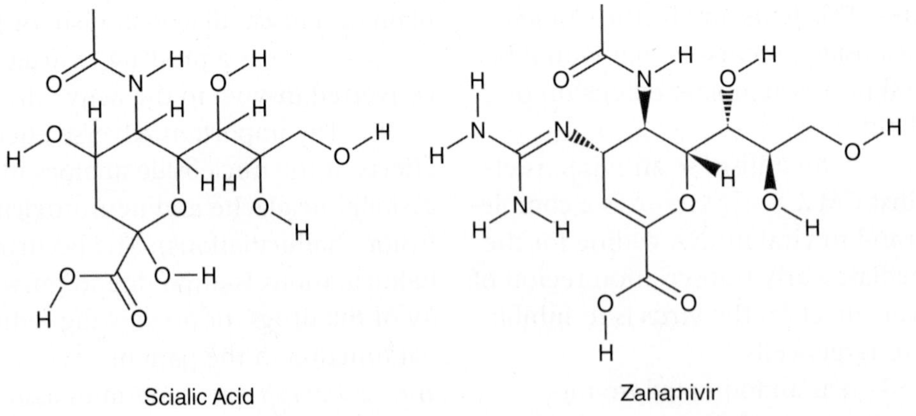

Scialic Acid

Zanamivir

FIGURE 16-15 Zanamivir structure.

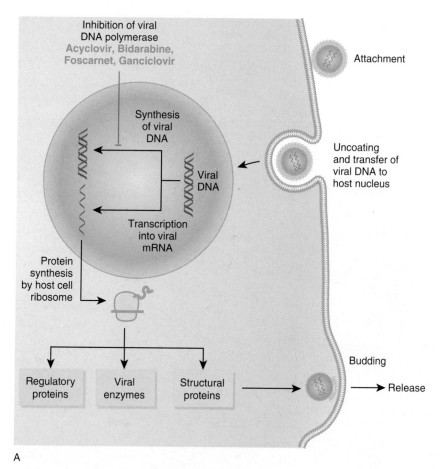

A

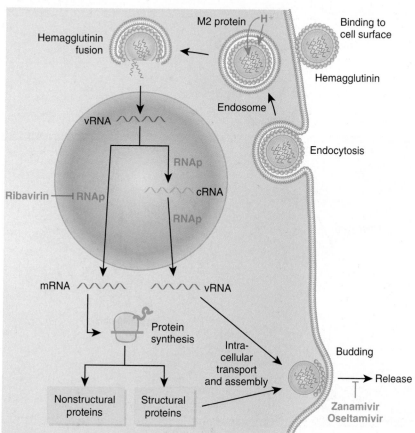

FIGURE 16-16 Herpesvirus (DNA) and influenza (RNA) virus replication cycles.

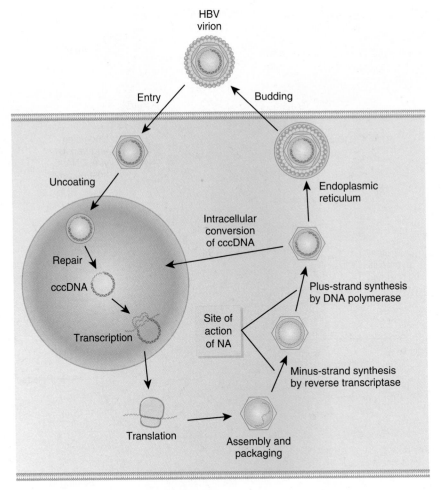

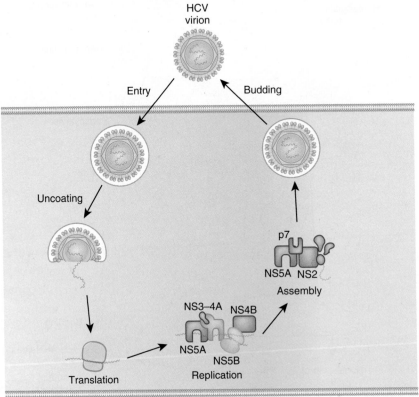

FIGURE 16-17 Lifecycles for hepatitis B and C.

Viruses
  A. DNA
  B. RNA
    1. Orthomyxoviruses and retroviruses
    2. Picornaviruses and most RNA viruses

IFN Effects

  ① Inhibition of transcription
  Activates Mx protein
  Blocks mRNA synthesis

  ② Inhibition of translation
  Activates methylase, thereby
  reducing mRNA cap methylation

  Activates 2'5'A oligoadenylate synthetase
  → 2'5'A → inhibits mRNA splicing and activates
  RNaseL → cleaves viral RNA

  Activates protein kinase P1 → blocks eIL-2a
  function → inhibits initiation of mRNA translation

  Activates phosphodiesterase → blocks tRNA function

  ③ Inhibition of post-translational processing
  Inhibits glycosyltransferase, thereby reducing
  protein glycosylation

  ④ Inhibition of virus maturation
  Inhibits glycosyltransferase, thereby reducing
  glycoprotein maturation

  ⑤ Inhibition of virus release
  Causes membrane changes → blocks budding

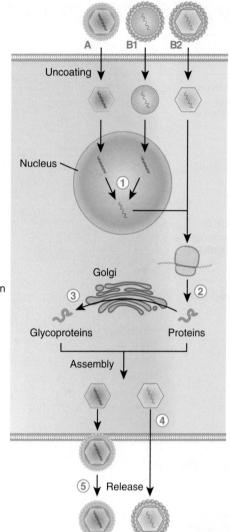

FIGURE 16-18 Cellular effects of interferons toward viral resistance.

textbook regarding the lifecycle and biochemistry of the hepatitis C viruses.

The patient's virus is first genotyped, so that the optimum combination of anti-hepatitis C drugs can be selected. The drugs within the three main anti-hepatitis C categories are shown in Table 16-14. All of these drugs interfere with the hepatitis C viral replication complex, including interference with RNA-dependent RNA polymerase (FIGURE 16-19).

Many antiviral medications compete with viral nucleosides or nucleotides during the viral replication cycles. They are not always devoid of effects in host cells but are so overwhelmingly biased toward their effects on viral replication that their effects (if any) in human cells are not normally problematic.

Adefovir (diprivoxil) is a prodrug of **adefovir**. **Adefovir** is phosphonate nucleotide analog of adenosine monophosphate (AMP). It acts as a competitive inhibitor of *viral* DNA polymerases and reverse transcriptases and causes viral DNA chain termination. Adverse effects include potential nephrotoxicity.

Entecavir is a guanosine nucleoside analog, competing with normal

TABLE 16-14	Antiretroviral Agents	
Antiretroviral Drug Class	Drug (Generic) Name	Abbreviation
Nucleoside Reverse Transcriptase Inhibitors (NRTIs)	Zidovudine	ZDV, AZT
	Didanosine	ddI
	Stavudine	d4T
	Zalcitabine	DDC
	Lamivudine	3TC
	Abacavir	ABC
	Tenofovir	TDF
	Emtricitabine	FTC
Non-Nucleoside Reverse Transcriptase Inhibitors (NNRTIs)	Nevirapine	NVP
	Efavirenz	EFV
	Delvirdine	DLV
	Etravirine	ETV
Protease Inhibitors (PI)	Saquinavir	SQV
	Indinavir	IDV
	Ritonavir	RTV
	Nelfinavir	NFV
	Amprenovir	APV
	Lopinavir	LPV
	Atazanavir	ATV
	Fosamprenavir	FPV
	Tipranavir	TPV
	Darunavir	DRV
Entry Inhibitors (EIs)	Enfuvirtide	T-20
	Maraviroc	MVC
Integrase Strand Transfer Inhibitors (ISTIs)/Integrase Inhibitors (IIs)	Raltegravir	RAL

deoxyguanosine triphosphate, inhibiting HBV reverse transcriptase. **Lamivudine** is a nucleoside analog that inhibits HBV DNA polymerase (and also HIV reverse transcriptase, see the following discussion). **Telbivudine, tenofovir,** and **ribavirin** are also nucleoside analogs effective against hepatitis B and/or C.

As discontinuation of some analog drugs can lead to severe acute hepatitis B exacerbations, liver functions should be followed closely in patients who are taking these drugs, but especially those who discontinue treatment.

Antiretroviral Agents

The agents used against retroviruses (Table 16-15) are all of recent discovery and have been developed primarily in response to the emergence of HIV in the late 1970s. Some of these agents are also used in the treatment of hepatitis C, and a few have been investigated for activity against protozoan infections such as *Plasmodium, Trichomonas,* and *Giardia* (Andrews et al., 2006; Dunn et al., 2007).

Therapeutic use of these agents for their principal indication, HIV/AIDS, is a complex, highly specialized topic and cannot be fully addressed here; the classes of medications that are selected and combined for treatment of any particular patient depend on a great many variables related to **host factors**, natural history of the infection, strain of HIV virus involved, comorbidities, and many other considerations. However, certain general information about the classes of drugs used for antiretroviral therapy can be described.

Retroviruses are single-stranded (positive sense) RNA viruses (they have RNA genomes). These viruses utilize a DNA intermediate, and reverse transcriptase

The normal "central dogma" of molecular biology is that DNA is transcribed to RNA, which is then translated to make useful proteins. Thus, we are accustomed to a DNA-based genome. Retroviruses utilize an RNA genome to create DNA, via reverse transcription, which can then be utilized to make necessary proteins. In order to produce proteins required by retroviruses to propagate, a unique enzyme, *reverse transcriptase,* is employed, to produce a *single-stranded* DNA chain from a RNA template, and host-supplied DNA bases. From there, a complementary DNA chain is made, resulting in double-stranded DNA. Therefore, approaches to treating retroviral infections (such as HIV), are multi-focal, focusing on the various steps of attachment, entry, enzyme usage, integration, and propagation, to achieve cure or remission from the virus.

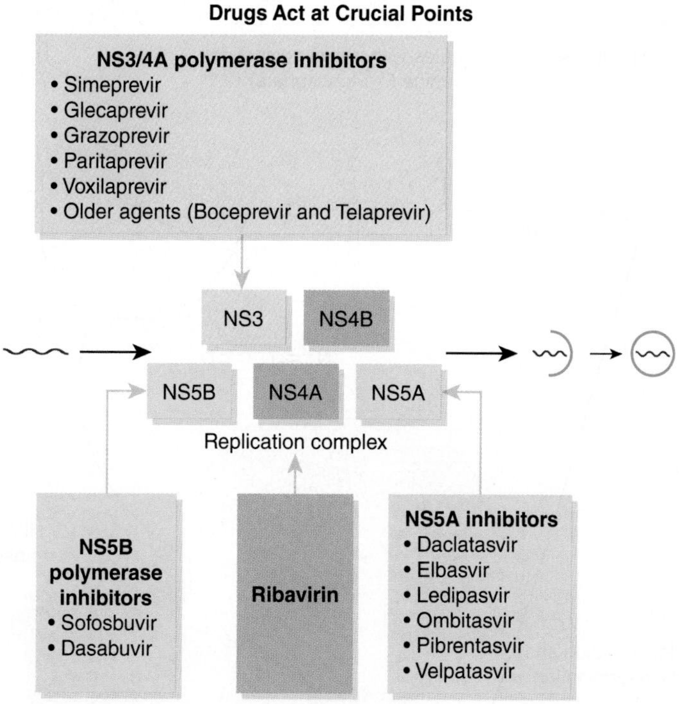

Drugs Act at Crucial Points

FIGURE 16-19 Antiretroviral interference with the hepatitis C viral replication complex.

Nucleoside Reverse Transcriptase Inhibitors (NRTIs)

NRTIs work by a fairly simple mechanism: They masquerade as a nucleoside—one of the building blocks of DNA and RNA—to fool the enzyme reverse transcriptase into using them for construction of viral DNA/RNA. Because they are not, in fact, the correct chemical, they stop the reproduction of viral genetic matter, thereby inhibiting the spread of the virus to uninfected cells.

As the category name implies, the NRTIs focus on disrupting viral reverse transcription. NRTIs include zidovudine, didanosine, stavudine, zalcitabine, lamivudine, abacavir, tenofovir, and emtricitabine. Viral RNA-dependent DNA polymerase (also called reverse transcriptase) converts viral RNA into proviral DNA. So far, drugs used to target this step are nucleoside-or nucleotide analogs (this section) or non-nucleoside inhibitors (next section). The nucleoside/nucleotide analogs lack a 3' hydroxyl group, and work by competitively inhibiting incorporation of natural nucleotides, thus stopping proviral DNA elongation (FIGURE 16-20).

As a group, NRTIs' adverse effects include fatigue, flatulence, nausea, headache, peripheral neuropathy, neutropenia, hypersensitivity (especially with abacavir), and pancreatitis—possibly from mitochondrial toxicity.

Drug Interactions and Contraindications

Hypersensitivity responses are most prominent in patients who have HLA-B*5701 and who take abacavir; before initiating abacavir therapy, therefore, antibody testing for the presence of HLA-B*5701 is warranted. Patients with positive results should not receive abacavir. Patients with negative results should be watched for hypersensitivity symptoms such as fever, skin rash, malaise, nausea, headache, myalgia, chills, diarrhea, vomiting, abdominal pain, dyspnea, arthralgia, and respiratory symptoms. Onset of hypersensitivity usually occurs within nine days of initiation of therapy but may develop at any point in the first six

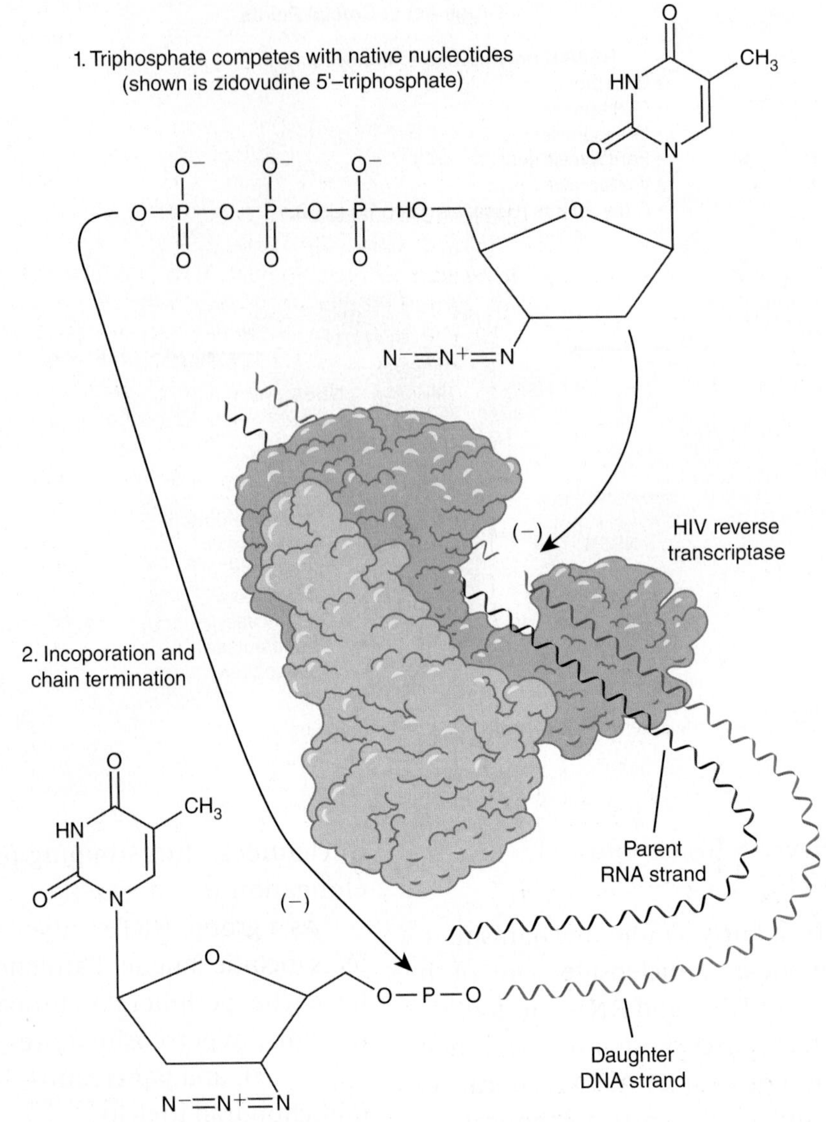

1. Triphosphate competes with native nucleotides
(shown is zidovudine 5'–triphosphate)

FIGURE 16-20 Nucleoside and nucleotide reverse transcriptase inhibition.

weeks; if such symptoms develop, the drug must be withdrawn.

Nursing Considerations

A 2008 study of NRTIs (D:A:D Study Group, 2008) found that specific agents in this class, abacavir and didanosine, produce a transient (six months post cessation) increase in risk of cardiovascular events. Two other drugs, the thymidine analogs stavudine and zidovudine, contribute to increased lipid levels and reduced glucose tolerance, potentially increasing the patient's risk of developing diabetes. Thus, a baseline assessment of

patients' cardiovascular health and glucose tolerance should be made prior to starting therapy, with monitoring of status continuing for the duration of therapy plus six months. Prolonged exposure to NRTIs has been linked to non-cirrhotic portal hypertension, with some patients developing esophageal varices.

Lactic acidosis is another serious potential risk of NRTI therapy, particularly in female and obese patients. Mortality in such instances is as much as 50%, so patients should be monitored for insidious-onset gastrointestinal prodrome, weight loss, and fatigue, which may rapidly progress to tachycardia, tachypnea, jaundice, muscular weakness, mental status changes, respiratory distress, pancreatitis, and organ failure (NIH/AIDSInfo, 2013).

Peripheral neuropathy, sometimes irreversible, may occur with **stavudine**, **zalcitabine**, or **didanosine**.

Non-Nucleoside Reverse Transcriptase Inhibitors (NNRTIs)

NNRTIs affect the same process as NRTIs, but in a different manner. Instead of "fooling" reverse transcriptase into creating nonviable genetic matter, NNRTIs work directly against the enzyme's activity to reduce its ability to perform its function. Unfortunately, microbes are reasonably resilient when it comes to dodging the direct approach, so resistance to these agents has developed fairly quickly. However, when used in combination with other antiviral and antiretroviral agents, they are still fairly effective against HIV (Zdanowicz, 2006).

Several drugs in this class are absorbed better when they are taken with food.

The NNRTIs include **nevirapine**, **efavirenz**, **delvirdine**, and **etravirine**. These drugs bind the HIV-1 reverse transcriptase enzyme in a hydrophobic pocket in the p66 subunit, changing the enzyme's structure, such that it becomes much less efficient. Because these drugs are not nucleoside or nucleotide analogs, no phosphorylation by intracellular enzymes is required for them to work (**FIGURE 16-21**). However, these drugs are strain-specific (i.e., for HIV-1, not HIV-2, or other retroviruses), and so should only be used for their specified strain (usually to-date, HIV-1). They are hepatically metabolized. Adverse effects include rash, elevated transaminases, CNS/psychiatric effects, and headache.

Drug Interactions and Contraindications

The NNRTI class interacts with numerous other drug classes and interaction potential should be thoroughly assessed before adding these drugs, or when adding new drugs to NNRTIs.

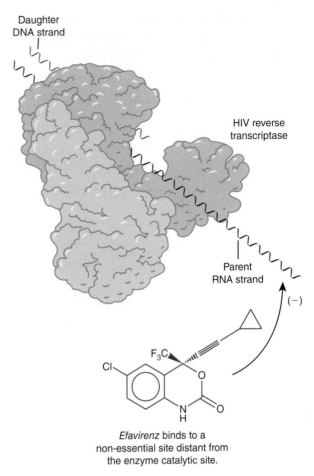

Efavirenz binds to a non-essential site distant from the enzyme catalytic site.

FIGURE 16-21 Non-nucleoside reverse transcriptase inhibition.

Nursing Considerations

Assess the patient's prescriptions for potential interactions. A history of hepatitis and other liver disease should be obtained, as liver damage may occur with any of the NNRTIs but is particularly significant in patients with prior liver disease. Rash and sores are common adverse effects.

Assess the patient's psychiatric history when **efivirenz** may be prescribed due to this medication's CNS effects. If the patient reports CNS symptoms, advise bedtime dosing of the medication and see if the symptoms subside or diminish after two to four weeks.

Protease Inhibitors (PIs)

The protease inhibitor class includes a variety of drugs. Members of this class act by suppressing the viral enzyme protease, which the retrovirus needs to replicate itself. They are rarely used alone, but are more often used in combination with other antiretroviral classes.

Protease inhibitors (PIs) include saquinavir, indinavir, ritonavir, nelfinavir, amprenovir, lopinavir, atazanavir, fosamprenavir (a prodrug for amprenovir), tipranavir, and darunavir. These drugs use diverse mechanisms to disrupt the viral enzyme aspartyl protease. Even though humans have aspartyl proteases

(renin, pepsin, gastricsin, to name a few), the viral aspartyl proteases have a different enzyme active site than human aspartyl proteases, and so viruses are preferentially inhibited. These drugs have diverse mechanisms including a transition state analog (TSA) of the enzyme substrate (saquinavir, FIGURE 16-22), enzyme active site complement molecules (ritinovir and lopinavir, atazanavir), binding to the enzyme's proteolytic

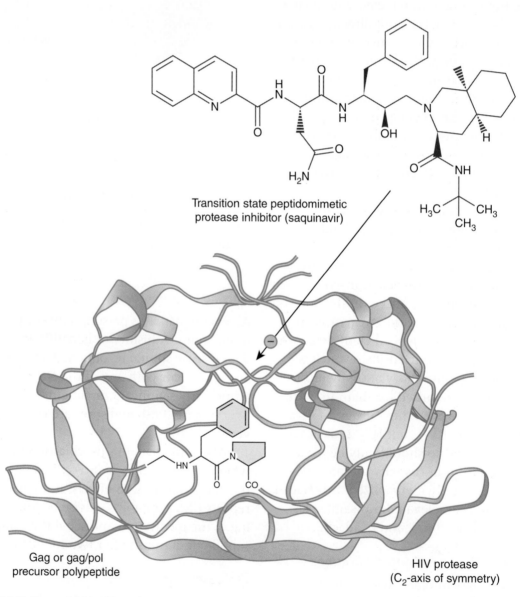

Transition state peptidomimetic protease inhibitor (saquinavir)

Gag or gag/pol precursor polypeptide

HIV protease (C_2-axis of symmetry)

FIGURE 16-22 Protease inhibitor (shown here, sequinavir) mechanism of action.

site (**darunavir**), or simply impeding the enzymatic binding site (**nelfinavir, tipranavir**). As these drugs vary slightly in their mechanisms, their adverse effects can also vary, including diarrhea, nausea vomiting, crystalluria and nephrolithiasis, hyberbilirubinemia, and hepatotoxicity.

Drug Interactions and Contraindications

Protease inhibitors in general are associated with an increased risk of hematuria and bleeding, and intracranial hemorrhage has been reported in some patients using **tipranivir**. Risk factors for bleeding include CNS lesions, trauma, surgery, hypertension, alcohol abuse, coagulopathy, and concomitant use of anticoagulant or antiplatelet agents, including vitamin E (NIH/AIDSInfo, 2013). All protease inhibitors increase the risk of liver dysfunction and hepatitis, for which the patient should be monitored. In addition, these drugs increase blood glucose levels, so patients with diabetes or prediabetes should be monitored for hyperglycemia and diabetic/cardiovascular complications.

Use of a protease inhibitor in a patient taking ergot-derived medications for migraine poses a risk of ergotism and vasospasm; discontinue use of the migraine medication before initiating protease inhibitor therapy. Coadministration of protease inhibitors with acid-reducing agents such as **omeprazole** or **ranitidine** may reduce the latter drugs' bioavailability (Klein et al., 2008).

Ritonavir has been shown to increase triglycerides, cholesterol, SGOT (AST), SGPT (ALT), GGT, CPK, and uric acid levels (Wang et al., 2007). These effects may occur with other drugs in this class as well, so regardless of the specific agent used, baseline values should be obtained before initiating therapy and updated at intervals or if any clinical signs or symptoms of hypercholesterolemia, uremia, or other imbalances occur during therapy. Patients should be advised to stay well hydrated due to risk of kidney stones, particularly if using **atazanavir**.

Nursing Considerations

Protease inhibitors are better absorbed when taken with food. Monitor patients for indications of cardiovascular complications (e.g., dyslipidemia), as these drugs are known to produce such effects (D:A:D Study Group, 2008). Patients prescribed protease inhibitors generally need close monitoring and follow-up, not merely because of the drug effects but also because of the nature of the illness for which they are receiving treatment (HIV/AIDS). Educate patients on the need for consistency in medication use and for prompt reporting of adverse effects and symptoms associated with medication use.

Entry Inhibitors (EI)

Enfuvirtide and **maraviroc** work by different mechanisms, but both inhibit viral fusion to the host cell membrane via gp1 and CD4 interactions. **Maraviroc** is a CCR5 (chemokine receptor) antagonist (FIGURE 16-23). It blocks the binding of viral gp120 to the chemokine receptor. **Enfuvirtide** is a 36 amino acid peptide that is analogous to part of the virus gp41. By interacting there, **enfuvirtide** blocks the ability for successful fusion of the virus to the host cell membrane.

Integrase Strand Transfer Inhibitors (ISTIs)

Raltegravir is a viral integrase inhibitor. It works by preventing the formation of covalent bonds between the host and viral DNA, which is required for successful integration of viral DNA into the host cell genome (FIGURE 16-24).

A summary of the retrovirus lifecycle and steps where the different drugs affect it is shown in FIGURE 16-25.

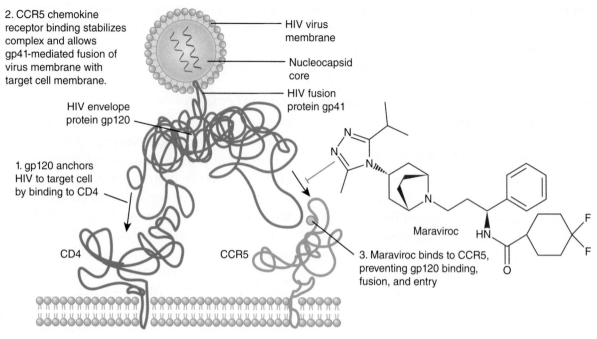

2. CCR5 chemokine receptor binding stabilizes complex and allows gp41-mediated fusion of virus membrane with target cell membrane.

HIV virus membrane

Nucleocapsid core

HIV fusion protein gp41

HIV envelope protein gp120

1. gp120 anchors HIV to target cell by binding to CD4

CD4

CCR5

Maraviroc

3. Maraviroc binds to CCR5, preventing gp120 binding, fusion, and entry

FIGURE 16-23 Mechanism of entry inhibitor (EI) maraviroc.

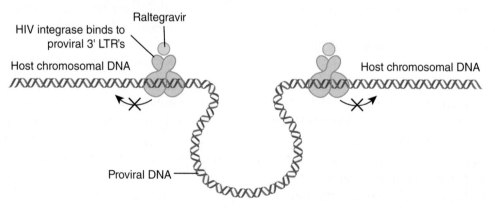

Raltegravir

Raltegravir binds to HIV integrase, prevents DNA strand transfer.

Raltegravir

HIV integrase binds to proviral 3' LTR's

Host chromosomal DNA

Host chromosomal DNA

Proviral DNA

FIGURE 16-24 Mechanism of raltegravir, an HIV integrase inhibitor.

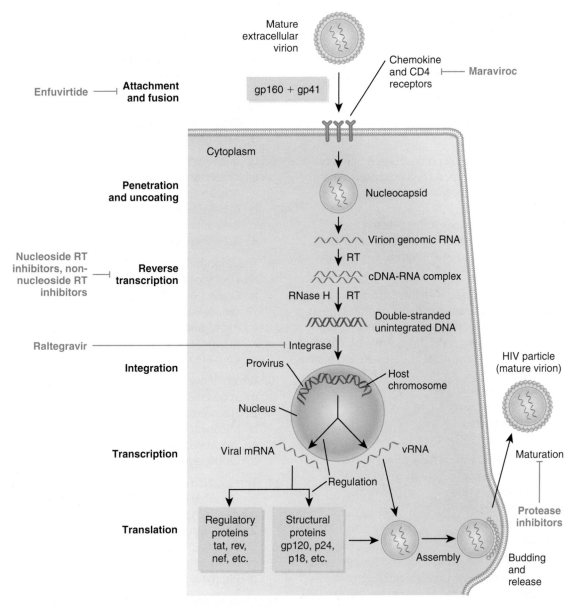

FIGURE 16-25 Summary of the antiretrovirus actions in the retrovirus lifecycle with HIV, a prototype retrovirus.

CHAPTER SUMMARY

Microbial life is extremely diverse, and, as has been true for a very long time, humans often have competitive interactions with these other forms of life. Historically, our immune systems have been our only defense against the infringement of microbes into our bodies, and their associated disease sequelae. A recent development in our competition has been the ability to investigate the mechanisms by which other forms of life live and function, and how they infect human tissue. This has provided us with a competitive advantage, as we can design drugs that hinder or destroy pathogens. However, as our competition has been ongoing and is always evolving, we are unable to remain complacent with regard to creating new drugs to combat infection. Our infectious opponents naturally tend to develop counter measures, to evade our best antimicrobials. Thus, the competition may well never be over.

This chapter has introduced the basic concepts of antimicrobial pharmacology, including drugs designed to combat bacteria, fungi, parasites, viruses, and other infectious agents. The interested reader is encouraged both to study more antimicrobial pharmacology in-depth and to keep abreast of new developments in the story of our struggle against microbial life.

1. Which group of anti-infective drugs acts by inhibiting protein synthesis in the bacterial cell?
   a. Fluoroquinolones
   b. Sulfonamides
   c. Aminoglycosides
   d. Penicillins

2. A third-generation cephalosporin is different from a first-generation cephalosporin in that the third-generation cephalosporin:
   a. Costs less.
   b. Has less resistance to beta-lactamases.
   c. Is unable to penetrate cerebral spinal fluid.
   d. Has increased activity against Gram-negative bacteria.

3. A patient diagnosed with infection with a non-drug-resistant Gram-positive organism reports that she has experienced a life-threatening allergic response to penicillin in the past. Which of the following is the most appropriate alternative medication?
   a. Cephalosporin
   b. Aminoglycoside
   c. Carbapenem
   d. Macrolide

4. Which class of antibacterial agent is used to cleanse the bowel before surgery?
   a. Aminoglycosides
   b. Macrolides
   c. Penicillins
   d. Lincosamides

5. Which of the following peak and trough levels are associated with gentamicin toxicity in aminoglycoside therapy?
   a. Peak levels >2.0 mcg/mL and trough levels >0.2 mcg/mL
   b. Peak levels >6.0 mcg/mL and trough levels >4 mcg/mL
   c. Peak levels >12.0 mcg/mL and trough levels >2 mcg/mL
   d. Peak levels >20.0 mcg/mL and trough levels >12 mcg/mL

6. The nurse should instruct the patient receiving an oral tetracycline to do which of the following?
   a. Take the medication with a full glass of milk.
   b. Stop the medication if he or she develop heart palpitations.
   c. Store the medication in a clear plastic bottle.
   d. Stay out of the sun while taking the medication.

7. A patient taking a fluoroquinolone should restrict the intake of:
   a. Dairy products.
   b. Coffee.
   c. Orange or lemon juice.
   d. Green, leafy vegetables.

8. IV vancomycin should be used cautiously in which of the following clients?
   a. An 18-year-old
   b. A 30-year-old
   c. A 50-year-old
   d. A 75-year-old

9. The antitubercular drugs are given in combination because they:
   a. Can act on different phases of the bacterial cell life cycle.
   b. Avoid causing microbial resistance.
   c. Are more cost-effective if given together.
   d. Cause fewer adverse effects.

10. Which of the following oral antifungal drugs must be taken on an empty stomach?
    a. Fluconazole
    b. Miconazole
    c. Ketoconazole
    d. Clotrimazole

11. There is an increased risk of renal toxicity if amphotericin B is taken with which of the following medications?
    a. Corticosteroid
    b. Digoxin
    c. Heparin
    d. Phenytoin

12. Chloroquine is contraindicated in patients with which of the following conditions?
    a. Liver disease
    b. Blood dyscrasias
    c. CNS diseases
    d. Retinal diseases

13. In a patient being treated with antiviral medications, which antiparasitic agent may become less effective as a result of a drug interaction?
    a. Mebenzadole
    b. Ivermectin
    c. Praziquantel
    d. Oxamniquine

CASE STUDIES

Case Scenario 1

A 24-year-old female presents to the walk-in clinic with complaints of increased urinary urgency and a burning sensation during urination, for the past three days. The patient relates that she has had a urinary tract infection in the past, about age 15, but denies any other problems with her urinary tract since then. She tells you that she recently began a new job as a second-grade teacher in the public school system, which required her to go three to four hours at a time without the opportunity to go to the bathroom, and this was new to her. She has been drinking cranberry juice, which she heard was helpful for UTIs, but it does not seem to have helped alleviate the symptoms.

Other than seasonal allergies, which she treats with diphenhydramine, she has no significant medical history. She is well developed and well nourished, and reported allergies include penicillin, when she was a child, but she does not recollect what reaction she had. Physical exam findings are as follows:

- Vital signs: Temperature 101.3°F, blood pressure 121/79, pulse 74, respirations 15.
- Weight: 135 lbs, height 64 inches
- Eyes and Ears: Appear normal.
- Neck & Lymph Nodes: Thyroid gland symmetrical, no nodules or lymphadenopathy.
- Chest: Clear to auscultation.
- Heart: Regular rate; S_1 and S_2 heart sounds present.
- Lungs: Clear to auscultation bilaterally anterior and posterior.
- Abdomen: Nontender, no organomegaly.
- Genitourinary: Normal external genitalia; no vaginal discharge.
- Rectal: No hemorrhoids.
- Labs: Normal, except urine is yellow and cloudy, and cultures positive for Gram-negative rods. 24 hours later, culture shows sensitivity to ampicillin, ciprofloxacin, and cefazolin.

Case Questions

1. Based on the exam findings, what are the possible reasons for the woman's urinary pain?
2. Based on the patient's history, which drug should be avoided?
3. How should the nurse educate the patient regarding UTIs?
4. What are the signs and symptoms for uncomplicated UTIs?

CASE STUDIES

Case Scenario 2

A seven-year-old boy presents to the clinician's office with his mother, with complaints of fever, headache, and cough. The mother states that her son has been sick since yesterday. When he first become ill, he had sudden onset of fever (at least 101°F), chills, and body aches. His head has ached off-and-on and seems worse when he coughs. His cough is non-productive, and he is fatigued and has little appetite, which is unusual for him. The patient has no significant medical history. Physical exam findings are as follows:

- Vital signs: Temperature 102.6°F, blood pressure 85/59, pulse 115, respirations 20.
- Weight: 86.7 lb (39.3 Kg); Height 57 inches.

CASE STUDIES (CONTINUED)

- Anterior cervical lymphadenopathy.
- Skin: No lesions or bruises.
- Cardiovascular: Slightly tachycardic, but regular.
- Lab: Positive nasopharyngeal swab for influenza A virus.

Case Questions

1. Based on the exam findings, what are the reasons for the boy's symptoms?
2. What is the treatment plan?
3. What are the signs and symptoms of influenza infection?

REFERENCES

AbbVie, Inc. (2017). *Biaxin (clarithromycin) professional prescribing information*. Retrieved from http://www.pdr.net/full-prescribing-information/biaxin?druglabelid=6#section-8.1

Albengres, E., Le Louët, H., & Tillement, J.P. (1998). Systemic antifungal agents: Drug interactions of clinical significance. *Drug Safety, 18*(2), 83–97.

Albin, S., & Agarwal, S. (2014). Prevalence and characteristics of reported penicillin allergy in an urban outpatient adult population. *Allergy and Asthma Proceedings, 35*(6), 489–494. http://doi.org/10.2500/aap.2014.35.3791

Andrews, K.T., Fairlie, D.P., Madala, P.K., Ray, J., Wyatt, D.M., Hilton, P. M., . . . McCarthy, J.S. (2006). Potencies of human immuno deficiency virus protease inhibitors in vitro against *Plasmodium falciparum* and in vivo against murine malaria. *Antimicrobial Agents and Chemotherapy, 50*(2), 639–648.

Annè, S., & Reisman, R.E. (1995). Risk of administering cephalosporin antibiotics to patients with histories of penicillin allergy. *Annals of Allergy, Asthma & Immunology, 74*(2), 167–170. Retrieved from http://europepmc.org/abstract/MED/7697478/reload=0;jsessionid=n5tGGXfRcYbVVOBGhU6r.10

Aschenbrenner, D., Cleveland, L., & Venable, S. (2006). *Drug therapy in nursing*. Philadelphia, PA: Lippincott Williams & Wilkins.

Bennett, N.J., Gilroy, S.A., & Rose, F.B. (2013). *Pneumocystis jiroveci* pneumonia: Overview of PCP. *Medscape E-Medicine*. Retrieved from http://emedicine.medscape.com/article/225976-overview

Boothe, D.M. (2018). Sulfonamides and sulfonamide combinations. *Merck Manual: Veterinary Manual*. Retrieved from http://www.merckvetmanual.com/pharmacology/antibacterial-agents/sulfonamides-and-sulfonamide-combinations.

Bouazza, N., Pestre, V., Jullien, V., Curis, E., Urien, S., Salmon, D., & Tréluyer, J.M. (2012). Population pharmacokinetics of clindamycin orally and intravenously administered in patients with osteomyelitis. *British Journal of Clinical Pharmacology, 74*(6), 971–977.

Campagna, J.D., Bond, M.C., Schabelman, E., & Hayes, B.D. (2012). The use of cephalosporins in penicillin-allergic patients: A literature review. *Journal of Emergency Medicine, 42*(5), 612–620. doi: 10.1016/j.jemermed.2011.05.035

Cox, H.S., Kalon, S., Allamuratova, S., Sizaire, V., Tigay, Z.N., Rusch-Gerdes, S., . . . Mills, C. (2007). Multidrug-resistant tuberculosis treatment outcomes in Karakalpakstan, Uzbekistan: Treatment complexity and XDR-TB among treatment failures. *PLoS One, 2*(11), e1126.

Cozzarelli, N.R. (1980). DNA gyrase and the supercoiling of DNA. *Science, 207*, 953–960.

D:A:D Study Group. (2008). Use of nucleoside reverse transcriptase inhibitors and risk of myocardial infarction in HIV-infected patients enrolled in the D:A:D study: A multi-cohort collaboration. *Lancet, 371*(9622), 1417–1426.

Depont, F., Vargas, F., Dutronc, H., Giauque, E., Ragnaud, J.M., Galperine, T., . . . Moore, N. (2007). Drug-drug interactions with systemic antifungals in clinical practice. *Pharmacoepidemiology and Drug Safety, 16*(11), 1227–1233.

Doi, Y. & Chambers, H.F. (2015). Penicillins and β-lactamase inhibitors. In J.E. Bennett, R. Dolin, and M. J. Blaser (Eds.). *Mandell, Douglas, and Bennett's Principles and Practice of Infectious Diseases*, 8th ed., 263–277. Elsevier Saunders: Philadelphia.

Drawz, S.M., & Bonomo, R.A. (2010). Three decades of β-lactamase inhibitors. *Clinical Microbiology Reviews, 23*(1), 180–201.

Dunn, L.A., Andrews, K.T., McCarthy, J.S., Wright, J.M., Skinner-Adams, T.S., Upcroft, P., & Upcroft, J.A. (2007). The activity of protease inhibitors against *Giardia duodenalis* and metronidazole-resistant *Trichomonas vaginalis*. *International Journal of Antimicrobial Agents, 29*(1), 98–102.

Eriksson, K., Larsson, P.G., Nilsson, M., & Forsum, U. (2011). Vaginal retention of locally administered clindamycin. *APMIS, 119*(6), 373–376.

Feng, Y., & Zhao, L. (2011). Zoonotic potential and molecular epidemiology of *Giardia* species and giardiasis. *Clinical Microbiology Reviews, 24*(1), 110–140.

Fiekers, J.F. (1999). Sites and mechanisms of antibiotic-induced neuromuscular block: A pharmacological analysis using quantal content, voltage clamped end-plate currents and single channel analysis. *Acta Physiologica, Pharmacologica, et Therapeutica Latinoamericana, 49*(4), 242–250.

Food and Drug Administration (FDA). (2011). FDA drug safety communication: Serious CNS reactions possible when linezolid (Zyvox) is given to patients taking certain psychiatric medications. Retrieved from http://www.fda.gov/drugs/drugsafety/ucm265305.htm

Gonzalez, M.E. (2018). Stevens-Johnson syndrome (SJS) and toxic epidermal necrolysis (TEN). *Merck Manual Professional Version.* Retrieved from https://www.merckmanuals.com/professional/dermatologic-disorders/hypersensitivity-and-inflammatory-skin-disorders/stevens-johnson-syndrome-sjs-and-toxic-epidermal-necrolysis-ten.

Hawkey, P.M. (2012). Carbapenem antibiotics for serious infections. *British Medical Journal, 344,* e3236.

Hempel, S., Newberry, S.J., Maher, A.R., Wang, Z., Miles, J.N., Shanman, R., . . . Shekelle, P. G. (2012). Probiotics for the prevention and treatment of antibiotic-associated diarrhea. *Journal of the American Medical Association, 307*(18), 1959–1969.

Herbert-Ashton, M., & Clarkson, N. (2008). *Quick look nursing: Pharmacology* (2nd ed.). Sudbury, MA: Jones and Bartlett.

Hickson, M. (2011). Probiotics in the prevention of antibiotic-associated diarrhoea and *Clostridium difficile* infection. *Therapeutic Advances in Gastroenterology, 4*(3), 185–197.

Karch, A. (2008). *Focus on nursing pharmacology.* Philadelphia, PA: Lippincott Williams & Wilkins.

Karumbi, J. & Garner, P. (2015). Directly observed therapy for treating tuberculosis. *Cochrane Database of Systematic Reviews, 5,* CD003343. doi: 10.1002/14651858.CD003343.pub4

Kim, G.K. (2010). The risk of fluoroquinolone-induced tendinopathy and tendon rupture: What does the clinician need to know? *Journal of Clinical and Aesthetic Dermatology, 3*(4), 49–54.

Klein, C.E., Chiu, Y.L., Cai, Y., Beck, K., King, K.R., Causemaker, S.J., . . . Hanna, G.J. (2008). Effects of acid-reducing agents on the pharmacokinetics of lopinavir/ritonavir and ritonavir-boosted atazanavir. *Journal of Clinical Pharmacology, 48*(5), 553–562.

Lass-Flörl, C. (2011). Triazole antifungal agents in invasive fungal infections: A comparative review. *Drugs, 71*(18), 2405–2419.

Lehne, R.A. (2012). *Pharmacology for nursing care.* Philadelphia, PA: Elsevier Health Sciences.

Loubatières-Mariani, M.M. (2007). The discovery of hypoglycemic sulfonamides. *Journal de la Société de Biologie, 201*(2), 121–125.

MacDougall, C. & Chambers, H.F. (2011a). Protein synthesis inhibitors and miscellaneous antibacterial agents. In L. Brunton, B. Chabner, & B. Knollman (Eds.). *Goodman & Gilman's The Pharmacological Basis of Therapeutics,* 12th ed. (1521-48). McGraw-Hill: New York.

MacDougall, C. & Chambers, H.F. (2011b). Aminoglycosides. In L. Brunton, B. Chabner, & B. Knollman (Eds.). *Goodman & Gilman's The Pharmacological Basis of Therapeutics,* 12th ed. (1505–20). McGraw-Hill: New York.

Mahesh, C.B., Ramakant, B.K., & Jagadeesh, V.S. (2013). The prevalence of inducible and constitutive clindamycin resistance among the nasal isolates of staphylococci. *Journal of Clinical and Diagnostic Research, 7*(8), 1620–1622.

Moore, D.E. (2002). Drug-induced cutaneous photosensitivity: Incidence, mechanism, prevention and management. *Drug Safety, 25*(5), 345–372.

Morar, M., Bhullar, K., Hughes, D.W., Junop, M., & Wright, G.D. (2009). Structure and mechanism of the lincosamide antibiotic adenyltransferase LinB. *Structure, 17*(12), 1649–1659.

National Institute of Allergy and Infectious Diseases (NIAID). (2011). Antimicrobial (drug) resistance: Causes. Retrieved from http://www.niaid.nih.gov/topics/antimicrobialresistance/understanding/pages/causes.aspx

National Institutes of Health (NIH)/AIDSInfo. (2013). Guidelines for the use of antiretroviral agents in HIV-1-infected adults and adolescents: Limitations to treatment safety and efficacy. Retrieved from http://aidsinfo.nih.gov/guidelines/html/1/adult-and-adolescent-arv-guidelines/31/adverse-effects-of-arv

Nunn, P. (2012). "Totally drug-resistant" tuberculosis: A WHO consultation on the diagnostic definition and treatment options. 4th Global Laboratory Initiative Partners' Meeting, Les Pensières, France. April 17–19, 2012. World Health Organization. Retrieved from: http://www.stoptb.org/wg/gli/assets/html/day%201/Nunn%20-%20Totally%20Drug-Resistant.pdf

Papp-Wallace, K.M., Endimiani, A., Taracila, M.A., & Bonomo, R.A. (2011). Carbapenems: Past, present, and future. *Antimicrobial Agents and Chemotherapy, 55*(11), 4943–4960.

Putignani, L., & Menichella, D. (2010). Global distribution, public health and clinical impact of the protozoan pathogen *Cryptosporidium. Interdisciplinary Perspectives on Infectious Diseases,* 753512. http://dx.doi.org/10.1155/2010/753512

Rogers, K. (2009). Aminoglycosides. In Encyclopedia Britannica. Chicago, IL: Encyclopedia Britannica.

Romano, A., Mondino, C., Viola, M., & Montushi, P. (2003). Immediate allergic reaction to β-lactams: diagnosis and therapy. *International Journal of Immunopathology Pharmacology, 16,* 19–23.

Rougier, F., Claude, D., Maurin, M., Sedoglavic, A., Ducher, M., Corvaisier, S., Jelliffe, R., & Maire, P. (2003). Aminoglycoside nephrotoxicity: Modeling, simulation, and control. *Antimicrobial Agents and Chemotherapy, 47,* 1010–1016. doi: 10.1128/AAC.47.3.1010-1016.2003

Sendzik, J., Shakibaei, M., Schäfer-Korting, M., & Stahlmann, R. (2005). Fluoroquinolones cause changes in extracellular matrix, signalling proteins, metalloproteinases and caspase-3 in cultured human tendon cells. *Toxicology, 212*(1), 24–36.

Spigaglia, P., Barbanti, F., Dionisi, A.M., & Mastrantonio, P. (2010). *Clostridium difficile* isolates resistant to fluoroquinolones in Italy: Emergence of PCR ribotype 018. *Journal of Clinical Microbiology, 48*(8), 2892–2896.

Strahilevitz, J., & Hooper, D.C. (2005). Dual targeting of topoisomerase IV and gyrase to reduce mutant selection: Direct testing of the paradigm by using WCK-1734, a new fluoroquinolone, and ciprofloxacin. *Antimicrobial Agents and Chemotherapy, 49*(5), 1949–1956. http://doi.org/10.1128/AAC.49.5.1949-1956.2005

Tabarsi, P., Chitsaz, E., Tabatabaei, V., Baghaei, P., Shamaei, M., Farnia, P., . . . Velayati, A.A. (2011). Revised Category II regimen as an alternative strategy for retreatment of Category I regimen failure and irregular treatment cases. *American Journal of Therapy, 18*(5), 343–349. doi: 10.1097/MJT.0b013e3181dd60ec

Takahashi, H.L., Hayakawa, I., & Akimoto, T. (2003). The history of the development and changes of quinolone antibacterial agents. *Yakushigaku Zasshi, 38*(2), 161–179.

Tan, A., Holmes, H. M., Kuo, Y.-F., Raji, M. A., & Goodwin, J. S. (2015). Coadministration of co-trimoxazole with sulfonylureas: Hypoglycemia events and pattern of use. *The Journals of Gerontology Series A: Biological Sciences and Medical Sciences, 70*(2), 247–254. http://doi.org/10.1093/gerona/glu072

Tanne, J.H. (2008). FDA adds "black box" warning label to fluoroquinolone antibiotics. *British Medical Journal, 337*(7662), 135. http://doi.org/10.1136/bmj.a816

Tedesco, F.J. (1977). Clindamycin and colitis: A review. *Journal of Infectious Disease, 135*(Suppl.), S95–S98.

Thong, B.Y.-H. (2010). Update on the management of antibiotic allergy. *Allergy, Asthma, and Immunology Research, 2*(2), 77–86.

Tortajada Girbés, M., Ferrer Franco, A., Gracia Antequera, M., Clement Paredes, A., García Muñoz, E., & Tallón Guerola, M. (2008). Hypersensitivity to clavulanic acid in children. *Allergologia et Immunopathologia (Madrid), 36*(5), 308–310.

Vandeputte, P., Ferrari, S., & Coste, A. T. (2012). Antifungal resistance and new strategies to control fungal infections. *International Journal of Microbiology,* 713687. doi: 10.1155/2012/713687. Epub December 1, 2011.

Vermes, A., Guchelaar, H.J., & Dankert, J. (2000). Flucytosine: A review of its pharmacology, clinical indications, pharmacokinetics, toxicity and drug interactions. *Journal of Antimicrobial Chemotherapy, 46*(2), 171–179.

Wang, X., Mu, H., Chai, H., Liao, D., Yao, Q., & Chen, C. (2007). Human immunodeficiency virus protease inhibitor ritonavir inhibits cholesterol efflux from human macrophage-derived foam cells. *American Journal of Pathology, 171,* 304–314.

World Health Organization (WHO). (2017). Guidelines for treatment of drug-susceptible tuberculosis and patient care, 2017 update. Geneva, Switzerland: Author.

Youngster, I., & Barnett, E.D. (2013). Traveler's health: Interactions among travel vaccines and drugs. *CDC Yellow Book 2018* (Ch. 2). Retrieved from http://wwwnc.cdc.gov/travel/yellowbook/2014/chapter-2-the-pre-travel-consultation/interactions-among-travel-vaccines-and-drugs

Zdanowicz, M.M. (2006). The pharmacology of HIV drug resistance. *American Journal of Pharmaceutical Education, 70*(5), 100–115.

Zonios, D.I., & Bennett, J.E. (2008). Update on azole antifungals. *Seminars in Respiratory and Critical Care Medicine, 29*(2), 198–210.

Glossary

5-HT₃ receptor antagonists: Drugs that are selective for the seronin 5-HT$_3$ receptor; used to prevent and treat nausea and vomiting.

5-HT₄ receptor: One of the receptors for serotonin, which is targeted by gastrointestinal drugs.

Absorption: The pharmacokinetic process of drug movement across a physiological barrier at the site of drug administration to enter the systemic circulation (bloodstream); the rate (how fast) of absorption is dependent upon the complexity of the physiological barrier.

ACE inhibitors: Drugs that prevent angiotensin-converting enzyme (ACE) from acting on angiotensin I to produce angiotensin II.

Acetylcholine: A neurotransmitter that stimulates receptors in the ganglia, somatic neuromuscular junction, and neuroeffector junction.

Acetylcholinesterase: A carboxylesterase enzyme that inactivates the neurotransmitter acetylcholine in neurons and in the neuromuscular junction by hydrolysis into choline and acetate.

Acid reflux disease: Disease caused by overproduction of gastric acid.

Acne: One of the most common skin conditions affecting children and adolescents; caused by sebaceous gland hyperplasia triggered by increased androgen levels, changes in the growth and differentiation of cells lining the hair follicles, bacterial invasion of the follicle by *Propionibacterium acnes*, and subsequent inflammation of the follicle epithelium.

Active ingredient: A component that affects the structure or function of the human body through pharmacological activity.

Active metabolite: A structurally changed drug that can elicit the same therapeutic response as the parent drug and retain its pharmacological activity.

Acute dystonia: A syndrome of abnormal muscle contractions that produces repetitive involuntary twisting movements and abnormal posturing of the neck, trunk, face, and extremities.

Acute otitis media (AOM): A type of ear infection that is usually painful and can have other symptoms such as redness of the tympanic membrane, pus in the ear, fever, pulling or tugging on the affected ear (in children), and irritability.

ADME: An acronym for the pharmacokinetic processes that characterize the rate of drug movement throughout the body: A, absorption; D, distribution; M, metabolism; and E, elimination.

Adrenal cortex: The outer part of the adrenal gland, which releases corticosteroids.

Adrenal glands: Glands that sit atop each kidney; made up of the adrenal cortex and the adrenal medulla. It releases corticosteroids (which help regulate metabolism, immune function, sexual function, and the balance of sodium and water) and catecholamines (which increase heart rate and blood pressure in response to physical and emotional cues).

Adrenal medulla: The region of the brain where the catecholamine norepinephrine is converted to a different catecholamine, epinephrine, by phenylethanolamine *N*-methyl transferase.

Adrenergic agonists: Drugs that stimulate the sympathetic nervous system, either by direct activation of receptors or by promoting the release of receptor-activating catecholamines.

Adrenergic antagonists: Drugs that blocks the activity of acetylcholine, norepinephrine, or other neurotransmitters.

Adrenergic nerves: Neuronal tissue in the sympathetic nervous system that secretes norepinephrine or epinephrine when stimulated.

Adrenergic receptors: Sensory nerve endings in the sympathetic nervous system that respond to norepinephrine and/or epinephrine. Categorized as alpha and beta receptors (with subtypes) according to the tissue in which they are located and the physiological effects that they exert on the body.

Adverse effect: An unintended drug effect that causes harm to the functioning of a body system (also called adverse event).

Adverse event: An unintended drug effect that causes harm to the functioning of a body system.

Afferent: Carrying sensory information.

Affinity: The strength, or tightness, of the "chemical binding attraction" between two molecules that bond to form a complex; the degree of the chemical attraction corresponds to the strength of the bond and the length of time the molecules remain bound before dissociating. For example, a drug- (or ligand-) receptor complex, or a drug–protein complex; measured in terms of the binding constant, k_A.

Affinity constant: The strength of the binding constant (k_A).

Agonist: A drug that binds to a biological receptor and initiates the same physiological response produced by the natural substance for that receptor (i.e., a neurotransmitter or hormone).

Agranulocytosis: A reduced white blood count and leukocyte count that can be caused by psychiatric medications.

Akathisia: Unpleasant sensations of "inner" restlessness that manifest as an inability to sit still or remain motionless.

Albumin: The most abundant protein in plasma, formed principally in the liver and constituting up to two-thirds of the 6% to 8% protein concentration in the plasma, and is integral for the transport of drugs to tissues.

Aldosterone: A steroid hormone produced by the adrenal glands.

Aldosterone antagonists: Medications that inhibit sodium resorption through the renal nephron collecting ducts.

Allergen: A substance that triggers a response by the body's immune system.

Alveoli: Air sacs in the lungs.

Alzheimer disease: A neurodegenerative disorder that is the most common form of dementia.

Amide: A class of local anesthetic, which includes lidocaine.

Aminosalicylates: Drugs containing 5-aminosalicylic acid (5-ASA or mesalamine).

Analgesics: Medications that provide pain relief.

Androgens: A class of gonadal steroids.

Anesthetic adjunct: Anesthesia used to limit the patient's pain and enhance the sedating effects of a maintenance anesthetic.

Anesthetics: Drugs that obstruct nerve impulses to prevent the transmission of pain signals; medications intended to reduce or eliminate sensation.

Angina pectoris: Chronic chest pain; generally a product of coronary artery disease that restricts blood flow to the heart.

Angiotensin I: An amino acid peptide hormone that causes vasoconstriction and an increase in blood pressure.

Angiotensin II: The product created by the conversion of angiotensin I by angiotensin-converting enzyme; it causes potent vasoconstriction and the release of aldosterone.

Angiotensin II receptor blockers: Drugs that block the receptors where angiotensin II binds to cells.

Angiotensin-converting enzyme (ACE): The enzyme that converts angiotensin I to angiotensin II.

Angle-closure glaucoma: A medical emergency, in which the fluid at the front of the eye, in the anterior chamber, cannot drain through the angle where the cornea and iris meet, and the angle gets blocked off by part of the iris, causing a sudden increase in eye pressure.

Antacids: The oldest drugs used to control gastric acidity.

Antagonist: A drug that binds to a biological receptor and blocks, or inhibits, the same physiological response produced by the natural substance for that receptor (i.e., a neurotransmitter or hormone).

Anterior chamber: A space in front of the eye from which clear fluid flows in and out to nourish the nearby tissues.

Anthelmintic: A drug that treats an infection by worms.

Antibacterial: A drug used to treat bacterial infection.

Antibiotic: A drug that targets any organism in the body, including symbiotic (nonpathogenic) microbes as well as micro- and macro-organismal pathogens.

Anticholinergics: Drugs that relieve painful cramping spasms by binding to muscarinic receptors in the gastrointestinal mucosa, and that inhibit intestinal gland secretion, thereby helping prevent severe diarrhea. Drugs that block muscarinic cholinergic receptors, thereby causing bronchodilation.

Antidiuretic hormone (ADH): Also called vasopressin, a hormone released by the pituitary gland that induces increased water resorption by the kidneys.

Antiemetic agents: Drugs that prevent and treat nausea and vomiting.

Antifungal: A drug used to treat fungal infection.

Antihistamines: Drugs that target receptors for histamine.

Antihypertensive: Having the effect of lowering blood pressure.

Anti-infective: A drug that treats an infection by an organism.

Antimicrobial: A drug that treats an infection by a microbial pathogen.

Antispasmodics: Centrally acting muscle relaxants used to relieve musculoskeletal pain and spasms, and to diminish spasticity in a variety of neurologic disorders; also called spasmolytics.

Antipsychotics: Medications that were developed to treat the symptoms of schizophrenia, psychosis, delusional disorders, bipolar disorder, and depression as well as other nonpsychiatric disorders.

Antiviral: A drug used to treat viral infection.

Anxiety: A normal reaction to stress that in some situations can be beneficial.

Area under the curve (AUC): A measurement of the total amount of drug that reaches the systemic circulation, derived from the plasma-level time curve; used to determine the extent of absorption of a drug (bioavailability).

Arrhythmias: Rhythmic disturbances of the heart's electrical impulses.

Assessment: Collecting subjective and objective data from the patient, significant others, medical records (including laboratory and diagnostic tests), and others involved in the patient's care.

Asthma: An immune system dysfunction that manifests in the respiratory system.

Ataxia: Unsteadiness when walking.

Atherosclerosis: The buildup of cholesterol and other fatty materials in the wall of a coronary artery.

Atony: Failure of muscles to contract.

Atopic dermatitis: A common inflammatory skin disorder that is characterized by a pruritic, scaling rash that flares and subsides at intervals.

Atopy: Type I hypersensitivity.

Atrophy: Thinning or depression of the skin often associated with application of a topical or injected steroid.

Atypical antipsychotics: Second-generation antipsychotic medications.

Auditory hallucinations: A psychotic symptom that causes sounds or voices to be heard. It can occur in schizophrenia or manic episodes.

Autonomic nervous system (ANS): A division of the peripheral nervous system that regulates involuntary or visceral bodily processes, particularly cardiac, smooth muscle, and glandular function. Subdivided into the sympathetic and parasympathetic nervous systems.

Axons: Part of a neuron.

β_2-receptor agonists: Long- and short-acting drugs that target beta receptors; used in treating respiratory diseases.

Bactericidal: An antimicrobial agent that kills the target bacterium.

Bacteriostatic: An antimicrobial agent that inhibits the target bacterium's reproduction or health, suppressing or weakening it sufficiently to allow the patient's immune system to complete the recovery process.

Bacterium: Singular form of *bacteria*, which are prokaryotic single-celled microorganisms, normally classified in the kingdom Monera that can be grouped as Gram-negative (possessing an outer membrane), Gram-positive (no outer membrane), or ungrouped.

Barbiturate: A class of CNS depressant medications that produce sleepiness and relaxation.

Benign prostate hyperplasia (BPH): A condition in which the enlarged prostate presses against the urethral canal and interferes with normal urination.

Benzodiazepines: A class of drugs that act primarily on the central nervous system and are often the first-line treatment for anxiety. They enhance the inhibitory effects of gamma-aminobutyric acid (GABA) and bind to benzodiazepine receptors at the GABA-a ligand-gated chloride-channel complex.

Beta blockers: Drugs that block the beta adrenoceptors in the heart so norepinephrine and epinephrine cannot bind to them.

Beta-receptors: Receptors located on the heart, bound by norepinephrine and epinephrine. When stimulated, the resultant effects lead to increased heart rate and myocontractility.

Beta-lactamase: An enzyme that breaks down the molecular integrity of beta-lactam antibiotics, thereby preventing them from entering the cell and destroying it.

Beta-mimetic drugs: Drugs that inhibit uterine activity by binding with beta-adrenergic receptors in the uterus.

Biguanides: A group of diabetes drugs that prevent the production of glucose in the liver.

Bioavailability: The total amount (the extent) of drug that reaches the systemic circulation; expressed as a fraction of an administered dose of unchanged drug that reaches the systemic circulation.

Biopharmaceutics: The study of (1) the physiochemical properties of a drug molecule that determine how the drug is formulated into its "dosage form" (e.g., capsule, tablet, solution, transdermal patch); (2) the ability of the drug dosage form(s) to deliver the chemically active form of the drug in a sufficient amount (dose); (3) the ability of the dosage form to withstand physiological conditions inside the patient's body; and (4) how the rate of active drug release from the dosage form is controlled (i.e., neither too slowly nor too quickly).

Biotransformation: Chemical modification (direct chemical change) of the drug structure, often by enzymatic processes in the body.

Bipolar disorder: A psychiatric disorder characterized by mood swings between depression and mania.

Blockers: Another name for antagonists.

Blood pressure: The measure of the amount of force that blood exerts upon blood vessel walls as it flows throughout the body.

Blood–retinal barrier: The barrier that separates the blood from the retina of the eye, through which medications must pass before entering the eye.

Bradykinesia: Slow movement and muscle rigidity.

Bradykinin: A substance that causes vasodilation in the cardiovascular system.

Brain stem: The midbrain and hindbrain.

Brand name: The drug name selected by the company requesting initial FDA approval for the drug; this identifies it as the exclusive property of that company.

Broad-spectrum: Effective against many strains of microorganisms.

Bronchioles: Small branches of the airway found in the lungs.

Bronchoconstriction: Constriction of the airway.

Buccal: Between the cheek and gum.

Butyrophenones: Dopamine-receptor antagonists traditionally used for antiemetic therapy.

Calcitonin: A hormone produced by the thyroid that inhibits bone resorption.

Calcium-channel blockers: A class of antihypertensive medications that act on the heart by blocking calcium channels, which helps lower cardiac output by both reducing the force of contraction and decreasing the frequency of contractions.

Cannabinoids: Drugs based on the psychoactive ingredient in marijuana; sometimes used as antiemetic agents.

Carbonic anhydrase inhibitor: A drug that prevents the production of the carbonic anhydrase enzyme. When carbonic anhydrase is inhibited, the formation of bicarbonate ions is slowed, with subsequent reduction in sodium and fluid transport.

Cardiac output (CO): The amount of blood the heart is able to pump in one minute.

Cardioselective: Exerting more effect on the heart than on other tissue.

Catecholamine: A compound, such as norepinephrine, epinephrine, and dopamine, whose underlying chemical structure is characterized by the presence of a catechol moiety. Also produced by the body and exerts important physiological effects in regulating the body's response to stress.

Central compartment: The circulatory system; the bloodstream.

Central nervous system (CNS): The brain and the spinal cord.

Central nervous system (CNS) stimulation: Activating effects produced by antipsychotic medications.

Cerebellum: Part of the hindbrain.

Cerebrum: Part of the forebrain.

Cerumen: Ear wax.

Chemical name: The description of the chemical composition and molecular structure of a compound.

Chemoreceptor trigger zone (CTZ): A subcortical center in the medulla that antiemetic drugs typically affect.

Chloride-channel activators: Drugs that activate the type 2 volume-regulated chloride channels found in gastric parietal cells and in small intestinal and colonic epithelia. Intestinal chloride secretion is critical for intestinal fluid and electrolyte transport.

Cholelithiasis: Obstruction by gallstone formation.

Cholesterol: A sterol form of lipid.

Cholinergic agonists: Medications or chemicals that interact with acetylcholine receptors to produce nicotinic or muscarinic responses at autonomic or neuromuscular synapses.

Cholinergic antagonists: A drug that acts against muscarinic acetylcholine receptors, where it caps and blocks the actions of acetylcholine.

Cholinergic mimetic agents: Drugs that are used for stimulating gastrointestinal motility, accelerating gastric emptying, and improving gastroduodenal coordination. They work by increasing the availability of the neurotransmitter acetylcholine.

Cholinergic nerves: Neuronal tissue that releases acetylcholine at the synapse. Includes preganglionic sympathetic and parasympathetic nerves, as well as somatic motor nerves and postganglionic sympathetic nerves.

Chronic bronchitis: A form of chronic obstructive pulmonary disease in which inflammation of the bronchi and mucus-producing glands leads to excessive mucus secretion, which in later stages of COPD can contribute to obstruction.

Chronic obstructive pulmonary disease (COPD): A disease in which patients struggle to breathe. It has an immunological component but is also characterized by the progressive breakdown of the mechanical processes of breathing due to damage to the bronchioles and alveoli in the lungs.

Ciliary muscle: A circular band of fibers located in the ciliary body and used for accommodation when it contracts by relaxing the suspensory ligament of the lens so that the lens becomes more convex.

Clearance: The fixed volume of fluid (containing the drug) cleared of drug per unit of time.

Clinical pharmacology: The application of the concepts and principles of pharmacology to properly evaluate patients, design individualized dosage regimens to achieve therapeutic drug levels, and ensure optimal clinical outcomes.

Cognitive symptoms: Symptoms of schizophrenia that include difficulties with the ability to pay attention and to focus, as well as the presence of significant learning and memory problems and disordered thinking.

Combination therapy: Use of multiple drugs concomitantly (e.g., use of more than one antibiotic to eradicate a superinfection).

Comedogenic: The description of a substance that clogs pores or fosters the formation of precursor acne lesions.

Comorbid: Co-occurring.

Compartmental model theory: A mathematical pharmacokinetic model used to describe the pattern of drug movement throughout the body; models describe the distribution of the drug into various "compartments," or groups of tissues with similar blood flow and drug affinity.

Competitive antagonist: An antagonist that binds to the same site as the agonist for that receptor, preventing the agonist or the receptor's ligand from binding to the receptor site.

Complicated UTI: A urinary infection occurring in a patient with a structural or functional abnormality of the genitourinary tract.

Conduction blockade: The means by which most local anesthetics work—that is, by interfering with nerve signaling, thereby reducing permeability of voltage-gated sodium channels. When sodium cannot pass through these channels, the ability of the channels to conduct signals is reduced, effectively interrupting the transmission of the nerve's "message" of pain to the brain.

Congestive heart failure (CHF): A progressive disease in which the heart is unable to pump with sufficient force to push blood through the blood vessels.

Conjunctivitis: An ocular infection in which the eye appears bright red, swollen, and painful.

Contraception: Prevention of pregnancy.

Controlled substances: Substances with a potential for abuse—specifically, narcotics, hallucinogens, stimulants, depressants, and anabolic steroids; they are categorized by schedule (Schedules I–V), based on their therapeutic use and potential for abuse.

Cornea: The transparent part of the coat of the eyeball that covers the iris and pupil and lets light into the interior.

Coronary artery disease: A condition that occurs when blood flow to the heart is restricted, or completely blocked, depriving cardiac muscle of oxygen.

Corpus cavernosum: A channel in the shaft of the penis.

Corticosteroids: Drugs that have glucocorticoid-receptor agonist action, resulting in several anti-inflammatory effects. They affect eicosanoid metabolism, inflammation, and edema.

Cortisol: A steroid hormone produced by the adrenal glands and released in response to stress.

Covalent bonds:

COX-2 inhibitors: Nonsteroidal anti-inflammatory drugs.

Craniosacral system: Another term for the parasympathetic nervous system, due to the origin of the nerve fibers in the cranial and sacral spinal nerves.

Cream: A dermatologic vehicle; a semi-solid emulsion of oil in water (soluble in water) or water in oil (not water soluble).

Culture: The intentional in-vitro cultivation of a tissue (e.g., blood, serum, urine, cells) sample, with the aim of detecting the presence of microbial infection.

Cyclic adenosine monophosphate (cAMP): A substance found in cell membranes. Decreased cAMP permits degranulation of the membrane, releasing primary and secondary mediators as part of the immune response.

Cyclooxygenase (COX): The enzymes that produce prostaglandins.

Cysteinyl leukotriene type-1 (CysLT-1) receptors: The binding targets for cysteinyl-leukotrienes; they are found in smooth muscle cells, airway macrophages, and eosinophils.

Cystitis: Uncomplicated lower urinary tract infection.

Cytochrome P450 3A4 (CYP3A4): An enzyme, primarily located in the liver and intestine, responsible for metabolizing substances in the body, aiding their removal.

Cytotoxic: Targeting fast-growing cells.

Deep vein thrombosis (DVT): The formation of blood clots in the deep veins of the legs, due to plaque buildup in the arteries.

Delusional disorder: Unreal, often unfounded thoughts that can include paranoia, grandiose, sexual, or somatic beliefs that are not found to be based in reality.

Delusions: False beliefs about one's self or other people or objects that persist despite the facts, occurring in some psychotic states.

Dendrites: Part of a neuron.

Dependence: The physical and behavioral need to continue a substance due to addiction and tolerance. Discontinuing the substance could cause physiological symptoms of withdrawal.

Depolarizing: A subclass of neuromuscular blocking drugs, which blocks the function of acetylcholine receptors on skeletal muscle via depolarizing the plasma membrane of the skeletal muscle fiber.

Depot preparations: Preparations of medications that are absorbed slowly over an extended period of time.

Depression: A common mental disorder that presents with a depressed mood, loss of interest in daily activities, lack of pleasure, feelings of guilt or low self-worth, disturbed sleep or appetite, low energy and poor concentration, and possibly, suicidal thoughts.

Dermatopharmacology: Pharmacology as it applies to dermatologic conditions.

Dermatophytosis: A fungal infection involving the hair, skin, and nails that may be treated systemically.

Diabetes mellitus: A disorder of glucose metabolism.

Diaphoresis: Excessive sweating.

Diastolic: Related to the force exerted while the heart muscle is relaxed between beats.

Dihydropterate synthetase: An enzyme that plays a role in the process by which bacteria synthesize their own folic acid using pteridine and para-aminobenzoic acid as building blocks for dihydropteroic acid, a precursor to folic acid.

Direct-acting: The ability to simulate a receptor without the need of intermediary compounds or processes.

Direct renin inhibitors: Drugs that reduce the availability of renin, thereby limiting the amount of angiotensin I available for conversion to angiotensin II.

Distorted thinking: Inaccurate thoughts, often including negative thinking, that result in a poor self-image.

Distribution: The pharmacokinetic process of drug movement out of the systemic circulation to the site of drug action, tissue compartments, and other peripheral sites; the chemical composition of the drug molecule governs its ability to diffuse out of the bloodstream and into tissues, organs, or other areas outside of the bloodstream.

Diuresis: The process of excess fluid excreted as urine.

Diuretics: Drugs that cause the kidneys to remove greater amounts of salt and water from circulation, which in turn lowers the fluid volume; also called "water pills."

Dopamine: A neurochemical that plays a key role in Parkinson disease; an endogenous catecholamine derivative.

Dopamine-receptor antagonists: A class of antiemetic agents that works by blocking dopamine receptors via receptor antagonism.

Dose: Amount of drug that is administered to a patient.

Dose-response curve: A dose-response curve is a graphical method used to characterize the relationship between the dose of a drug and the amount of drug required to produce the maximum physiological (therapeutic) effect; often used to compare the effectiveness of two drugs, or characterize the degree of drug responses.

Dosing interval: The amount of time between doses of medication; the time span separating when the second dose is given in relation to the first.

Drug: A substance or chemical capable of altering a biochemical or physiological process(es) in the body.

Drug action: An alteration in a physiological or biochemical process that takes place because of the drug's interaction with a specific site within the body.

Drug activity profile: A graphical representation of the concentration of drug in the body over a given period of time.

Drug classifications: Categorization of drugs based upon their mechanism of drug action; drugs can be classified based on how they affect certain body systems, such as *bronchodilators*; by their therapeutic use, such as *antinausea*; or based on their chemical characteristics, such as *beta blockers*.

Drug name: The trade name of a drug, which is assigned by the pharmaceutical company that manufactures the drug, and the generic name, which is the official name and is not protected by trademark.

Drug resistance: Alteration of an organism's genetic structure, following repeated exposures to a drug, that enables the organism to withstand the effects of that drug; an adaptive mechanism when organisms encounter adverse conditions.

Dry-powder inhaler (DPI): A device used to deliver an inhaled medication to the lungs in the form of a dry powder.

Dual innervation: In the autonomic nervous system, refers to the presence of both sympathetic and parasympathetic receptors in body organs or tissue.

Duration of action: The length of time a drug exhibits a therapeutic effect after the drug is administered.

Dyspepsia: Upset stomach; indigestion.

Dyspnea: Shortness of breath.

Dyssomnias: Sleep disorders characterized by a disturbance in the amount or quality of sleep.

Early response: In the immune system, a reaction that occurs within minutes to hours after exposure to an allergen.

Eclampsia: Seizures during pregnancy.

Eczema: A skin condition characterized by a pruritic, scaling rash that flares and subsides at intervals (see atopic dermatitis).

Effector organs: Organs that respond to stimulation of the nerve receptors that they contain.

Efferent: Carrying motor information.

Efficacy: How well a drug works.

Elimination: Removal of a drug from the body.

Elimination rate constant: The first-order rate constant that characterizes the rate (how fast) of drug elimination of from the body.

Emesis: Vomiting.

Emollient: A substance that soothes the skin.

Emphysema: A form of chronic obstructive pulmonary disease in which the alveoli walls are damaged so that the alveoli lose their shape and elasticity, which makes it both more difficult for the sacs to fill with air and more difficult for gas exchange to occur over the damaged areas.

Endocrine system: A complex body system composed of hormone-secreting glands including the hypothalamus, anterior and posterior pituitary, pineal body, thyroid, parathyroid, thymus, adrenals, pancreas, and reproductive glands (ovaries or testes).

Endogenous: Refers to substances that are produced naturally within the body or body systems.

Enteral: Introduction of a medication into the body through the gastrointestinal tract.

Enteric nervous system (ENS): Part of the autonomic nervous system that carries out key functions in support of systemic neurologic and immunologic well-being, and is highly responsive to both physical and emotional stimuli.

Enterohepatic circulation: The cycle in which a drug is absorbed, excreted into the bile, and reabsorbed as part of biliary elimination.

Epidural: A route of medication administration via the epidural space surrounding the spinal cord.

Epidural anesthesia: Anesthesia used during labor as well as delivery for management of pain. Under local anesthesia, a catheter is inserted into the epidural space; an opioid drug and a local anesthetic are then injected into the catheter.

Epilepsy: A brain disorder in which clusters of neurons sometimes signal abnormally in the brain.

Epinephrine: A direct-acting adrenergic agonist that stimulates α- and β-adrenergic receptors in the sympathetic nervous system.

Erectile dysfunction: Inability to sustain an erection adequate for sexual satisfaction.

Eructation: Belching.

Ester: A class of local anesthetic; more likely to produce an allergic reaction than amides.

Estrogen: A hormone produced by the reproductive system.

Exogenous: Produced outside of the body.

Extrapyramidal symptoms (EPS): Adverse effects associated with use of first-generation antipsychotic medications; acute dystonia, Parkinsonian symptoms, mask-like facies, shaking palsy, trembling palsy, akathisia, and tardive dyskinesia.

Feedback loop: A means of maintaining homeostasis of the body.

Fetotoxic: Harmful to a fetus.

FEV$_1$: FVC ratio: The ratio of forced expiratory volume in 1 second (how much air a patient can blow into the spirometer tubing in 1 second) to forced vital capacity (the total volume of air expired after a full inspiration).

First-dose effect: Severe hypotension that occurs the first time an alpha-blocker drug is administered.

First-order kinetic drugs: Drugs that have a rate of elimination that is a function of (dependent upon) the amount of drug remaining in the body.

First-pass effect: The metabolism of an orally administered drug into a pharmacologically inactive form before it enters the systemic circulation; extensive first-pass metabolism can result in a loss of up to 80% of the oral dose of the drug; also called presystemic elimination.

Fluid volume: The volume of blood passing through the blood vessels.

Follicle-stimulating hormone (FSH): Gonadotropin hormone released from the anterior pituitary.

Forebrain: Part of the brain containing the thalamus, hypothalamus, and cerebrum; it is responsible for functions such as receiving and processing sensory information, thinking, perceiving, producing and understanding language, and controlling motor function.

Fungus (fungi): Unicellular or multicellular saprophytic and parasitic eukaryotic organisms.

Gallstones: Acute cholecystitis.

Gamma-aminobutyric acid (GABA): One of the principal inhibiting chemicals in the brain; it causes chloride channels for negatively charged ions to open and flood into excited neurons.

Ganglia: Masses of nerve tissue and nerve synapses that form part of the autonomic nervous system.

Gastric reflux: Regurgitation of stomach contents back into esophagus.

Gastritis: The inflammatory reaction of the swollen lining of the stomach.

Gastroesophageal reflux disease (GERD): Chronic acid reflux.

Gastroparesis: Also called delayed stomach emptying. A medical condition that stops or slows the movement of food from the stomach to the small intestine.

Gastroprokinetic drugs: A class of drugs that act by increasing the frequency of contractions in the small intestine without disrupting their rhythm, ultimately resulting in enhanced gastrointestinal motility.

Gel: A dermatologic vehicle; a transparent, semi-solid, non-greasy emulsion of propylene glycol and water.

Generalized anxiety disorder: A disorder of excessive anxiety and worry often including physiological symptoms and depression.

Gestational diabetes: A variant of type 2 diabetes in which insensitivity to insulin signaling develops in response to some of the endocrine changes of pregnancy; glucose intolerance of varying severity first appearing in pregnancy.

Gestational hypertension: Systolic blood pressure equal to or greater than 140 mm Hg and/or diastolic blood pressure equal to or greater than 90 mm Hg on at least two occasions at least 6 hours apart after the 20th week of gestation in a woman who was previously normotensive.

Glands: Hormone-secreting organs.

Glaucoma: A group of diseases that damage the optic nerve because of elevated intraocular pressure, which can result in vision loss and blindness.

Glucagon: A hormone that helps to regulate blood glucose.

Glutamate: A major excitatory mediator in the brain that binds to receptors that open channels for sodium, potassium, and calcium into the cell.

Goals: The expected behaviors or results of drug therapy, usually identified in the form of broad statements for achievement of more specific outcome criteria.

Gonadotropin: Any of the hormones secreted by the pituitary gland that stimulate the female gonads or reproductive organs.

Gonadotropin-releasing hormone (GnRH): A hormone secreted by the hypothalamus.

Gram negative: A descriptor for bacteria that do not take up the Gram stain.

Gram positive: A descriptor for bacteria that take up the Gram stain.

Half-life: The amount of time required to eliminate one-half of the amount of a drug in the body.

Heart rate (HR): The number of times that the heart beats, measured by unit of time, most often number of beats per minute.

Helminth: Worm.

High-density lipoprotein (HDL): "Good" cholesterol; an increase in HDL correlates with a decrease in the risk of coronary heart disease.

Hindbrain: Part of the brain stem that extends from the spinal cord and contains the pons and cerebellum; it assists in maintaining balance and equilibrium, as well as movement coordination and conduction of sensory information.

Histamine: A chemical compound involved in local immune response, physiological function in the gut, and action as a neurotransmitter associated with gastrointestinal function and local immune responses.

Histamine-2 (H$_2$) receptor antagonists: Drugs that decrease gastric acidity by blocking the H$_2$ receptors, thereby decreasing gastric acid production.

Homeostasis: The process of maintaining physiological stability.

Hormone: A chemical substance produced by endocrine glands that regulates certain physiological functions.

Host factors: Factors that play major roles in the effectiveness of an antimicrobial agent. Some of these factors are client age, pregnancy status, genetic characteristics, drug allergy history, site of the infection, state of the patient's immune system, and status of the liver and kidneys.

Human placental growth hormone: A pregnancy-related hormone that causes an increased resistance to insulin.

Human placental lactogen (hPL): A pregnancy-related hormone.

Huntington's chorea: Continuous involuntary, jerky movements of the limbs or facial muscles that can be associated with the long-term use of antipsychotic medications.

Hyperglycemia: Elevated blood glucose level.

Hyperkalemia: An electrolyte imbalance caused by high potassium levels.

Hyperkeratotic: Hypertrophy or excess production of the keratin or horny layer of the skin. This causes a rough, thick, or wart-like texture of the affected skin.

Hyperlipidemia: High cholesterol and/or triglyceride levels.

Hypersensitivity reaction: An inappropriate immune response against innocuous, non-pathogenic antigens involving the humoral and/or cell-mediated branches of the immune system, and which may or may not be exaggerated when compared to reactions to pathogenic antigens.

Hypertension: High blood pressure.

Hypertensive crisis: A life-threatening side effect of MAOIs caused by eating tyramine-containing foods and beverages. High levels of tyramine cause a significant increase in the neurotransmitter norepinephrine in the gut, leading to excessively high blood pressure.

Hypertensive emergency: A condition in which the patient has both severe hypertension and a risk of end-organ damage.

Hypnotics: Drugs that produce sleep, and if used as an anesthetic agent, can induce either sedation or a complete loss of consciousness for purposes of accomplishing procedures.

Hypoglycemia: Lower than normal blood glucose level.

Hyponatremia: Abnormally low sodium level.

Hypothalamic–pituitary–thyroid axis: The body systems that regulate almost every endocrine function in the body.

Hypothalamus: Part of the forebrain.

Immunoglobulin E (IgE): A type of immunoglobulin that mediates the immune response to contact with allergens.

Impaction: A condition of the ear in which cerumen dries and hardens to form a plug in the external ear canal, which is difficult and painful to remove.

Inactive metabolite: A drug's metabolite that is unable to elicit a therapeutic response.

Indirect-acting: The impact of a substance that requires intermediate processes or agents to achieve its effect.

Induction anesthesia: The process of creating a state of unconsciousness or semi-consciousness (sedation) prior to a painful or unpleasant procedure.

Infiltrative anesthesia: Anesthesia delivered via direct injection to the nerves that require blockade.

Inflammatory bowel disease (IBD): Ulcerative colitis and Crohn's disease.

Inhalational anesthetic: An inhaled drug most often used for general or partial anesthesia, used for a patient undergoing surgery or other invasive, stressful, or complex procedure that require the patient to remain still for long stretches of time.

Inhibitors: Another name for antagonists.

Injectable pen: A pen-like device containing a premeasured amount of medication.

Insulin: A hormone secreted by the pancreas that helps to regulate blood glucose.

Insulin resistance: Decreased ability of cells to use insulin due to antagonistic effects of hormones produced in pregnancy.

Integumentary system: The three layers of the skin, the associated glandular structures, plus the mucous membranes, hair, and nails that make up the human body's largest organ system.

Intralesional injection: Direct delivery of medication to the site of a lesion so as to treat a local condition without systemic effects.

Intramuscular (IM): Within the muscle.

Intraocular pressure (IOP): Pressure within the eye.

Intraosseous (IO): Into the marrow cavity of the bone.

Intrathecal: Into the cerebrospinal fluid.

Intravenous (IV): Into the vein.

Intravitreal: Into the eye.

Involuntary movements: Uncontrollable twitches and jerks and movements of the limbs, trunk, or facial muscles associated with use of antipsychotic medications.

Iris: The opaque contractile diaphragm perforated by the pupil and forming the colored portion of the eye.

Iris sphincter: Smooth muscle surrounding the iris.

Iritis: Inflammation of the iris of the eye.

Irreversible receptor antagonists: Chemically reactive compounds in which after covalent binding, the physiological response is completely blocked and cannot be undone.

Irritable bowel syndrome (IBS): A functional gastrointestinal disorder, characterized by unexplained abdominal pain, discomfort, and bloating in association with altered bowel habits.

Keratoconjunctivitis sicca: Chronic dry eye.

Keratolytic: A substance that softens, loosens, or removes rough, horny, hyperkeratotic skin.

Lacrimation: Watering of the eyes.

Lag-time: The time it takes for a drug to enter the bloodstream.

Laryngospasm: A spasm of the vocal cords that can occlude the airway, making ventilation impossible.

Late response: In the immune system, a reaction that occurs hours after exposure to an allergen and requires specialized (emergency department) treatment.

Laxatives: Drugs to control constipation.

Leukotrienes (LT): Inflammatory molecules that are products of phospholipid breakdown via arachidonic acid metabolism, usually from host cells, including mast cells and eosinophils.

Leukotriene receptor blocker: Also called *leukotriene receptor antagonist (LTRA)*; a class of anti-inflammatory drugs that interfere with the leukotriene-mediated inflammatory process by blocking (antagonizing) natural ligand (leukotriene) binding.

Leukotriene synthesis blockers: Anti-inflammatory drugs that inhibit leukotriene formation, especially those inhibiting 5-lipooxygenase, which converts arachidonic acid to prostaglandins.

Ligand: Naturally occurring compounds that are specific to receptor molecules.

Lipids: A class of molecules that include a variety of substances: fatty acids, sterols (including cholesterol), certain fat-soluble vitamins (A, D, E, and K), and glycerides.

Local anesthetic: Medication used to block pain or other sensations in a specific area of the body when complete or partial sedation is not desired or is contraindicated.

Lotion: A dermatologic vehicle; a clear spray, foam, or free-flowing solution.

Low-density lipoprotein (LDL): "Bad" cholesterol; an increase in LDL correlates with an increase in the risk of coronary heart disease.

Low- or normal-tension glaucoma: Glaucoma without any increased intraocular pressure.

Luteinizing hormone (LH): Gonadotropin hormone released from the anterior pituitary.

Magnesium sulfate: A mineral used to stabilize hypokalemia (low potassium levels).

Maintenance anesthesia: The use of anesthetic agents to prolong an unconscious or sedated state for procedures that require a time frame longer than an induction agent usually lasts.

Mania: A mental disorder that presents with the following symptoms: being easily distracted, reduced need for sleep, poor judgment, loss of temper, reckless behavior, poor impulse control, hyperactivity, excessive energy, grandiose thoughts, racing thoughts, excessive talking, and agitation or irritability. Psychotic symptoms, such as auditory and visual hallucinations and delusional thoughts, may also be present.

Margin of safety: The difference between the minimum effective concentration and the minimum toxic concentration.

Maximum tolerable concentration: The highest concentration of a substance (medication) that can be tolerated and not cause death.

Mechanism of action: How and where in the body a drug works, as well as the biological molecule to which the drug binds.

Medication administration error: A mistake related to the dispensing or administration phase of drug distribution.

Medication errors: Mistakes (or preventable events) in medication prescribing, ordering, labeling, distributing, dispensing, administering, or monitoring that may lead to patient harm or the inappropriate use of medication.

Medulla oblongata: The part of the midbrain that is responsible for autonomic functions such as breathing, heart rate, and digestion.

Meglitinides: A type of insulin secretagogue that inhibits adenosine triphosphate-sensitive potassium channels of the beta cell membrane.

Melena: Dark stools that occur with gastrointestinal bleeding.

Mesolimbic: An area of the brain associated with dopamine activity, located in the midbrain.

Metabolic syndrome: The combination of obesity, diabetes, and dyslipidemia.

Metabolism: The pharmacokinetic process of chemically changing the structure and chemical properties of the "parent" (original) drug, by enzymatic processes in the body.

Metabolite: A drug molecule that has undergone a chemical change to its structure; a metabolite may or may not be pharmacologically active.

Metered-dose inhaler (MDI): A device used to deliver a precise dose of an inhaled medication to the lungs.

Microcomedone: Precursor acne lesions.

Midbrain: The part of the brain stem that connects the forebrain and the hindbrain; it is involved in auditory and visual responses as well as motor function.

Middle ear: A small membrane-lined cavity that is separated from the outer ear by the tympanic membrane and that transmits sound waves from the tympanic membrane to the partition between the middle and inner ears through a chain of tiny bones.

Minimum alveolar concentration (MAC): In regard to inhalational anesthesia, the alveolar concentration that prevents patient movement in 50% of patients in response to surgical stimulation.

Minimum effective concentration (MEC): The amount of drug it takes to produce the intended pharmacological response of the drug.

Minimum inhibitory concentration: The lowest concentration of drug at which an organism's growth is inhibited.

Minimum toxic concentration (MTC): The drug dose that no longer produces the intended therapeutic response but produces the first signs of drug toxicity.

Miosis: Constriction of the pupil secondary to the contraction of the iris sphincter.

Mixed obstructive/restrictive airway disease: A complex respiratory disease, such as chronic obstructive pulmonary disease, that has characteristics of both mixed airway disease and restrictive airway disease.

Monoamine oxidase inhibitor (MAOI): Drugs that block the breakdown of monoamine oxidase; used for the treatment of depression and anxiety.

Monoclonal anti-IgE antibody: A recombinant humanized IgG$_k$ monoclonal antibody that binds IgE antibodies, reducing the amount of IgE available to bind to high-affinity IgE receptor (FceRI) on the surface of mast cells and basophils.

Mood stabilizers: A class of medications used to treat bipolar disorder. They stabilize the patient's mood and eliminate mood swings, or make them less frequent and less severe.

Motility: Movement (as through the digestive tract).

Motor tics: Sudden contractions of muscle groups often involving the face or upper arms. They often are associated with a dopamine overload.

Mucosal membranes: Membranes with many mucous glands, especially those that line body passages and cavities that connect directly or indirectly with the exterior that protect, support, and absorb nutrients, and secrete mucus, enzymes, and salts.

Mucosal-protective agents: Drugs that shield the gastric mucosa from harmful effects of gastric acid via a variety of mechanisms.

Muscarinic acetylcholine receptors: The principal cholinergic end-receptors stimulated by acetylcholine in postganglionic parasympathetic nerves.

Muscarinic M$_3$ antagonists: Antimuscarinic anticholinergic agents used to reduce bowel motility and prevent painful cramping spasms in the intestines.

Muscle relaxants: Medications that seek to ease painful and involuntary contraction of injured or overstimulated muscle cells.

Muscle spasm: A sudden involuntary contraction of one or more muscle groups; usually an acute condition associated with muscle strain or sprain.

Myocardial infarction: Heart attack.

Narcotic: Opioid; a type of analgesic derived from the Asian poppy.

Narrow-spectrum: Effective against only a few strains of microorganisms.

Negative chronotrope: A drug that alters impulse conduction in the heart.

Negative symptoms: Symptoms of schizophrenia that include poor insight and judgment, lack of self-care, emotional and social withdrawal, apathy, agitation, blunted affect, and poverty of speech.

Nerve processes: Finger-like projections of neurons that consist of axons and dendrites.

Neuroleptic malignant syndrome: Adverse effects associated with use of first-generation antipsychotic medications; characterized by high fever, stiffness of the muscles, altered mental status (paranoid behavior), wide swings of blood pressure, excessive sweating, and excessive secretion of saliva.

Neuromuscular blockers: Medications that act by preventing neuromuscular transmission at the neuromuscular junction, causing paralysis of the affected skeletal muscles.

Neurons: The basic units of the nervous system.

Neuropathic pain: Chronic pain resulting from nervous system injury, either in the CNS (brain and spinal cord) or PNS (periphery).

Neurotonin-1 receptor antagonists: A new class of antiemetic agents; they act through the inhibition of substance P involved in the emesis reflex both centrally and peripherally.

Neurotransmission: The transmission of nerve signals in the brain caused by the release of brain chemicals dopamine, serotonin, and norepinephrine.

Nicotinic acetylcholine receptors: Acetylcholine-responsive receptors on postsynaptic parasympathetic ganglionic membranes.

N-methyl-D-aspartate (NMDA): A type of receptor found in the brain and spinal column.

Nociceptive: Related to pain.

Noncompetitve antagonist: A drug that binds to a site different from the endogenous ligand's binding site but is still able to block the receptor's "normal" physiological response.

Nondepolarizing: A subclass of neuromuscular blocking drugs, which blocks the function of acetylcholine receptors on skeletal muscle without activating them, causing flaccid paralysis of skeletal muscles.

Nonprogressing labor: Labor that appears to have halted or is progressing only very slowly.

Nonretrovirus: One of the two major types of viruses.

Nonsteroidal anti-inflammatory drugs (NSAIDs): A class of drugs that provides both analgesic and antipyretic effects.

Norepinephrine: A potent vasopressor and cardiac stimulant that acts directly on α- and β-adrenergic receptors of the sympathetic nervous system.

Nosocomial: Hospital acquired.

Nucleoside: One of the building blocks of DNA and RNA.

Nucleoside reverse transcriptase inhibitors: A class of antiviral drugs used to treat HIV infection, AIDS, and sometimes hepatitis B.

Nursing diagnoses: Statements of patient problems, potential problems, or needs.

Nursing process: A systematic, rational, and continuous method of planning, providing, and evaluating individualized nursing care, to include the administration of medications.

Obsessive-compulsive disorder: An anxiety disorder characterized by recurring, intrusive thoughts that lead to repetitive (compulsive) behaviors.

Obstructive airway disease: A respiratory disease, such as asthma and emphysema, in which the major abnormality is decreased airflow into the lungs; manifests in patients as difficulty completely *exhaling* air.

Offset: The time needed for an effect to dissipate.

Ointment: A dermatologic vehicle; a semi-solid grease or oil with little or no water (insoluble in water).

One-compartment model: A model of drug movement throughout the body in which the drug enters and stays in the systemic circulation (central compartment), does not move into other tissues, and is eliminated.

Onset: The time of the first measurable response to the drug.

Open-angle glaucoma: An eye condition at which the angle where the cornea and the iris meet remains open, but the fluid passes too slowly through the drain, causing the fluid to build up and increase the pressure in the eye to the point that the optic nerve may be damaged.

Ophthalmic: Relating to the eye.

Opioids: Narcotics; a type of analgesic derived from the Asian poppy. Medications that act on opioid receptors in the brain and nervous system to provide pain relief or sedation.

Opioid receptors: Receptors found in the brain and nervous system; designated as delta, kappa, and mu.

Optic nerve: Either of the second pair of cranial nerves that pass from the retina to the optic chiasma and conduct visual stimuli to the brain.

Oral: By mouth.

Orthostatic hypotension: A rapid drop in blood pressure that can occur after moving from the lying to standing position resulting in dizziness and light headedness.

Otalgia: Pain in the ear.

Otic: Relating to the ear.

Otitis externa: "Swimmer's ear"; an infection of the inner ear and the outer ear canal that can cause the ear to itch or become red and swollen to the point that touching it or even applying pressure to the ear is quite painful.

Otitis media with effusion (OME): The buildup of fluid in the middle ear without the signs and symptoms of pain, redness of the eardrum, pus, or fever.

Otorrhea: Drainage of fluid from the ear.

Ovaries: The female reproductive glands.

Ovulation: Release of an egg by the ovaries as part of the menstrual cycle.

Palsy: A condition involving uncontrollable body tremors of one or multiple parts of the body.

Pancreas: A gland located behind the stomach that has both endocrine and exocrine functions.

Panic disorder: A severe anxiety attack that can include tremors, tachycardia, shortness of breath, diaphoreses, and fear of dying. Persistent fear of reoccurring attacks can cause significant changes in behavior.

Paranoia: A delusion involving suspiciousness or a belief that others are out to harm you. Often the delusion triggers self-protective actions.

Parasite: An organism that lives in or on a host, depending on the host for its survival, without benefitting the host, possibly causing disease in the host.

Parasomnias: Sleep disorders characterized by abnormal nervous system behavior.

Parasympathetic nervous system (PNS): Part of the autonomic nervous system that activates passive functions such as stimulating the secretion of saliva in the mouth or digestive enzymes into the stomach or small intestines.

Parathyroid: Two small pairs of glands embedded in the back of the thyroid gland that secrete parathyroid hormone (PTH), which helps regulate calcium absorption and release in the blood and bones.

Parathyroid hormone: A hormone secreted by the parathyroid gland that helps regulate calcium absorption and release in the blood and bones.

Parenteral: Introduction of a medication into the body directly into the circulatory system.

Parietal cells: Specialized cells that produce gastric acid in response to stimulation of histamine, acetylcholine, and gastrin receptors released from the surrounding antral G cells and enterochromaffin-like cells.

Parkinson's disease: A neurologic disorder in which nerve cells in the area of the brain that involve muscle movement (corpus striatum and substantia nigra) are affected.

Parkinsonian symptoms: Rhythmic muscular tremors, rigidity of movement, and droopy posture.

Peak expiratory flow rate (PEFR): A measurement of how fast a patient can exhale a volume of air (measured in liters/minute).

Peak flow (PF): The patient's maximum airflow; a measure of respiratory status.

Peak flow meter: A respiratory device used at the bedside that registers, in cubic centimeters, how much airflow is present.

Peptic ulcer disease: Infection with a microbe, *Helicobacter pylori*, that promotes harmful overproduction of gastric acid and lesions on the stomach lining.

Peptidoglycan: An important layer of bacterial cell walls.

Peripheral dopamine-1 agonists: A class of medications that promote vasodilation and thereby relieve high blood pressure during an acute crisis.

Peripheral nervous system (PNS): The parts of the nervous system other than the brain and the spinal cord.

Peripheral vision: The ability to see objects to the side and out of the corner of the eyes.

Pharmaceutical: A chemical substance that has medicinal properties; a chemical that works in such a way as to correct an abnormal biochemical or physiological function (including restoration of functions that are absent, intermittent, or subnormal).

Pharmacodynamics: The study of the "molecular mechanism of drug action" or how the drug interacts at its "active" site to produce the intended drug response; also characterizes the amount of drug needed at the site of action to produce a biological response.

Pharmacokinetics: The study of the rate of drug movement throughout the body; focuses on the amount of drug in the body and how fast the drug moves throughout the body; specifically, at the processes of drug absorption, distribution, metabolism, and elimination (ADME).

Pharmacologic activity: The therapeutic response induced by a medication, including how and where in the body a drug produces such a response.

Pharmacology: The study of the actions, chemistry, effects, and therapeutic uses of drugs; incorporating pharmacokinetics, pharmacodynamics, pharmacotherapeutics, and toxicology.

Phenothiazines: Dopamine-receptor antagonists traditionally used for antiemetic therapy.

Pheochromocytoma: A neuroendocrine tumor usually located in the medulla of the adrenal gland that is capable of producing large and dangerous amounts of catecholamines in the body.

Phobic disorders: An irrational, illogical fear of an object or situation.

Phosphodiesterase-5 (PDE-5) inhibitors: Pharmacologic agents used to treat penile erectile problems.

Pineal body: A gland located above and behind the pituitary gland that secretes melatonin in response to dark and light, and helps regulate the body's daily biological clock (circadian rhythm) and sleep/wake cycles.

Pituitary: A gland that has significant involvement in multiple endocrine functions.

Plasma-level time curve: A graph of the concentration of a drug measured in a series of blood samples over time.

Plasma proteins: Proteins present in the bloodstream, to which some drugs bind.

Pons: Part of the hindbrain.

Positive inotrope: A drug that increases the force of the heart's contraction.

Positive symptoms: Symptoms of schizophrenia that include distortion of reality thinking. Paranoia, auditory and visual hallucinations, and delusions may be present.

Postganglionic neuron: Any of the nerves of the autonomic nervous system originating in the ganglia and terminating in the effector organs.

Postoperative nausea and vomiting (PONV): Nausea, vomiting, or retching that occurs post-surgery, generally within the first 24-48 hours.

Postpartum: After birth.

Post-traumatic stress disorder (PTSD): An anxiety disorder caused by a severe traumatic experience that includes symptoms of intrusive memories, flashbacks, nightmares, hyper vigilance, and avoidance of certain stimuli.

Potassium-channel blockers: A group of antiarrhythmics that interfere with cardiac action via inhibition of potassium outflow.

Potency: A comparison measure of the relative concentration of drug required to achieve a given magnitude of response.

Pre-eclampsia: Gestational hypertension is accompanied by proteinuria.

Preganglionic neuron: Any of the nerves of the autonomic nervous system originating in the central nervous system and terminating in the ganglia.

Prehypertension: A precursor condition for hypertension that is associated with an increased risk of myocardial infarction and coronary artery disease.

Prenatal vitamins: Supplements taken prior to conception to ensure adequate amounts of essential vitamins and minerals for the mother and fetus.

Prescription drugs: Drugs ordered by a licensed provider, such as a physician, dentist, or nurse practitioner.

Presystemic elimination: A first-pass effect.

Preterm labor: Premature onset of labor.

Preventive medications: In respiratory conditions, drugs that restrict the disease; they include antagonists of primary mediators or primary mediator effects.

Primary mediators: Substances released during degranulation of the cell membrane that cause overt respiratory symptoms, including bronchoconstriction, vasodilation, and increased mucus secretion.

Prodrug: A chemical compound (drug) that is pharmacologically inactive in its dosage form; following administration, it requires the body to metabolize the drug into its pharmacologically active chemical structure.

Progesterone/progestin: A gonadal steroid.

Prolactin: A protein hormone released by the pituitary gland that is involved with the secretion of milk, stimulates testosterone synthesis, and is involved in the immune system.

Prostaglandin: Chemicals produced by the body that promote inflammation, pain, and fever. These lipid compounds derived from arachidonic act as chemical messengers throughout the body.

Prostate: A gland that is part of the male reproductive system that produces part of the seminal fluid that carries the sperm from the testes to the outside of the body.

Prostatitis: Inflammation of the prostate gland, often caused by an infectious process.

Proteinuria: Elevated urine protein level—300 mg or greater in 24 hours.

Proton-pump inhibitors (PPIs): Drugs that inhibit the action of the proton pump in the stomach, which directly blocks gastric acid production.

Protozoan: Unicellular eukaryotic organisms, of the kingdom Protista, that live in water or as parasites.

Pruritic/pruritus: Itching.

Psychosis: Delusional disorder.

Psychotropic drugs: Drugs used to treat psychiatric disorders.

Pupil: The contractile aperture in the iris of the eye.

Pyelonephritis: Acute, complicated urinary tract infection.

Rate process: The process of drug movement–either zero or first-order.

Receptor: A specific molecule on a cell with which a drug interacts.

Recurrent UTI: A urinary tract infection that follows resolution of a previous infectious episode. The recurrent UTI could indicate a relapse from the same organism that caused the previous episode or it could indicate reinfection with a different organism.

Relapse: Return of symptoms of a disease.

Remission: Diminution of symptoms of a disease.

Renal clearance: The volume of plasma that is cleared of drug per unit time through the kidneys.

Renin: The molecule responsible for the conversion of angiotensinogen to produce angiotensin I.

Renin–angiotensin–aldosterone system (RAAS): Part of the system that regulates blood pressure. Its end products are angiotensin II and aldosterone, which elevate blood pressure through vasoconstriction of arterioles and volume expansion caused by increased sodium.

Rescue medications: In respiratory conditions, drugs that are used when symptoms progress, or for patients whose symptoms are not well controlled. They act more rapidly than preventive medications.

Resistant: In regard to pathogens, being invulnerable to the effects of a particular drug.

Respiratory distress syndrome: A lung disorder sometimes observed in premature neonates, caused by insufficient production of the surfactant coating the inner surface of the lungs, leading to the inability of the lungs to expand and contract properly during breathing, often progressing to lung collapse, accompanied by accumulation of a protein-containing film lining the alveoli and their ducts; this leads to grunting respirations, use of accessory muscles, and nasal flaring appearing soon after birth.

Restrictive airway disease: Conditions, such as pulmonary fibrosis, where patients experience difficulty expanding their lungs with air (*inhaling*), though usually with normal flow through the larger respiratory components, resulting in decreased airflow, lung volume, and blood oxygenation.

Retina: The sensory membrane that lines the eye, is composed of several layers including one containing the rods and cones, and functions as the immediate instrument of vision by receiving the image formed by the lens and converting it into chemical and nervous signals that reach the brain by way of the optic nerve.

Retrovirus: A subdivision of viruses that includes human immunodeficiency virus (HIV).

Salicylates: Nonsteroidal anti-inflammatory drugs.

Saturable-binding kinetics: When concentration of a drug is high, and the enzymes become saturated so can no longer metabolize the drug; also known as Michaelis-Menten pharmacokinetics.

Schizophrenia: A delusional disorder associated with three types of symptoms: positive, negative, and cognitive.

Second messengers: Systems that are activated upon stimulation of the receptor.

Secondary mediators: Substances released during degranulation of the cell membrane that cause overt respiratory symptoms, including bronchoconstriction, vasodilation, and increased mucus secretion.

Sedation: A state of unconsciousness or semi-consciousness.

Selective α_1-blockers: Medications that block only α_1-receptors without affecting β-receptors.

Selective serotonin reuptake inhibitor (SSRI): The first-line antidepressant and anxiolytic medication class. SSRIs work by blocking the serotonin reuptake pump in the synaptic space, thereby increasing the concentration of serotonin in the brain.

Sensitivity: Degree of microbial susceptibility to a drug, measured by the effectiveness at inhibiting microbial growth.

Serotonin: 5-hydroxytryptamine (5-HT); an important neurotransmitter of the gastrointestinal tract system.

Serotonin 5-HT receptor: One of the receptors for serotonin that is targeted by gastrointestinal drugs.

Serotonin/norepinephrine reuptake inhibitor (SNRI): The first-line antidepressant and anxiolytic medication class. They work by blocking both the serotonin and norepinephrine pumps in the synaptic space, thereby boosting the availability of serotonin and norepinephrine in the brain.

Serotonin reuptake pump: A type of monoamine transporter protein that returns serotonin from the synaptic cleft to the presynaptic neuron; the chemical method by which serotonin is transported within the cell synapse at the cell body and the dendrites. It is associated with the mechanism of antidepressant medications.

Serotonin syndrome: A condition that develops when suppression of serotonin reuptake (e.g., from medications) causes an excess concentration of serotonin in the brain stem and spinal cord. Symptoms include alterations in mental status and coordination, diaphoresis (excessive sweating), tremor, rapid heartbeat, muscle spasms, blood pressure fluctuations, and fever.

Sexually transmitted infection (STIs): Any bacterial, fungal, parasitic, and viral infection that can be transmitted to sexual partners.

Side effects: Responses in tissues where a drug's effects are neither needed nor wanted, often causing problematic symptoms such as rash, itching, muscle pain, headache, and so on.

Signal transduction: The process of transmitting cell signals, which can be amplified by activating the second-messenger system within a cell.

Slow-reacting substance of anaphylaxis (SRSA): A group of three leukotrienes (C4, D4, E4) that induces smooth muscle contraction and bronchoconstriction, similar to the action of histamine, but acts in minutes rather than seconds, and with longer duration than histamine.

Sodium-channel blockers: A group of antiarrhythmics (Class I) that interfere with cardiac action via impairment of sodium ion conduction.

Somatic nervous system: Part of the peripheral nervous system consisting of peripheral nerve fibers that send sensory information to the central nerve system and motor nerve fibers that project to skeletal muscles.

Spasmolytics: Centrally acting muscle relaxants that are used to relieve musculoskeletal pain and spasms, and to diminish spasticity in a variety of neurologic disorders; also called antispasmodics.

Spasticity: A state of increased muscular tone with amplification of the tendon reflexes; often associated with disease states, illness, or injury such as multiple sclerosis, stroke, and spinal cord injury.

Specificity: (1) Relative degree of microbial selectivity of an antimicrobial drug, for purposes of selecting optimum antimicrobial therapy. (2) The degree of confidence with regard to pathologic microbial identification for purposes of diagnosis.

Spinal column: A series of bones that extends from the neck to the lower back and that protects the spinal cord.

Spinal cord: A cylindrical bundle of nerves that is connected to the brain, running down the protective spinal column, extending from the neck to the lower back.

Spirometer: A device that measures both volume and airflow in the lungs.

Statins: The most widely prescribed medications for hyperlipidemia; the most effective drug class available in terms of ability to lower cholesterol levels.

Steady-state drug levels: The concentration of drug in the body remains constant over time, given a consistent dosage regimen; the amount of drug going into a patient roughly equal to the amount being eliminated by the body.

Subcutaneous: Between the dermis and muscle layer.

Sublingual: Under the tongue.

Substituted benzamides: Dopamine-receptor antagonists traditionally used for antiemetic therapy.

Sulfonylureas: A type of insulin secretagogue that inhibits adenosine triphosphate-sensitive potassium channels of the beta cell membrane.

Superinfection: The development of a new infection while therapy for the initial infection is under way.

Susceptible: In regard to pathogens, being vulnerable to the effects of a particular drug.

Sympathetic nervous system (SNS): A division of the autonomic nervous system that regulates activity related to the body under conditions of stress.

Sympathomimetic: A drug that stimulates sympathetic nervous action, simulating normal transmitter actions, in physiological effect.

Synapse: The junction between the axon terminal of a nerve and an adjacent nerve, muscle end plate, or effector organ.

Synaptic space: The space between nerve cells that are involved with nerve transmission.

Systemic administration: Introduction of a medication into the body directly into the circulatory system.

Systemic vascular resistance: The resistance to blood flowing that is present in the body from the vasculature after the exit from the left ventricle (not including the pulmonary vasculature).

Systolic: Related to the force of blood pressing against vessel walls while the heart is contracting during a beat.

Tardive dyskinesia (TD): Involuntary movement of the facial muscles and tongue.

Teratogen: A compound that interferes with the normal developmental process in the fetus.

Testes: The male reproductive glands.

Testosterone: An androgen that is the only biologically active hormone.

Thalamus: Part of the forebrain.

Therapeutic drug monitoring (TDM): The close monitoring of drug plasma levels to ensure that the drug concentration levels remain within therapeutic limits.

Therapeutic index: The ratio of the minimum concentration of drug that produces toxic effects and the minimum concentration that produces the desired effect.

Therapeutic response: An interaction in which a chemical (medication) produces a therapeutic, or intended, response by or within the organism (patient).

Therapeutic window: The span of concentration between the minimum concentration of drug that produces toxic effects and the minimum concentration that produces the desired effect.

Thiazolidinediones: Insulin-sensitizing agents that cause the body to need less insulin and to use available insulin more effectively.

Thoracolumbar system: Another term for the sympathetic nervous system, due to the origin of the nerve fibers in the thoracic and lumbar regions of the spinal cord.

Thromboxanes (TXAs): Eicosanoids (lipids) derived from arachidonic acid, but from the prostaglandin-producing side of the cascade.

Thymosin: A hormone produced by the thymus gland that triggers the creation of T-cells.

Thymus: A gland located in the upper chest behind the sternum that plays a role in immune function. It produces the hormone thymosin and is most active during childhood; it atrophies after adolescence.

Thyroid: A butterfly-shaped gland located in the front, lower part of the neck that releases the hormones l-triiodothyronine (T_3) and l-thyroxine (T_4), which affect all organs and cellular metabolism and assist in controlling functions such as heart rate, blood pressure, and muscle tone.

Thyroid-stimulating hormone (TSH): A hormone that controls the release of T_3 and T_4 through a negative feedback loop to the anterior pituitary gland.

Tocolytic drugs: Drugs that are prescribed to stop labor and allow pregnancy to continue until the fetus reaches full term.

Tolerance: The state whereby a medication loses its effectiveness and higher doses are needed to produce the same pharmacologic effect. It is associated with physical dependence to certain drugs or medications.

Topical anesthetic: Medication provided in a cream, ointment, gel, or other vehicle for use on superficial skin conditions that cause pain or itching.

Tourette syndrome: A neurologic disorder of children involving multiple involuntary motor and vocal tics and the utterance of words or phrases. It can be caused by the use of neuroleptics or stimulant medications.

Toxicity: Drug poisoning.

Toxicology: The study and characterization of the adverse effects caused by excessively high concentrations of drug in the body and the harmful, potentially fatal results that may result.

Transdermal: Applied topically to the skin as in a patch.

Transmucosal: Applied topically to mucous membranes.

Treatment-resistant: A descriptor for those disorders that do not respond to or only partially respond to multiple trials of medications and continue to be problematic.

Tricyclic antidepressant (TCA): A group of antidepressant medications, all of which inhibit the reuptake of norepinephrine and treat a broad range of depression and anxiety disorders.

Triglycerides: A type of lipid; a high triglyceride level is a risk factor for heart disease.

Tympanic membrane: Eardrum.

Type I hypersensitivity: An excessive response of the immune system to an encounter with a substance to which it has been sensitized, specifically associated with IgE antibodies.

Typical antidepressants: First-generation antipsychotic medications.

Tyramine: An amino acid involved in the chemical function of the MAOI antidepressants.

Uncomplicated UTI: Urinary tract infection generally considered to occur in healthy, nonpregnant, ambulatory females with no functional or anatomic abnormalities of the urinary tract.

Urethra: The outlet to the bladder.

Urethritis: A bacterial or viral-induced inflammation of the urethra, which is the conduit carrying urine from the bladder to the outside of the body; characterized by painful urination.

Urinary incontinence: Inability to control urination; it can range from "leaking" of small amounts of urine to a complete inability to restrain urine flow via maintenance of voluntary muscle control.

Urinary tract: Part of the genitourinary system that handles waste elimination.

Urinary tract infection (UTI): Pathogenic invasion of the urinary tract.

Uveitis: Inflammation of the uvea.

Vasodilation: Opening of blood vessels.

Vasodilators: Drugs that dilate blood vessels.

Vasopressin antagonists: Medications that interfere (antagonize) vasopressin receptors.

Vasopressor: The ability of a substance to cause vasoconstriction of blood vessels and resultant increases in blood pressure.

Vehicle: A carrier for a pharmaceutical agent that transports the medication across the skin barrier and into the body.

Very low-density lipoprotein (VLDL): A lipid that serves as the principal transporter for other lipids, including triglycerides.

Vesicoureteral reflux (VUR): A disorder in which urine flows back from the bladder into the ureters.

Virus: A parasitic microbe.

Visual hallucinations: A psychotic symptom that distorts reality and causes a person to see objects or persons that cannot be seen by others. It can occur in schizophrenia or manic episodes.

Volume of distribution (V_D): A measurement of the fluid volume in which the drug is "dissolved" or contained; the amount of fluid necessary to account for the "concentration" of drug in the body.

Withdrawal: Refers to the symptoms after stopping an addicting substance by an individual in whom dependence has been present. It often includes craving to restart the addicting substance.

Zero-order kinetic drugs: The rate of elimination for a drug remains constant irrespective of the amount of drug remaining in the body.

Index

Note: Page numbers followed by *f* and *t* indicates figures and tables.